LOW VISION

PRINCIPLES AND MANAGEMENT

LOW VISION
PRINCIPLES AND MANAGEMENT

Christine Dickinson

Professor
Division of Pharmacy and Optometry
University of Manchester
Manchester, United Kingdom

Ana Hernández Trillo

Senior Lecturer
Division of Pharmacy and Optometry
University of Manchester
Manchester, United Kingdom

Michael D. Crossland

Senior Research Fellow
Institute of Ophthalmology
University College London
London, United Kingdom;
Specialist Optometrist
Low Vision Clinic
Moorfields Eye Hospital NHS Foundation Trust
London, United Kingdom

ELSEVIER

ISBN: 978-0-323-87634-6

Content Strategist: Kayla Wolfe
Content Development Manager: Somodatta Roy Choudhury
Content Development Specialist: Shilpa Kumar
Publishing Services Manager: Shereen Jameel
Project Manager: Maria Shalini
Cover and Design Direction: Ryan Cook
Marketing Manager: Belinda Tudin

Printed in India.
Last digit is the print number: 9 8 7 6 5 4 3 2 1

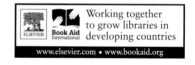

Low-vision care must be one of the widest-ranging topics in clinical optometry, spanning as it does ocular pathology, epidemiology, lighting, optical design, psychological adaptation to the disorder, devices for sensory substitution, and many other aspects. It draws upon the expertise of a multidisciplinary team of professionals, each with their own contribution to make to the life of the person with vision impairment. Many experienced low-vision practitioners find the interaction of this wide range of disciplines the major appeal of clinical and research work in this field. It should not be surprising that the topic is so diverse, since the individual with vision impairment has a right to expect a comprehensive service to address all their needs, including appropriate medical and surgical care; comprehensive and accurate description of the visual impairment; early access to state-of-the-art devices and instruction in their use; full visual and functional assessment; choice in whether to use vision or other methods to carry out a task; and freedom from ridicule and discrimination, particularly in work and education. This book describes all aspects of this process in a logical sequence. Although we hope the book will interest all professionals working in vision impairment, it is primarily aimed at student and practicing optometrists so that the role of the optometrist in delivering this service is emphasised. Part IV of the book (Clinical Procedures) assumes that the reader will be actively using the techniques described.

Whereas rehabilitation specialists have 'clients' or 'service users', and researchers have 'subjects' or 'participants', optometrists see 'patients', and the latter terminology has been used throughout for consistency. A general grounding in optometric and ophthalmological topics is assumed, so the terminology and procedures of routine eye examination are not explained, and ocular pathology is not discussed in detail: these matters are only dealt with as they relate specifically to low-vision care. Benefits and other services available for people with vision impairment are correct at the time of writing. Although the details of these are subject to intermittent change, their general framework is expected to remain unaltered. Few details have been given of specific models of low vision aid, since these are frequently updated. Examples and photographs have been used to illustrate particular points, but this is not to suggest that the aid described is the only, or the best, appliance available.

Following the practical routines described in this book will allow the interested practitioner to offer assistance to individuals with visual impairment, and their families, and to understand the theory behind the procedures used. We hope that both optometrists and patients will benefit, with low vision established in the mainstream of optometric practice, and the patient gaining the same access to the world which the rest of the population enjoys.

ACKNOWLEDGEMENTS

The authors wish to thank the many clinicians and researchers who have passed on their enthusiasm for, and knowledge and experience of, low vision in its many aspects. We are also grateful to the many patients who have given us an insight into what is meant by 'living with low vision'. We hope that we have captured the valuable information learned from all these sources in this book.

CONTENTS

What Is Low Vision?

Low vision, partial sight and visual impairment are synonyms for the same state: reduced vision, with both eyes open, even with the best optical correction. The definition does not include those who are monocular: these patients have different problems and are rarely considered in this category. The term also implies that some form vision (i.e. the ability to recognise shapes, no matter how close they must be placed) remains, and that vision is not simply confined to light perception. 'Regular lenses' in this context include required distance refractive corrections and reading additions up to +4.00 DS. The latter forms a somewhat arbitrary dividing line, whose origin is historical: it has been assumed that the closest distance at which a patient would normally read is 25 cm, for which the normally sighted presbyope would require a +4.00 DS addition.

DISORDER, IMPAIRMENT, ACTIVITY LIMITATION AND PARTICIPATION RESTRICTION

Whilst impairment describes the clinical status of the individual, different terminology is required to describe the effect on the individual in their everyday life. The International Classification of Functioning, Disability and Health (ICF) attempts to standardise the description of the functional consequences of disease at various levels. Thus, *visual impairment*, *activity limitation* and *participation restriction* are in fact used to describe the consequence to the bodily organ affected (the impairment) and the consequence to the patient, both in terms of their practical abilities (activity limitation) and the interaction with the society in which they live (participation restriction), of some disease or disorder of the anatomical structure or physiological function of the eye, which may be congenital, acquired or due to trauma.

Thus, clinical tests of physiological function, such as visual acuity or visual fields, are measures of visual impairment: on a recognised and standardised test, the patient does not perform as well as 'normal'. Activity limitation is the lack, loss or reduction of an individual's ability to perform certain tasks. Whether impairment causes activity limitation depends on the task to be performed or the practical skills to be exercised: if the impairment is the loss of one leg, for example, then this definitely limits the activity of walking, but the loss of one eye would usually cause very little limitation for watching television, even though there is no doubt that an impairment is present.

In the context of individuals with low vision, it is the so-called instrumental activities of daily living (IADLs) which are most significant, as they are important in order to live independently in the community. The mnemonic for the list of relevant activities is SHAFT[2], representing the following list:

Shopping
Housekeeping
Accounting (managing money)
Food preparation (including medication)
Transportation (or travel)
Technology (including telephones)

TABLE 1.1   **The Relationship Between Disease, Impairment, Activity Limitation and Participation Restriction for Ocular Pathology**

Level	Disease/disorder	Impairment: consequence at level of the organ		Activity limitation: consequence at level of patient	Participation restriction: consequence in the wider social environment
Definitions	Ophthalmological diagnosis	A change in the structure or function of the eye or visual pathway		A problem in the performance of daily activities	Social disadvantage: the inability, or need for exceptional effort, to fulfill role in society considered appropriate for that individual
		Anatomical structure	Physiological function		
Examples	Age-related macular degeneration	Photoreceptor degeneration	Central scotoma: central vision patchy and distorted	Recognising faces	Fear of rejection by friends not acknowledged in the street
	Cataract	Crystalline lens opacity	Poor contrast sensitivity: inability to detect low-contrast edges	Falling on steps and kerbs	Unable to go out alone

Whether the activity limitation becomes a participation restriction depends on how the patient reacts to it. If the patient feels, or actually is, at a disadvantage in society and cannot live their life as they expect or would choose to do (or at least not without making an enormous effort), that is participation restriction. The areas of life in which the individual may perceive that they are disadvantaged include, for example, education, employment, recreation and leisure, and personal relationships.

To apply these definitions in the case of the disorder of age-related macular degeneration (AMD), this can be identified as progressive degeneration of the photoreceptors in the macular area, causing a loss of acuity and partial central field loss. This would be detected as an impairment on a clinical test of the central field, such as the Amsler Grid, when the patient would notice distortion. This distortion would affect the visibility of anything the patient fixated centrally and may be noticed in the everyday task of recognising faces, on finding that only the outline and not the fine detail can be seen. This may become participation restriction if the patient worries about unwittingly ignoring, and thus alienating, a friend passed in the street. Some further examples are given in Table 1.1, which illustrates the ICF as applied to ocular disease, showing the wide-ranging consequences at all levels.

LOW VISION DEFINED BY VISUAL ACUITY

Low vision can therefore be defined either in terms of the visual impairment which is created or the extent of the visual activity limitation, and both are used according to the particular situation. It may be decided to use the visual impairment to classify low vision and set a threshold visual standard which is considered 'normal' with any value below that representing 'low vision'. There are difficulties in deciding on a suitably simple and repeatable visual test and determining exactly where the pass/fail boundary should be set. The most familiar test of spatial vision is the resolution task of Snellen acuity, which involves the ability to discriminate the smallest possible letters at maximum contrast (nominally 100%), and 'normal' performance is taken as 6/6 (0.0 logMAR). The test has the advantage that is in common usage, is easily performed, and the result is described by a single value.

The International Classification of Diseases 11th Revision (ICD-11) (World Health Organization [WHO], 2018) classifies vision impairment (VI) into two groups, based on presenting visual acuity for distance or near.

Distance vision impairment:
- Mild—visual acuity worse than 6/12 to 6/18
- Moderate—visual acuity worse than 6/18 to 6/60
- Severe—visual acuity worse than 6/60 to 3/60
- Blindness—visual acuity worse than 3/60 (or a visual field diameter <10°)

Near vision impairment:
- Near visual acuity worse than N6 or M 0.8 at 40 cm

These definitions of VI and blindness have changed considerably over time (WHO, 2019). When first introduced in 1972, they were based on 'best corrected' visual acuity. This would still be a conventional definition to use for low-vision rehabilitation in high-income countries where refractive correction and medical treatment are widely available. In 2010, the change was made to 'presenting' visual acuity to reflect the considerable contribution of uncorrected refractive error to the everyday functioning of many individuals. The 'mild' category includes those people who may be considered to have 'socially significant' vision loss: this is a group who would not be permitted to drive in many countries.

LOW VISION DEFINED BY THE NEED FOR REHABILITATION

As far as patients are concerned, however, they are more likely to identify their visual difficulties in terms of functional limitations, complaining of an inability to perform everyday tasks, such as reading, driving or recognising faces. It is extremely difficult to quantify such problems, or to relate them to a particular level of visual acuity (a particular degree of impairment). It is common in a low-vision clinic to encounter a patient with, for example, very constricted visual fields who navigates easily, whilst another patient with more moderate loss needs to use touch instead of vision to get around.

There is an ongoing search for a simple clinical test of impairment which can be easily and quickly performed in the consulting room and gives an accurate prediction about how limited a patient will be when carrying out a practical task such as reading or navigating in unfamiliar places: as suggested earlier, that correlation may not exist. It is certainly true that distance visual acuity has been found to be a poor predictor of mobility, face recognition and reading. Other tests, such as contrast sensitivity and visual field measurement, have been found to increase the accuracy of predictions, but often the only solution is to test the patient on the actual task—this is of course done routinely for reading, where samples of print paragraphs of various sizes are used. It can be argued that trying to link impairment and activity limitation is irrelevant: regardless of the patient's acuity, if they are having visual difficulties with a task then they need rehabilitative help to allow them to perform it. Equally, the exact level of acuity which constitutes impairment is variable: if patients have a hobby or occupation which requires 6/4 acuity and they only have 6/9, then they will consider themselves to be visually impaired; someone whose main interests are watching television and going to the pub may be satisfied with 6/18 visual acuity. For this reason, it is important that low-vision services should be accessible to anyone who may benefit from them. World Health Organization (WHO) consultants emphasised that arbitrary visual acuity levels should not be used to determine whether the patient should have access to rehabilitation (Barry & Murray, 2005; Hyvarinen, 1992), and this is a conclusion that would be endorsed by many service providers.

LOW VISION DEFINED IN LEGISLATION

Most high-income countries have a system of social care where certain groups become identified to receive financial benefits or have access to appropriate services. The visually impaired and blind are one such group, and they are 'registered' in order to show their eligibility for special attention. Registration is undertaken with the aim to:
- assess what health and social work resources will be needed for the number of visually impaired people in a particular area and

- act as the patient's passport to appropriate welfare benefits.

This leads to definitions of 'legal' blindness: a level of visual acuity and/or extent of visual field which the patient must not exceed if they are to be certified officially as 'blind'; it is felt that such standards are required to prevent fraud.

There are problems in achieving a consistent definition of blindness as the WHO (1966) identified 65 different definitions of blindness worldwide, although the UK appears to be unique in having the dual categories of Sight Impairment (SI; previously called 'Partially Sighted') and Severely Sight Impairment (SSI; previously 'Blind'). Even if a particular level of impairment could be (SI; previously called 'Partially Sighted') and Severely Sight Impairment (SSI; previously 'Blind'). Even if a particular level of impairment could be universally agreed, this can still cause difficulties in interpretation (Mokhles et al., 2017). A patient may, for example, have a 'real' acuity of 6/48, but this is not a letter size which is available on most standard Snellen charts. On the standard chart, when presented with a letter of '6/60' and the next size of '6/36', the patient's vision will only be recorded as '6/60'. If the level of acuity required in order to be registered was chosen as 6/60, they would qualify, and yet a more accurate measure would have revealed that they were not eligible (Gresset et al., 1993). Similar difficulties arise when a particular extent of visual field is quoted as the registration criterion. It is possible to envisage a pathological condition where there is a very small island of central vision, but a much larger isolated peripheral crescent of functional visual field. In this case, patients are unlikely to be able to use the peripheral island of vision for useful navigation, yet officially their visual fields may be too large for them to be registered (Fischer, 1993; Mokhles et al., 2017). There is also doubt whether a measurement of the impairment by standard clinical tests would yield exactly the same measurement if repeated: there is evidence that performance (especially for contrast sensitivity) can be improved following an interview with an empathetic and encouraging clinician (Duckworth et al., 1994).

Even if the vision test result is unequivocal, two patients with the same acuity might perform very differently, and more discriminating tests of vision (such as glare disability or contrast sensitivity) might offer a better indication of how the patient functions in everyday life. Some countries choose not to set a level of impairment to define 'blindness', but instead rely on a measure of activity limitation. In these terms, blindness might be determined as inability to walk across an unfamiliar room unaided. Of course, this brings its own complications: if a different task had been chosen, the patient may have performed much better, and there will be no standardisation in the type and size of 'room', its lighting or the arrangement and colour of its furniture.

In the UK, there is an attempt to use both impairment and activity limitation to define SSI (previously 'blindness') and SI (previously 'partial sight'). The legal definition of blindness was based on being 'so blind as to be unable to do any work for which eyesight is essential'. As this is based on ability it allows for individual discretion and interpretation, although there are recommended acuity and visual field levels to try to ensure consistency. The introduction of a category of 'sight impairment' in the UK in 1948, with acuity levels which are higher and which only allows access to some of the benefits available to the severely sight impairment, is another way to offer help to patients who require it but do not meet the 'blindness' criterion (although it will still not include all those who the WHO identifies as suffering from mild or moderate vision loss where a visual acuity standard of less than 6/12 is adopted).

Registration will therefore not identify all those in need. Silver et al. (1978) concluded that for a group of visually impaired patients of whom only 10 would be classified as blind when tested in the hospital clinic, 20 are functioning as blind because of their lower acuity under the generally poorer lighting levels in the home. The results of an Office of Population Census and Surveys (OPCS) survey (Martin et al., 1988) suggested that 1,668,000 people in the UK suffered visual difficulties, including 25% of all those aged over 75 years, and 45% of over 85-year-olds in the UK had reported difficulties with their eyesight when completing their census return in 1980. In 2018, updated estimates suggest 1.93 million people in the UK have visual acuity <6/12 (Pezzullo et al., 2018).

The UK Registration System

In the UK, the *Blind Persons Act 1920* legislation provided specific welfare facilities for the blind, and a definition of blindness was introduced (little changed to the present day) which established eligibility for those benefits (Abel, 1989). The sight impairment (partial sight) category was added by the *National Assistance Act* in 1948.

The functional definitions are as follows:

- Severe Sight Impairment (SSI)—'so blind as to be unable to do any work for which eyesight is essential'
- Sight Impairment (SI)—'substantially and permanently handicapped by defective vision caused by congenital defect or illness or injury'

Despite the worthwhile nature of a definition related to activity limitation, there is obviously much scope for interpretation here, so an attempt has been made to quantify the corresponding impairment (Dementia and Disability Unit, 2017; Quartilho et al., 2016), with the patient fully corrected and using both eyes: there is no provision for consideration of a loss in only one eye.

- Severe Sight Impairment (SSI)
  - 3/60 or worse
  - 6/60 or worse with field contraction
  - 6/60 or better with contracted field causing functional impairment (e.g. reduction of inferior field or bitemporal hemianopia)
- Sight Impairment (SI)
  - 3/60 to 6/60, full fields
  - 6/24 to 6/60, with moderate field contraction (superior or patchy loss), media opacities or aphakia
  - 6/18 or better if marked field defect such as hemianopia

It is difficult to apply any of these definitions to young children because of the inaccuracy in acuity measurement using a Snellen chart. It is therefore recommended that children are registered as sight impairment until the age of 4 years, unless obviously totally blind. When they reach this age they can be tested using an optotype chart with optimum refractive correction and registered in the same way as adults.

The patient is registered with the Local Authority, but the process starts with certification, which can only be carried out by an ophthalmologist using a form known as the Certificate of Vision Impairment (CVI) in England and Wales, the CVI (Scotland) in Scotland and the A655 in Northern Ireland. The CVI replaced the previous BD8 in England in September 2005 and Wales in April 2007 and replaced the BD1 in Scotland in April 2018. It is normally the ophthalmologist who will suggest registration and discuss it with the patient: social workers, eye clinic liaison officers, optometrists or other professionals may ask the ophthalmologist to consider this when appropriate. Note that people who are not currently under the care of a hospital eye clinic will need to be re-referred to an ophthalmologist for this to be done. If patients disagree with their registration category (e.g. so they can obtain the enhanced benefits associated with SSI registration), they can appeal for independent assessment to the Ophthalmic Referee Service. Patients can have their registration category changed, or even be deregistered if vision improves. Despite this, patients often perceive registration (particularly as SSI) as 'the end of the road' and assume there is no longer any hope of treatment: earlier and more recent surveys suggest that ophthalmologists perhaps consider it in much the same way, with patients receiving active treatment being least likely to be registered (Barry & Murray, 2005; Boyce et al., 2014; Robinson et al., 1994).

The CVI Form

This is the 'Record of Examination to Certify a Person as Severely Sight Impairment or Sight Impairment'. It is divided into four parts.

- Part 1 (to be completed by the ophthalmologist)—Patient details (name, address, telephone number, email address, date of birth, sex, NHS number), certificate of sight Impairment or severely sight Impairment, which indicates the registration category, and gives the date the form was completed: this is the date on which the patient becomes entitled to any associated benefits, name of the ophthalmologist who signs the document and hospital address.
- Part 2 (to be completed by the ophthalmologist)—Aspects of visual function including aided/unaided visual acuity, category of field defect (extensive loss of peripheral visual field—including hemianopia), and if the patient has been referred for low-vision services.
  Part 2a—Diagnosis of the disorder or disease causing the visual impairment for patients 18 years of age or over
  Part 2b—Diagnosis of the disorder or disease causing the visual impairment for patients under the age of 18
- Part 3 (to be completed by the patient (or parent/guardian if the patient is a child) and eye clinic staff (e.g. Eye Clinic Liaison Officer [ECLO]/Sight Loss Advisor))—Additional information for the patient's local council including living circumstances (e.g. lives alone), support, physical

mobility difficulties, hearing difficulties, learning disabilities, dementia, employment status, if in full-time education or if they are a baby, child, or young person, and are they known to the specialist visual impairment education service. Any additional relevant information can also be added here (e.g. risk of falls, medical conditions, emotional impact of sight loss, urgent support needed and the reasons why, or benefits of vision rehabilitation). Finally, the patient's information and communication needs are added here (preferred method of contact, preferred method of communication, preferred format of information and preferred language).

- Part 4 (to be completed by the patient [or parent/guardian if the patient is a child] and eye clinic staff [e.g. ECLO/ Sight Loss Advisor])—Consent to share information (declaration of permission for a copy of the CVI to be sent to the patient's GP, the local council, and the Royal College of Ophthalmologists, Certifications Office at Moorfields Eye Hospital) and a declaration confirming that the patient has been informed that they must not drive.

In addition to renaming the BD8 as CVI, in 2003 two other new forms were introduced:

- The Hospital Eye Service Referral of Vision Impaired Patient for Social Needs Assessment (RVI)
- The Low Vision Letter or Low Vision Leaflet (LVL) (LVI previously)

The eye clinic staff member completes the RVI if they think that a patient would benefit from an assessment of their needs, even if registration is not appropriate at present. This form highlights the areas of concern (e.g. cooking unaided, getting about safely). The patient may not yet be eligible for registration, may be in the middle of treatment which might alter their status, or may have refused registration. Once completed, the RVI is sent to Social Services and one copy is kept in the patient's hospital notes, another copy is sent to the GP and a third copy will be kept by the patient.

The second form (LVL) is used when a community optometrist identifies a person with significant sight problems. This form is distributed from Social Services to local optometrists or can be downloaded by the optometrist. This form is to be given to the patients with sight problems whom the optometrist feels would benefit from advice and assessment. The patient should send the form to Social Services, giving details of their age, circumstances (e.g. living alone) and problems (as on the RVI).

The Legislative Background

Section 29 of the *National Assistance Act 1948* lays down the responsibilities of the local authority for those registered as blind and partially sighted.

Mandatory functions are as follows:

- Keeping the registers of the people who are severely sight impairment and sight impairment.
- Providing a social work service, advice and support for those living in their own home or elsewhere.
- Making available facilities for social rehabilitation and for adjustment to the disability: this includes teaching

techniques for communication (such as Braille) and mobility.
- Providing facilities for social, recreational, occupational and cultural activities.

Additional services which can be provided include accommodation, transport and holiday homes.

The *Chronically Sick and Disabled Persons Act 1970* provides for a wider range of services to be offered by the local authority, when it identifies a need for them, such as:

- Practical help and adaptations in the home
- Supply of radio, television, library or similar recreational facilities
- Provision of, or assistance in obtaining, a telephone and any special equipment necessary to enable the use of a telephone
- Holidays
- Recreation and education away from the home, and transport to them
- Meals in the home, or elsewhere

Some local authorities interpret need more generously than others, and this may not be in the same way as the potential recipient who feels that a particular service is essential to him or her.

The *Care Act 2014* legislates to provide those persons with visual impairment with care services and support, tailored to their own individual needs (a 'care plan'), which will allow them to live independently in their own homes (if possible). Any individual can request an assessment of their needs, which in the case of VI, will be carried out by a specialist team within Adult Social Services which may specialise in VI, or combine hearing and vision care within a broader Sensory Team.

If a need is identified which the local authority does not have the staff to provide, then it is required to buy in the services of, for example, a voluntary society or a freelance consultant. The recipient may have to make some contribution to the cost of some services: there is no uniform policy on charging, but it is usually based on the individual's income and savings.

The rights of visually impaired children are specified in the *Children and Families Act 2014*, which was intended to achieve a better integration of health, education and social care provision. Each local authority must publish its 'Local Offer' which describes the provision it makes for the young people in its area. It provides information for young people, their parents and carers, and professionals regarding education, health and care services, leisure activities and support groups. The Local Offer should also be responsive to the needs of the individuals using the services, who are encouraged to provide feedback about what is needed.

The local authority draws up a register of disabled children within its area, but this is not the same as the SSI and SI registers, and it is not necessary for the child to be registered as visually impaired in order for their needs to be assessed. For the purposes of this list, disability (defined by the *Equality Act 2010*) is 'a physical or mental impairment which has a long term (i.e. a year or more) and substantial adverse effect on their ability to carry out everyday activities'. Local Education Authorities (LEAs) identify children from 2 years of age (up to the age of 25 if they are still in full-time education) who are likely to have 'special educational needs' (SEN) or are disabled. A child has SEN if they 'have a disability which prevents/hinders them from making use of educational facilities usually provided for children of that age'. So-called 'special' schools now usually cater for pupils with additional nonvisual disabilities and health needs. Regardless of the degree of visual impairment, most children with VI in the UK attend mainstream schools.

The SEND Code of Practice 2015 covers the provision for children (0–25 years old) with SEN, and each mainstream school has a SENCO (SEN Coordinator). If the school does not have the resources to support the child from its SEN budget (e.g. if the child requires specialist equipment or one-to-one classroom support) then an assessment can be carried out by the Local Authority to determine if it is necessary to provide an Education, Health, and Care Plan (EHCP) for the child, which is reviewed annually.

Children with VI should have access to the full National Curriculum, but may also need some formal training in the 'life skills' which normally sighted children may pick up from observing peers and parents, and in independent mobility. These will ideally be taught by a Registered Qualified Habilitation Specialist (RQHS), who will work with the child within the school. Children with VI in a mainstream school may be withdrawn from classes for a few hours each week in order to have special tuition from a Qualified Teacher of the Visually Impaired (QTVI) such as in Braille or touch-typing. Some schools have an attached unit for children with VI. The QTVI can also visit the parents and the child at their home and in an early years setting, providing advice, guidance and support. The QTVI is a key person in the educational development of the child with visual impairment and will remain supporting the child throughout their school years,

These professionals may be based within the local authority's specialist service for children and young people with visual or hearing impairment which might be called the Inclusion Team (IT), Children's Sensory Service or VI service. This service will:

- offer support and advice to families about their child's sensory impairment;
- provide assessments regarding the child or young person's sensory impairment;
- write advice and provide strategies to support children and young people in their learning and development;
- provide specialist equipment when needed;
- teach Braille and British Sign Language as appropriate;
- train teachers and other professionals about sensory impairment;
- liaise with parents and other professionals;
- provide awareness-raising sessions for peers;
- attend meetings and reviews; and
- signpost families to other services.

All children should be referred to this service directly from the hospital eye department when the eye condition is diagnosed. Any parent or professional can contact this service directly in the event that the expected referral has not taken place correctly.

University students (undergraduate and postgraduate) can get help with the extra costs they incur because of their disability, via the Disabled Students Allowance. This could cover specialist equipment (such as computer software or an Electronic Vision Enhancement System [EVES]); nonmedical help (e.g. a note-taker or reader); and the extra travel costs (perhaps taxi fares where public transport is not available). Extra costs related to their accommodation are covered by the university if the student is in a hall of residence.

Finding employment is a major problem for people with low vision and unemployment is far higher in the visually impaired population. The employment benefits which are available are linked to the patient being registered as 'disabled'. This is not automatic and should be requested by the visually impaired person at their local Jobcentre. It is likely that any person registered as severely sight impairment and sight impairment will be eligible for registration as disabled. Work Coaches based in the Jobcentre Plus are trained to help the person with disabilities to find work or to gain new skills for a job. They will conduct an employment assessment to understand what type of work would suit the person best and can help with work preparation, recruitment, interview coaching and even confidence building. The length of time an employment assessment takes depends on the person's individual needs and can last from half a day to a few days or longer. After the assessment, the person will agree to a plan of action with the Work Coach, which may include training or taking part in a programme such as Access to Work, Residential Training or Work Choice. The Work Coach can also provide referrals to a specialist work psychologist, if necessary, for a more detailed employment assessment (JobcentrePlus, 2021).

Residential training courses can help people with visual impairment to get a job, gain more experience to keep a job or become self-employed. People who are severely sight impairment or sight impairment and unemployed can apply for residential training if there are not any suitable training courses available locally. Courses are run by the Jobcentre or the Royal National College for the Blind (RNC) (Royal National Institute for the Blind [RNIB], 2021). The World Blind Union (WBU) have recently developed Project Aspiro (World Blind Union, 2021)—a career planning and employment website for people who are severely sight impairment and sight impairment (as well as service providers, friends and family, and employers). The website includes information and helpful tools that address the career planning process, including living independently, learning and education, preparing for work, and working life. There are explanatory videos and audio clips as well as profiles of organisations, programmes, services and useful websites around the world.

'Access to Work' is a scheme to enable employed or self-employed people with a visual impairment to work more efficiently, or to increase their capacity for work. The specific types of help may include: the cost of a taxi to work if public transport is inappropriate; special equipment, or modifications to existing equipment; adaptations to the premises or working environment; a personal reader or assistant at work. For the visually impaired person this may well be the route by which an electronic magnifier, text-to-speech, or Braille device, could be obtained for work. Financial limits to the aid available depend on if the person is employed or self-employed, how long they have been in their job, the size of the employer and the type of help they need. The Access to Work scheme normally pays the full cost of any adaptations if the person has been in the job for less than 6 weeks, if the person is self-employed, and if the person needs funding for a support worker, travel to work or interviews and communication support at interviews. If the person applies for the scheme after having been in the role for more than 6 weeks, the employer might need to contribute towards the cost of adaptations and gadgets paid for by Access to Work. Funding is ongoing and will be reviewed every 3 years or if the person's condition changes. The employer owns the equipment bought through Access to Work and is also responsible for the maintenance, insurance and disposal costs (SCOPE, 2020). Some of the adaptations required in the workplace to make it accessible to an employee with VI would be considered as reasonable adjustments under the Equality Act, and funding would not be available for these. Disability Confident (DC) is a government scheme to encourage employers to make their working environment, practices and recruitment process as inclusive as possible: for example, guaranteeing an interview to any disabled applicant who has the essential qualifications.

Advantages of Registration

Legislation is largely concerned with specifying the provision by the local authorities, but the exact form which this takes will vary depending on the geographical area in which the visually impaired person lives. This variation is inevitable as local authorities may be buying in rehabilitation services from a variety of different sources, including voluntary societies. Local authorities offer services according to need rather than registration, but registration is likely to be a passport to obtaining the most appropriate help with the minimum difficulty, and it acts as a trigger or catalyst in the awareness and receipt of services. Registered individuals are always proportionately more aware of available services and gadgets, and use them more: to take a simple example, 31% of people registered visually impaired, but only 2% of people who were unregistered with the same vision, owned a talking clock or watch (Bruce et al., 1991).

Under the provisions of the Care Act, anyone can request an assessment by their local authority Social Services Department to determine what would be required to allow them to live as full and independent lives as possible in their own homes. This often takes the form of Home Care Services (a home help to assist with cleaning, cooking and shopping), and Meals on Wheels. Many social services departments employ rehabilitation workers/officers to work with the visually impaired to meet their particular needs to perform daily living tasks, and to have safe mobility and travel. This may involve advice on specialist equipment, or adaptations to the home (such as improved lighting, or handrails). If the

person is registered as SSI, the Blue Badge scheme, run by local authorities, allows drivers to park in spaces reserved for disabled people. The Blue Badge scheme does not fully apply in the City of London but allocated parking is provided for people with disabilities in the Square Mile.

Although the details vary depending on the locality, there are usually concessions for public transport. For example, in Greater Manchester, a person registered as SSI is eligible for a free travel pass on buses and trains and those who are registered SI are eligible for a concessionary travel permit. People who are registered SSI or SI in Merseyside are eligible for an English National Concessionary Travel Pass which offers free travel on all buses, trains and Mersey Ferries river crossings. In London, everyone whose vision is too poor to qualify for a driving licence can apply to their local borough council for a Freedom Pass for free travel on all bus, tram, Tube, Docklands Light Railway (DLR), London Overground and Transport for London (TfL) Rail services in all zones. Several areas also provide vouchers for discounted taxi fares for those registered as SSI. Everyone who is registered as SI or SSI can apply for a disabled persons' railcard which gives one-third off all rail fares for the holder and an accompanying person.

Other sources of help available to people with visual impairment are central government, (national) voluntary agencies, and commercial organizations. Within these categories, the benefits may be available only to those who are registered as SSI, to any registered person, or also to those who are not eligible for registration. Registration is necessary to qualify for most financial benefits and for help from a number of voluntary agencies and commercial organisations.

Financial benefits come within the remit of central government, and are limited to:

1. An addition to the personal allowance (the amount of money that can be earned before starting to pay income tax) of a SSI person in work (Blind Person's Allowance). This can be transferred to a spouse if the registered person is unemployed.
2. A 50% discount on the television licence if the person is registered as SSI (a SSI person could also purchase a sound-only receiver for which no licence is required).
3. Disabled Living Allowance (DLA, for those under 16 years) and Personal Independence Payment for older individuals. These are not automatic and not means-tested. There are 'care' and 'mobility' components in each benefit, if the individual can give evidence of their need in these areas (and the RNIB provide detailed guidance on how to present a claim). It is expected that all children need care from their parents, but DLA is designed to recognise the additional care needed by a child with VI compared to a child of the same age without VI.

There is no other benefit which is given because of visual impairment, but there are some general benefits which operate with special conditions for those with disabilities. Most are on the basis of financial need and are 'means-tested': a calculation is made of the minimum amount which is considered necessary to live on, and there is an entitlement to benefit if the amount of income and savings does not reach this level. Benefits and allowances are not always cumulative, however, and receipt of one payment can be deducted from another entitlement: specialist individual advice must be sought by applicants, and a number of organisations operate telephone helplines. More up-to-date information is provided by the charities, the RNIB (2020), Henshaws Society for the Blind People (Henshaws, 2019), or www.sightadvicefaq.org.uk.

Both SI and SSI people qualify for:

4. A free General Ophthalmic Services (GOS) Sight Test (also including payment to the optometrist of the fee for a domiciliary visit if that is necessary), although there is no special eligibility for a GOS Spectacle Voucher to be used for the supply of spectacles. People registered as SSI and SI cannot have their prescriptions dispensed by an unregistered supplier.

It is worth noting that optical (but not electronic) low-vision aids are prescribed through the Hospital Eye Service (HES), and supplied free on permanent loan at the discretion of the optometrist to anyone who needs them: registration is not required. There is no formal provision for the supply of aids through the GOS by high-street optometrists, although it may be possible to use a GOS Spectacle Voucher towards the purchase of some spectacle-mounted aids (see Chapter 22). Throughout Wales, optometrists, ophthalmic medical practitioners (OMPs) and dispensing opticians (DOs) based in high-street practices provide Low Vision Service Wales (LVSW), through which the low-vision aids are available on loan and free of charge. The scheme additionally offers (free of charge) an electronic pocket magnifier and spectacle-mounted low-vision aids (Charlton et al., 2013). In England, there are commissioned enhanced clinical pathways in some local areas which allow community practitioners to participate in similar schemes (see Chapter 22).

5. Exemption from VAT (value added tax) when buying products designed and manufactured exclusively for the use of disabled: an example of such device might be an EVES.

The national voluntary organisations are open to anyone seeking information and advice: the RNIB, for example, has an online shop on its website. Registration gives extra entitlements, however, because those who are registered get some items free of VAT. A radio and/or a portable smart device can be supplied by the British Wireless for the Blind Fund, but only to those who are registered SSI, SI, over the age of 8 years and in receipt of a means-tested benefit. Commercial organisations also offer concessions: BT makes no charge for directory enquires for a registered SSI or SI person who registers with the service in advance: they are given a Personal Identification Number to quote when requesting a number. Bank and Building Societies websites and apps should be fully accessible to SSI and SI people and will ensure that the person has a fully accessible way of obtaining their account details or provide the person with equipment to enable access to their account. Braille, large print or audio statements and information leaflets are usually provided on request.

Although an enormous range of benefits and services exist, they are extremely complex and diverse and, individually, quite small. It takes a great deal of persistence in seeking out information by people with visual impairment in order to find out what might be of benefit to them, and all possible measures need to be taken to publicise available services. Some selected findings from the RNIB survey (Bruce et al., 1991) highlight problems in several areas. Although those registered as visually impaired tend to be proportionately more aware than the unregistered, the lack of knowledge is surprising: although many have very low incomes and are often dependent on state benefits, only 29% had received any expert advice on their entitlements; only 11% had received practical advice on daily living skills from Social Services staff; and over one-third could not name a single voluntary organisation involved in helping those with sight problems. The low-vision practitioner can play a significant role by pointing out the possible benefits of registration, and encouraging this whenever possible.

EQUALITY AND ACCESSIBILITY

In 1993, the United Nations adopted the 'Standard Rules on the Equalization of Opportunities for Persons with Disabilities' (United Nations, 1993) which showed a shift in concepts of disability from the 'medical model' to the 'social model'. The so-called medical model looks at what is 'wrong' with the disabled person. It creates low expectations, and stereotypes, with pathways being decided for them (e.g. blind people being directed to work as basket weavers or piano tuners). The social model acknowledges that much disability is caused by the way that society is organised. The focus is on removing barriers (physical and attitudinal) to allow individuals who are different to be equal in society, with control over their own lives. The prevailing terminology uses words such as 'independence' 'choice' 'empowerment' 'enablement'.

In the UK, the *Equality Act 2010* superseded the requirements of the *Disability Discrimination Act 1995* which stated that individuals should not be discriminated against on the basis of disability (or eight other 'protected characteristics'). Any service provider (i.e. a public or private organisation) must not treat a person with disability 'less favourably', whether providing a free service or one for which a charge is made. They are required to make 'reasonable adjustments' in order to ensure that the disabled individual does not encounter any barriers to accessing services. A very simple 'reasonable adjustment' is the provision of documents in large print by banks and utility companies.

One of the services which individuals with visual impairment often experience great difficulty in accessing is healthcare. There are several barriers which have been identified, such as the difficulties and cost of travelling, and safety when out and about (Tan et al., 2018).

As well as physical access to healthcare, there is also a lack of access to information (Beverley et al., 2011). Since 2016 there has been a requirement that all healthcare information should be accessible in a suitable format (Marsay, 2005) so the provider should discuss this with each of their service users. However, when a review of this implementation was carried out in 2017 (NHS; England, 2017) over 40% of respondents had not heard anything about the standard, and only 20% had noticed any improvement. Reading medication labelling is another often-reported difficulty, and guidance is available as to how this should be done appropriately (NPSA & NHS, 2006).

THE ICF

As noted previously, the ICF attempts to standardise the description of the functional consequences of disease at various levels.

Obviously there are many differences between individuals in lifestyle, which will influence the activities they wish to undertake, but there are environmental and personal factors which can also affect how successfully the impairment can be managed.

The environment includes the individual's home, workplace or school (for example), and the people they interact with in those settings ('local'). However, it also includes the society in which they live: the voluntary agencies and public services, and the prevailing attitudes, awareness and legislation about disability ('global').

Personal factors refer to the characteristics of the individual with visual impairment: their race, age, sex, religious beliefs, upbringing, coping strategies, mental and physical health and education. In a mixed low-vision population, physical and mental health were found to be the most important of these factors in determining rehabilitative outcomes (Hernandez Trillo & Dickinson, 2012). In an AMD population, the personality trait of neuroticism (a tendency to anxiety and pessimism) was a significant predictor of successful outcomes (Rovner et al., 2014).

Fig. 1.1A shows how these components fit within the theoretical model, and Fig. 1.1B gives a simple example. This is a patient who finds that their reading is now very difficult due to AMD. They are very determined and keen to be independent, because they have no family close by. The patient attends the hospital low-vision clinic and is provided with a magnifier to assist with reading correspondence. They are also registered as SI and receive a visit from the Social Services Department who provide a reading lamp. The patient contacts the bank who arrange to provide all correspondence in large print.

TACKLING THE DISABILITY

The lay perception of blindness is 'no perception of light', but it is clear that legal definitions allow patients who have considerably better vision than that to be registered as blind. In fact, a survey by Riley (1970) showed the typical range of acuities in those registered as blind (in a US sample) during a typical year, suggesting that over 75% do have some measurable form of vision (Table 1.2).

A UK survey of reading vision showed that 55% of people registerable as SSI reported being able to read newspaper headlines, whilst only 4% had no perception of light (Bruce et al., 1991). The percentage of total blindness among those registered as blind in infancy is much higher, however, reaching 46% in some studies (Mitry et al., 2013). Some people do have no useful vision, or even no perception of light. These patients can be described as 'functionally blind', which Genensky (1971) defined as:

- unable to read or write visually;
- unable to manoeuvre or orientate visually;
- unable to recognise objects visually.

For such people, help would involve a strategy of sensory substitution (see Chapter 15): a replacement of the visual sense by a tactile or auditory stimulus, such as Braille. The remaining population of people who are registered as SI or SSI have low vision, and will be helped with the strategies described in Parts II and III of this book, allowing them to develop their own personal 'toolkit' of resources.

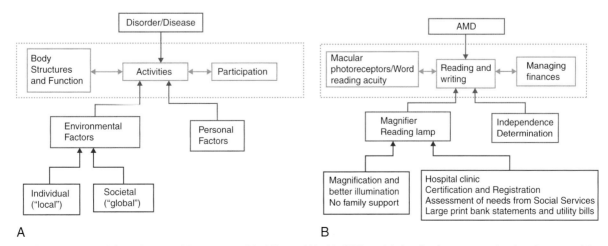

A   B

Fig. 1.1 (A) The International Classification of Functioning, Disability and Health (ICF) model showing how personal and environmental factors can influence activity limitation and participation restriction. (B) An example of the ICF completed for an individual patient. *AMD*, Age-related macular degeneration.

TABLE 1.2 The Distribution of Visual Impairment in a Blind Population

Visual Impairment	% of Blind Population
Absolute blindness (no perception of light)	5.2
Perception of light	9.1
Perception of light with detection of direction	1.2
6/240	15.7
6/240 to 6/120	9.9
6/120 to 6/60	18.2
6/60	27.7
Restricted visual field with acuity >6/60	5.7
Unknown	7.3

From Riley, L. H. (1970). The epidemiology of partial sight. American Journal of Optometry and Archives of American Academy of Optometry, 47(8), 587–600.

The Multidisciplinary Approach to Low-Vision Care

The consequences of visual impairment affect many aspects of the individual's life, and care of the patient requires much more than simple 'vision enhancement'. Jose (1983, p. 62) defined the concept of an integrated model of low-vision rehabilitation which:

> 'must include a comprehensive look at all the individual's needs (vocational, educational, social, psychological, financial, optometric and medical). Such a service mandates the interaction of several disciplines … Simply stated, low vision care is a philosophy that promotes the maximal use of vision, and the vision rehabilitation service is a commitment by an interdisciplinary group of professionals to help low vision persons fulfill that philosophy'.

The low vision service should be a rehabilitative or habilitative process which provides a range of services for people with low vision to enable them to make use of their eyesight to achieve maximum potential:

- addressing psychological and emotional needs of patient and carer;
- assessing function and providing aids and training; and
- facilitating modification to home, school and work environments.

In the context of low vision, carers are often family members (spouse, parent, sibling or child) and are perhaps better described as 'informal caregivers'. They can be adversely affected in this situation and experience stress and anxiety, and often require practical advice and information, and emotional support (Enoch et al., 2021).

The concept is gaining acceptance, although the UK was slower than many countries in realising its potential. There is still little agreement about where the boundaries should be placed between the roles of particular professions, and it must be accepted that the scope of services provided by a given 'profession' will vary between practitioners,

depending on that individual's experiences, geographical location and local resources. Much is made of just how great the range of professionals involved in a 'model' low-vision service can be—an educationalist, employment specialist, physiotherapist, occupational therapist, social worker, lighting engineer, orthoptist, psychologist and audiologist, among others, may be called into the 'vision team' for particular patients. It is usual, however, to have a 'core' of an ophthalmologist, an optometrist (carrying out refraction and prescribing), a 'low-vision trainer' and a rehabilitation officer (although this would be an occupational therapist in some countries).

Low-vision training may be carried out by a separate individual, or this role can be fulfilled by another member of the team, but this person has a pivotal role in translating the ability to, for example, 'see to read' (reach a threshold performance for letters of newsprint size) into regularly and comfortably reading the newspaper for pleasure. It is clear that satisfying acuity requirements does not necessarily guarantee efficient reading by the low-vision individual, if training and 'rehabilitation' are lacking. If patients are left to their own devices to learn to use an aid, this may not occur spontaneously as the optimum method is not always obvious. The patient needs to be taught how to apply the aid to the particular task in which they are interested, and this training is an essential part of the rehabilitation process. In the UK, low-vision services are organised in several different ways, but there are few examples of truly multidisciplinary clinics (Dickinson et al., 2011). More typically, all the professionals mentioned previously are available but in different places. There is therefore a multiagency approach to providing the full range of rehabilitation, which means that there needs to be excellent interagency communication to make this work properly and effectively. This has the potential to be very confusing for the patient, as all these communications are happening in the background (if they are happening at all), and the patients tend not to appreciate the way in which the provision is organised. The possibility that individuals will not be aware of, or not gain access to, the full range of resources, is much greater in such a system.

Fig. 1.2 shows the components of a comprehensive multidisciplinary service, much of which could be delivered by several different professionals. There is often an impression that rehabilitation has to wait until treatment of a condition is completed. The circular diagram helps to illustrate that there is no fixed entry point to the service, or any specific patient pathway. Several stages can occur simultaneously—even whilst a condition is under active treatment the patient could be referred for (perhaps temporary) aids and assistance. If appropriate to the individual, access to all the professionals in this multidisciplinary team should be available. Different interactions may be appropriate at different stages of the sight loss journey, and some facilities will be revisited several times.

Tables 1.3 and 1.4 give examples of how particular individuals might interact with such a system, and how different the patient journey can be. The emphasis is on patient-centred

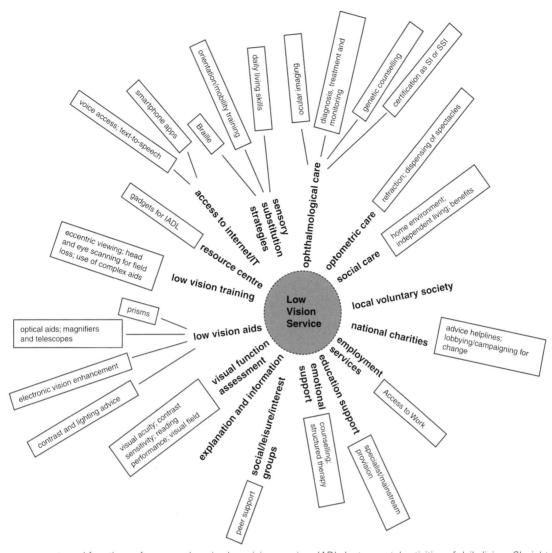

Fig. 1.2 The components and functions of a comprehensive low vision service. *IADL*, Instrumental activities of daily living; *SI*, sight impairment; *SSI*, severe sight impairment.

care, with provision guided by the patient's requirements and choices. From a UK perspective, the different professionals and organisations who may be involved in the patient management at different stages have been identified. However, there are some services which could be delivered in a variety of different ways: for example, information about the eye disease might come from the optometrist, ophthalmologist, ECLO or a charity website, and signposting to other services can happen in many ways. Unfortunately, awareness of the full range of services available (by both professionals and patients) is not as good as it should be, and opportunities for signposting are often missed.

Patient 1 (Table 1.3) attended their local optometry practice for a routine eye examination, but complaining of visual difficulties with TV and reading. The optometrist identified dry AMD, and offered practical advice about improved contrast and lighting around the home; advised sitting closer to the TV; and provided reading spectacles with a higher reading addition than the habitual progressive lenses which the patient used. The patient was advised to go the RNIB online

shop to purchase a suitable reading lamp, and was given details of the Macular Society. From the Macular Society newsletters and website the patient learned about monitoring their vision with the Amsler grid, and, a few years later, did identify central distortion in one eye and attended the hospital, where treatment was given. Several years later, the condition had progressed in both eyes to the extent that the patient was eligible for registration, and the ECLO discussed this with the patient, and they agreed that this would be beneficial. In conversation with the patient, the ECLO realised that the patient had been restricting their social activities recently, and suggested they contact the local society for the blind. The patient was able to join a singing group, and get advice about how to make their home computer easier to see. They saw several gadgets to help with household tasks in the Resource Centre, and when the Rehabilitation Worker came to assess them at home, several of these were provided for them. The optometrist in the hospital low-vision clinic provided optical magnifiers to the patient for reading, but these were tiring to use for long periods. When the patient

TABLE 1.3   The Interaction of an Example Patient (Patient 1) With Low-Vision Services

Timeline			
	Community optometrist	Identification of dry AMD	Vision enhancement advice 'bigger, bolder, brighter'
	Signposting to ➡	RNIB (online shop)	Task lamp
	Signposting to ➡	Macular society	Information about AMD
			Lifestyle advice
	Patient identifies visual distortion and attends Emergency Eye Centre		
	Ophthalmologist	Anti-VEGF treatment	
	Ophthalmologist	Certification and forms sent to Local Authority for registration	
	ECLO	Benefits of registration	
	Signposting to ➡	Local society for the blind	Advice on IT accessibility
			Resource Centre for demo of IADL gadgets
			'Singing' special interest/peer support group
	Hospital Optometrist	Optical aids for TV and reading	
	Rehabilitation Officer (makes contact with patient as part of registration process)	Assessment of need	Adaptations around the home
			Provision of symbol cane
			Advice on audio reading and Talking Books
			Benefits advice
	Macular Society	Information about electronic magnifiers	
	Supplier	Advice and purchase of electronic magnifier	

AMD, Age-related macular degeneration; *ECLO*, eye clinic liaison officer; *IADL*, instrumental activities of daily living; *IT*, information technology; *RNIB*, Royal National Institute for the Blind; *VEGF*, vascular endothelial growth factor.

TABLE 1.4   The Interaction of an Example Patient (Patient 2) With Low-Vision Services

Timeline			
	Community optometrist	Identification of retinal abnormality, annular field loss	Lighting, glare and contrast advice; computer accessibility options; driving advice
	Signposting to ➡	University Disability and Student Support Service	
	Ophthalmologist	Diagnosis of RP	
	Genetic testing		
	Electrodiagnostic testing		
	ECLO	Emotional support	
	Signposting to ➡	Retina UK	Peer support Facebook group
	Ophthalmologist	Registration	
	Hospital optometrist	Optical aids for field loss	
	Community optometrist	Spectacles and tints	
	ECLO		
	Signpost to ➡	Disabled Students Allowance	Text-to-speech software
	Signpost to ➡	Blind in Business	Employment training: Access to Work
	Social services	Long cane mobility	
	Signposting to ➡	Disability Snowsport UK	Skiing with guide

ECLO, Eye clinic liaison officer; *RP*, retinitis pigmentosa.

attended the Macular Society conference, they were able to see the many different types of electronic magnifiers: they arranged with a supplier to purchase one, after having a home demonstration.

Patient 2 (Table 1.4) is a university student who attended their community optometry practice complaining of difficulties with night vision, and discomfort in bright light. The optometrist advised the patient how to reverse the contrast on the computer, and advised on tinted lenses and using a baseball cap to avoid glare. The patient was referred to the ophthalmologist who confirmed the diagnosis of retinitis pigmentosa. The ECLO supported the patient as they came to terms with this diagnosis, and signposted them to Retina UK, where they would be able to access peer support from others in a similar situation. As the condition progressed, the patient was eligible for certification and registration. The hospital optometrist discussed optical and electronic aids with the patient, but they decided not to go ahead because of the unusual cosmetic appearance. The ECLO told the patient that they could get help via the Disabled Students Allowance to purchase text-to-speech software since they found reading visually very tiring. The patient was concerned about how they would find employment after graduation, so they were signposted to Blind in Business to get individual guidance. Although the patient had rejected contact with Social Services when they were first registered, they later realised that they would benefit from mobility training and contacted the Rehabilitation Worker. The patient had given up on skiing as their vision deteriorated, but the Rehabilitation Worker told them that this was one of many sports which are adapted for individuals with VI, and put them in contact with the relevant organisation.

The Role of the Optometrist

There are two areas in which the optometrist has a particular role in low vision. The first is in prevention and health education. If pathology can be detected at an early stage before the patient experiences obvious symptoms, then treatment may be possible, and is likely to be more effective. The aim is to successfully treat such conditions so that permanent impairment does not result. Advice on the use of suitable protective eyewear can also prevent VI due to trauma.

If impairment is not avoided, then optometric intervention to prescribe low-vision aids (LVAs) can take place. The aim now is to prevent activity limitation—the impairment itself cannot be altered. There is a certain amount of overlap of all the strategies involved in care of the low-vision patient, and there will be occasions when suitably experienced professionals move beyond their usual remit. It is perfectly possible, for example, for the optometrist to suggest how the patient might enhance the dial markings on a domestic appliance if the patient has not seen a rehabilitation officer to obtain this advice. Increasingly there are enhanced services delivered in community practices (see Chapter 22). At the very least, the optometrist should be aware of the different organisations who could help the patient, be prepared to offer advice to the patient and their families, and know where to direct them for further information on the help to which they are entitled. Community optometrists could look in the Sightline directory (by postcode) (www. sightlinedirectory.org.uk) to find information about the different local organisations that there are in their area. Another responsibility of community optometrists is to hand out and explain the LVL to those patients who they feel would benefit from advice and assessment from social services (but are not ready or eligible for registration).

The Role of the Patient

A final point which has not yet been considered in this scheme is the role of the patient and their family and friends. The process of low-vision care is not something which happens whilst patients passively observe. They have to participate, being willing to discuss their difficulties, and then consider and try out possible solutions. Patients must be motivated to want to play an active part and must feel able to do so. From a naive viewpoint, the situation seems obvious; of course, patients must want to improve their visual performance—it is only natural that they should do so, and they would not have sought advice otherwise. It does not take long to realise that this is not necessarily true for a whole variety of reasons.

To consider just a few examples:

- The use of a magnifier may require patients to hold the reading material closer to them, which they may not be prepared to do.
- The patient may feel a fraud having been registered SSI but now being able to see to read.
- Older people living alone may feel that children and grandchildren will not call in so frequently if a magnifier allows them to read their own correspondence, or a child may not take them to the supermarket if their shopping is delivered online.
- The patient's family may not like the patient drawing attention to them by reading the restaurant menu with a magnifier.
- The patient may only be interested in trying to find some new surgical or medical treatment which offers a complete cure of the visual impairment.

These factors will need to be identified and addressed in order for useful advice to be given to the patient.

REFERENCES

Abel, R. A. (1989). Visually impaired people, the identification of the need for specialist provision: A historical perspective. *British Journal of Visual Impairment, VII*, 47–51.

Barry, R. J., & Murray, P. I. (2005). Unregistered visual impairment: Is registration a failing system. *British Journal of Ophthalmology, 89*(8), 995–998. https://doi.org/10.1136/bjo.2004.059915.

Beverley, C. A., Bath, P. A., & Barber, R. (2011). Health and social care information for visually-impaired people. *Aslib Proceedings: New Information Perspectives, 63*(2–3), 256–274. https://doi.org/10.1108/00012531111135691.

Boyce, T., Leamon, S., Slade, J., et al. (2014). Certification for vision impairment: Researching perceptions, processes and practicalities in health and social care professionals and patients. *British Medical Journal Open, 4*(4), 1–7. https://doi.org/10.1136/bmjopen-2013-004319.

Bruce, I., McKennell, A., & Walker, E. (1991). *Blind and partially sighted adults in Britain: The RNIB survey* (Vol. 1). HMSO.

Charlton, M., Jenkins, D., Rhodes, C., et al. (2013). The Welsh Low Vision Service—A summary. *Optometry in Practice, 12*(1), 29–38.

Dementia and Disability Unit. (2017, Aug 17). *Certificate of Vision Impairment: Explanatory notes for consultant ophthalmologists and hospital eye clinic staff in England.* Department of Health. https://assets.publishing.service.gov.uk/government/uploads/system/uploads/attachment_data/file/637590/CVI_guidance.pdf.

Dickinson, C., Linck, P., Tudor-Edwards, R., et al. (2011). A profile of low vision services in England: The low vision service model evaluation (LOVSME) project. *Eye, 25*(7), 829–831. https://doi.org/10.1038/eye.2011.112.

Duckworth, K., Overbury, O., Conrod, B., et al. (1994). Effects of health workers' behaviour on low vision patients' anxiety levels and visual performance. *Investigative Ophthalmology & Visual Science, 35*, 1414.

England, N. H. S. (2017). *Accessible Information Standard: Post-implementation review-report* (1–22). www.england.nhs.uk/accessibleinfo.

Enoch, J., Dickinson, C., & Subramanian, A. (2021). What support do caregivers of people with visual impairment receive and require? An exploratory study of UK healthcare and charity professionals' perspectives. *Eye.* https://doi.org/10.1038/s41433-021-01821-6.

Fischer, M. L. (1993). "Legal gray areas" in low vision: The need for clarification of regulations. *Journal of the American Optometric Association, 64*(1), 12–14.

Genensky, S. M. (1971). A functional classification system of the visually impaired to replace the legal definition of blindness. *American Journal of Optometry and Archives of American Academy of Optometry, 48*(8), 631–642.

Gresset, J., Vachon, N., Simonet, P., et al. (1993). Discrepancy in the evaluation of visual impairment of elderly low-vision patients by general eye care practitioners and by low-vision practitioners. *Optometry and Vision Science: Official Publication of the American Academy of Optometry, 70*(1), 39–44. https://doi.org/10.1097/00006324-199301000-00008.

Henshaws. (2019). *Benefits and support.* https://www.henshaws.org.uk/knowledge-village/benefits-support/.

Hernandez Trillo, A., & Dickinson, C. M. (2012). The impact of visual and nonvisual factors on quality of life and adaptation in adults with visual impairment. *Investigative Ophthalmology and Visual Science, 53*(7), 4234–4241. https://doi.org/10.1167/iovs.12-9580.

Hyvarinen, L. (1992). Rehabilitation and world blindness. *Current Opinion in Ophthalmology, 3*(6), 793–795. https://doi.org/10.1097/00055735-199212000-00018.

JobcentrePlus. (2021). How to get a job when you have a disability. https://www.jobcentreguide.co.uk/jobcentre-plus-guide/34/about-disability-employment-advisors.

Jose, R. T. (1983). *Understanding low vision.* American Foundation for the Blind.

Marsay, S. (2005). Accessible information: Specification V1.1. *Nursing, 35*(7), 10. https://doi.org/10.1097/00152193-200507000-00008.

Martin, J., Meltzer, H., & Ellit, D. (1988). *The prevalence of disability among adults. Office of Population Censuses and Surveys.* HMSO.

Mitry, D., Bunce, C., Wormald, R., et al. (2013). Causes of certifications for severe sight impairment (blind) and sight impairment (partial sight) in children in England and Wales. *British Journal of Ophthalmology, 93*, 1431–1436. https://doi.org/10.1136/bjophthalmol-2013-303578.

Mokhles, P., Schouten, J. S. A. G., Beckers, H. J. M., et al. (2017). Does the World Health Organization criterion adequately define glaucoma blindness. *Clinical Ophthalmology, 11*, 473–480. https://doi.org/10.2147/OPTH.S129605.

National Patient Safety Agency (NPSA) & NHS (2006). *A guide to the graphic design of medication packaging* (76).

Pezzullo, L., Streatfeild, J., Simkiss, P., et al. (2018). The economic impact of sight loss and blindness in the UK adult population. *BMC Health Services Research, 18*(1), 1–13. https://doi.org/10.1186/s12913-018-2836-0.

Quartilho, A., Simkiss, P., Zekite, A., et al. (2016). Leading causes of certifiable visual loss in England and Wales during the year ending 31 March 2013. *Eye, 30*(4), 602–607. https://doi.org/10.1038/eye.2015.288.

Riley, L. H. (1970). The epidemiology of partial sight. *American Journal of Optometry and Archives of American Academy of Optometry, 47*(8), 587–600.

RNIB. (2021). *Employment support and benefits.* RNIB.

Robinson, R., Deutsch, J., Jones, H. S., et al. (1994). Unrecognised and unregistered visual impairment. *British Journal of Ophthalmology, 78*(10), 736–740. https://doi.org/10.1136/bjo.78.10.736.

Rovner, B. W., Casten, R. J., Hegel, M. T., et al. (2014). Personality and functional vision in older adults with age-related macular degeneration. *Journal of Visual Impairment and Blindness, 108*(3), 187–199.

Royal National Institute for the Blind. (RNIB). (2020). *Benefits, concessions and registration: About this guide.* RNIB.

SCOPE. (2020). *Access to Work grant scheme.* https://www.scope.org.uk/advice-and-support/access-to-work-grant-scheme/?gclid=Cj0KCQjwjbyYBhCdARIsAArC6LIl0iDJzVoVGyPEvk-v-SknarUcspVqZaqphnUS59PETBIxQ2Ulve8aAiP6EALw_wcB.

Silver, J., Gould, E. S., Irvine, D., et al. (1978). Visual acuity at home and in eye clinics. *Transactions of the Ophthalmological Societies of the United Kingdom, 98*, 262–266.

Tan, A. C. S., Man, R., Wong, C. W., et al. (2018). Randomized controlled trial evaluating a novel community eye care programme for elderly individuals with visual impairment. *Clinical and Experimental Ophthalmology, 46*(6), 593–599. https://doi.org/10.1111/ceo.13140.

United Nations. (1993). Standard Rules on the Equalization of Opportunities for Persons with Disabilities. General Assembly on 20 December 1993 (resolution 48/96 annex). https://www.un.org/development/desa/disabilities/standard-rules-on-the-equalization-of-opportunities-for-persons-with-disabilities.html.

WHO. (1996). Blindness information collected from various sources. *Epidemiology Vital Statistics Reports, 19*, 437–511.

WHO. (2019). *World report on vision* (Vol. 214). World health Organization.

World Blind Union. (2021). *Project Aspiro.* http://www.projectaspiro.com/en/Pages/default.aspx.

World Health Organization (WHO). (2018). *International classification of diseases* (11th ed.). https://icd.who.int/en.

Prevalence and Causes of Low Vision

THE WORLD-WIDE SITUATION

The prevalence of visual impairment (VI) is the percentage of the general population who have the condition at a given point in time. Usually, the prevalence of VI in a selected but representative sample is determined, and then extrapolated to the entire population. If comparisons are to be made between countries, and over time, then a consistent definition of VI is required, and the World Health Organization (WHO) definitions have been discussed in Chapter 1. These definitions, part of the 11th revision of the *International Classification of Diseases (ICD-11)*, have changed considerably over time, leading to significant increases in the reported prevalence. This means that comparisons to surveys in earlier years should be made with caution.

The priority for the WHO is to determine the Global Burden of Disease. VI is one of 291 different diseases and injuries (Keeffe & Resnikoff, 2018) which are investigated to establish the cost on the population in terms of the years of life lost (less relevant for VI than some other diseases) or years lived with a disability. These data can be used to advocate for resources to be allocated to the particular diseases by member states. Monitoring changes over time is necessary to judge the effectiveness of the healthcare infrastructure which has been put in place.

If all age groups in the population are not equally affected, this could be expressed in the form of an 'age blindness burden' (ABB). This can be found by dividing the proportion of the blind in the age group, by the proportion of the region's population which is of the same age.

So,

$$ABB = \frac{\% \text{ of blind in that age group}}{\% \text{ of total population in that age group}}$$

$$= \frac{\dfrac{\text{number of blind in age group}}{\text{total number of blind}}}{\dfrac{\text{number of population in age group}}{\text{total population}}}$$

If not all countries/geographical regions are equally affected, it is possible to express this difference in terms of a regional blindness burden (RBB), found by dividing the proportion of the total world blind in that region, by the proportion of the world population which inhabits that area.

So,

$$RBB = \frac{\% \text{ of blind in the region}}{\% \text{ of total population in the region}}$$

$$= \frac{\dfrac{\text{number of blind in region}}{\text{total number of blind}}}{\dfrac{\text{number of population in region}}{\text{total population}}}$$

If the region has its 'fair share' of the world blind population—for example, it might have 10% of the world's population and 10% of the world blind amongst that population—it would have an RBB of 1.0. A RBB >1.0 indicates that the region needs to prioritise blindness prevention and treatment when deciding how to divide limited resources. However, it is likely that each region has a different age profile within its population, so the 'age adjusted' prevalence could be used to make the regional comparison more realistic. This compares each population as if they had the same age profile.

Prevalence of Visual Impairment

The most recently published data suggest that the age-adjusted prevalence of moderate/severe VI and blindness globally is 4.34%, based on over 338 million cases (Bourne et al., 2021; Steinmetz et al., 2021) (Table 2.1) (It should be borne in mind that including mild impairment and uncorrected presbyopia increases this figure to 2.2 billion).

This can be broken down by geographical region (Pascolini & Mariotti, 2012) to show the prevalence and regional burden of both blindness and moderate/severe VI (Table 2.2). It can be seen that the regional differences for more severe loss are relatively small but would be much greater if mild impairment and uncorrected presbyopia were included. Rates of unaddressed near vision impairment are estimated to be greater than 80% in western, eastern and central sub-Saharan Africa, while comparative rates in high-income regions of North America, Australasia, Western Europe and Asia-Pacific are reported to be lower than 10% (Bourne et al., 2021; Steinmetz et al., 2021).

TABLE 2.1 Age-Adjusted Prevalence of VI and Blindness Globally in 2020

	Blind	Moderate/Severe VI	Mild VI
Globally	0.53%	3.58%	3.2%
	43.3 million	295 million	

VI, Visual impairment.
Reprinted with permission from Elsevier. Causes of blindness and vision impairment in 2020 and trends over 30 years, and prevalence of avoidable blindness in relation to VISION 2020: the Right to Sight: an analysis for the Global Burden of Disease Study. *The Lancet Global Health, 9*(2), e144–e160.

Fig. 2.1 shows the difference in prevalence by age, which is much more dramatic. As shown in Table 2.3, throughout the world it is older adults within the population who bear the burden of significant VI, with the global prevalence rising from 10 in every 1000 children to 140 in every 1000 adults over 50 years of age.

Causes of Visual Impairment

Many of the most common causes of moderate or severe distance vision impairment or blindness globally could be treated or prevented: these are uncorrected refractive error, cataract, glaucoma, corneal opacities, diabetic retinopathy, and trachoma.

A more detailed analysis (Flaxman et al., 2017) shows the relative importance of the major causes of blindness and moderate/severe VI in the different economic/geographical regions in 2015 (Table 2.4).

It can be clearly seen that refractive error is responsible for over half of all VI, and cataract is responsible for more blindness than any other condition, despite the management of cataract being straightforward. This is particularly the case in low-/middle-income countries where surgical treatment is not readily available. A recent study (Resnikoff et al., 2020) showed that the estimated global number of ophthalmologists was 232,866 in 2015, ranging from 0 in some small Pacific Island countries (Cook Islands, Micronesia, Nauru, Niue and Tuvalu) to 36,342 in China. Approximately 17% of the global population in 132 countries have access to less than 5% of the global ophthalmologist population. Two-thirds of the global ophthalmologist population were located in 13 countries (China, USA, India, Japan, Brazil, Russia, Germany, Italy, Egypt, France, Mexico, Spain and Poland). Fourteen countries had less than 1 ophthalmologist per million people and 13 countries had more than 100 ophthalmologists per million population. The data also showed a dramatic relationship with income, with those countries with higher income presenting a greater density of ophthalmologists: 76.2 per million population, compared

TABLE 2.2 Number of People Blind and With Moderate/Severe VI, and Corresponding Share of Global Impairment, by Region, in 2010

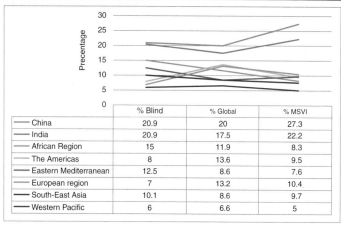

	% Blind	% Global	% MSVI
China	20.9	20	27.3
India	20.9	17.5	22.2
African Region	15	11.9	8.3
The Americas	8	13.6	9.5
Eastern Mediterranean	12.5	8.6	7.6
European region	7	13.2	10.4
South-East Asia	10.1	8.6	9.7
Western Pacific	6	6.6	5

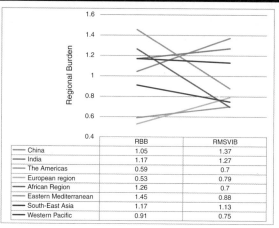

	RBB	RMSVIB
China	1.05	1.37
India	1.17	1.27
The Americas	0.59	0.7
European region	0.53	0.79
African Region	1.26	0.7
Eastern Mediterranean	1.45	0.88
South-East Asia	1.17	1.13
Western Pacific	0.91	0.75

(Left) The percentage of the global population (% Global), the percentage of the blind population (% Blind), and the percentage of the population with moderate and severe visual impairment (% MSVI), by world region, in 2010. (Right) A calculation of the Regional Blindness Burden (RBB) and Regional Moderate and Severe Visual Impairment Burden (RMSVIB) as described in the text.
Based on data from Pascolini and Mariotti, 2012.

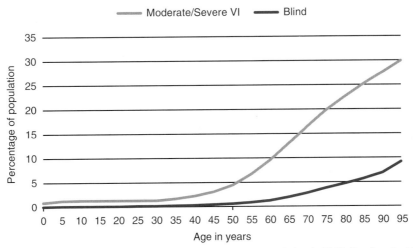

Fig. 2.1 The prevalence (%) of distance vision impairment *(VI)* by age in the global population in 2020. Reprinted with permission from Elsevier. Trends in prevalence of blindness and distance and near vision impairment over 30 years: An analysis for the Global Burden of Disease Study. *The Lancet Global Health*, *9*(2), e130–e143; Reprinted with permission from Elsevier. Causes of blindness and vision impairment in 2020 and trends over 30 years, and prevalence of avoidable blindness in relation to VISION 2020: the Right to Sight: an analysis for the Global Burden of Disease Study. *The Lancet Global Health*, *9*(2), e144–e160.

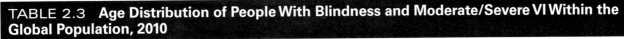

TABLE 2.3 Age Distribution of People With Blindness and Moderate/Severe VI Within the Global Population, 2010

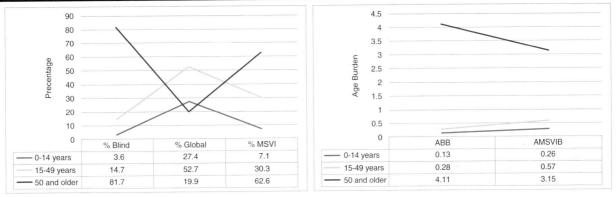

	% Blind	% Global	% MSVI
0-14 years	3.6	27.4	7.1
15-49 years	14.7	52.7	30.3
50 and older	81.7	19.9	62.6

	ABB	AMSVIB
0-14 years	0.13	0.26
15-49 years	0.28	0.57
50 and older	4.11	3.15

(Left) The percentage of the global population (% Global), the percentage of the blind population (% Blind), and the percentage of the population with moderate and severe visual impairment (% MSVI), by age group, in 2010. (Right) A calculation of the Age Blindness Burden (ABB) and the Age Moderate and Severe Visual Impairment Burden (AMSVIB) as described in the text.
Based on data from Pascolini and Mariotti, 2012.

with 3.7 per million in low-income countries. Surprisingly, the study found that the density of ophthalmologists was very weakly correlated with the prevalence of blindness. There are many factors that could contribute to this: the proportion of ophthalmologists who carry out cataract surgery, the age range and urban/rural mix of the population, and variable access to healthcare based on socioeconomic status.

Trachoma is caused by the Gram-negative bacterium *Chlamydia trachomatis*, which produces a chronic follicular conjunctivitis, characterised by lesions of the tarsal conjunctiva. A single infective episode, often occurring first in the preschool child, is self-limiting and unlikely to cause blindness, but repeated re-infection leads to conjunctival scarring. This leads to trachomatous trichiasis (TT) in some people and results in mechanical abrasion of the cornea, and secondary bacterial infection, leading to ulceration, scarring and vascularisation with eventual blindness due to viewing through an opaque cornea. Trachoma can be eliminated as a public

health problem through use of a package intervention known as the 'SAFE strategy', comprising surgery for TT, antibiotics to clear ocular *C. trachomatis* infection, facial cleanliness and environmental improvement (access to clean water and sanitation) to reduce *C. trachomatis* transmission (WHO, 2020b). Nine countries (Cambodia, China, Ghana, Islamic Republic of Iran, Lao People's Democratic Republic, Mexico, Morocco, Nepal and Oman) have been officially validated as having eliminated trachoma as a public health problem. Another four countries (Gambia, Iraq, Myanmar and Togo) have reported achievement of the prevalence targets for elimination.

Onchocerciasis is caused by the parasite *Onchocerca volvulus* for which humans are the only natural host. The parasite larvae and the adult worms can be found throughout the body, particularly the eyes and skin. Infection often occurs in childhood and leads to significant VI (due to the keratitis, uveitis and choroiditis caused by direct invasion of the tissues) in about 10% of those infected. The disease occurs mainly in

TABLE 2.4 **Mean Estimated Percentage[a] of the Major Causes of Blindness (Upper Figure) and Moderate/Severe VI (Lower Figure), in Each Economic/Geographical Region in 2015**

Region	Uncorrected Refractive Error	Cataract	Glaucoma	AMD	DR	Corneal Opacity	Trachoma
High-income Asia Pacific	13.13	20.32	13.51	16.66	3.87	2.38	0
	49.36	14.66	3.6	11.60	4.07	0.79	0
Central Asia	12.85	25.94	14.17	14.01	3.60	3.58	0
	48.26	18.11	4.05	10.05	4.06	1.41	0
East Asia	12.90	43.58	7.06	5.33	0.51	4.26	1.81
	47.08	32.54	1.56	3.39	0.57	1.54	1.33
South Asia	36.43	36.58	5.81	1.44	0.16	2.43	0.04
	66.39	23.62	1.09	1.31	0.15	0.74	0.03
Southeast Asia	12.57	45.0	6.99	5.24	0.59	4.39	0.13
	46.14	33.95	1.57	3.46	0.71	1.63	0.07
Australasia	13.11	19.65	13.48	16.52	4.48	2.35	0
	49.26	14.1	3.59	11.36	4.72	0.78	0
Caribbean	12.59	25.74	9.61	5.64	0.79	1.65	0
	47.85	18.09	2.25	3.76	0.89	0.52	0
Central Europe	12.98	25.42	14.08	15.92	3.10	3.63	0
	49.40	18.16	3.95	10.85	3.12	1.38	0
Eastern Europe	13.00	20.91	14.33	19.53	4.91	3.43	0
	48.53	14.84	4.13	13.39	5.06	1.32	0
Western Europe	13.12	21.42	13.50	15.39	3.30	2.43	0
	49.61	15.49	3.58	10.68	3.48	0.81	0
Andean Latin America	12.62	27.48	9.40	3.84	0.39	1.60	0
	46.07	20.23	2.22	2.44	0.42	0.53	0
Central Latin America	12.71	23.97	9.99	6.19	0.95	1.62	0
	47.90	17.03	2.34	3.96	1.02	0.52	0
Southern Latin America	13.00	21.68	13.61	14.34	3.51	2.41	0
	48.20	15.95	3.71	10.11	3.93	0.82	0
Tropical Latin America	12.90	21.88	10.45	7.39	1.33	1.54	0
	49.26	15.27	2.41	4.68	1.38	0.49	0
North Africa and Middle East	12.34	28.11	6.89	3.16	1.39	4.47	2.62
	44.58	21.37	1.62	2.16	1.61	1.67	1.90
High-income North America	13.08	20.13	13.45	15.85	4.33	2.39	0
	49.53	14.39	3.56	10.86	4.55	0.79	0
Oceania	12.61	47.29	6.72	3.08	0.31	4.24	0
	47.76	34.60	1.43	2.07	0.34	1.55	0
Central sub-Saharan Africa	12.72	43.62	14.14	5.18	0.47	4.01	0.27
	46.50	34.41	3.63	3.42	0.51	1.55	0.21
East sub-Saharan Africa	12.16	44.67	11.70	3.16	0.23	3.76	7.02
	46.79	32.35	2.90	2.37	0.31	1.36	5.78
Southern sub-Saharan Africa	12.38	35.18	15.47	11.75	1.56	4.05	0.51
	48.05	26.94	4.12	8.01	1.77	1.53	0.31
West sub-Saharan Africa	12.36	43.56	13.27	3.98	0.29	3.85	3.43
	46.35	34.14	3.29	2.54	0.38	1.49	2.46
World	**20.28**	**35.15**	**8.49**	**5.93**	**1.06**	**3.21**	**0.97**
	52.34	**25.15**	**2.05**	**4.38**	**1.30**	**1.14**	**0.64**

[a]Percentage on each row do not add to 100% since 'other' causes omitted.

AMD, Age-related macular degeneration; *DR*, diabetic retinopathy; *VI*, visual impairment.

Reprinted with permission from Elsevier. Global causes of blindness and distance vision impairment 1990–2020: a systematic review and meta-analysis. *The Lancet Global Health, 5*(12), e1221–e1234.

West Africa but there are endemic regions across the African continent, and some small foci in Central and South America: in these areas, onchocerciasis used to overtake cataract as the major cause of blindness. According to WHO (2020a), currently, around 218 million people live in areas known to be endemic for onchocerciasis. However, for many there is little risk for onchocerciasis-related blindness or skin disease as long as mass drug administration (MDA) with ivermectin continues. Four countries have been verified for the interruption of transmission of human onchocerciasis, and many others have finished MDA, completed posttreatment surveillance, or both, in at least one transmission area in their territory.

The chronic age-related conditions of diabetic retinopathy, glaucoma and age-related macular degeneration (AMD)

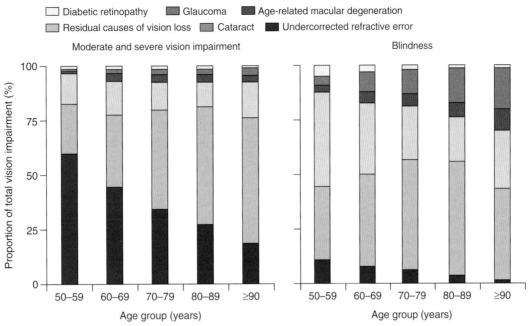

Fig. 2.2 The relative amount of moderate/severe visual impairment and blindness attributable to each cause, by age group. Reprinted with permission from Elsevier. Causes of blindness and vision impairment in 2020 and trends over 30 years, and prevalence of avoidable blindness in relation to VISION 2020: the Right to Sight: an analysis for the Global Burden of Disease Study. *The Lancet Global Health, 9*(2), e144–e160.

are relatively less important contributors to the prevalence of significant visual loss globally (Fig. 2.2). However, they are important because (1) they are less likely to be treatable because relatively sophisticated instrumentation and regular monitoring are required to manage the conditions (and to diagnose glaucoma initially), and (2) the prevalence is likely to increase as overall life expectancy improves (as they are more common in the older age groups).

Both glaucoma and AMD are less likely to be identified in population surveys because any coexisting uncorrected refractive errors or cataracts are more likely to be listed as the cause of the visual loss (Keeffe & Resnikoff, 2018).

VISUAL IMPAIRMENT IN THE UK

Prevalence of Visual Impairment From Registration Data

Registration of the visually impaired not only serves as a passport to various benefits on an individual basis (see Chapter 1) but can also give information on the prevalence and causes of severe sight impairment (SSI) and sight impairment (SI) in the UK. Prevalence is given by the total number of individuals on the registers on a particular date each year. The incidence can also be found: this is the percentage of those who were newly registered within the preceding year who have a particular status. A decrease in the incidence of the number of people whose sight has been lost to a particular pathology is obviously encouraging, but it must be remembered that it is a relative figure: an apparent fall in one condition may be due to a rise in the number of those registered due to other conditions.

This epidemiological information cannot easily be compared with data from other countries, as the criteria used for certification are unique. In addition, certification and registration are both voluntary, and there are many reasons why a patient may choose not to be registered: lack of financial benefit (especially for SI registration), the social stigma of disability, poor patient acceptance of 'blindness', and others.

It might be expected that under-registration is also due to some individuals not being under the care of an ophthalmologist. However, Robinson et al. (1994) found that amongst those attending ophthalmic clinics, only 48.4% of those eligible were registered. It appears that active treatment tends to mitigate against registration, with registration most likely to take place when the patient is due for discharge. Ophthalmologists based their decisions on offering certification on the visual acuity (VA) rather than the patient's functioning, and regarded certification as the 'final stage' in the medical management of a patient's condition, only offering it at the end of the treatment (Boyce et al., 2014). This means that many do not get help when it would be useful, and this contributes to the negative feeling they have of registration: a last resort when nothing else can be done. It is important that health professionals and patients are well informed about the purpose and benefits of certification and registration, both to improve support for these patients who are severely sight impaired and sight impaired, and to provide important epidemiological data.

Table 2.5 suggests that since the year 2000, the number of people registered severely sight impaired has steadily decreased to a small extent, whilst the number on the register for SI has remained constant overall. These figures seem surprising, particularly in view of the increasing life expectancy in the population, although improved treatment for exudative AMD may be one cause. There are also considerable (and unexplained) regional variations in registrations, which suggest that they represent an incomplete picture. It appears intuitively incorrect that there should be similar numbers registered in each category as one would expect the lower degrees of impairment to predominate (e.g. see the worldwide figures for blindness compared to VI). However, many individuals who would be categorised as visually impaired on WHO criteria fall below the threshold for SI certification.

It is interesting to look at the age variation in these figures: the 2017 data suggested a total visually impaired population in England of more than 290,475, with over 65% of those affected aged over 75 years of age (Table 2.6). In contrast, the number of visually impaired children is very low, yet they form a much larger proportion of the general population.

Around one-third of those registered also experience at least one additional disability (Table 2.7), with physical disabilities being most common. The extent of those disabilities may be underestimated: if an individual has multiple disabilities, only one is recorded.

Causes of Visual Impairment From Registration Data

Despite its imperfections, the registration process produces a considerable body of data which can be further analysed to look at the different diseases which cause VI. It must be emphasised that the results do not indicate how common a particular pathology is, but only how commonly it causes permanent and serious VI (Evans & Wormald, 1993).

Table 2.8 shows the percentage of cases of registered as SSI and SI by cause, where that cause was identified as the single factor, for the year between April 2012 and March 2013.

The usefulness of this aetiological data rests in reasonably regular comparisons, and on consistent definitions of the registration categories and disease descriptions. Since 1991 when the data were first collected from the revised BD8 forms, to date, when data are collected from the new Certificate of Vision Impairment (CVI) forms, 'degeneration of the macula and posterior pole' was, and still is, the leading cause of registration as SSI and SI, even though certifications due to AMD have reduced due to increasing availability of anti-vascular endothelial growth factor (VEGF) drugs. Glaucoma and AMD account for nearly 75% of all new registrations of those aged over 75 years, and over 50% of those in the 65 to 74 year age group.

TABLE 2.5 Total Number of Those Registered as Severely Sight Impaired and Sight Impaired in England Between the Years 2000 and 2017

Year	Total Number of Severely Sight Impaired	% Change	Total Number of Sight Impaired	% Change
2000	157,820		148,680	
2003	156,675	−0.8	155,230	+4.4
2006	152,455	−2.7	155,200	<−0.01
2008	152,980	+0.3	156,285	+0.7
2011	147,810	−3.0	151,000	−3.0
2014	143,385	−3.0	147.700	−2.0
2017	141,525	−1.3	148,950	+0.8

The percentage increases in these numbers between the stated dates are also given.
From Government Statistical Service. (2017). *Registered blind and partially sighted people as at 31 March 2017*, England. HMSO.

TABLE 2.6 Registration Figures for the SSI and SI in England on 31 March 2017 in Each Age Group, Expressed as an Absolute Number, and as a Percentage of the Total Registered Group

		Age Groups (Years)						
		0–4	5–17	18–49	50–64	65–74	75+	Total
SSI	Number	615	4495	19,495	18,080	14,765	84,075	141,525
	%	0.4	3.2	13.7	12.7	10.4	59.4	
SI	Number	555	5380	18,610	16,165	15,260	92,980	148,950
	%	0.4	3.6	12.5	10.8	10.2	62.4	

SI, Sight impaired; *SSI*, severely sight impaired.
From Government Statistical Service. (2017). *Registered blind and partially sighted people as at 31 March 2017*, England. HMSO.

TABLE 2.7 Percentage of Individuals Registered as SSI or SI in England on 31 March 2017 With the Additional Identified Primary Disability

Deaf	Hard of Hearing	Physical Disabilities	Mental Health	Learning Disabilities	All
1.2%	7.2%	21.1%	1.5%	2.7%	33.8%

SI, Sight impaired; *SSI*, severely sight impaired.
From Government Statistical Service. (2017). *Registered blind and partially sighted people as at 31 March 2017*, England. HMSO.

TABLE 2.8 Percentage of Registrations as SSI and SI Due to the Conditions Listed, Based on Registrations Attributed to a Single Cause, in England and Wales for the year April 2012 to March 2013

Diagnosis	SSI	SI
Degeneration macular and posterior pole	57.4	58.6
Glaucoma	11.9	8.4
Hereditary retinal disorders	8.9	5.6
Diabetic retinopathy/ maculopathy	5.8	7.0
Optic atrophy	5.3	4.0
Cerebrovascular disease	2.9	7.1
Disorders of the visual cortex	2.8	4.4
Retinal vascular occlusion	2.2	1.9
Keratitis, corneal opacity and other disorders of cornea	1.6	1.7
Myopia	1.2	1.3
Total	100%	100%
	(n = 8085)	(n = 10184)

SI, Sight impairment; *SSI*, severe sight impairment.
From Quartilho, A., Simkiss, P., Zekite, A., Xing, W., Wormald, R., & Bunce, C. (2016). Leading causes of certifiable visual loss in England and Wales during the year ending 31 March 2013. *Eye, 30*(4), 602–607. https://doi.org/10.1038/eye.2015.288.

The infective anterior segment disorders seen in global data, such as trachoma, are almost unknown. The vast majority of cataracts are treated and the patient suffers no permanent impairment. Overall, the percentage of preventable and treatable 'anterior segment' causes of blindness is low: the incidence of generally nonremediable posterior segment conditions is much higher. Macular disease, which is so significant in the UK statistics, appears to have very low incidence in low- and middle-income countries: there are 10.4 million cases of blindness due to age-related macular disease worldwide, in comparison to over 65 million caused by cataract (WHO, 2019).

The number of certifications due to diabetic eye disease in the UK is falling. Liew et al. (2014) reported in their study that, for the first time in five decades, diabetic retinopathy/maculopathy was no longer the leading cause of certifiable blindness among working age adults in England and Wales. In the population of working age, the ocular complications of diabetes are now the second most common cause of blindness (14.4%) (preceded by hereditary retinal disorders [20.2%] and followed by optic atrophy [14.1%]).

One of the reasons proposed for this reduction is better diabetic screening: the NHS Diabetic Eye Screening Programme (DESP) offers an annual fundus photograph to all people with diabetes aged 12 years and over. Screening is important because the patient is rarely aware of problems until the condition is well-advanced, and comprehensive screening programmes are needed to regularly examine this at-risk but asymptomatic population. The WHO and the International Diabetes Federation have supported the introduction of screening programmes globally (Kohner, 1991). The National Health Service in England (NHS, 2013) and Diabetic Eye Screening Wales (DESW) (Public Health Wales [PHW], 2018) screen almost 2 million and 150,000 diabetic patients annually, respectively. If retinopathy is identified, there are new and effective treatments, with the development of multidisciplinary teams to deliver intravitreal therapies, and new imaging technology to aid with diagnosis and following up progression of disease (Rahman et al., 2020).

Frequently, diagnosis of glaucoma is late in the disease progression due to the asymptomatic nature of the condition. Rahman et al. (2020) highlighted in their study the importance of patients' education and awareness to avoid the advancement of the disease, particularly in those patients with higher risk factors (i.e. family history of glaucoma, African or Asian ethnicity). Their research also supports the need to build stronger collaborations between community optometrists and hospital care in order to encourage take-up of annual community eye examinations which will enable early diagnosis of glaucoma and avoid VI.

Although the industrialised countries do not suffer the shortage of ophthalmological care of the developing world, it is not inevitable that all patients gain equal access to it. Javitt (1994) drew attention to the fact that 67% of blindness in Black Americans arose from preventable causes, whereas the equivalent percentage for White people was only 33%: the pattern is the same in elderly subjects who have access to free eye care, so the reasons are not wholly economic. Muñoz et al. (2000) found that African Americans had a disproportionate number of blinding diseases and were less likely to have seen an eye-care provider in the past year compared to White patients (50% vs 69%). Robinson et al. (1994) found proportionately fewer Asian and Afro-Caribbean patients attending hospitals for treatment than would be expected from the frequency of these ethnic groups in the general population. Scase and Johnson (2005) recognise the underuse of eye-care services and lower receipt of rehabilitation among ethnic minorities, particularly among Asian and Afro-Caribbean people. The review highlights the need for more cultural relevance, sensitivity and linguistic competence among eye-care providers, and more accessible and appropriate material for Asian communities regarding information about relevant eye health issues. Patel and Baker (2006) have suggested several reasons for the reluctance of the Indian population interviewed to access the eye-care system. These include misconceptions about diseases, its management and fear, as well as the negative experiences of individuals such as dissatisfaction with the outcome, long waiting lists and difficulties with appointments. These findings suggest that health education publicity needs to be presented in a form which is appropriate to the particular population group.

For the hereditary retinal disorders, the genetic code or predisposition to the condition exists from birth, but serious impairment is typically delayed until adult life. Most common among these dystrophies is retinitis pigmentosa (RP), the general name for a large group of hereditary retinal diseases which are characterised by a degeneration of the photoreceptors and retinal pigment epithelium. The inheritance of RP can be autosomal recessive, autosomal dominant or X-linked recessive, with the latter often being described as clinically the most severe. Stargardt disease is the most prevalent inherited macular dystrophy. At present, although work on possible gene therapies is ongoing, only genetic counselling could reduce the numbers of cases of inherited blindness.

Information From Population Surveys

The number of individuals with VI in the UK based on surveys is considerably higher than the number who are registered, partly due to the inclusion of mild VI. The Life Opportunities Survey (2011) (Vine et al., 2011), in which participants self-declared difficulty with vision, put the figure at 3% of the population over 16 years of age in Great Britain. Based on the population at the time, this would have been 1.5 million individuals. The prevalence varied from 1% of the 16 to 34 age group to 11% in those aged over 75 years. Pezzullo et al. (2018) estimated that 1.93 million individuals in the UK are visually impaired. Their calculations were based in part on the data obtained as part of the MRC Trial of the Assessment and Management of Older People in the Community (Evans et al., 2002, 2004). This study invited participants aged 75 and over to attend their GP practice, and their presenting VA was measured. Those with a VA of <6/18 were considered to have VI, and <3/60 was defined as blind. Table 2.9 shows the prevalence found overall and in each age group. The marked increase in prevalence in the over-85s and over-90s suggested that grouping older populations together as a single group underestimates these effects (Evans et al., 2002).

In a follow-up study, the cause of the VI was identified and this is shown in Table 2.10. This was mostly identified from GP and hospital records, but uncorrected refractive error was assigned as the cause for those whose acuity improved with a pinhole.

For those with low vision, the commonest reasons are conditions which ought to be relatively easily managed: uncorrected refractive error and cataract. For those who are categorised as blind, then AMD and glaucoma are most common. These findings emphasise the importance of regular eye examinations in this age group. Perhaps surprisingly, in a systematic review, there was no evidence that screening programmes in this age group were effective when compared with not screening (Clarke et al., 2018). The authors felt that this was because many of the participants did not take up the offer of an eye examination/ophthalmic intervention when their visual problems were revealed in a screening, and many of those not screened were able to seek an eye examination independently.

VISUAL IMPAIRMENT IN CHILDREN

Global Comparisons

There are approximately 1.4 million blind children in the world, while 17.5 million have low vision (World Health Organization WHO, 2012). Compared with the situation in adults, blindness prevalence is much lower in children: in high-income countries, around 0.03%, although rising to 0.15% in some low- and middle-income countries (Khanna et al., 2019). Approximately 75% of the world's blind children live in the poorest areas of Africa and Asia (Gilbert & Foster, 2001). For children, the number of years spent as blind is disturbingly high, leading to a great emotional, social and economic cost for these children, their families and societies (Gilbert & Foster, 2001; Gogate et al., 2009). In fact, it has been suggested that the number of 'blind years' due to all

TABLE 2.9 Prevalence of Low Vision and Blindness in Different Age Groups, Plus Estimated Overall Population Numbers Based on the mid-2001 UK Population

	Low Vision <6/18 to 3/60		Blindness <3/60	
	%	Estimated Number	%	Estimated Number
All ages	10.3	506,000	2.1	103,000
75–79 years	5.6		0.6	
80–84 years	9.6		2.3	
85–89 years	19.2		4.3	
90+ years	30.0	128,000	6.9	29,000

Data from Evans, J. R., Fletcher, A. E., Wormald, R. P. L., Ng, E. S., Stirling, S., Smeeth, L., et al. (2002). Prevalence of visual impairment in people aged 75 years and older in Britain: Results from the MRC trial of assessment and management of older people in the community. *The British Journal of Ophthalmology, 86*(7), 795–800.

TABLE 2.10 The Percentage of Cases of Low Vision and Blindness[a] Attributed to the Different Causes in Each Age Group

Causes	Refractive Error		AMD		Cataract		Glaucoma		Diabetes	
Age group (years)	LV	B	LV	B	LV	B	LV	B	LV	B
75–79	46.5	0	18.0	51.4	23.7	8.6	5.1	17.1	2.9	11.4
80–84	41.7	1.1	26.7	70.0	25.3	5.6	8.1	13.3	2.5	3.3
85–89	32.7	0	33.5	72.0	32.3	15.9	7.5	13.4	2.0	0
90+	25.8	0	44.5	88.4	30.3	9.3	4.5	14.0	0.7	0

[a]Low vision (LV: <6/18 to 3/60) and blindness (B: <3/60).
From Evans, J. R., Fletcher, A. E., & Wormald, R. P. L. (2004). Causes of visual impairment in people aged 75 years and older in Britain: An add-on study to the MRC Trial of Assessment and Management of Older People in the Community. *British Journal of Ophthalmology, 88*, 365–370.

causes for children, is almost equal to the number of 'blind years' due to cataract in adults (Gilbert & Foster, 2001). Education is a basic human right, yet about 50% of children with disabilities in low and middle-income countries are excluded from education, and the problem affects girls more than boys (Humanity & Inclusion, 2020).

As the prevalence of VI in children is low, it is very difficult to carry out population surveys and obtain meaningful results. Therefore, information on causes of VI is often gathered from targeted populations, such as children in schools for the blind, and this can be incomplete.

Considering the causes by country, it is notable how much childhood blindness is avoidable (either preventable or treatable) in low-income countries, compared with high-income countries (Table 2.11). In the poorest countries of the world, corneal scarring due to vitamin A deficiency, measles infection, ophthalmia neonatorum, and the effects of harmful traditional eye remedies prevail (Gilbert & Foster, 2001). A common cause of childhood blindness worldwide is xerophthalmia, which is primarily a disease of preschool children resulting from vitamin A deficiency. In 2002, it was reported (West, 2002) that there were 127 million and 4.4 million preschool children in the world with vitamin A deficiency and xerophthalmia, respectively. In some countries, more than 50% of preschool children have the deficiency, and concurrent acute infections, such as measles, make the child particularly vulnerable to the corneal complications which can lead eventually to opacification and blindness. Each year 5 to 10 million children are affected worldwide, with about 10% of these becoming blind. Due to the susceptibility of the child to systemic infection, there is an 80% mortality of those children who are blind, within 1 year. A 2008 study (Black et al., 2008) reported that vitamin A deficiency in newborn babies,

infants and children resulted in about 6% of under-5 deaths, 5% of under-5 disability-adjusted life-years (DALYs), and 1.7% of total DALYs. The management of the condition is simple, with a single capsule of vitamin A (200,000 IU) rapidly reversing any ocular manifestations of the disease within 2 days, and conferring protection for up to 6 months. In fact, many foodstuffs rich in vitamin A (such as breast milk, tropical fruits and green leafy vegetables) are available but they are not readily consumed (Narita & Taylor, 1993), so dietary supplements will be required until education achieves the required improvement in diet (Mayo-Wilson et al., 2011).

Retinopathy of prematurity (ROP) is rare in low-income countries because these premature babies do not survive, and ROP does not cause much VI in high-income countries because there are well-established and effective neonatal screening and treatment protocols in operation. In high-income countries, much of childhood blindness is currently 'unavoidable', and due to cerebral VI or to inherited conditions (e.g. albinism, Leber Congenital Amaurosis).

Visual Impairment in Children in the UK

Some information is available from registration data and, as in the adult population, there is probably considerable under-registration (Keil et al., 2017). As mentioned previously, certification and registration are voluntary and there is no statutory requirement for it to be offered, although it is considered good practice to offer it by the Royal College of Ophthalmologists. In some cases, vision improves with age and when diagnosis and prognosis are uncertain, some ophthalmologists may wait months or even years before offering certification (Bunce et al., 2017). Other challenges include the certification of children with cognitive impairment which may result in certification delays (Boyce et al., 2015). In

---

TABLE 2.11 The Prevalence of Avoidable and Unavoidable Cases of Children With Severe Visual Impairment and Blindness[a] by Socioeconomic Development

Aetiology		Bangladesh (LIC)	Ethiopia (LIC)	Malaysia (MIC)	UK (HIC)
Unavoidable		38.8	33	49.5	82
Avoidable (treatable and preventable)		61.2	67	50.5	18
Treatable		33.9	17.3	42.9	12.0
	ROP	1.3	0.0	17.4	3.0
	Cataract	27.3	6.8	17.2	5.0
	Glaucoma	4.3	1.7	7.6	3.0
	Uveitis	1.1	8.8	0.7	1.0
Preventable		27.3	49.7	7.6	6.0
	Infections	7.7	13.9	0.0	4.0
	Ophthalmia neonatorum	0.7	3.0	0.4	0.0
	Vitamin A deficiency	17.7	30.8	0.0	0.0
	Trauma	0.8	2.0	2.5	1.0
	Adverse drug reactions	0.4	0.0	4.7	1.0

HIC, High-income country; LIC, low-income country; MIC, middle-income country; ROP, retinopathy of prematurity.
[a]Severe visual impairment (<6/60 to 3/60); blindness (<3/60).
From Koay, C. L., Patel, D. K., Tajunisah, I., Subrayan, V., & Lansingh, V. C. (2015). A comparative analysis of avoidable causes of childhood blindness in Malaysia with low income, middle income and high income countries. *International Ophthalmology*, *35*(2), 201–207. https://doi.org/10.1007/s10792-014-9932-x.

addition, certification occurs in eye clinics and there is evidence of poor uptake of hospital eye care for children identified with significant visual needs (Pilling & Outhwaite, 2017).

Certification and registration are not a direct route to early educational and developmental support (Keil et al., 2017), which decreases the uptake. In the UK, the lead professional in supporting infants and children with VI is usually the local authority specialist qualified teacher for children and young people with vision impairment (QTVI). QTVIs offer and deliver support in the home as well as in education settings. Referral to the VI service should be made as soon as possible after a VI has been identified and should not depend on certification status or process (Keil et al., 2017). Educational needs are met, whenever possible, in mainstream schools, and registration does not influence this choice: only a minority of visually impaired children identified by the Local Education Authority are registered (Walker et al., 1992). Even this is not the full story, because there are marked differences between geographical regions of the UK as to the prevalence of children identified as visually impaired by their LEA: from 0.018% to 0.26% of the school population, with an average slightly above 0.1%. There are data from an Office of Population Censuses and Surveys (OPCS) survey (Bone & Metzler, 1989) which suggests that the higher figure may be more accurate.

The major causes of blindness in the 0- to 15-year-old age group are distinctly different from those in the adult population. Analyses of the CVI data in 2009/10 (Mitry et al., 2013) found that cerebral VI was the most common cause of both SI and SSI registration (21.8%). Based on 2014/15 data (Bunce et al., 2017), the most common single cause of both SSI and SI were hereditary retinal dystrophies. Cerebral VI was the next most common single cause of SSI, and the third most common single cause for SI. It seems clear that prenatal factors (including genetic causes) are involved in the majority of cases, and in only about 10% to 20% does the cause appear to arise later than the perinatal period. This percentage was 16% in the BCVIS2 study (Teoh et al., 2021), which gathered information directly from paediatricians and ophthalmologists of all the children aged under 18 who were newly diagnosed with VA of logMAR 0.5 or worse from October 2015 to November 2016 in the UK. Of the total of 784 cases identified, 72% had additional non-ophthalmic disorders (13% hearing impairment, and 21% speech and language difficulties), and 4% died within the year. Only 44% had an ophthalmic condition which affected a single ocular site; 48% had cerebral VI, and these children were much more likely to have the additional disabilities. Half of the total number of cases were identified in their first year of life, and 62% of cases were due to hereditary causes. Although this study included milder degrees of visual loss than an earlier similar study (Rahi & Cable, 2003), the same associations of VI with an ethnic minority (especially South Asian), low socioeconomic status, and low birthweight/premature birth were found.

This high incidence of other mental or physical impairments among children with VI has been extensively reported in other countries (Drews et al., 1992; Dale & Sonksen, 2002;

Dale & Salt, 2007; Sonksen & Dale, 2007; Tadić et al., 2009), and is perhaps due to the increased survival of profoundly brain-damaged children. Despite the additional problems (or even, in fact, because of them), it is important to try to provide as much assistance as possible to such children in order to maximise their quality of life. The more severe levels of VI are also more commonly found in those impaired from birth: it is extremely rare for an acquired defect to lead to 'no perception of light'.

PROJECTIONS FOR THE FUTURE

The population is an increasingly ageing one, suggesting ever increasing numbers of visually impaired patients in the future. In 2016, there were 11.8 million UK residents aged 65 years and over, representing 18% of the total population. In 2041, it is predicted that there will be 20.4 million residents aged 65 years and over, making up 26% of the total population. The fastest increase will be seen in the 85 years and over age group. In mid-2016, there were 1.6 million people aged 85 years and over (2% of the total population); by mid-2041 this is projected to double to 3.2 million (4% of the population) and by 2066 to treble, and at that time there will be 5.1 million people aged 85 years and over making up 7% of the total UK population. Coupling these figures with the dramatic increase in the prevalence of blindness with increasing age shows that the numbers of visually impaired people is bound to rise. Geographically, within the UK, there is a higher proportion of older population living in rural and coastal areas, with the highest percentage of the population aged 65 years and over living in the South West region of England (more than 21.6% of the population are aged 65 years or over) (Office for National Statistics [ONS], 2018). This presents significant challenges in the provision of eye-care services: most specialist ophthalmology centres are currently in larger cities. The Public Health Outcomes Framework (PHOF) was first published by the Department of Health in the UK in 2012. This uses health indicators to understand improvements, identify areas which need resourcing, and highlight potential inequalities. The CVI data is used as the health indicator for sight loss, and can hopefully be used as a basis for improving services, both locally and nationally (Rahman et al., 2020). The challenge will be to maintain the current decreases in CVI registration due to AMD as the number of older people in the population increases. The PHOF can also be used to monitor the effect of programmes designed to ensure equal access to eyecare by all ethnic communities (particularly those at increased risk of glaucoma).

The older person with deteriorating vision is likely to have other chronic health problems which may influence the way in which vision affects lifestyle. The incidence of heart disease, hearing difficulties and arthritis (to name just a few) will be at least as high as in the general population, although some studies suggest that the incidence is higher among the blind population (Court et al., 2014; Rosenbloom, 1992). In addition there may be other negative lifestyle changes such as bereavement, social isolation and lower income.

The ageing of the world population is causing great concern about an ever-increasing backlog of untreated eye disease. Currently, at least 2.2 billion people have a near or distance vision impairment. In at least 1 billion—or almost half—of these cases, vision impairment could have been prevented or has yet to be addressed. Between 2015 and 2050, the proportion of the world's population over 60 years of age will nearly double from 12% to 22%. The pace of the population ageing is much faster than in the past; by 2050 the world's population aged 60 years and older is expected to total 2 billion, up from 900 million in 2015. Currently, there are 125 million people aged 80 years old or older in the world. By 2050, there will be 120 million living in China alone, and 434 million people in this age group worldwide and 80% of older people will be living in low- and middle-income countries (WHO, 2018). Approximately 75% of the global population who are blind are aged 50 years or older (Bourne et al., 2017). A recent study (Steinmetz et al., 2021) indicates that the prevalence of vision impairment has increased with age globally since 1990 till today, with cataract being the principal cause for global blindness for ages 50 years and older, followed by uncorrected refractive error, glaucoma and AMD. The contribution of glaucoma and AMD is higher in the older groups, while the contribution of diabetic retinopathy decreases with age. An interesting fact is that diabetic retinopathy was the only cause of blindness that showed a global increase in age prevalence between 1990 and 2020. It is projected that more than 600 million people will be living with diabetes by 2040 (Ogurtsova et al., 2017), and as people with diabetes live progressively longer, the number of people with diabetic retinopathy and the resulting VI is projected to increase quickly (Teo et al., 2020; Wong et al., 2018).

In high-income countries, the prevalence of VI due to AMD has declined by almost 30% from 1990 to 2020, probably associated with the introduction of anti-VEGF treatment for neovascular AMD (Steinmetz et al., 2021). However, in low- and middle-income countries, the cost of these drugs is prohibitive for most, and the medical infrastructure for delivering them does not exist.

For childhood blindness in low-income countries, provision of basic eye- and healthcare services to reduce avoidable blindness will gradually change the pattern of diseases to that currently seen in high-income countries. As healthcare infrastructure improves, there will also be the opportunity to offer low-vision rehabilitation services, which currently have a minimal role. The education of healthcare professionals and parents to overcome barriers of lack of awareness and misconceptions, and of parents to prevent over-protection and isolation of children, will be important. Throughout the world, it appears that the number of visually impaired adults is inevitably set to rise: the demand for low-vision services, appropriate to the particular environment in which the patient lives, is also set to grow at an ever-increasing rate.

REFERENCES

Black, R. E., Allen, L. H., Bhutta, Z. A., et al. (2008). Maternal and child undernutrition: Global and regional exposures and health consequences. *The Lancet, 371*(9608), 243–260. https://doi.org/10.1016/S0140-6736(07)61690-0.

Bone, M., & Meltzer, H. (1989). *OPCS surveys of disability in Great Britain, Report 3. The prevalence of disability among children.* HMSO.

Bourne, R. R. A., Flaxman, S. R., Braithwaite, T., et al. (2017). Magnitude, temporal trends, and projections of the global prevalence of blindness and distance and near vision impairment: A systematic review and meta-analysis. *The Lancet Global Health, 5*(9), e888–e897. https://doi.org/10.1016/S2214-109X(17)30293-0.

Bourne, R. R. A., Steinmetz, J., Flaxman, S. R., et al. (2021). Trends in prevalence of blindness and distance and near vision impairment over 30 years: An analysis for the Global Burden of Disease Study. *The Lancet Global Health, 9*(2), e130–e143. https://doi.org/10.1016/S2214-109X(20)30425-3.

Boyce, T., Leamon, S., Slade, J., et al. (2014). Certification for vision impairment: Researching perceptions, processes and practicalities in health and social care professionals and patients. *BMJ Open, 4*, 1–7. https://doi.org/10.1136/bmjopen-2013-004319.

Boyce, T., Dahlmann-Noor, A., Bowman, R. (2015). Support for infants and young people with sight loss: A qualitative study of sight impairment certification and referral to education and social care services. *BMJ Open, 5*(12), 1–8. https://doi.org/10.1136/bmjopen-2015-009622.

Bunce, C., Zekite, A., Wormald, R., et al. (2017a). Is there evidence that the yearly numbers of children newly certified with sight impairment in England and Wales has increased between 1999/2000 and 2014/2015? A cross-sectional study. *BMJ Open, 7*(9), 1–7. https://doi.org/10.1136/bmjopen-2017-016888.

Clarke, E. L., Evans, J. E., & Smeeth, L. (2018). Community screening for visual impairment in older people. *The Cochrane Database of Systematic Reviews, 2018*(2), CD001054. https://doi.org/10.1002/14651858.CD001054.pub3.

Court, H., McLean, G., Guthrie, B., et al. (2014). Visual impairment is associated with physical and mental comorbidities in older adults: A cross-sectional study. *BioMed Central Medicine, 12*(1), 1–8. https://doi.org/10.1186/s12916-014-0181-7.

Dale, N., & Salt, A. (2007). Early support developmental journal for children with visual impairment: The case for a new developmental framework for early intervention. *Child: Care, Health and Development, 33*(6), 684–690. https://doi.org/10.1111/j.1365-2214.2007.00798.x.

Dale, N., & Sonksen, P. (2002). Developmental outcome, including setback, in young children with severe visual impairment. *Developmental Medicine and Child Neurology, 44*(9), 613–622. https://doi.org/10.1017/S0012162201002651.

Drews, C. D., Yearginallsopp, M., Murphy, C. C., et al. (1992). Legal blindness among 10-year-old children in metropolitan Atlanta: Prevalence, 1985 to 1987. *American Journal of Public Health, 82*, 1377–1379.

Evans, J. R., & Wormald, R. P. L. (1993). Epidemiological function of BD8 certification. *Eye, 7*, 172–179.

Evans, J. R., Fletcher, A. E., Wormald, R. P. L., et al. (2002). Prevalence of visual impairment in people aged 75 years and older in Britain: Results from the MRC trial of assessment and management of older people in the community. *British Journal of Ophthalmology, 86*(7), 795–800.

Evans, J. R., Fletcher, A. E., & Wormald, R. P. L., et al. (2004). Causes of visual impairment in people aged 75 years and older in Britain: An add-on study to the MRC Trial of Assessement and Management of Older People in the Commuity. *British Journal of Ophthalmology, 88*, 365–370.

Flaxman, S. R., Bourne, R. R. A., Resnikoff, S., et al. (2017). Global causes of blindness and distance vision impairment 1990–2020: A systematic review and meta-analysis. *The Lancet Global Health, 5*(12), e1221–e1234. https://doi.org/10.1016/S2214-109X(17)30393-5.

Gilbert, C., & Foster, A. (2001). Childhood blindness in the context of VISION 2020—The right to sight. *Bulletin of the World Health Organization, 79*(3), 227–232. https://doi.org/10.1590/S0042-96862001000300011.

Gogate, P., Kalua, K., & Courtright, P. (2009). Blindness in childhood in developing countries: Time for a reassessment? *Public Library of Science Medicine, 6*(12), 12–15. https://doi.org/10.1371/journal.pmed.1000177.

Government Statistical Service. (2017). *Registered blind and partially sighted people at 31 March 2017 England*. HMSO.

Humanity, & Inclusion. *Report November 2020—Let's break silos now! Achieving disability-inclusive education in a post-COVID world*. https://reliefweb.int/report/world/let-s-break-silos-now-achieving-disability-inclusive-education-post-covid-world?gclid=Cj0KCQjwntCVBhDdARIsAMEwACnptVyGyckXMDxgkL0rGtHUzXyTrmkYrpEWnT-wM2Ci6cju4hwDDz8aAuplEALw_wcB.

Javitt, J. C. (1994). Universal coverage and preventable blindness. *Archives of Ophthalmology, 112*, 453.

Keeffe, J., & Resnikoff, S. (2018). Prevalence and causes of vision impairment and blindness: The global burden of disease. In R. Khanna, G. Rao, & S. Marmamula (Eds.), *Innovative approaches in the delivery of primary and secondary eye care. Essentials in ophthalmology*. Springer. https://doi.org/10.1007/978-3-319-98014-0_2.

Keil, S., Fielder, A., & Sargent, J. (2017). Management of children and young people with vision impairment: Diagnosis, developmental challenges and outcomes. *Archives of Disease in Childhood, 102*(6), 566–571. https://doi.org/10.1136/archdischild-2016-311775.

Khanna, R. C., Rao, G. N., & Marmamula, S. (2019). *Innovative approaches in the delivery of primary and secondary eye care*. Springer. https://doi.org/10.1007/978-3-319-98014-0.

Kohner, E. M. (1991). A protocol for screening for diabetic retinopathy in Europe. *Diabetic Medicine, 8*, 263–267.

Liew, G., Michaelides, M., & Bunce, C. (2014). A comparison of the causes of blindness certifications in England and Wales in working age adults (16-64 years), 1999-2000 with 2009-2010. *BMJ Open, 4*(2), 1–6. https://doi.org/10.1136/bmjopen-2013-004015.

Mayo-Wilson, E., Imdad, A., Herzer, K., et al. (2011). Vitamin A supplements for preventing mortality, illness, and blindness in children aged under 5: Systematic review and meta-analysis. *BMJ (Online), 343*(7822), 1–19. https://doi.org/10.1136/bmj.d5094.

Mitry, D., Bunce, C., Wormald, R., et al. (2013). Causes of certifications for severe sight impairment (blind) and sight impairment (partial sight) in children in England and Wales. *British Journal of Ophthalmology, 97*(11), 1431–1436. https://doi.org/10.1136/bjophthalmol-2013-303578.

Muñoz, B., West, S. K., Rubin, G. S., et al. (2000). Causes of blindness and visual impairment in a population of older Americans: The Salisbury Eye Evaluation Study. *Archives of Ophthalmology, 118*(6), 819–825. https://doi.org/10.1001/archopht.118.6.819.

Narita, A. S., & Taylor, H. R. (1993). Blindness in the tropics. *The Medical Journal of Australia, 159*, 416–420.

National Health Service in England (NHS). (2013). *NHS Diabetic Retinopathy Screening Programme* (17). https://assets.publishing.service.gov.uk/government/uploads/system/uploads/attachment_data/file/256492/22_nhs_diabetic_eye.pdf.

Office for National Statistics (ONS). (2018). Living longer: How our population is changing and why it matters.

Ogurtsova, K., da Rocha Fernandes, J. D., Huang, Y., et al. (2017). IDF Diabetes Atlas: Global estimates for the prevalence of diabetes for 2015 and 2040. *Diabetes Research and Clinical Practice, 128*, 40–50. https://doi.org/10.1016/j.diabres.2017.03.024.

Pascolini, D., & Mariotti, S. P. (2012). Global estimates of visual impairment: 2010. *British Journal of Ophthalmology, 96*(5), 614–618. https://doi.org/10.1136/bjophthalmol-2011-300539.

Patel, D., & Baker, H. M. I. (2006). Barriers to uptake of eye care services by the Indian population living in Ealing, West London. *West London Health Education Journal, 65*(3), 267–276.

Pezzullo, L., Streatfeild, J., Simkiss, P., et al. (2018). The economic impact of sight loss and blindness in the UK adult population. *BMC Health Services Research, 18*(1), 1–13. https://doi.org/10.1186/s12913-018-2836-0.

Pilling, R. F., & Outhwaite, L. (2017). Are all children with visual impairment known to the eye clinic. *British Journal of Ophthalmology, 101*(4), 472–474. https://doi.org/10.1136/bjophthalmol-2016-308534.

Public Health Wales (PHW). (2018). *Diabetic eye screening Wales Annual Statistical Report 2019-20*. https://phw.nhs.wales/services-and-teams/screening/diabetic-eye-screening-wales/diabetic-eye-screening-wales-annual-statistical-report-2018-191/.

Rahi, J. S., & Cable, N. (2003). Severe visual impairment and blindness in children in the UK. *Lancet, 362*(9393), 1359–1365. https://doi.org/10.1016/S0140-6736(03)14631-4.

Rahman, F., Zekite, A., Bunce, C., et al. (2020). Recent trends in vision impairment certifications in England and Wales. *Eye, 34*(7), 1271–1278. https://doi.org/10.1038/s41433-020-0864-6.

Resnikoff, S., Lansingh, V. C., Washburn, L., et al. (2020). Estimated number of ophthalmologists worldwide (International Council of Ophthalmology update): Will we meet the needs? *British Journal of Ophthalmology, 104*(4), 588–592. https://doi.org/10.1136/bjophthalmol-2019-314336.

Robinson, R., Deutsch, J., Jones, H. S., et al. (1994). Unrecognised and unregistered visual impairment. *British Journal of Ophthalmology, 78*, 736–740.

Rosenbloom, A. A. (1992). Physiological and functional aspects of aging, vision, and visual impairment. In A. L. Orr (Ed.), *Vision and aging: Crossroads for service delivery* (pp. 47–68). American Foundation for the Blind.

Scase, M. O., & Johnson, M. R. D. (2005). Visual impairment in ethnic minorities in the UK. *International Congress Series, 1282*, 438–442. https://doi.org/10.1016/j.ics.2005.05.085.

Sonksen, P. M., & Dale, N. (2007). Visual impairment in infancy: Impact on neurodevelopmental and neurobiological processes. *Developmental Medicine & Child Neurology, 44*(11), 782–791. https://doi.org/10.1111/j.1469-8749.2002.tb00287.x.

Steinmetz, J. D., Bourne, R. R. A., Briant, P. S., et al. (2021). Causes of blindness and vision impairment in 2020 and trends over 30 years, and prevalence of avoidable blindness in relation to VISION 2020: the Right to Sight: an analysis for the Global Burden of Disease Study. *The Lancet Global Health, 9*(2), e144–e160. https://doi.org/10.1016/S2214-109X(20)30489-7.

Tadić, V., Pring, L., & Dale, N. (2009). Attentional processes in young children with congenital visual impairment. *British Journal of Developmental Psychology, 27*(2), 311–330. https://doi.org/10.1348/026151008X310210.

Teo, Z. L., Tham, Y. C., Yu, M., et al. (2020). Do we have enough ophthalmologists to manage vision-threatening diabetic retinopathy? A global perspective. *Eye, 34*(7), 1255–1261. https://doi.org/10.1038/s41433-020-0776-5.

Teoh, L. J., Solebo, A. L., & Rahi, J. S. (2021). Visual impairment, severe visual impairment, and blindness in children in Britain (BCVIS2): A national observational study. *The Lancet Child & Adolescent Health, 5*(3), 190–200.

Vine, L., Willitts, M., Farmer, M., et al. (2011). *Life Opportunities Survey, wave 1*. Health Statistics Quarterly. www.odi.gov.uk/los.%0Ahttp://search.proquest.com/docview/859022644?accountid=12037%5Cnhttp://linksource.ebsco.com/linking.aspx?sid=ProQ:envscijournals&fmt=journal&genre=unknown&issn=14651645&volume=&issue=49&date=2011-04-01&spage=4&title=Health+Statistics.

Walker, E., Tobin, M., & McKennell, A. (1992). *Blind and partially sighted children in Britain: The RNIB Survey (Vol. 2)*. HMSO.

West, K. P. (2002). Proceedings of the XX International Vitamin A Consultative Group Meeting. *Extent of Vitamin A Deficiency among Preschool Children and Women of Reproductive Age, 75*(0022), 2857–2866S.

WHO. (2012a). Control and prevention of blindness and deafness. https://www.emro.who.int/entity/blindness/index.html.

World Health Organization (WHO). (2012b). *Global data on visual impairment* 2010 (17). http://www.emro.who.int/control-and-preventions-of-blindness-and-deafness/announcements/global-estimates-on-visual-impairment.html.

WHO. (2018). Ageing and health. https://www.who.int/news-room/fact-sheets/detail/ageing-and-health.

WHO. (2019). *World report on vision*. World Health Organization. https://www.who.int/publications/i/item/9789241516570.

WHO. (2020a). *Elimination of human onchocerciasis: Progress report, 2019–2020* (WER No. 45, 2020, 95, 545–554). https://www.who.int/publications/i/item/who-wer9545-545-554.

WHO. (2020b). *WHO alliance for the global elimination of trachoma by 2020: Progress report, 2019* (WER No. 30, 2020, 95, 349–360). https://www.who.int/publications/i/item/who-wer9530.

Wong, T. Y., Sun, J., Kawasaki, R., et al. (2018). Guidelines on Diabetic Eye Care: The International Council of Ophthalmology recommendations for screening, follow-up, referral, and treatment based on resource settings. *Ophthalmology, 125*(10), 1608–1622. https://doi.org/10.1016/j.ophtha.2018.04.007.

Clinical Measures of Visual Performance

There is a plethora of vision tests available, including both tests designed for general clinical use and those specific to low vision. Even within the 'low vision' category the tests are not universally applicable and no single test can fulfil all requirements, although some tests have more than one use. The strengths and weaknesses of the particular test need to be acknowledged and understood, and tests should be selected carefully after considering why visual performance is being measured.

WHY DO WE TEST VISUAL PERFORMANCE?

For what purposes might visual performance be measured in a patient with visual impairment?

1. For the early detection, or to monitor progression, of an ocular disorder. Usually the earlier that diagnosis occurs, the more likely that any treatment that is available will be successful. This could mean that the disorder could be treated before it causes permanent impairment; that is, before it leads to 'low vision'. There is increasing interest, particularly in tests which monitor progression, that these could be self-administered by the patient at home. Delivering such tests on a personal electronic device (tablet or smartphone) makes this more feasible but brings a new set of challenges in calibration of screen luminance, viewing distance, room illumination, and in digital exclusion.
2. To compare with 'normal' performance, or with an accepted standard; for example, the Department for Transport test

for drivers where a car number plate of standard size must be read at a fixed distance. When defining the category of vision impairment (VI) (e.g. when using the *International Classification of Diseases 11th Revision* (*ICD-11*) or when completing a Certificate of Vision Impairment (CVI) form (see Chapter 1), or classifying for disabled sport (see Chapter 15) it is important to have simple, internationally recognised visual acuity (VA) and visual field tests.
3. To measure improvement and decline in performance with specific aids and devices; this might be between consecutive visits, with and without spectacle lenses, or with two different types of magnifier.
4. To quantify the patient's own subjective impression of their visual performance in everyday circumstances. A very simple example might be a test of VA in the presence of a bright light to try to measure just how significant are the patient's complaints of poor vision on a sunny day.
5. To predict the outcome of a medical or surgical treatment, or a rehabilitation programme. There are always some risks with surgery, no matter how commonplace, and rehabilitation can have enormous costs (financial, and in the time involved). It is therefore sensible for the patient and practitioner to have as much information as possible in order to decide whether the potential benefits outweigh the risks, and to allow expectations to be managed.
6. Predicting visual function for everyday tasks. This is the most important consideration for low-vision rehabilitation. Although patients are usually well aware of the activity

limitations caused by their impairment, it is often necessary to quantify this. Unfortunately, there may be no direct correlation between functional performance and standard clinical tests: a patient may achieve a high score on an acuity test and yet perform poorly on a practical task like reading, or a patient may be able to navigate alone in a busy street despite a very constricted visual field. This was discussed in a feature issue of *Ophthalmic and Physiological Optics* (Wood et al., 2011). It is important for the patient that the low-vision practitioner should be able to interpret their performance in terms such as 'can cross a road safely' rather than 'can identify the 1.0 logMAR line on a chart'. It is difficult to devise simple clinical tests which relate directly to task performance, not least because there are many different visual and nonvisual skills interacting. Success in crossing the road, for example, may combine the extent of visual field, movement and contrast perception, hearing ability, experience, confidence and the amount of training received. As this problem has proved so difficult, there has been a shift to asking patients to describe their own functional difficulties in a structured and quantifiable way. These functional measures of performance (Patient Reported Outcome Measures or PROMs) are discussed in Chapter 4.

ASSESSING THE PERFORMANCE OF VISION TESTS

In most of the situations described, if the test is to be useful, it must produce results which are both repeatable (reproducible) and sensitive. To put this in a clinical context, if the VA of a patient was measured twice in quick succession, the result produced should be identical on both occasions (the test is repeatable), even if the test was carried out by two different practitioners in two different settings (the test is reproducible). If the patient received some treatment in between these two measurement sessions which did improve their ocular condition, it would be expected that this would be reflected in a noticeable difference in the two measurements (the test is sensitive).

If repeated use of the same test is required, especially over a short time period, then the test must also be available in multiple versions which have been shown to be equivalent to each other, and this is not a trivial problem. Despite the care taken by the developers, it may only be when extensive data are collected by later researchers that differences between versions are revealed.

Vision tests designed to be displayed on computer screens have become very popular in recent years. They have the advantage that the controlling software (and therefore the entire test design) can be changed without needing new hardware. This means that 'improvements' can be made to the test almost continuously, but also means that the version currently in use may be different from that which was included in a validation study. The use of electronic displays seems to solve the technical difficulties of having a large number of versions of a particular test, but this masks the fact that these versions are unlikely to have been rigorously tested. For some tests, insufficient attention is given to the effect of screen resolution (pixel density) and luminance variations; in particular electronic screens may not be able to measure contrast sensitivity (CS) (Thayaparan et al., 2007).

It would be unusual for a completely novel test of visual performance to be introduced, but if a new format for an established measure is developed (e.g. a new VA chart) it is necessary to validate such a test by comparison with a 'gold standard' measurement technique that has already been shown to have the required repeatability and sensitivity. To evaluate this agreement, the mean difference (or bias) and the limits of agreement (LoA) are required. It should be decided in advance of the study what results would be clinically acceptable: for example, a difference in VA of 'two letters' between two letter charts would be clinically insignificant, whereas a difference of 'two lines' may be unacceptable. Deciding these limits can also allow the researcher to determine the required number of participants that will be needed in the study (power calculation). Bland and Altman (2010) describe how the analysis to compare the tests should be carried out, once the two measurements have been obtained appropriately (e.g. in randomised order; matched viewing conditions).

Fig. 3.1 shows an example 'Bland–Altman plot' from such a study, with each data point representing the acuity of one eye from one participant.

This particular plot shows a systematic difference between the two tests (the mean difference (bias) is not zero) and the subjects on average read about three more letters on the New Test than on the Gold Standard. Considering the individual differences, the standard deviation (SD) was 6.5 letters. Therefore, we would expect 95% of the differences to lie within 1.96 (or approximately 2) SD of the mean. So nearly all differences between pairs of measurements will be within the boundary of mean + 2 SD (3 + 13 = 16) to mean − 2 SD (3 − 13 = −10), and these are called the 95% LoA. It is the LoA which are often much more indicative of the limitations of a technique than the bias, which even for a test giving very variable results, can be close to zero. In this example, we can see that the New Test can give acuity results which differ by several lines (both better and worse) compared to the Gold Standard, and the two tests would certainly not be interchangeable.

Note that the simpler method of performing a linear regression between the two tests is not appropriate: although this will show whether the two tests are related, it will not show any differences in scoring between the two tests.

DISTANCE VISUAL ACUITY

The most familiar test of spatial vision is the resolution task presented by a distance acuity chart (traditionally a Snellen design), which determines the ability to discriminate the smallest possible symbols (optotypes) at the highest contrast. Contrast is $(L_{max} - L_{min})/(L_{max} + L_{min})$ where L_{max} and L_{min} are respectively the maximum and minimum luminances in the target: for black optotypes on a white background (or vice versa) this is recommended to be at least 75%: the letters should have luminance no greater than 15% of the background level (British Standards Institution [BSI], 2018). The standard optotype is the Landolt ring (or 'C') with a choice of at least four gap positions, but it is more common to use letters as optotypes. In discriminating a letter the viewer is detecting the gap between adjacent limbs that make up the letter. Performance is defined in terms of the angular subtense of the 'gap': 1.75 mm at 6 m subtends 1 minute arc (min arc), which is taken to be 'normal' performance. The symbols, or optotypes, have standardised shapes, being drawn within a 5-unit × 5-unit square with limb widths equal to 1 unit, and the overall letter height equal to 5 units (Fig. 3.2).

There are several ways in which the acuity measured with optotypes can be expressed, and these are illustrated in Table 3.1. The Snellen fraction (which for 'normal' vision is often taken as 6/6) has the viewing distance as the numerator, and the denominator is the distance from which the stroke width of the letter would subtend an angle of 1 min arc at the eye (the angular subtense of the complete letter would be 5 min arc): the lines of letters on commercially produced charts are labelled with this latter distance. *Snellen (6 m)* defines the standard viewing distance as 6 m, and *Snellen (20 ft)* simply

converts this into feet. The 6/6 acuity standard can therefore be described as requiring a *minimum angle of resolution (MAR)* of 1 min arc. *Decimal notation* expresses the Snellen fractions as a decimal, or alternatively it is the reciprocal of the MAR. *LogMAR* is the logarithm to base 10 of the MAR in min arc. In the logMAR system each step (line) is 0.1 log units, and this is equal to an approximate multiplication factor of 1.25, and this represents the size difference between the limb widths making up the corresponding letters. Each additional 0.3 logMAR represents a doubling in optotype size: on a conventional chart this means letters on each line are twice the size of letters on the row three lines below, and half the size of optotypes on the row three lines above.

Acuity notations can be converted between these different systems, but this is based solely on letter size and the angular subtense of the limb widths. It does not take into account any variation between charts in the shape of letters, recognition difficulty of letters chosen, letter spacing and line separation, and number of letters on each row. All of these factors could affect an individual patient's measured acuity. In general, it

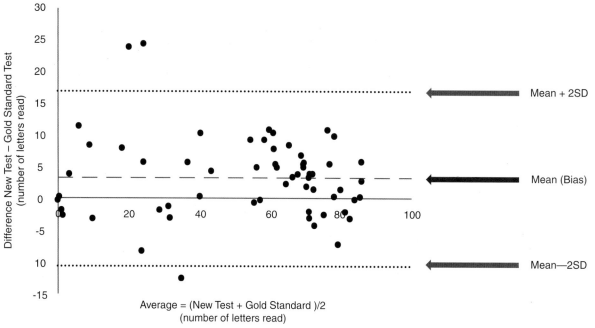

Fig. 3.1 The Bland–Altman plot shows (on the *y*-axis) the difference between the numbers of letters read on the new acuity chart (New Test) and the traditional acuity chart (Gold Standard), and on the *x*-axis the average of the two results. The dashed line shows the mean difference (bias) and the dotted lines show the limits of agreement (mean ± 2 SD). *SD*, Standard deviation.

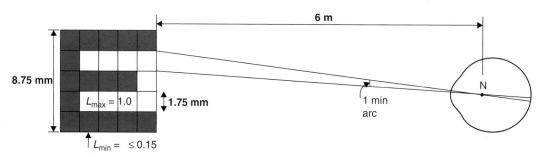

Fig. 3.2 A schematic illustration of normal visual acuity, where the optotype which can just be resolved, has a distance between adjacent limbs of 1.75 mm, which subtends an angle of 1 min arc at the nodal point of the eye (N) when viewed from 6 m.

TABLE 3.1 The Interrelationship Between the Different Acuity Notations

MAR (min arc)	logMAR	Snellen (6 m)	Snellen (20 ft)	Decimal Notation
100	2.0	6/600	20/2000	0.01
79	1.9	6/480	20/1600	0.0125
63	1.8	6/380	20/1250	0.016
50	1.7	6/300	20/1000	0.02
40	1.6	6/240	20/800	0.025
32	1.5	6/190	20/630	0.032
25	1.4	6/150	20/500	0.04
20	1.3	6/120	20/400	0.05
15.8	1.2	6/95	20/320	0.063
12.5	1.1	6/75	20/250	0.08
10.0	1.0	6/60	20/200	0.1
8.0	0.9	6/48	20/160	0.125
6.3	0.8	6/38	20/125	0.16
5.0	0.7	6/30	20/100	0.2
4.0	0.6	6/24	20/80	0.25
3.2	0.5	6/19	20/63	0.32
2.5	0.4	6/15	20/50	0.4
2.0	0.3	6/12	20/40	0.5
1.58	0.2	6/9.5	20/32	0.63
1.25	0.1	6/7.5	20/25	0.8
1.0	0.0	6/6	20/20	1.0
0.8	−0.1	6/4.8	20/16	1.25
0.63	−0.2	6/3.8	20/12.5	1.6
0.5	−0.3	6/3	20/10	2.0

MAR, Minimum angle of resolution.

is not appropriate to express acuity measured in Snellen as logMAR values, although Snellen equivalents can be given for measurements made on a logMAR chart (Elliott, 2016).

The standard for 'normal' acuity (6/6) is the ability to correctly resolve and identify letters whose limb width subtends an angle of 1 min arc at the eye. However, a high proportion of young subjects can achieve a performance which is considerably better than 6/6 (Elliott et al., 1995). High-contrast VA is widely used by optometrists because it is an excellent way to take 'baseline' measurements: to compare performance, for example, with and without the use of spectacle lenses, as it is extremely sensitive to blur. It can also be used to confirm that a magnifying device is producing the expected improvement in performance: if, for example, the patient uses an aid labelled as '2×' magnification, the retinal image will be twice the size. This means that the patient will be able to recognise letters from the test chart in which the detail has one-half the angular subtense. Acuity should therefore improve by a factor of 2: for example, an acuity of 6/36 would be expected to improve to 6/18 with a 2× telescope. A factor of 2 is a change of 0.3 log units, so 2× magnification would increase logMAR VA from, for example, 0.7 to 0.4.

In determining a baseline acuity level for a low-vision patient, however, standard Snellen charts are not the most suitable test, as they are designed to measure normal or near-normal acuity. This means that the ratio of letter size between adjacent rows is much smaller as the higher acuity levels are approached; there is, for example, a 1.2× increase in size from 6/5 to 6/6, compared to the 1.67× change from 6/36 to 6/60. The number of letters per line also varies from one to eight in moving down the chart. It is well-known that spatial resolution for letters is influenced by the presence of adjacent contours which are closer than a letter-width distance away (Flom et al., 1963). This 'contour interaction' effect is not well controlled in the Snellen chart because of the different letter spacings on each line, and an optimal design would demand that the spacing between letters and rows be proportional to the letter size throughout. The presence of surrounding contours around the target letter may be particularly confusing in the case of a patient with central scotoma: with an isolated letter the patient can search and locate it more accurately.

Early attempts to produce an acuity chart for people with low vision concentrated on providing very large targets—the Feinbloom chart uses numbers up to a '210 m' size (i.e. the detail in the letter subtends 1 min arc at 210 m, and it could be seen by someone with 6/6 vision at that distance). The Sloan chart uses a constant size progression from row to row (1.25×, or 0.1 log unit), but the number of letters and their spacing varies at each level (Bailey, 1978; Sloan, 1980).

The Bailey-Lovie chart was the earliest attempt to fulfil all the requirements to measure 'low vision' in a commercially available design. It can easily be used at different working distances, has equal numbers of letters per line (5), equivalent line and letter spacing throughout, the 10 letters used have approximately equal legibility and there is a standard ratio of size between adjacent rows (1.25×, or 0.1 log units) (Bailey & Lovie-Kitchin, 1976). The scoring of VA on a Snellen chart is often on a row-by-row basis, with the patient given credit for a row if they read the majority of letters on it (although results such as '6/18 + 2' are sometimes recorded). This grading is relatively coarse and insensitive to change (the patient may read an extra half-line but achieve the same score), and letter-by-letter scoring is preferred. On a logMAR chart, the 0.1 'credit' for reading a full row of (usually) five letters can be subdivided into 5 × 0.02 steps for reading each individual letter. Remembering that logMAR scores decrease for an improvement in performance, reading the line labelled 0.7 plus 3 out of the 5 (smaller) letters on the 0.6 line would lead to a final score of 0.64.

In low-vision work, the Snellen chart is frequently presented at different viewing distances, leading to recorded acuities such as '2/36' or '1/60'. The numerator expresses the actual viewing distance used, with the denominator giving the distance from which a 'normal' observer would be able to recognise the letter: in fact it would be labelled with this latter value on the chart. In the logMAR system, the viewing distance does not form part of the notation, and must be accounted for separately: the chart must also be labelled with the viewing distance for which it is calibrated. If the viewing distance from the chart decreases by a factor of 0.1 log units, then all the letters on the chart should be effectively magnified by that same factor. If the patient could read the line labelled 0.7 at 6 m, his acuity now (at a 4.8 m viewing distance) should be 0.6. If the viewing distance decreased by 0.2 log units (to 3.8 m) the acuity should improve to 0.5 logMAR. Although the patient's acuity is now apparently 0.5, this has been enhanced by the closer viewing distance, and must be compensated to give a correct acuity assessment. Thus, if you decrease the viewing distance by 0.2 log units, the logMAR acuity recorded should **increase** by 0.2 log units: as in the example given, a logMAR acuity of 0.5 recorded at 3.8 m is 'really' 0.7. The sequence of viewing distances that represent progressive 0.1 log unit steps does not need to be committed to memory, as it is given in the Snellen notation labelling on the chart. The distances from which the detail in the letters subtends 1 min arc are labelled for successive rows as 60, 48, 38, 30, 24, 19, 15, 12, 9.5, 7.5, 6, or by dividing by 10: 6, 4.8, 3.8, 2.4, 1.9, 1.5, 1.2, 0.95, 0.75 and 0.6. To take an example, suppose a patient has an acuity recorded as 0.5 logMAR at a viewing distance of 3.0 m. This represents a 0.3 log unit change in viewing distance from 6 m (3 steps of 0.1 log unit each on the scale given), so the acuity must be compensated by adding 0.3 to the recorded acuity:

the patient's VA is therefore actually 0.5 + 0.3 = 0.8 logMAR. A 0.3 log unit decrease of the viewing distance (or to put it more simply, a halving of the viewing distance) and a subsequent increase in the recorded VA by 0.3 is in practice usually sufficient to deal with the majority of acuities encountered. If not, a further halving of the viewing distance (to one-quarter its original value) and an increase in the measured logMAR acuity by 0.6 (0.3 + 0.3) can be used.

The number of letters presented at each size on the Bailey-Lovie chart is illustrated in Fig. 3.3, in comparison to a standard Snellen chart. It can be seen that a patient with an acuity of logMAR 0.6 (6/24) would have had the opportunity to read 25 letters on the Bailey-Lovie chart, compared with only 6 on a standard Snellen chart. As well as giving a more accurate assessment of acuity, this must increase the confidence of the patient, and allow better comparisons of the clarity of letters during subjective refraction. The letters used are those chosen by the British Standards Institution for the 1968 Standard for Test Charts, and there is no 'O' or 'C': this can lead to difficulties in finding a target for the subjective confirmation of astigmatic correction. The chart is also larger and of different shape to the more traditional Snellen chart, and therefore requires a specific internally illuminated cabinet.

More commonly used at the present time is the ETDRS chart (Fig. 3.4).

This was developed due to a need to have several equivalent versions of the same chart design which could be used when taking multiple measurements during a clinical trial: it is named after the 'Early Treatment Diabetic Retinopathy Study', for which it was developed (Ferris et al., 1982). These charts use combinations of the 10 Sloan letters (S, O, C, D, K, V, R, H, N, Z) which have similar, although not identical, recognition difficulty. The letter combinations for each line on the chart are therefore chosen so that the summed difficulty for the five letters combined, differs by less than 1% between lines. The standard viewing distance of the chart is 4 m, and this can be halved to 2 m or 1 m as required (for visually impaired observers). If refraction is carried out with letter charts at these distances, then the subjective prescription will be over-plussed by an amount equal to the dioptric distance of the chart. At 2 m, the prescription would be +0.50 D (reciprocal of 2 m) relative to a correction for infinity (as determined by retinoscopy) (e.g. −2.00 DS rather than −2.50 DS). Similarly, to obtain the optimum acuity using a chart at a closer distance may require the 'distance' refractive correction to have a compensating plus lens added (e.g. add +1.00 to the distance prescription to measure the VA at 1 m).

Although many charts are now available based on these principles (including those designed for presentation on electronic screens), care must be taken in describing them as Bailey-Lovie or ETDRS charts. In most cases it is true that they are logMAR charts, but they may not share other important design features (number and spacing of letters; letter shapes; range of letters used).

The Bailey-Lovie and ETDRS charts were very specifically designed to standardise the effect of surrounding contours (crowding) on visual perception. It is therefore important that extra contours are not introduced by the practitioner pointing

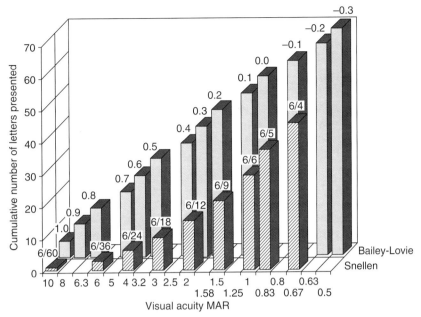

Fig. 3.3 The cumulative number of letters which will have been presented to, and read correctly by, a patient achieving a given acuity level on a standard Snellen or Bailey-Lovie/ETDRS (Early Treatment Diabetic Retinopathy Study) letter chart. The fixed geometric decrease (0.1 log unit, 0.8×) in letter size on adjacent rows reading down the chart for the Bailey-Lovie/ETDRS chart is also shown. *MAR*, Minimum angle of resolution.

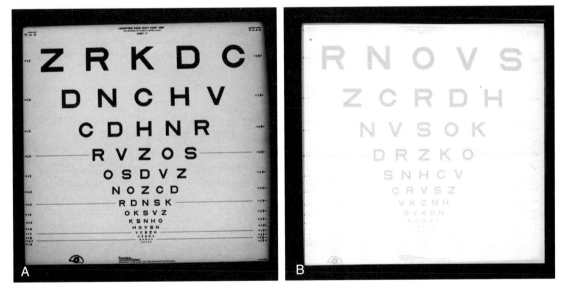

Fig. 3.4 (A) High-contrast ETDRS chart and (B) Low-contrast ETDRS chart, in illuminated cabinet. (The appearance of a low-contrast chart has been created photographically for illustration purposes.)

to letters to orientate the patient. Requiring the patient to find 'the first letter' or 'the third line' also gives the practitioner the opportunity to find out about the patient's localisation ability: poor performance can suggest the presence of scotomas. The presence of a scotoma which stops the patient from reading a large part of the chart also creates problems for scoring logMAR acuity, because the VA recorded with the missing letters accounted for does not give an accurate representation of the resolution ability of the patient. For clinical purposes, it would be more accurate to record VA descriptively such as 'only left half of chart seen, first three letters of logMAR 0.3 correct'. Some practitioners, especially within clinical trials,

use a letter-counting method to quantify VA by the total number of letters read, but this is very difficult to interpret without detailed knowledge of the measurement protocol (Elliott, 2016).

In the same way that the Bland-Altman method can be used to assess agreement of two different tests, it can also be used to assess the agreement of a test with itself—that is, its repeatability. In this case, the mean difference (bias) can again be measured (e.g. the patient may perform better on the second attempt due to familiarity), and the variability is expressed as the 'coefficient of repeatability'. For patients with normal acuity it can be 0.07 logMAR (3.5 letters better or worse on second attempt) (Camparini et al., 2001), whereas for those with macular degeneration it may be as much as two (Patel et al., 2008) or three (Aslam et al., 2014) lines.

ASSESSING ULTRA-LOW VISION

With a conventional letter chart which can be moved close to the patient, the poorest level of VA which can be quantified with a Snellen chart designed for 6 m would be 0.5/60 (6/720 or logMAR 2.08), by bringing the chart to 50 cm. For a 4 m ETDRS chart at 50 cm, the poorest VA recordable would be about logMAR 1.9. Note that in both cases, any potential defocus from the close viewing distance would be very unlikely to impact VA of this level. If the chart is not resolved at this distance, the traditional optometric approach to describe vision is to use 'hand movements', 'perception of light with/without projection' (projection being the ability to determine the direction from which a light is shining), and then 'no perception of light'. Such 'tests' of performance are nonstandardised, and can also be psychologically demoralising for the patient, suggesting their vision is so poor that methods to measure it do not exist. The Berkeley Rudimentary Vision Test is a simple clinical test which has been proposed to attempt to quantify these very low levels of visual performance, once the limits of a letter chart have been reached (Bailey et al., 2012). The test is presented manually by the clinician on double-sided cards, where the visual tasks get progressively easier. First single letters are used (consisting of a single letter 'E' of four different sizes, whose orientation can be changed to alter the task), firstly at 1 m, and if not seen then at 25 cm. If this test is not possible, the target is changed to a square-wave grating of four different stripe widths, whose orientation must be identified at 25 cm. The next grade of vision is tested with 'white field projection' using a card which is half black and half white, or all black with a white quadrant. Finally, 'black-white discrimination' is tested using a card which is white on one side and black on the other. For each of the tests, rotating the cards allows many different target presentations to be made by the clinician.

If the acuity drops below the level measurable with a letter chart, it is very unlikely that vision enhancement will be possible. However, recently a new area of rehabilitation of this 'ultra-low vision' has begun to develop involving individuals who have undergone various forms of visual restoration. This restoration may involve, for example, gene therapy, or an ocular or cortical 'bionic implant', often for an individual with a hereditary retinal degeneration. In these cases, it may be important to carefully document visual performance before and after the procedure. The way in which those with bionic implants learn, or are taught, how to access and use the novel visual information available, is a field which is still in its infancy.

CONTRAST SENSITIVITY

Despite the usefulness of VA as a performance measure, it is not a complete description of visual performance as it does not deal with the ability to detect large objects and low contrasts. CS does test the ability to detect such objects. As these are important components of the 'real' visual world, it is claimed to provide a better assessment of the patient's true functional vision. The contrast sensitivity function (CSF) represents the reciprocal of the contrast detection threshold for sine-wave gratings (alternate light and dark bars) of variable spatial frequency (cycles/degree) and contrast. Sine waves are used because they are the simplest spatial stimulus, and more complex luminance distributions can be Fourier-analysed into a series of sine-waves: the response of the visual system to a complex pattern can be predicted from its response to the component sine-wave stimuli.

CS for gratings is a much more fundamental, lower-level visual task, involving simple *resolution* of the presence of the grating, compared to the higher-level *recognition/identification* task which is required when letters have to be named in a traditional VA test. Nonetheless, the angular subtense of the two tasks can be equated. If the patient is able to detect a grating then they can distinguish that the black bars are separate, so the gap between them (i.e. the white bar) will subtend 1 min arc at the eye (by analogy with the threshold for logMAR 0.0 [6/6] letter acuity). Thus, 1 cycle of the grating would subtend 2 min arc or 1/30 degree, and 30 cycles would subtend 1°. Thus, a patient with 6/6 vision for high contrast Snellen letters should be able to detect a 30 cycle/degree grating at maximum contrast: this highest spatial frequency which can be detected represents the cut-off or limit to detection ability where CS becomes minimal (and equal to 1, the reciprocal of the maximum grating contrast which also equals 1). In the same way, logMAR 0.3 (6/12) would be equivalent to 15 cycles/degree, for example, and this letter target can be schematically represented on the same axes as the CSF. Changes in target size are indicated by shifts along the x-axis (spatial frequency), whilst different contrast levels are represented on the y-axis. The peak sensitivity usually occurs around 3–5 cycles/degree with a lower sensitivity for both higher and lower spatial frequencies. This gives a characteristic inverted-U-shaped curve, shown in Fig. 3.5.

Having a low contrast threshold for detection of the grating (being able to see it even when presented with minimal contrast, which could be approximately 0.5% for a grating of the optimal spatial frequency) indicates a very high CS (1/0.005 = 200; log CS = 2.3). Clinically the CSF has been used to detect patients with normal/near-normal VA yet complaining of subjective visual difficulties: such a case is illustrated in Fig. 3.5 (Arden, 1978, 1983; Bodis-Wollner & Comisa, 1980). The two curves represent the response of two different patients, who obviously have different contrast sensitivities. Although Patient 1 has a reduced sensitivity to low spatial frequencies, the higher frequencies can be detected almost normally, and acuity is high. Nonetheless this subject may have significant visual problems due to the marked differences in the ability to detect large low-contrast objects. Similarly, it is possible to envisage patients with almost equal functional ability (as the detection of low-spatial-frequency, low-contrast targets is equivalent), yet very different acuity

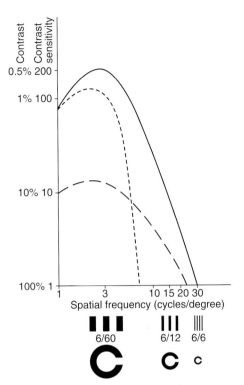

Fig. 3.5 The *solid line* represents a 'normal' contrast sensitivity function. The *dashed line* shows the theoretical response of Patient 1 with a loss of sensitivity to low- and medium-spatial frequencies, but normal sensitivity to high-spatial frequency (and therefore near-normal visual acuity). The *dotted curve* indicates a loss of high-spatial frequency sensitivity (resulting in poor acuity) in Patient 2 but normal sensitivity for low-spatial frequency targets.

for high contrast optotypes (as the high-contrast threshold for high-spatial-frequency targets is different).

In the presence of *refractive* blur created by uncorrected ametropia, the acuity loss is equivalent for both high- and low-contrast targets, since the blurred image has the same contrast as the target which created it. This is not equally true, however, of the *diffusive* blur produced by media opacity (such as cataract) (Ho & Bilton, 1986). Here there is scattering of light within the eye, and the effect of this is to increase the luminance of the retinal image in both the light and the dark areas, thus reducing the effective contrast. These patients often complain of 'faded' or 'washed-out' vision due to scattering of light within the eye reducing image contrast. These complaints are often out of proportion to the VA which is still relatively good: as this is a high-contrast target, the patient can still recognise the letters despite a reduction in contrast. The same contrast attenuation applied to a low-contrast target is likely to take it below threshold. Thus, the low-contrast performance is likely to be more representative of 'everyday' visual complaints than that of high-contrast, and CS is a very useful clinical test.

Despite its potential usefulness, measurement of the full CSF is fraught with difficulties in the clinical setting (Legge & Rubin, 1986). Traditional methods are time-consuming, and it can be difficult to decide what constitutes 'abnormality' (because it is difficult to combine the results for all spatial frequencies into a single score). Computer-based methods such as the 'quick-CSF' (Lesmes, Lu, Baek, & Albright, 2010; Dorr, Lesmes, Lu,

& Bex, 2013) are impressive, but are not yet widely adopted in clinical practice. A further problem is that there is a marked effect of the field-of-view on the CSF (Estevez and Cavonius, 1976; Howell and Hess, 1978). The work of Hess (Hess, 1987) suggested that CSF results in low vision must be interpreted with great care. It appears that if the patient has a field defect that obscures part of the grating display, this alone is enough to produce a characteristic loss of CS. With a simulated central scotoma in a normally sighted subject, a loss of sensitivity to high spatial frequencies is induced; peripheral field loss gives a low spatial frequency loss, and a mid-peripheral annular scotoma induces a loss at medium spatial frequencies, whilst high and low spatial frequencies are unaffected.

Clinical Tests

There have been a number of attempts to produce practical CS tests suitable for use in clinical practice. These clinical tests generally restrict the range of spatial frequencies over which testing is carried out, so a full CSF is not obtained. In patients with visual impairment such tests are very useful for what they can suggest about functional performance of everyday tasks. However, such tests are also used clinically as a screening device to detect the early stages of pathology before the acuity is impaired.

Available clinical tests fall into three categories:

1. *Sinusoidal gratings at limited number of frequencies*

This approach to testing the CSF is illustrated schematically in Fig. 3.6A which shows how the test targets sample the CSF curve, with the chart appearance shown in Fig. 3.6B. This was the design used in the Vistech Vision Contrast Test System (VCTS) chart (Ginsburg, 1984) and the related Functional Acuity Contrast Test (FACT).

Each row of the chart represents one spatial frequency, with the columns representing decreasing contrast levels moving from left to right. The gratings are oriented vertically, or tilted right or left. The patient 'reads' along each row from left to right, progressing from high-contrast to low-contrast targets, reporting on the orientation of the grating pattern in each disc. This 'forced choice' procedure is a robust psychophysical task, designed to minimise the effect of different patient criteria, as some patients would not report the direction or presence of a grating unless they were absolutely sure, whereas others respond positively when much less certain. Such a test is much simpler, quicker (because only a limited number of spatial frequencies are tested), and cheaper than electronically generated sinewave stimuli. However, in this case, the high chance of a correct guess (33%), combined with only one presentation of each target, leads to variability in results (Pesudovs et al., 2004): Reeves et al. (1991) found that significant changes in performance occurred on successive sessions that were due to chance rather than to real changes in the patient's vision. A further disadvantage is the limited number of contrast levels which can be presented, leading to a risk of 'ceiling' or 'floor' effects: individuals with subtle CS defects can see all the targets, whereas those with moderate CS loss cannot see any targets (Pesudovs et al., 2004).

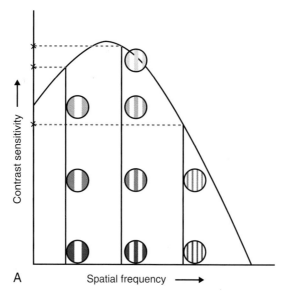

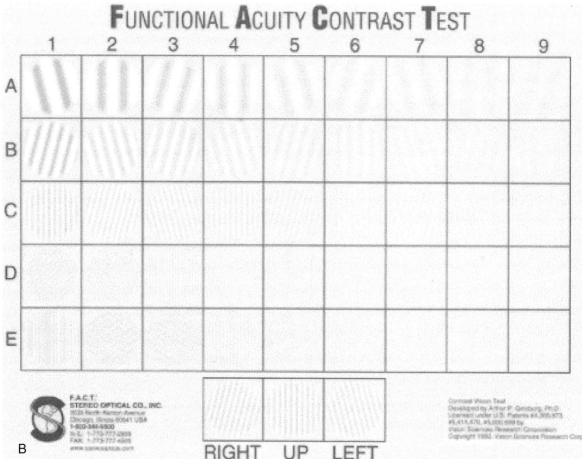

Fig. 3.6 (A) A schematic representation of the way in which contrast sensitivity is measured by a test such as (B) the FACT (Functional Acuity Contrast Test) chart. From Hitchcock, E.M., Dick, R.B., & Kreig, E.F. (2004). Visual contrast sensitivity testing: a comparison of two F.A.C.T. test types. *Neurotoxicology and Teratology, 26*, 271–277.

2. *Low-contrast VA*

In this case the patient is required to read letters of decreasing size at one or more fixed levels of contrast (Fig. 3.7).

The smallest letter size which can be read at a given contrast level is representative of the cut-off spatial frequency at that level—the point where a horizontal line representing that contrast level intersects with the CS curve. The characteristic

shape of the CSF (especially the slope of right-hand edge), is apparent as a difference in acuity at two different contrast levels. Bailey (1993) used 100% and 10% contrast, whereas Regan and Neima (1984) recommended 96% and 7% (see Fig. 3.4). Even people with good vision show a predictable reduction in VA at the lower contrast level. The presence of a visual loss which changes the slope of the high-frequency

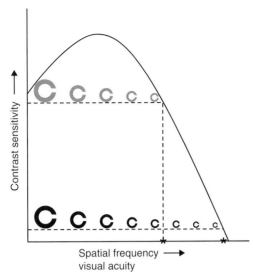

Fig. 3.7 A schematic representation of the way in which contrast sensitivity is assessed by a test comprising letters of variable size in a high-contrast and a low-contrast version. An example of such charts is shown in Fig. 3.4.

portion of the CSF would be detected by a disproportionately poorer acuity for the low-contrast letters. Regan (1988) describes such responses in patients with glaucoma and multiple sclerosis, even though their high-contrast acuity remains normal. This type of test has therefore been recommended as useful for screening for eye disease during routine eye examinations. The Colenbrander Mixed Contrast Card Set is a near vision chart with adjacent high- and low- (10%) contrast letters and sentences presented at progressively decreasing sizes. The patient is asked what is the smallest print that can be read in black text, and the smallest print that can be read in grey text (which is expected to be bigger). A two- to three-line difference in VA is typical of normal subjects, but differences up to 10 lines have been identified in some patients (Colenbrander & Fletcher, 2005).

3. Test of peak CS

To measure peak CS, the patient views large, easily seen detail (to be near the spatial frequency corresponding to peak sensitivity) at variable contrast to establish the detection threshold (Fig. 3.8). The aim is to determine a single value which represents the minimum contrast required in order for a target to be visible. The best known tests in this category are the Pelli-Robson (PR) Low Contrast Letter Chart (Pelli et al., 1988; Reeves, 1991) and Mars Letter Contrast Sensitivity Test (Arditi, 2005). These are both tests which are printed (rather than being backlit in an illuminated cabinet) and therefore they rely on the correct amount and uniformity of illuminance from an external source in order to create the labelled contrast levels: the instructions in the user manuals supplied with these tests should be followed carefully to ensure accurate results. Rather than gratings, both use letters as their targets (and the Mars test is also available with numbers in order to be language neutral). Provided the letters are large, the peak spatial frequencies are well-represented in the image.

It has been claimed that letters are more appropriate than gratings, as they are more familiar to the patient, are

relatively easy to produce in comparison to sine-wave gratings, and they allow simultaneous testing of detection at all orientations (whereas gratings only test at one, usually vertical). There is, however, a major difference between the task of *detection* of (large field) gratings compared to *recognition* of isolated letters, so the two are not directly comparable. The general design of both the PR and Mars tests is the same, with the Mars specifically being designed to overcome some of the disadvantages of the PR. The Mars chart is small enough to be hand held and is designed to be viewed from 50 cm with the habitual reading correction. The PR is wall mounted, so exposure to light and dust change the contrast over time. It is viewed from 1 m (although it was originally intended to be at 3 m), and some clinicians recommend using a +0.75 add for people with advanced presbyopia. Each test displays eight rows of letters. There is only one version of the PR test, but the Mars test has three versions, so providing an easy means to test both eyes monocularly, and binocularly. The latter can be stored in a protective case to keep it clean, and the smaller size makes it easier to achieve even illumination.

The tests are calibrated to measure log CS.

$$\log CS = \log \frac{100}{\text{contrast threshold (\%)}} \text{ or } \log CS = -\log C$$

where contrast threshold is the contrast of the faintest letter which can be recognized. Contrast here is Weber contrast:

$$\text{Contrast} = \frac{L_{target} - L_{background}}{L_{background}}$$

To take an example, contrast threshold C = 0.021 (2.1%), CS = 47.6, log CS = 1.68

Different ways to score the PR test have been recommended over the years. Each triplet of letters differs by 0.15 log units from the preceding triplet: to achieve the score for that triplet the patient has to read two out of the three letters correctly. However, some clinicians have scored it 'by letter' and counted 0.05 log units for each letter. For the Mars test each successive symbol decreases in contrast by 0.04 log units reading from the top left of the chart, so genuine scoring by letter is used.

Because CS testing involves detection rather than recognition, it is customary to allow patients to read 'O' for 'C', and vice versa (Thayaparan et al., 2007). The different nature of the task must be explained to the patient: near threshold they should be encouraged to blink and move their eyes, and guess the symbol if any shape is vaguely seen. This is very different to threshold for VA, when the black letter is still clearly detected, but its internal detail cannot be discriminated.

There is also a CS test available as part of the Thomson Test Chart 2000 Software (Thomson Software Solutions, Welham Green, UK), based on the PR, but only displaying one triplet of letters at a time. This may give different, and less repeatable results than either the PR or the Mars test: it is thought this may be due to the higher screen luminance, and the difficulty of displaying low contrasts accurately on a computer monitor which tends to artificially boost low-contrast features (Thayaparan et al., 2007).

Other contrast detection tests which seek to determine a single 'peak sensitivity' are the so-called 'edge' tests. The first of these was the Melbourne Edge Test (Verbaker & Johnston, 1986; Grey & Yap, 1987). The patient is presented with a circular target which is divided across the middle and has a different intensity on each side of the border: the orientation of the border must be detected and it may be oriented vertically or tilted slightly to right or left. Contrast is progressively reduced until the border can no longer reliably be distinguished. Here the stimuli are back-illuminated on a light box, and the results obtained do depend on the luminance of the test.

CS tests whose repeatability has been confirmed experimentally, can be used to monitor changes in performance with time, or interocular differences, which may not have been detected by high-contrast VA tests. The tests may also, for example, be used to confirm the patient's subjective impression that their vision has deteriorated, despite the preservation of optotype acuity; or to decide which eye might perform most effectively when viewing through a magnifier when the monocular VAs are equal. A further use of CS tests is to demonstrate to relatives and carers the difficulties which the person with low vision experiences: for example, it can be very useful to show that they can only see high-contrast letters on a PR chart and then explain that faint objects will be invisible to them.

In summary, CS is a very useful descriptor of the visual status, and provides distinct information compared to that offered by other tests. Although it is a threshold test, it may help to quantify and explain the patient's functional difficulties. A lowered CS is likely to impair the patient's ability to see steps, curbs, and irregularities in the pavement, for example, because their recognition depends on the detection of relatively small contrast differences between features with large angular subtense (Fig. 3.9).

Seeing faces is a task of great practical significance to the patient: this applies both for recognising friends in the street, but also for its role in face-to-face communication where gestures, eye contact and mouth shapes corresponding to letters are all useful cues, especially to an older person whose hearing may also be impaired. Erber and Osborn (1994) found

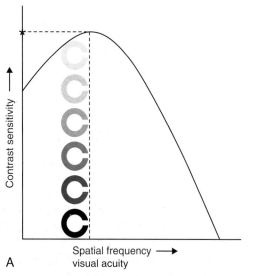
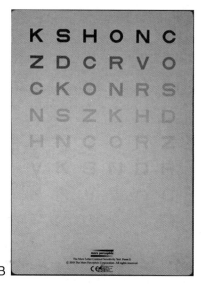

Fig. 3.8 (A) A schematic representation of the way in which contrast sensitivity is assessed by a test consisting of letters of fixed size and variable contrast. (B) The Mars Letter Contrast Chart is an example of a test of this design.

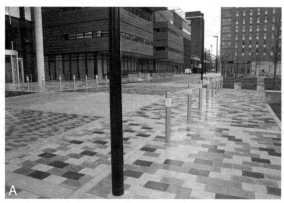
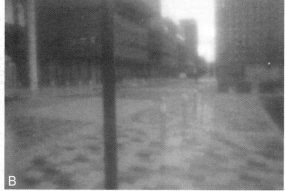

Fig. 3.9 (A) The low-contrast posts at this pavement edge are difficult to detect, particularly when contrast sensitivity is impaired (as in (B)). The lamp-post is easier to detect because of its greater contrast with the background.

that for acuity less than 6/180, even the most robust facial cues (head nodding and shaking) could not be seen with a 1 m viewing distance: but with acuity better than 6/24, even subtle facial cues such as eye contact were seen by all subjects. However, faces are low-contrast targets, and Dickinson and Taylor (2011) found that speechreading ability was impaired by even subtle losses of CS (a simulated log CS of 2.0 relative to the normal level of 2.3). On a practical level, in the consulting room, auditory and tactile back-up to visual gestures must be used: where the patient's attention would usually be engaged by eye contact, this might be backed up by a gentle touch on the hand; encouragement during history-taking might be given by both head nodding and verbal signals. Reduced CS also has a considerable effect on reading performance (see Reading Section), which may seem counter-intuitive as this task usually involves small detail at relatively high contrast. In fact there are very few everyday tasks whose performance is not impacted by reduced CS: from competitive rifle shooting (Allen et al., 2018) to judging the location and distance of objects (Subramanian & Dickinson, 2006), to take just two examples.

PREDICTING THE OUTCOME OF CATARACT SURGERY

Just because the patient has one pathology which is treatable (cataract) does not mean that there is no other disease present. Either corneal or retinal comorbidity could mean that on removal of the cataract only limited improvement in vision will be achieved. In some cases, the surgery is required as part of treatment (e.g. in glaucoma management) or to allow monitoring of retinal disease, even if vision is not improved. However, in some cases, the patient will undergo the inconvenience and potential risks of the surgical procedure, with the possibility of a disappointing visual result. If resources are limited, it may be necessary to restrict treatment to those patients with a realistic prospect of visual improvement, or to determine which of their two affected eyes has the best visual prognosis. For both the surgeon and the patient, then, a realistic assessment of the 'potential vision' is required and a wide range of subjective and objective visual tests has been proposed (Hurst & Douthwaite, 1993; Vianya-Estopà et al., 2006).

Some of these methods have been devised to try to 'bypass' the opacity. The Potential Acuity Meter (PAM) is a slit-lamp attachment in which an optical system is used to project the image of a Snellen chart directly onto the macula (Minkowski et al., 1983). A lens forms an image of the illuminated letter chart which has an area only 0.15 mm in diameter in the plane of the patient's pupil, and the examiner directs this to an observable 'window' in the opacity. The patient (wearing their refractive correction) sees the chart when they look down the beam and reports the lowest line which can be read. In laser interferometry, two coherent laser beams are directed through 'windows' in the opacity (Green, 1970; Faulkner, 1983). When these coincide on the retina they interfere, with coincident troughs in the wave forming dark areas, and peaks creating light zones. The result

is a grating of light and dark bars whose spatial frequency can be varied by altering the separation of the laser beams. Unfortunately, it does require windows in the opacity (and at different spacings depending on the spatial frequency to be created), and the image is very bright and large, so it can often be detected even if a macular scotoma is obscuring or distorting part of it.

If two grating patterns of black-and-white stripes are overlapped, a regular pattern of dark stripes is seen in a different direction to those in the original pattern. By varying the relative orientation of the two patterns, the spatial frequency of the resultant 'Moiré fringes' can be altered: a threshold can be determined if this is increased until the patient can no longer detect it. Lotmar (1980) used this method in his 'Visometer' to measure acuity for a fringe pattern produced on the retina when white light was projected via two rotatable gratings through apertures in the opacity.

The idea of allowing image-forming rays to pass through a window in the opacity has led to suggestions of using a form of pinhole acuity to assess potential vision. The standard pinhole test used routinely in subjective refraction is unlikely to help because the loss of light limits performance. However, a modified version has been developed which has been called the 'potential acuity pinhole', 'super pinhole' or 'illuminated near chart'. In each case, the requirements are that the patient has a dilated pupil (and that in itself may be beneficial in revealing improvement), an occluder with multiple 1-mm pinhole apertures to place close to the eye, and a very brightly illuminated test chart (usually at near) (Hofeldt & Weiss, 1998; Melki et al., 1999). The patient can move the pinholes to 'search' for the best acuity; the test is quick, inexpensive, and easy for the patient to carry out (Chang et al., 2006); and optimum refractive correction is not required.

The clinical usefulness of any of these tests lies of course in how well they can predict the postoperative acuity, and none are particularly effective: it should be emphasized that the majority of research in this area has involved predicting acuity in patients with no additional eye disease (Kessel et al., 2016). Vianya-Estopa et al. (2009) found that for eyes with moderate cataract and comorbidity, only their super-illuminated pinhole test (a white-on-black distance letter chart) was a better predictor of the outcome than the clinical judgement of experienced cataract surgeons. In all techniques, the predictions become less accurate as the lens opacity becomes more dense, but these are precisely the cases where the fundus cannot be visualised and the techniques would have greatest value. However, it does seem that these techniques rarely overestimate the potential acuity in such cases, so a good preoperative result is unlikely to be due to artefact and does suggest a successful outcome.

VISUAL FIELD TESTING

Peripheral Visual Fields

At its most basic, visual field testing determines the total extent of the peripheral vision of the patient, and their ability to detect an object whose image is falling on peripheral retina. There are various 'qualitative' visual field measures which rely on practitioner judgement (Eperjesi, 2010). In the low-vision context, the most useful is one described as 'kinetic boundary perimetry', using a bead (5–10 mm in diameter, and red or white in colour [whichever gives the best contrast with the surrounding walls]) on top of a black rod about 30 cm in length. The examiner sits opposite the patient, and the patient views the examiner's eye which is directly ahead: testing can be binocular, or monocular with the fellow eye well covered. The examiner brings the target around from behind the patient who reports when the bead target is first seen, as it moves from non-seeing to seeing, and then if it disappears as it is brought radially towards the direction of gaze. Bringing the target from above, below, temporal and nasal allows these extremes of the field to be determined. Because defects which respect the vertical and horizontal midlines are relatively likely (e.g. hemianopia, or quadrantanopia), it is better for the examiner to move the target slightly 'off' these meridians, rather than directly along them (e.g. to move the target from '11 o'clock' and '1 o'clock', rather than from '12 o'clock'). Although there are many automated visual field instruments (e.g. the Humphrey, Henson, Medmont, and Dicon ranges), these are not well suited to measuring functional visual fields. These instruments concentrate visual field testing within the central 30°, are designed to test monocularly, and, most importantly, are designed to pick up small changes in threshold sensitivity. If such a device is to be used in low-vision rehabilitation, the best option is to use a suprathreshold binocular test such as the binocular Esterman programme, which is usually included as it is used to assess compliance with the visual field requirements for driving in the UK. This test is considerably suprathreshold (targets are around 100× brighter than threshold), and 120° extent of the horizontal field is explored. Any automated programme is, however, best avoided for individuals with very severe reduction in visual field (e.g. tunnel vision): they can spend several minutes during the test when they are not responding, as targets are repeatedly presented to non-seeing areas of their visual field, which they can find very distressing. An accurate extent of the visual field for such patients is best obtained using the Amsler chart, which covers the central 20° of the visual field.

One would expect the visual field extent to be related to the ability of individuals to navigate their environment. Lovie-Kitchin et al. (1990) used a real obstacle course to find out which areas of the visual field were necessary for safe mobility and orientation. They found that the central 37° radius, and the right, inferior and left annulus between 37° and 58° were the most significant zones. The integrity of the extreme periphery of the field was not particularly significant. Marron and Bailey (1982) and Long et al. (1990) also found that visual field, and (grating) CS, were good predictors of orientation and mobility performance. Central and peripheral fields are both related to self-reported visual function, with the peripheral field (beyond 30°) being a slightly better predictor of mobility function (Subhi et al., 2017).

Central Visual Fields

Central field loss is very common in people with low vision, and this will affect multiple aspects of visual function. Although the automated visual field screeners described previously can be used to measure central visual fields, there are many limitations with using them to assess field loss (as opposed to subtle threshold variation). The most significant is that people with central field loss are likely to use a preferred retinal locus (PRL) so the test grid will not necessarily be centred on the fovea (see Chapter 13). They also typically have far poorer fixation stability, so the accuracy of each stimulus position will be low. This will reduce the sensitivity, repeatability and accuracy of the visual field test (Crossland et al., 2005). Even with specific targets (four pericentral spots, or a diamond) designed to aid fixation, and careful instruction of the patient, there is no guarantee that fixation is stable and central (Bellmann et al., 2004)

Traditional kinetic perimetry using a 2- or 3-mm white target on a Bjerrum (tangent) screen viewed from 1m is considered to be accurate (Achard et al., 1995), although extremely time-consuming, and demanding for the patient. Fixation again cannot be easily controlled, although an experienced clinician may be able to observe fixation changes, or notice if the plotted blind spot is not in its expected location.

The most accurate way to measure the central visual field is to use a microperimeter, although these instruments remain relatively uncommon in clinical practice. Microperimetry was originally a term used to describe perimetry using extremely small targets, which could identify the scotomas caused by the retinal blood vessels in normal eyes. Nowadays it is the term used for a technique which would be better described as 'fundus perimetry' or 'fundus-related perimetry' (Crossland et al., 2012). In this technique, the stimulus presented to the patient is simultaneously seen imaged on the fundus, and so its location can be clearly identified, and does not depend on the patient's fixation. The first commercial instrument to be used in this way was the Rodenstock Scanning Laser Ophthalmoscope (SLO), although linking the successive target presentations/fundus images together had to be performed manually. Several microperimeters are now available which carry out this process automatically, each with advantages and disadvantages, including the MP-1, MP-3 and MAIA devices. If the instrument is to be used to investigate severe central field loss, it must have the ability to present very bright targets: if very clear fundus images are required this is likely to require a scanning laser rather than camera-based system (Fig. 3.10). A microperimeter can also be used to identify the location and stability of the PRLs for an individual with a central scotoma, and this may be helpful in eccentric viewing (EV) training (see Chapter 13). Microperimetry is time-consuming, requires a skilled operator, and can only be performed monocularly, reducing its relevance to everyday life under binocular conditions. In contrast, nonautomated tests such as kinetic boundary perimetry can all be performed quickly, easily and binocularly.

A more familiar test of central field function is the Amsler chart. The most commonly used version (although

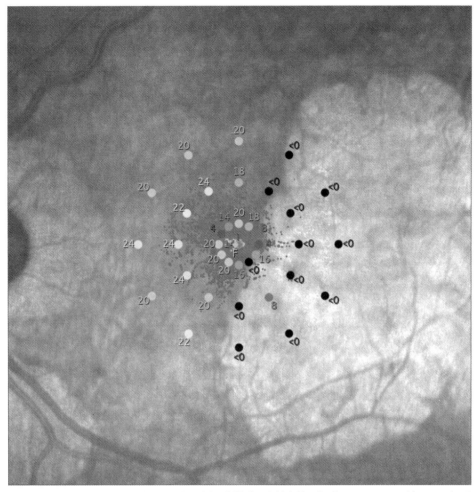

Fig. 3.10 Sensitivity values (dB), fixation points (blue dots) and the PRL (I = initial, F = final) over a zoomed-in scanning laser ophthalmoscope image (Figure courtesy of iCare).

the manual contains a range of different plate designs which are rarely used) presents a white grid of squares subtending 20° × 20° degrees on a black background. There is an alternative plate which has two diagonal lines added, forming a cross which aids fixation. The test is designed to be viewed from 28.5 cm such that each 5-mm square in the grid subtends an angle of 1°. It can be very sensitive, even showing distortion in early macular disease when VA is still good. On occasions, however, it shows an entirely spurious false negative response: the patient may have severe macular pathology with poor acuity, yet report the grid as complete, clear and undistorted. Sometimes patients arc given a copy of the chart to monitor their vision at home, and this is often a black-on-white grid, which is found to be less sensitive (Augustin et al., 2005). The problem has been investigated in detail by Schuchard (1993) who compared both threshold and suprathreshold Amsler grid testing with an illuminated white grid, and a red grid produced by an SLO. When the grid subtended 15° × 15° around the primary position, no normal subject was able to detect their own blind spot; 77% of scotomas of 6° or less in abnormal eyes were not found. Even if scotomas are reported, they are probably inaccurate as 66% of patients with a foveal scotoma used an eccentric retinal location to fixate the centre

of the grid, and each of the grids tended to underestimate the size of the scotoma. Some patients, however, reported larger scotomas, perhaps because of eye movements. Schuchard calls for a redesign of the familiar Amsler Grid to one in which missing areas are not so easily 'filled in' perceptually. Intuitively, it seems reasonable to try to make the test more sensitive by using lower-contrast red-on-black grids, or by viewing the white-on-black grid through crossed polaroids: as the angle between the polaroids is varied, the perceived contrast of the chart will progressively reduce (Wall & May, 1987; Swann & Lovie-Kitchin, 1991). In fact, such attempts have been unsuccessful, and Achiron et al. (1994) suggest that in fact an illuminated high-contrast version of the grid is more sensitive, and just as good as automatic perimetry. When being used as a screening device, simply detecting the presence of a central abnormality may be sufficient, but to use the information for rehabilitation, an accurate size and location of the scotoma, and its relationship to the PRL, will be required. The California Central Visual Field Test (CCVFT; Fig. 3.11) (www.mattinglylowvision.com) which explores the central 15° diameter of the visual field works well for this purpose. It was originally designed by Fletcher, and modified by Cole (2008).

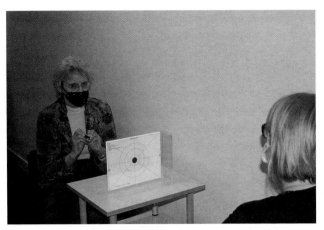

Fig. 3.11 The California Central Visual Field Test (CCVFT) in use to identify the presence of a central scotoma.

Three different laser pointers are used to provide the variable red spot stimuli for detection by the patient: small (1 mm) and dim (laser #1), small and brighter (#2), and large (3 mm) and bright (#3). Using each in turn can determine the depth as well as size of the scotoma. The CCVFT differs from other visual field tests in that the subject is not required to fixate foveally. Instead, they are asked to maintain their best fixation and attention on the central fixation spot, and so they are likely to use their PRL. This then allows scotoma location relative to habitual fixation to be determined.

The recording chart is placed in a clear plastic holder, which is placed upright on a table, 57 cm from the subject. There are three different charts, each with a different sized central fixation spot: the chart with the smallest target which can be seen comfortably by the patient is chosen. The clinician faces the patient, in order to observe eye position and stability of fixation, and views the recording chart from the back. The laser is briefly flashed in random locations onto the back of the recording chart, asking the patient to tap the table when they see the target. 'Seen' and 'not seen' locations are pencilled on the back of the chart, and transferred to the front at the end of the test. Trials for false positives can be introduced by pointing the laser towards the floor intermittently; false negatives can be determined by repeating previously seen locations.

ASSESSING POTENTIAL ACUITY IN THE PRESENCE OF A CENTRAL SCOTOMA

As noted previously, patients with bilateral central scotoma often use a PRL for fixation in place of the damaged fovea. Acuity would be expected to be lower than at the fovea, due to the well-known decline of VA towards the periphery of the retina, so preferably the area of preserved vision should be close to the fovea. The patient may already have developed the optimum PRL, but it may be that there is another retinal location that would be more favourable, and use of this could be trained. As training in EV can be time-consuming and difficult, it would be useful to have some indication of

likely success, and an indication of which area of the retina would best serve to replace the fovea, and become the 'Trained Retinal Locus' (TRL). Harris et al. (1985) described a near acuity test consisting of a two-dimensional array of identical letters. The test allows the same letter to be imaged on foveal and parafoveal retina, even if the patient fixates centrally, thus assessing whether potentially useful vision is present anywhere within the central visual field. If an eccentric point would perform better than the fovea, acuity for this letter array will be better than that measured for the same letter presented singly. However, this test only indicates that such a location exists but does not locate it. Visual field testing (as discussed earlier) could assist, but this uses a detection test for the presence of single light spots, whereas the TRL to be developed will be required to recognise letters and, if used for reading, it will be necessary to image several letters simultaneously in order to achieve an acceptable reading speed.

MacKeben (2008) has attempted to apply a more relevant 'Macular Mapping' test in which the 'topography of residual vision' is plotted by presenting letter targets to be recognised at 33 locations within the central visual field. The best candidate to become the TRL can then be determined in terms of its acuity, location, and size. As with other perimetry, the patient fixation must be controlled. MacKeben and Colenbrander (1992) suggest that their particular fixation target (eight radial spokes) stabilises gaze, but their technique does not allow objective confirmation of the patient's fixation (Trauzettel-Klosinski et al., 2003)

COLOUR VISION

As approximately 8% of the male and 0.4% of the female population (of Northern European ancestry) have colour vision defects (CVDs) (Cole, 2007), many people with VI will have an incidental congenital CVD. Only in the case of rare inherited retinal disease (e.g. rod monochromatism) is this CVD the cause of their visual impairment. Most visually impaired individuals are likely to have an acquired CVD, as these can arise from diseases at all stages of the visual pathway, and this may be mild or severe. These CVDs are difficult to classify, but those that affect acuity must be affecting the midget cell pathway which is specialised for spatial discrimination, and this would be expected to create R-G defects (Simunovic, 2016). Overall, however, acquired CVD which affect the B-Y pathway are twice as common as R-G defects, even though the short-wavelength cones are not involved in spatial discrimination. Measurement of colour vision in low-vision rehabilitation has not been considered as an important topic. The size of targets within tests such as the Ishihara plates is equivalent to approximately logMAR 1.6 (6/240), so it is a loss of CS which would be more likely to prevent the test being used with a patient.

Only one test has been specifically recommended for low vision, which is the Panel 16 Colour Vision Test. This is based on the Farnsworth D-15, but each of the caps is larger (3.3 cm), compared to the D-15 (1.2 cm). This changes the angle subtended at the eye (and a decreased viewing distance is also suggested in the instructions to increase it still further), which changes the area of retina over which the test is conducted. Any increase in area is likely to make the test easier to perform, because it may allow the image to fall on some better-functioning retinal area (unfortunately, this increase in size also changes the nature of the test, and helps those with a congenital CVD to make more accurate matches). The standard D-15 could also be adapted in the same way by using shorter working distances. The unique feature of the Panel 16 test is that it contains two separate sets of caps, and this allows it to be used more easily with those with a very severe CVD (or young children) who do not understand the task of arranging the caps 'in colour order'. They can, for example, be asked to make a series of individual cap matches: for example, the patient is given each cap in turn from set A and for each is asked to choose a match from a selection of the Set B caps (including the exact correct match) randomly arranged (http://www.lea-test.fi/index.html?start=en/vistests/instruct/pv16/testingp.html). Even an individual with no colour vision (such as someone with achromatopsia) can make matches on the Panel 16/D-15 tests, because the caps do differ in luminance. Arranging them based on this criterion (as different shades of grey) creates characteristic errors which are distinct from those typical of single cone defects.

Even if formal colour-vision testing is not carried out, it is helpful to question the patient about their colour vision. This can explore their ability to discriminate (can you tell black socks from brown socks?) or to detect (can you see a red rose on a bush?) certain colours. An acquired loss of such abilities could suggest loss of foveal vision, and a possible central scotoma: conversely, a preservation of colour discrimination would suggest a better prognosis for vision enhancement. Identifying CVDs is important for students: teachers can be asked to avoid colour coding school exercises (e.g. 'replace the red word with a different word').

READING

Reading is one of the major goals of people with low vision and difficulty with reading is such a common complaint in visual impairment that it has been suggested that low vision should be defined as the inability to read a newspaper at a normal working distance (40 cm) with the best refractive correction (Legge, 1991). Reading is an extremely complex visual task, requiring not only good vision but also accurate control of eye movements and the cognitive interpretation of the meaning of the text. For the majority of those with acquired VI, however, we usually assume that those aspects of reading were not an issue before the onset of VI, and concentrate on the visual aspects of the task.

Reading acuity does not correlate well with distance VA, and it is easy to think of a number of reasons why this may be the case: reading may be made more difficult by pupil constriction during near viewing enhancing the influence

of a central media opacity or the patient may be confused by the presence of adjoining letters within a word, whereas single targets can be resolved. Of course, reading acuity is rarely measured as the ability to read a line of letters one at a time, but rather as the ability to read words of the required print size, and this may sometimes be easier because the patient 'guesses' missing words or letters from the context of a meaningful sentence. In the everyday use of their reading ability, it will also be important for patients to achieve a certain reading rate (usually measured in words per minute [wpm]): very slow reading can impair understanding of the message conveyed and is extremely frustrating for the patient.

Gordon Legge and his group have considerably enhanced understanding of reading as a visual task in their research of reading over many years. They have found no reliable link between simple clinical measures and reading ability (Legge et al., 1992) and have suggested that in order to know how well someone will read, one actually has to perform a test of reading speed. They used a technique in which words are scrolled across a screen and the patient attempts to read as quickly as possible. The speed of presentation is then increased until the patient begins to make mistakes, and this maximum speed defines the threshold performance. Stimulus parameters (such as letter size, contrast and colour) can then be systematically altered in order to determine their effect on reading. Of course, this removes the influence of a number of important factors: the pattern of eye movements used during scrolling is different from that used in text reading, we do not know if comprehension of the text is maintained, and the reading rate is a maximum rather than the habitual rate. Nonetheless it has allowed the influence of field-of-view, letter size and contrast on reading speed to be determined, and Whittaker and Lovie-Kitchin (1993, 1994) offered a clinical interpretation of these data (see also Rumney, 1995).

Visual Requirements for Reading

Whittaker and Lovie-Kitchin (1993) proposed that the final reading rate achieved by the patient will determine what the patient can do with their reading ability: They suggest that to read for leisure or occupation (e.g. paperback novels) one needs 'high fluent' reading at maximum speed (approximately 160 wpm if possible, although 'fluent' reading of at least 80 wpm will be acceptable for some). To 'spot' read (perhaps price tags or cooking instructions) needs only 40 wpm. The latter, described as 'survival' reading by some researchers, may be sufficient for some patients: other patients may just want to read a single page of a familiar novel to send them off to sleep, and thus would not require 'high fluent' reading. Taking the results of experiments which have investigated the change in reading rate with stimulus parameters, Whittaker and Lovie-Kitchin (1993) argue that reading speed is slow when the stimulus is close to threshold but increases as the print size and contrast become progressively suprathreshold. This has led to the concepts of acuity reserve and contrast reserve becoming fundamental considerations in reading rehabilitation. Acuity reserve is the ratio of the size of the print which the individual is able to read comfortably (and so the size that will need to be achieved by magnification), relative to their acuity threshold. The contrast reserve is the contrast of the print which the patient wishes to read, relative to their contrast threshold, to achieve the required reading speed. As might be expected, the size of any central scotoma, and the field-of-view (the number of characters visible at any one time) also influence the reading rate. The optimum stimulus requirements are summarised in Table 3.2.

The importance of contrast reserve means that it is highly desirable to measure CS in any low-vision assessment. Whittaker and Lovie-Kitchin (1993) suggest, for example, that high fluent reading requires the letter contrast of the task to be 10× that of the lowest contrast the patient can detect. Letters in a paperback novel might have a contrast around 70%, so if the patient has a contrast threshold above 7%, they will not be able to read it fluently no matter what magnification system is introduced.

Conveniently, the contrast reserve needs little calculation, and can be determined direct from the PR or Mars tests. Table 3.3 shows the contrast reserve that would be achieved by a patient who could read each row of the Mars chart, assuming that the print they were reading had a contrast of 85%

(which is a reasonable expectation for black-on-white printed text, although an electronic display may be better).

Unfortunately, the contrast of a task cannot be easily manipulated, so if the contrast reserve is too low, the patient's expectations need to be managed, and alternative strategies such as audio-reading may be recommended if appropriate. A patient who read Row 3 or 4 on the Mars chart may benefit by listening to books for their leisure, although they might still perform 'survival' reading of their personal correspondence using an optical magnifier.

Table 3.2 also suggests that patients with a large central scotoma (>4°) will not read quickly, regardless of how much the task is magnified, or how well the patient learns to use an optimum PRL.

The most contentious finding (based on the work of Legge's group) was that a field-of-view of only four characters can support optimal reading speeds when the text is presented in scrolling mode. This is surprising because other studies on both low-vision patients and normally sighted subjects have suggested that more than 20 characters are needed (Rayner, 1983; Lowe & Drasdo, 1990), but the discrepancy may be largely explained by the difference in experimental methods: Beckmann et al. (1993) found that when the subject had to manipulate the text position by hand, reducing the

TABLE 3.2	The Stimulus Requirements to Achieve Different Reading Speeds		
Visual Requirement	**Optimum Reading of Normally Sighted Subject (~300 wpm)**	**Fluent Reading (>80–160 wpm)[a]**	**Spot or Survival Reading (40 wpm)**
Acuity reserve	6:1	2:1 (at least 2.5× and up to 7× for children)	1.3:1
Contrast reserve	30:1	10:1	3:1
Scotoma diameter	0 degrees	4 degrees	30 degrees
Field of view (characters)	4–6	4–6	1

[a]For children, this maximum would be about (10 wpm × (18 - age in years)) less than 160 wpm.
(Based on Lovie-Kitchin et al. [2001], Whittaker & Lovie-Kitchin [1993], Cheong et al. [2002], Lovie-Kitchin [2011]).
wpm, words per minute.

TABLE 3.3	The Contrast of the Letters Presented on Each Row of the Mars Test, With the Contrast Reserve Which the Patient Would Achieve for 85% Contrast Letters, and the Clinical Significance of This			
Row of Chart	**Log CS**	**Contrast Threshold (%)**	**Contrast Reserve**	**Clinical Implications**
1	0.04–0.24	91.2–57.5	0.9:1 to 1.5:1	Survival reading not achievable: consider nonvisual methods
2	0.28–0.48	52.5–33.1	1.6:1 to 2.6:1	
3	0.52–0.72	30.2–19.1	2.8:1 to 4.5:1	Survival reading achievable but not fluent reading
4	0.76–0.96	17.4–11.0	4.9:1 to 7.7:1	
5	1.00–1.20	10.0–6.3	8.5:1 to 13.5:1	Fluent reading achievable, optimise lighting and contrast
6	1.24–1.44	5.8–3.6	14.7:1 to 23.6:1	
7	1.48–1.68	3.3–2.1	25.8:1 to 40.5:1	Normal reading if print size adequate
8	1.72–1.92	1.9–1.2	44.7:1 to 70.8:1	

CS, Contrast sensitivity.

field size slowed reading considerably. This difference then can be attributed to 'page navigation' problems—that is, the difficulty of finding the beginning of the next line.

Considering Table 3.2 in combination with the findings of the clinical assessment of a low-vision patient can give very clear guidance regarding possible management strategies, and likely prognosis.

Reading Acuity

The three most common notations to specify print size are logMAR, Sloan M and N-point systems (Table 3.4), each used on different types of reading test.

The table shows the size of the lower-case letters (x-height) in different notations—the Sloan M-notation, the Point System and logMAR. The lower-case letter size in each case is the overall size in millimetres of a letter which has neither ascending or descending limbs (e.g. o, x, n)—this is often represented by the 'x-height' and this can be different for different fonts that are ostensibly the same 'size'. The comparison to distance acuities must be interpreted cautiously; there are marked differences in the visual tasks of reading single letters compared to reading words, but the comparison here simply relates to the total angular subtense of the component letters. In addition, the letters in reading print are not carefully shaped with a limb width equal to 1/5th of the letter height, so the discrimination task is not so clearly defined as it is when reading distance optotypes. Print contrast, word and line spacing, word length and difficulty could each affect performance as much as letter size.

The *Sloan M System* charts were originally designed to be used at a standard distance of 40 cm. Each letter size bears the notation 'x M' where x = the distance in metres at which the overall height of the lower-case letter subtends 5 min arc. Thus, 1 M print size is approximately equivalent to newsprint. Patient performance could be written as, for example, '2 M at 40 cm', but should more accurately be designated '0.40/2' (viewing distance in metres/print size read) in a way analogous to the Snellen distance acuity notation. The 'M' notation is the standard US terminology for print size, and its use is generally accepted in a wide variety of reading chart designs.

The *point notation* uses printing terminology for the size of letters, 1 point being 1/72 inch. Text which is labelled as 'x-point' was set on printing blocks x/72 inches high: this is therefore the distance from the top of an ascending limb to the bottom of a descending limb. The typeface used (Times Roman) in charts produced in the UK has been standardised and text is therefore labelled as 'Nx': N to indicate 'near vision standard test' followed by the number which indicates the point size of the print. This is the most common system in use in the UK, and is employed in a variety of different charts, the most common of which is the *Faculty of Ophthalmologists* booklet which consists of meaningful paragraphs of print.

As part of a low-vision assessment, it may be necessary to calculate, for example, the acuity required by a patient to read a sample of computer print-out. In such a case, the height of a lower-case letter on the sample can be measured: looking this up in the table then allows an acuity standard to be assigned for this.

Reading Tests

There are many different word reading charts available, and they differ in both the format of the test and the notation used to specify print size: the range of word lengths used often varies, and some use meaningful sentences and paragraphs whilst others employ unrelated words. Radner (2019) has emphasized the importance of standardization of charts to allow meaningful results to be reported, particularly in clinical trials. Choosing a test within the clinical context may be different from those for research purposes. It is important to have variations of word length when testing patients with macular problems, because they usually read short words accurately but cannot manage long words, or read only part of them. The use of meaningful paragraphs of print means that the patient's performance may be aided by astute guesswork as they attempt to fill in letters or words they cannot see by interpreting the likely meaning of the sentence. If assessing reading speed, a longer text (several sentences) may be required to reduce the effect of a brief but unrepresentative period of fast or slow reading. For example, a patient may have had a very long hesitation over just one word, and this is more likely with meaningful text as the patient suddenly realises it does not make sense and goes back (even if instructed not to!) to try to identify their mistake. A longer paragraph is more representative of everyday leisure reading, and may help to judge whether reading performance can be sustained. If a test is to be used repeatedly, different but equivalent versions are required, so the text cannot be remembered by the reader. In summary, the characteristics of the tests available should be matched to the requirements of the situation, bearing in mind the time constraints of the clinical assessment, and the stamina of the patient!

Some tests, including the Radner and MNREAD charts, are available in multiple languages. Comparing reading rates in different languages is not straightforward, due to differences in word length, information density and alphabet type. Some authors suggest using syllables-per-minute as a way to compare reading speed across languages, but more research is needed in this area. There are several tests which have been designed specifically for the assessment of low-vision patients. The most commonly used are probably the Bailey-Lovie word reading chart, the MNREAD test and the Radner charts.

The original Bailey-Lovie Word-Reading Chart (which is no longer produced) (Bailey & Lovie, 1980) had letters of sizes logMAR 1.6 to 0.0 (6/240 to 6/6 equivalent) at 25 cm in steps of approximately 0.1 log units: this translates in point notation to sizes of 80 point to 2 point (or 10 M to 0.25 M). There were between two and six unrelated words per line depending on the letter size, and word lengths between 4 and 10 letters were used. A weakness of the chart design was the limited number of words at large sizes, which makes reading speed hard to calculate. The current Bailey-Lovie Word Reading Chart has 10 words at each size, arranged over two lines, but the maximum size is now

TABLE 3.4   The Interrelationship of Reading Acuity Notations

Letter Size (x-height) (mm)	Sloan M-Notation	Point System	Equivalent logMAR VA for Letters Viewed at 40 cm	Approximate Snellen VA for Letters Viewed at 40 cm	Equivalent logMAR VA for Letters Viewed at 25 cm	Approximate Snellen VA for Letters Viewed at 25 cm
0.36	0.25	2	−0.21		0.00	6/6
0.45	0.32	2.6	−0.11		0.09	
0.55	0.4	3.2	−0.02	6/6	0.18	
0.71	0.5	4	0.09		0.29	6/12
0.83	0.6	4.8	0.15		0.36	
0.89	0.63	5	0.18	6/9	0.39	6/15
1.06	0.75	6	0.26		0.46	
1.1	0.8	6.4	0.28		0.48	6/18
1.4 newsprint	1	8	0.38		0.59	6/24
1.6	1.1	9	0.44		0.64	
1.75	1.25	10	0.48	6/18	0.68	
2.15	1.5	12	0.57		0.77	6/36
2.5	1.75	14	0.63		0.84	
2.7	1.9	15.4	0.67		0.87	
2.8	2	16	0.68	6/30	0.89	
3.2	2.3	18	0.74		0.94	
3.4	2.4	19.3	0.77		0.97	
3.5	2.5	20	0.78	6/36	0.98	6/60
4.2	3	24	0.86		1.06	
5.3	3.8	30	0.96		1.16	
5.6	4	32	0.98	6/60	1.19	
6.4	4.5	36	1.04		1.25	
6.6	4.7	37.5	1.05		1.26	
7.1	5	40	1.09		1.29	6/120
8.3	5.9	47	1.15	6/85	1.36	
8.5	6	48	1.16		1.37	6/150
9.7	7	56	1.22		1.43	
10.3	7.3	58.4	1.25		1.45	
11.1	8	64	1.28	6/120	1.48	
12.5	9	72	1.33		1.54	
12.9	9.1	73	1.35		1.55	
13.9	10	80	1.38	6/144	1.58	6/240
16.1	11.5	92	1.44		1.65	
20.2	14.5	116	1.54	6/208	1.74	6/350
25.2	18	143	1.64		1.84	

MAR, Minimum angle of resolution; *VA*, visual acuity.

44 point (Fig. 3.12A). There is also a version which uses sentences rather than unrelated words.

The most well-known reading chart for people with low vision is the MNREAD (https://legge.psych.umn.edu/mnread-acuity-charts) (available and validated in several languages), which consists of a meaningful (but unrelated) sentence at each size from logMAR 1.3 to −0.5 at 40 cm in steps of 0.1 log units (Fig. 3.12B). This equates to 8 M to 0.13 M, or 64 point to 1 point. The sentences are arranged over two sides of a large card printed in black on white (although white on black versions are

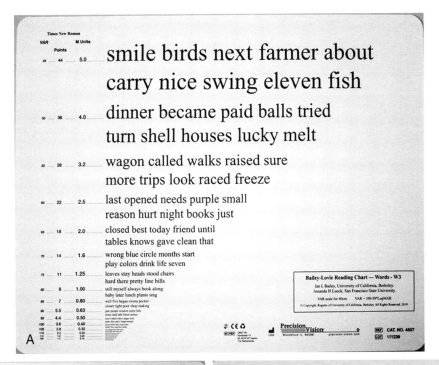

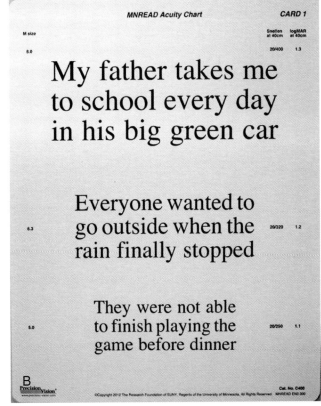

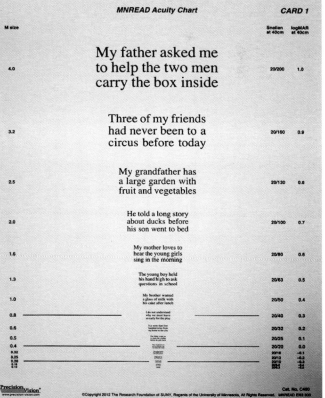

Fig. 3.12 (A) A Bailey-Lovie Word Reading Chart and (B) an MNREAD chart (two-sided).

available) with 85% contrast. Each sentence is arranged over three justified lines, is of equal linguistic complexity, contains 60 characters, and is scored as if it is made up of 10 six-letter words. There is a recommended protocol for how the test should be used. The chart should be placed at a 40 cm viewing distance, with the reader wearing an appropriate reading aid, and the sentences covered. Each sentence is revealed in turn, starting with the largest print: a stopwatch is started as the cover is removed, and stopped when the individual stops reading. The reader is asked to read as quickly and accurately as

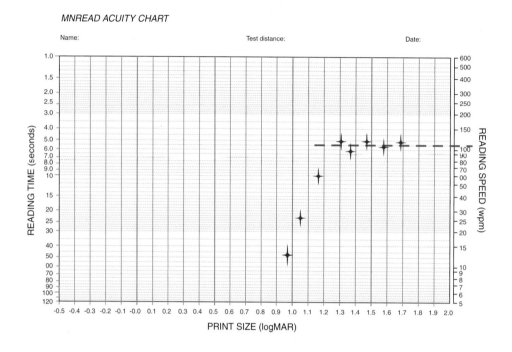

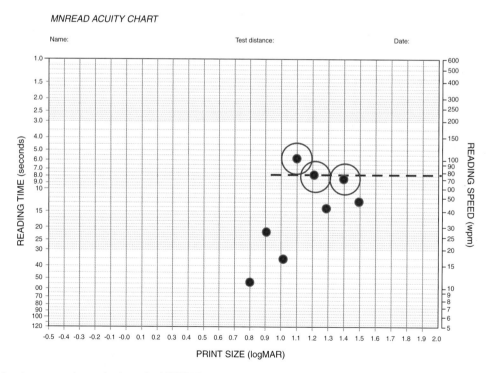

Fig. 3.13 The graphs show example results from the MNREAD test for two different patients: the **x**-axis shows print size (larger to the right) and the two **y**-axes show reading time and reading speed. (*Top*) The expected pattern with a horizontal line through the highest speeds to determine the maximum reading speed (MRS: 110 wpm) and critical print size (CPS: logMAR 1.3). (*Bottom*) An example of more variable results as seen in some low-vision patients. The MRS is determined as the average of the three fastest speeds (circled: 83 wpm) and the horizontal dashed line is drawn at 90% of MRS (75 wpm) to allow CPS to be determined (logMAR 1.1). *MAR*, Minimum angle of resolution, *wpm*, words per minute.

possible, and just to continue if they make a mistake. A two-sided score sheet is provided. One side contains a record of the sentences for the observer to mark off any words which were read incorrectly or missed: this is also where the duration of reading each sentence is recorded. The reader should be encouraged to attempt each sentence until the print is too small to allow them to read any words correctly. In practice it is often easier to audio record the patient reading the chart and to then score it retrospectively.

The measurement of threshold print size (TPS: the smallest size which can be read) is obtained by the formula:

$$TPS = 1.4 - (number\ of\ sentences\ read \times 0.1)$$
$$+ (number\ of\ words\ incorrect \times 0.01)$$

When counting the 'number of sentences read' any sentences where 10 or more words were missed/incorrect should be ignored and not included in the scoring (of either words or sentences).

The results are also plotted on the graph on the opposite side of the score sheet, which shows the reading time for each sentence on the y-axis, and the print size on the x-axis.

Reading speed is given on the opposite y-axis of the graph but is calculated as:

$$Reading\ speed = \frac{(10 - words\ missed)*60}{time\ taken\ in\ seconds}$$

In normally sighted readers, the points on the graph form a characteristic pattern (Fig. 3.13, top).

This plot allows the calculation of two more important parameters: the maximum reading speed (MRS) and the critical print size (CPS), which is the smallest print size which can be read at the MRS. To obtain the MRS, a horizontal line of best fit is drawn through the points representing the fastest speeds, and the value can be read off the y-axis. In the clinical context, the print size corresponding to the final point on this line can be read off the x-axis. This is the CPS. In readers with VI, the results can sometimes be difficult to interpret, because the plot does not fit the standard pattern. In these cases a reasonable approximation is to calculate the MRS to be the mean of the three fastest speeds obtained, and for the CPS to be the smallest print size allowing a reading speed of at least 90% of MRS (see Fig. 3.13 for an example), although other algorithms are possible (Patel et al., 2011).

Actually conducting the MNREAD test accurately (revealing the sentences, recording mistakes, handling a stopwatch, plotting the graph) is quite challenging, so various digital versions to automate some of the processes are available. App versions of MNREAD are available, with timing registered by operator taps on the screen, and errors entered manually (Calabrèse et al., 2018). This test is quick and easy to use, the display can be simply changed to reversed contrast, and it can be performed in multiple languages. Digital versions of various reading charts have been combined with automatic recognition of both the speaking duration of the reader (Labiris et al., 2020),

and the viewing distance of the reader (Hirnschall, Motaabbed, & Dexl, 2014)

It is worth pointing out that MNREAD acuity values are expressed in logMAR units, based on a viewing distance of 40 cm. When considering print size with magnification, these are not useful concepts. It is better to think of print sizes in terms of the physical size of the printed letters that the individual is able to access, and for this to be considered independent of the viewing distance required. The use of the three discreet parameters derived from the MNREAD has been considered both too complex, and yet still providing insufficient information. Calabrèse et al. (2016) introduced the concept of the Reading Accessibility Index, which is abbreviated to ACC, to capture more complete reading performance information in a single index. This aims to use a single value to express reading speed across the range of print sizes encountered in everyday life.

$$ACC = \frac{mean\ RS\ across\ the\ 10\ print\ sizes\ from\ 1M\ to\ 8M}{200}$$

Dividing by 200 normalizes the reading speed relative to young normally sighted individuals, so 'normal' performance would be expected to be an ACC = 1.0. Any of the print sizes which cannot be read at all will contribute RS = 0 to the mean.

The Radner Reading chart, firstly designed and validated in a German version (Stifter et al., 2004), and subsequently available in several languages, is similar in purpose to the MNREAD, and is able to test the same parameters. However, the way the sentences are constructed (they are always 14 words long), laid out, and selected (Radner & Diendorfer, 2014) is different.

As will be seen from the previous discussion, most reading tests concentrate on single sentences, and the testing of extended paragraphs is rare in a clinical setting. An exception is the IReST which uses paragraphs of meaningful text which are approximately 132 words in length (Trauzettel-Klosinski & Dietz, 2012). Unfortunately it is only available in a single print size (10 point, to equate to newsprint) so many low-vision readers cannot attempt the task at all (even with a magnifier).

Even with the wide range of tests available, there are still aspects of reading performance which are not routinely tested. The accuracy of reading (the percentage of words correct) will be extremely important if everyday tasks are to be accomplished effectively, and the reader is not to become frustrated. Surprisingly, this is rarely measured directly, and incorrect words just lead to a reduction in the calculated reading speed (because fewer correct words are read per minute). Another important factor for leisure reading is the duration of reading which is possible. This is too time-consuming to measure routinely and is best evaluated using a questionnaire such as the Manchester Low Vision Questionnaire (MLVQ) (Harper et al., 1999).

The Pepper Visual Skills for Reading Test (VSRT) (Baldasare et al., 1986; https://www.lowvisionsimulators.com/) was designed to test the performance of patients with macular scotomas in terms of both reading speed and the text presentation which caused them difficulty. It can also be used to investigate the reading difficulties of patients with homonymous hemianopia which is close to fixation (Blaylock, et al., 2016). The test is available in three versions, and in print sizes 1 M to 4 M (8 point to 32 point) with each page having print of a single size. Within the page there are 41 single letters and 69 words arranged over 13 lines of print, beginning with single letters, then on successive lines progressing to two- and three-letter and finally larger unrelated words (Fig. 3.14).

The spacing between the words and the lines also progressively decreases. The Pepper VSRT is not designed to measure the threshold acuity, but rather to determine reading speed as a measure of reading performance. It is suggested that the test is administered in a print which is the next larger size than the patient's threshold, and the result would then form a baseline value before the patient is, for example, trained to use their magnifier more effectively. The layout of the test is designed to create specific mistakes, through which the practitioner can identify how the patient might be trained to overcome these. For example, the lines becoming closer together will test the ability of the reader to make efficient return sweep eye movements from the end of one line to the beginning of the next; words which can still be read with either the beginning or the end missing will show whether the patient is fixating in the best location relative to a central scotoma. An alternative test with a similar rationale is SK Read (MacKeben et al., 2015) which has blocks of text of decreasing size (8 M to 0.4 M), and a variety of word lengths (unrelated) from one letter to six letters within each block.

A more meaningful test in terms of the true goal of reading might be to measure comprehension of the material: can the reader actually extract the correct meaning from the text. This must be as significant for the low-vision patient as for any other reader. Watson et al. (1992) tested the comprehension of low-vision patients who had previously been good readers, but now had macular loss and were using a magnifier which allowed them to read small print. Some individuals had very low comprehension for the material, demonstrating that just because reading speed is restored, comprehension may not follow. Nonetheless, some patients had very good comprehension, indicating that central vision loss and use of a magnifier do not preclude 'good' reading. These wide variations in the comprehension level of readers shows, however, that it does not correlate directly with reading speed or acuity. The Morgan Low Vision Reading Comprehension Assessment (https://www.lowvisionsimulators.com/products/morgan-reading-assessment-lvrca) is a test which uses the cloze procedure: comprehension of the text is assessed by the ability of the reader to fill in the missing word in each of a series of meaningful sentences. It is available in different print sizes (9 point to 24 point; 1 M to 3 M) to match the reading acuity and likely reading tasks of the patient.

VISUAL PERFORMANCE MEASUREMENT IN CHILDREN WITH VISUAL IMPAIRMENT

There are many tests for children's vision which can be used in the low-vision clinic (Saunders, 2010).

To measure VA of people who cannot name letters, there are three major types of test which can be used (McDonald, 1986). The simplest test is *detection acuity* which determines the ability to detect the presence of a stimulus against a background: this is usually in the form of a small black or white ball against a contrasting background and can be used from about 6 months of age. The examiner must judge the smallest target size which reliably elicits a reaction (typically a fixation or

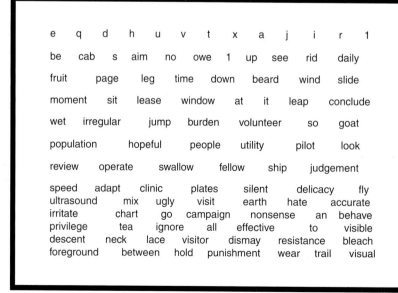

Fig. 3.14 A reading test in the format of the Pepper Visual Skills for Reading Test (VSRT) (Baldasare et al., 1986).

pursuit eye movement) from the child. Such tests are difficult to quantify but can be useful to also test the ability to localize and reach out to pick up the objects which have been seen: this ability is often impaired in cerebral visual impairment.

Resolution acuity is measured by the ability to discriminate a black-and-white striped grating from a homogeneous grey field with the same average luminance. In the form of a Preferential Looking (PL) test this can be used between birth and 1 year of age, and a resolution limit can be determined as the child will prefer to fixate the grating target which can be resolved rather than the homogeneous grey field. These two targets are presented simultaneously in front of the child and the observer watches the child's eyes to judge to which target an eye movement is made. In the clinical setting, the Teller or Keeler cards use the same strategy, with the grating and blank-field targets adjacent on a large card, which has a small observation hole in the centre (Teller et al., 1986). The observer holds up the card in front of the child and watches the eye movements of the child through the peep-hole as the target is presented. Resolution threshold is set at the spatial frequency to which the observer judges the child to be correctly responding consistently. An indirect measurement of resolution acuity can also be obtained by observing the optokinetic nystagmus which is induced by a moving grating. If the grating cannot be resolved, then the eye movement is not elicited.

From 1 year of age, it can be difficult to gain the child's cooperation for a PL procedure, as they easily become bored. It may however be possible to modify this to an operant PL procedure, where the child is encouraged to turn towards the displayed grating. If they respond correctly, they receive a reward in the form of the display of a moving musical toy (Mayer & Dobson, 1982). Woodhouse et al. (1992) adopted a different strategy in the Cardiff Acuity Test in which they attempt to make the stimulus more interesting than a grating. The test cards have a familiar outline shape (such as a fish, dog or house) in the upper or lower part of an otherwise uniform grey card. The outline is created by a white band, flanked on either side by black bands which are one-half the thickness of the white band: the angular subtense of the white band defines the resolution limit. If the target is beyond the child's resolution limit it becomes invisible, vanishing into the background. The clinician presents the card to the child and watches the direction of the eye movement response: although not required as part of the procedure, asking the child to name and point at the object can increase cooperation.

Recognition acuity is the third possibility, and the most perceptually demanding task. It requires the child to be able to recognise (and often name) a letter or picture from amongst a competing group of stimuli on the display. Reading a letter chart is an example of such a task. Attempts to test VA at the earliest age begin using picture or symbol tests, which the child can be asked to name, or to match by pointing to the same symbol on a hand-held card: the range of possible tests is reviewed by Saunders (2010). The Kay, LEA and Auckland tests use symbols and objects rather than letters, where the

optotypes are constructed using the same principles of angular subtense as are employed in the letter chart (Kay, 1983). Recognition of the importance of using crowded targets has led to children's vision tests being produced with the letters surrounded by contours (e.g. the Glasgow acuity cards [McGraw & Winn, 1995]). A low-contrast acuity test for children is available which uses the LEA symbols, and contrast levels ranging from 25% down to 1.25%, which would allow the difference between high and low contrast acuity to be used to assess the slope of the CSF.

No matter how cooperative a child is, it is impossible to use recognition tasks at earlier than 20 to 24 months: the necessary naming or matching skills are not present. From the age of 3 years, an attempt should be made to use letters in order to increase the reliability of measurements. The traditional letter-matching test for children was the Sheridan-Gardner Test which uses single-letter targets: this is now largely discredited for use in routine practice because of the absence of contour interaction. However, single letters can be useful in some cases to assess the vision of visually impaired children and adults, some of whom can perform very poorly with multiple targets.

By the age of 4, it is probable that a conventional linear letter chart can be used, and it is certainly recommended that registration status should be determined in this way: prior to this age it is suggested that children are certified as sight impaired rather than severely sight impaired, unless they obviously have no perception of light. The advantages of using a chart of Bailey-Lovie/ETDRS design rather than Snellen have already been discussed. In the youngest age group, the subjective response to the letters can be by matching, although it may be difficult to persuade a young child to match large numbers of letters. One letter per line may be identified until the approximate threshold is reached, and then the full line presented at that size. Matching may be difficult for a visually impaired child because a field defect may mean that the two symbols cannot be seen simultaneously. The incidence of severe visual impairment amongst adults and older children with learning disabilities is quite high, and a number of these methods of acuity measurement intended for infants can be adapted for these cases.

Although the grating resolution tasks have parallels to the adult CSF, the use of gratings as opposed to letters is simply determined by the type of test with which the child can be expected to cooperate. Gratings are used because they can be incorporated into a technique suitable for the youngest infant: typically, they will only be used at a nominal 100% contrast and thus only the high spatial frequency cut-off of the CSF will be determined.

To measure CS in children, or patients with learning difficulties who cannot respond to letters or numbers, the Hiding Heidi Low Contrast Test can be used (Fig. 3.15) (www.goodlite.com).

The test consists of six schematic faces with contrasts of 100%, 25%, 10%, 5%, 2.5% and 1.25% (approximate equivalent log CS values 0.1, 0.6, 1.0, 1.3, 1.6, 1.9) and a blank card. Normal room lighting is used, and the viewing distance

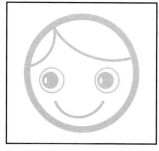 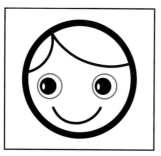

Fig. 3.15 Two example plates from The Hiding Heidi Low Contrast Test.

can be selected to be that which is relevant to the tasks the patient wishes to perform. Two cards are presented to the patient, one of which is the blank card, and the patient is asked to point towards the card with the visible face. The test should start with the 100% contrast card, and progressively decrease, being careful that a lack of response is only occurring when the target is below threshold, rather than because the patient has lost interest. With children, the test can be turned into a game ('Where's Heidi?') to capture their attention. However, Lovie-Kitchin et al. (2001) suggest that children with VI are less likely to have reduced CS than are adults with acquired loss.

The McClure Reading Test Type for Children has letters of different sizes to measure word reading acuity, and this reading material is also graded by difficulty appropriate for those of different ages. The font designed to test the younger children is also a simpler sans serif version, before switching to Times Roman for the older ages. Without such a specific test, it can be difficult to know whether a child is hesitant and slow because of their inability to resolve the print, or because of a difficulty in the reading process itself. Of course, care needs to be taken because 'easier' text tends to contain few long words and so it does not offer the same versatility in testing performance.

In addition to the Panel 16 Colour Vision test mentioned earlier, there are various colour vision tests designed for children that could be used (Tekavčič Pompe, 2020). There are various pseudoisochromatic plate tests which use pictures (Matsubara Color Vision Test) or symbols (Colour Vision Testing Made Easy) for children unable to read letters. However, both these tests only investigate R-G defects. The MRM test (Mollon-Riffin Minimalist test) (Mollon et al., 1991) is based on the D-15 and so does test all three colour axes. In this test, the child is presented with a mixed assortment of five caps in various shades of grey, and one coloured cap, The task is to pick out the coloured cap: this is repeated with coloured caps of decreasing saturation to make the task progressively more difficult. Pfäffli et al. (2020) tested children aged 3 to 10 years, with logMAR VA between 0.1 and 0.7, and found the Ishihara or Matsubara plates, and the MRM test, to be feasible to use in this population. Children with a VI which has an effect on their colour vision can benefit from practical advice regarding its effect on daily activities and their education (Cole, 2007), as can normally sighted children with a congenital CVD.

VISUAL PERCEPTUAL PROBLEMS: INVESTIGATING EXTRASTRIATE PATHWAYS

Clinicians are familiar with the type of visual problems that result from damage to the visual pathway from the retina to the visual cortex (V1), with the particular type of loss (e.g. homonymous quadrantanopia, bitemporal hemianopia) giving a good indication of the site of the lesion. However, signals are transmitted further, on to the extrastriate areas, which are specialised for processing of, for example, colour or motion. It is possible for these pathways to be affected alone, and so VA and visual field are relatively unaffected. There is no associated ocular pathology, and this condition is called cortical or cerebral visual impairment. In adults, the most likely cause of this damage is a stroke, or traumatic brain injury (TBI). In children, it may be due to prenatal (e.g. exposure of mother to drugs or alcohol), perinatal (e.g. oxygen deprivation during birth), or postnatal (e.g. nonaccidental injury) damage. In both age groups, the damage may spread beyond the visual areas, and there will be other neurological issues (e.g. effects on movement, word reading or speech), including effects on binocular vision and eye movements (which should also be carefully investigated). People may be able to read letters and not words, or in some cases be able to identify objects but not pictures of objects. Clinicians should be alert for 'unusual' visual concerns and should consider injury to higher visual areas if these problems are reported. In adult patients, there may also be memory, attention, concentration or fatigue issues. These perceptual problems can also be experienced in patients with Alzheimer disease, particularly in Posterior Cortical Atrophy (Schott & Crutch, 2019).

The two pathways are illustrated in Fig. 3.16, with both their location in the brain, and their functions being shown schematically. The ventral/temporal lobe and dorsal/parietal lobe processing streams are also known respectively as the 'what' and 'where' pathways. Lesions here mean that the individual can 'see' images formed on the retinae, but they cannot interpret those images appropriately. Typical 'where' problems include difficulty in reaching out to pick up or put down an object; inability to distinguish changes in floor level, or steps; or difficulty in interpreting an object amongst multiple other objects (simultagnosia). This latter problem can make it distressing for the individual to be in crowds; or difficult to find an item on a supermarket shelf, or clothes in a wardrobe. It can also cause problems with reading when confronted with a page full of words. Sometimes a typoscope with the slit held vertically can be used to assist by blocking out the excess information. Disruption of the 'what' pathways causes difficulty in recognising objects, words, or faces: the latter is termed prosopagnosia, and can mean the individual has difficulty recognising their own family or recognising where they are (topographical disorientation) (Corrow et al., 2016). It also makes it difficult to watch TV because they cannot recognise the characters and cannot interpret facial expressions.

Neglect (or hemispatial neglect) is also a consequence of a parietal lobe lesion. It is more common in injury to the right parietal lobe, leading to neglect of the left hemi-field. Neglect

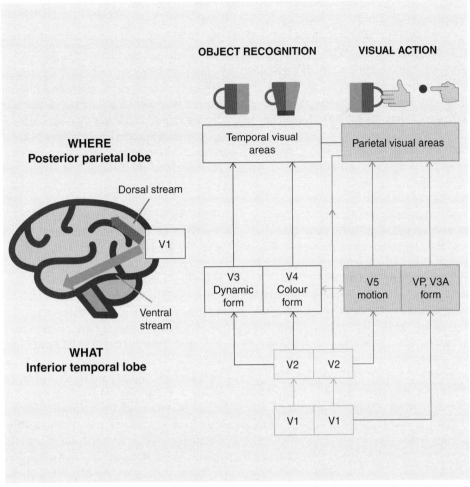

Fig. 3.16 A schematic illustration of the location (*left*) and function (*right*) of the dorsal/parietal and temporal/ventral extrastriate pathways. Images from Freepik at www.flaticon.com.

is a lack of awareness of one half of the visual field: there may also be hemianopia, but this is not always the case: the person 'forgets that this part of the world exists'. If asked to draw the numbers on a circular clock face, the individual may misplace or mis-space them (put them all to one side); they may only shave or apply make-up to one side of their face, or ignore food on one side of the plate.

It should be emphasised that in the context of a low-vision clinic, tests with high diagnostic accuracy are not necessary: the aim is to discover whether there are functional consequences of such a defect. Neglect can be identified as part of the routine low-vision history taking, or by directly asking whether they ignore food on one side of their plate. There are also several simple 'home-made' tests of neglect which could be carried out in practice, adapted from those used formally in neurology clinics (Ferber & Karnath, 2001). In each case, the targets must be large and bold enough to ensure that any acuity or contrast deficit is not affecting performance. The practitioner also needs to be aware if the patient has dexterity problems that may affect the hand movements required for some of the tasks.

Some possible 'visual perception tests' which can be used in the clinic are described in the following paragraphs.

The line bisection test: About 10 horizontal lines of 20 to 30 cm in length are drawn on an A4 sheet of paper, and the patient is asked to make a cross at the midpoint of each line. Any inaccuracies are diagnostic: in hemianopia, the midpoint is drawn towards the defective field, but in neglect it is positioned away from the affected field (Barton & Black, 1998).

The spacing test: An A4 sheet of paper is placed on the table directly in front of the patient, with long edge horizontal, and the patient is not permitted to move it to one side. They are given about 15 to 20 small objects (e.g. buttons or coins) and asked to space these out evenly across the sheet of paper: in the absence of neglect, they should place an equal number to the left and right of the midpoint.

Cancellation tests: A variety of letters and shapes (about 40 to 50 in total, up to 10 of each design) can be printed in random positions across an A4 page, presented in landscape format. Selecting one of the shapes, the patient is asked to locate and cross-out (cancel) each example of this on the page. If they only identify those on one side of the page, this indicates neglect.

Checking for difficulties the patient may experience in locating objects and coordinating movements to them (the functioning of the 'where' pathway) can be performed with similar tests. The cancellation test can be used, but this time the patient would have difficulty locating the required targets across the entire field, rather than only on one side. In fact, even if the target is located, the patient may have difficulty actually knowing how to put the pen onto the paper to cross it out.

An adaptation of the spacing test can also be used. At the start of the test, half of the objects should have already been positioned by the practitioner, evenly spaced across the paper. The patient is given the remaining objects, and asked to place one on top of each of those on the table. A similar test can be carried out with a chess or draughts board, and a selection of the pieces. The patient is asked to place the pieces just on the white spaces down one line of squares.

Subjective questionnaires and objective tests of face discrimination (Logan et al., 2016), have been devised to diagnose cases of prosopagnosia, but both would also show effects in patients with ocular disease (Logan et al., 2020).

Professionals should be aware that individuals with visual perceptual problems may be unaware of the nature of their vision loss, and even if they do have insight, they often find it very difficult to describe exactly what they are experiencing. It can require very careful questioning by the clinician to elicit this important information. It is even more challenging for the clinician when there is a simultaneous loss of VA, visual field and CS as well as the perceptual problems as some of the difficulties described will also be characteristic of visual problems (e.g. recognising faces, missing steps). However, the possibility of visual perceptual problems should be considered in patients with cortical lesions, if the functional difficulties described do not seem adequately explained by the results of clinical visual tests. The therapeutic and rehabilitative options are limited in these cases, but they must be identified so that the patient is not subjected to a frustrating and unsuccessful attempt to use a magnifier: referral to a neurologist is indicated in the first instance.

A PRAGMATIC VIEW OF VISUAL PERFORMANCE TESTING—THE FUNCTIONAL APPROACH

Of the whole range of visual tests discussed, all of which have been used in cases of low vision, which should be performed as part of a low-vision assessment on a given patient? (There are also additional tests described in Chapter 10 relating to performance in different lighting conditions.)

This depends on what information is required, and this may be a useful point to go back and revisit the section "Why Do We Test Visual Performance?" in this chapter. The time available to carry out a low-vision assessment is also limited, and the patient will rapidly become tired by extensive testing of their vision. It must also be remembered that these tests are (usually) describing impairments, whereas the patient is more interested in (overcoming) activity limitations, although one of the goals of rehabilitation is to help the patient understand their eye condition as well as possible.

The basic tests to be performed in the majority of cases will be best-corrected distance VA, near word acuity, and CS, with others added as required. Taking an effective history of the condition, and its effect on the patient's everyday abilities, may allow a number of formal quantitative tests of visual performance to be bypassed: these tests would determine the impairment, but the patient can identify the activity limitation which this causes, and its significance in areas of everyday life (participation restriction). Patients will of course be seen at all stages of the condition, but likely problem areas can be explored and atypical responses noted. The common effects of some ocular pathologies on visual performance (at the stage when the patient is likely to be requiring the help of a low-vision clinic) are listed in Table 3.5. These are given in terms of the impairment—the performance on a particular psychophysical test of vision—and the possible activity limitation—how it affects the patient performing activities in everyday life. Using a vision-related quality of life questionnaire may be one way to tackle this (see Chapter 4). However, in a clinical context, it can also be assessed by using precisely targeted questions to the patient, or carefully exploring and interpreting their complaints. For example, age-related macular degeneration (AMD) causes central scotomas which obscure some parts of an image, so the patient could be asked whether they notice missing letters in words, or sometimes read a sequence of numbers incorrectly; diffuse media opacities cause light scatter and reduction of contrast, so when the patient with cataract complains of difficulty in seeing at night, questioning reveals that this is in fact due to the presence of street-lights and car head-lights causing glare, rather than a true difficulty in low-light conditions. Cataract would only be expected to cause problems with dark adaptation when it became very dense and markedly reduced the amount of light transmitted to the retina. If necessary, a clinical test could be used to confirm the problem: in the first example this might be microperimetry, whilst in the second case, CS might be measured. These measurements do, however, only confirm what the patient has already described, although they may be useful in quantifying performance before and after the use of some intervention, or over a period of time. A knowledge of a particular disease allows the likely impairments caused by the condition to be anticipated, and this helps in targeting questions about activity limitations. For example, knowing the likely progression of retinitis pigmentosa (RP) suggests questions (at various stages) about travelling at night, with general mobility, with bright light, and eventually with reading long words. Although all patients are different, if the disease follows an unexpected pattern (e.g. sudden monocular vision loss is reported in RP) this raises the possibility of misdiagnosis or the presence of a second disease. More rigorous quantitative tests might be helpful in such cases, or in cases where subjective reports are inconsistent or contradictory.

The subjective nature of vision will cause each patient to experience different phenomena, even amongst individuals with the same pathology. Of course, there will be exceptions, and it is impossible to be too dogmatic: each patient also

TABLE 3.5 A Simplified Summary of Visual Impairments and Activity Limitations Which Are Likely to Result From Common Ocular Pathologies

Impairment	Activity Limitation	DISORDER					
Visual Performance Measure	Likely Functional Difficulty/ Patient Presentation	AMD	Diabetic Eye Disease	Cataract/ Diffuse Media Opacity	Glaucoma	RP	Corneal Scarring/ Irregularity/ Keratoconus
High-contrast VA	Seeing fine detail, reading small print; reading TV subtitles or bus numbers	Moderate loss, better if recorded with single letters	Moderate loss, may be better for single letters	Mild loss	Good in early stages	Good in early stages	Severe loss
Peripheral field	Bumping into people and obstacles, unable to orient/ navigate in unfamiliar environment, poor night vision	Unaffected	Mild effect if panretinal photocoagulation (greater if binocular)	Slight peripheral contraction	Severe peripheral loss if advanced	Marked peripheral loss	No effect
Central field	Recognising faces; seeing print even of large size; missing letters or number	Central distortion and metamorphopsia, progressing to loss	Patchy loss and distortion	No defect	No defect	Mid-peripheral field loss gradually encroaching into centre	Some distortion
Contrast sensitivity	Detecting obstacles, steps, low contrast objects reading coloured print on coloured backgrounds	Mild loss if scotoma not extensive, progressing to moderate/ severe loss	Moderate loss if maculopathy	Marked loss	Moderate loss if advanced	Severe loss	Marked loss
Effect of glare	See better (or be more comfortable) on cloudy day rather than bright and sunny	Moderate effect on vision, severe discomfort	Marked discomfort and visual effect if maculopathy	Severe effect on vision, mild/ moderate discomfort	Mild effect	Moderate effect on vision, severe discomfort	Moderate visual effect
Colour vision	Discriminating colours with similar luminance (especially low), e.g. navy blue and black	Poor due to loss of foveal cones	Early blue defect— patient subjectively unaware	Overall fading of colours/ loss of discrimination	Early blue defect— patient subjectively unaware	Early blue defect— patient subjectively unaware	Normal
Night vision/dark adaptation	Navigating after dark	Delayed dark adaptation in early stages, but patient may not be aware	Usually good unless extensive binocular panretinal photocoagulation	Good until dense cataract; glare and dazzle may be more severe than in daylight	Poor when peripheral field lost	Very poor	Normal
Progression	Deciding which eye is better; or which spectacles are most effective	Slow if 'dry' type, very fast if 'wet'	Phases of fast deterioration alternate with stable periods	Slow	Fast if not controlled	Slow	Usually slow, depending on pathology
Binocular or monocular	Worry about second eye following the course of very poor first eye	Initially monocular, marked binocular risk	Initially monocular, but binocular risk	Usually binocular, but one eye more severely affected	Usually binocular, because patient unaware until both eyes affected	Binocular, highly symmetrical	Depends on cause

AMD, Age-related macular degeneration; *RP*, retinitis pigmentosa; *VA*, visual acuity.

reacts differently to the impairments created by the pathology. Vision simulation spectacles (or smartphone apps), with lenses designed to create fogging, blurring or missing areas within the visual field, are often used, particularly in visual awareness training, to try to gain some insight. The information gathered from the assessment of visual performance and function will begin the process of suggesting ways to prevent the impairment from causing activity limitation and participation restriction in that particular patient's life.

REFERENCES

Achard, O. A., Safran, A. B., Duret, F. C., et al. (1995). Role of the completion phenomenon in the evaluation of Amsler grid results. *American Journal of Ophthalmology, 120*(3), 322–329. https://doi.org/10.1016/S0002-9394(14)72162-2.

Achiron, L. R., Witkin, N. S., McCarey, B. E., et al. (1994). An illuminated high contrast grid for assessing visual function in low vision patients. *Investigative Ophthalmology & Visual Science, 35*, 1953.

Allen, P. M., Ravensbergen, R. H. J. C., Latham, K., et al. (2018). Contrast sensitivity is a significant predictor of performance in rifle shooting for athletes with vision impairment. *Frontiers in Psychology, 9*, 1–10. https://doi.org/10.3389/fpsyg.2018.00950.

Arden, G. B. (1978). The importance of measuring contrast sensitivity in cases of visual disturbance. *British Journal of Ophthalmology, 62*, 198–209.

Arden, G. B. (1983). Recent developments in clinical contrast sensitivity testing. In G. M. Breinin & I. Siegel (Eds.), *Advances in diagnostic visual optics*. Springer.

Arditi, A. (2005). Improving the design of the Letter Contrast Sensitivity Test. *Investigative Ophthalmology & Visual Science, 46*(6), 2225–2229. https://doi.org/10.1167/iovs.04-1198.

Aslam, T., Mahmood, S., Balaskas, K., et al. (2014). Repeatability of visual function measures in age-related macular degeneration. *Graefe's Archive for Clinical and Experimental Ophthalmology, 252*(2), 201–206. https://doi.org/10.1007/s00417-013-2421-5.

Augustin, A. J., Offermann, I., Lutz, J., et al.(2005). Comparison of the original Amsler grid with the modified Amsler grid: Result for patients with age-related macular degeneration. *Retina, 25*(4), 443–445. https://doi.org/10.1097/00006982-200506000-00008.

Bailey, I. L. (1978). Visual acuity measurement in low vision. *Optometric Monthly, 69*, 116–122.

Bailey, I. L. (1993). New procedures for detecting early vision losses in the elderly. *Optometry and Vision Science, 70*, 299–305.

Bailey, I. L., Jackson, A. J., Minto, H., et al. (2012). The Berkeley Rudimentary Vision Test. *Optometry and Vision Science, 89*(9), 1257–1264. https://doi.org/10.1097/OPX.0b013e318264e85a.

Bailey, I. L., & Lovie, J. E. (1980). The design and use of a new near-vision chart. *American Journal of Optometry and Physiological Optics, 57*, 378–387.

Bailey, I. L., & Lovie-Kitchin, J. E. (1976). New design principles for visual acuity letter charts. *American Journal of Optometry and Physiological Optics, 53*, 740–745.

Baldasare, J., Watson, G. R., Whittaker, S. G., et al. (1986). The development of a reading test for low vision individuals with macular loss. *Journal of Visual Impairment and Blindness, 80*, 785–789.

Barton, J. J. S., & Black, S. E. (1998). Line bisection in hemianopia. *Journal of Neurology Neurosurgery and Psychiatry, 64*(5), 660–662. https://doi.org/10.1136/jnnp.64.5.660.

Beckmann, P. J., Legge, G. E., & Rentschler, C. A. (1993). The page-navigation problem in low-vision reading. *Investigative Ophthalmology & Visual Science, 34*, 789.

Bellmann, C., Feely, M., Crossland, M., et al. (2004). Fixation stability using central and pericentral fixation targets in patients with age-related macular degeneration. *Ophthalmology, 111*(12), 2265–2270. https://doi.org/10.1016/j.ophtha.2004.06.019.

Bland, J. M., & Altman, D. G. (2010). Statistical methods for assessing agreement between two methods of clinical measurement. *International Journal of Nursing Studies, 47*(8), 931–936. https://doi.org/10.1016/j.ijnurstu.2009.10.001.

Blaylock, S. E., Warren, M., Yuen, H. K., et al. (2016). Validation of a reading assessment for persons with homonymous hemianopia or quadrantanopia. *Archives of Physical Medicine and Rehabilitation, 97*(9), 1515–1519. https://doi.org/10.1016/j.apmr.2016.02.022.

Bodis-Wollner, I., & Comisa, J. M. (1980). Contrast sensitivity measurements in clinical diagnosis. In S. Lessell & J. T. W. van Dalen (Eds.), *Neuro-ophthalmology* (Vol. 1). Excerpta Medica.

British Standards Institution (BSI). (2018). *BS EN ISO 8596 : Ophthalmic optics—Visual acuity testing—Standard and clinical optotypes and their presentation* (p. 2017). BSI Standards Publication. ISO 8596.

Calabrèse, A., et al. (2018). Comparing performance on the MNREAD iPad application with the MNREAD acuity chart. *Journal of Vision, 18*(1), 1–11. https://doi.org/10.1167/18.1.8.

Calabrèse, A., Owsley, C., McGwin, G., et al. (2016). Development of a reading accessibility index using the MNREAD acuity chart. *JAMA Ophthalmology, 134*(4), 398–405. https://doi.org/10.1001/jamaophthalmol.2015.6097.

Camparini, M., Cassinari, P., Ferrigno, L., et al. (2001). ETDRS-fast: Implementing psychophysical adaptive methods to standardized visual acuity measurement with ETDRS charts. *Investigative Ophthalmology & Visual Science, 42*(6), 1226–1231.

Chang, M. A., Airiani, S., Miele, D., et al. (2006). A comparison of the potential acuity meter (PAM) and the illuminated near card (INC) in patients undergoing phacoemulsification. *Eye, 20*(12), 1345–1351. https://doi.org/10.1038/sj.eye.6702106.

Cheong, A. M. Y., Lovie-Kitchin, J. E., & Bowers, A. R. (2002). Determining magnification for reading with low vision. *Clinical and Experimental Optometry, 85*(4), 229–237.

Cole, B. L. (2007). Assessment of inherited colour vision defects in clinical practice. *Clinical and Experimental Optometry, 90*(3), 157–175. https://doi.org/10.1111/j.1444-0938.2007.00135.x.

Cole, R. J. (2008). Modifications to the Fletcher Central Field Test for patients with low vision. *Journal of Visual Impairment and Blindness, 102*(10), 659. https://doi.org/10.1177/0145482x0810201011.

Colenbrander, A., & Fletcher, D. C. (2005). The mixed contrast reading card, a new screening test for contrast sensitivity. *International Congress Series, 1282*, 492–497. https://doi.org/10.1016/j.ics.2005.05.212.

Corrow, J. C., Corrow, S. L., Lee, E., et al. (2016). Getting lost: topographic skills in acquired and developmental prosopagnosia. *Cortex, 76*, 89–103. https://doi.org/10.1016/j.cortex.2016.01.003.

Crossland, M. D., et al. (2005). Preferred retinal locus development in patients with macular disease. *Ophthalmology, 112*(9), 1579–1585. https://doi.org/10.1016/j.ophtha.2005.03.027.

Crossland, M., Jackson, M.-L., & Seiple, W. H. (2012). Microperimetry: a review of fundus related perimetry. *Optometry Reports, 2*(1), 2. https://doi.org/10.4081/optometry.2012.e2.

Dickinson, C. M., & Taylor, J. (2011). The effect of simulated visual impairment on speech-reading ability. *Ophthalmic and*

Physiological Optics, *31*(3), 249–257. https://doi.org/10.1111/j.1475-1313.2010.00810.x.

Dorr, M., Lesmes, L., Lu, Z-L., et al. (2013). Rapid and reliable assessment of the contrast sensitivity function on an iPad. *Investigative Ophthalmology & Visual Science*, *54*(12), 7266–7273. https://doi.org/10.1167/iovs.13-11743.

Elliott, D. B. (2016). The good (logMAR), the bad (Snellen) and the ugly (BCVA, number of letters read) of visual acuity measurement. *Ophthalmic and Physiological Optics*, *36*(4), 355–358. https://doi.org/10.1111/opo.12310.

Elliott, D. B., Yang, K. C. H., & Whitaker, D. (1995). Visual acuity changes throughout adulthood in normal healthy eyes: Seeing beyond 6/6. *Optometry and Vision Science*, *72*, 186–191.

Erber, N. P., & Osborn, R. R. (1994). Perception of facial cues by adults with low vision. *Journal of Visual Impairment & Blindness*, *88*, 171–175.

Eperjesi, F. (2010). *Qualitative visual field analysis opticianonline.net.* Retrieved July 30, 2022, from https://www2.aston.ac.uk/migrated-assets/applicationpdf/lhs/62105-Aston%20Perimetry%20Tool%20Optician%20Article.pdf.

Estevez, O., & Cavonius, C. R. (1976). Low-frequency attenuation in the detection of gratings: sorting out the artefacts. *Vision Research*, *16*, 497–500.

Faulkner, W. (1983). Laser interferometric prediction of postoperative visual acuity in patients with cataracts. *American Journal of Ophthalmology*, *95*, 626–636.

Ferber, S., & Karnath, H. O. (2001). How to assess spatial neglect—Line bisection or cancellation tasks? *Journal of Clinical and Experimental Neuropsychology*, *23*(5), 599–607. https://doi.org/10.1076/jcen.23.5.599.1243.

Ferris, F. L., Kassoff, A., Bresnick, G. H., et al. (1982). New visual acuity charts for clinical research. *American Journal of Ophthalmology*, *94*, 91–96.

Flom, M. C., Heath, G., & Takahaski, E. (1963). Contour interaction and visual resolution: contralateral effects. *Science*, *142*, 979–980.

Ginsburg, A. P. (1984). A new contrast sensitivity vision test. *American Journal of Optometry and Physiological Optics*, *61*, 403–407.

Green, D. G. (1970). Testing the vision of cataract patients by means of laser-generated interference fringes. *Science*, *168*, 1240–1242.

Grey, C. P., & Yap, M. (1987). Edge contrast sensitivity in optometric practice: an assessment of its efficacy in detecting visual dysfunction. *American Journal of Optometry and Physiological Optics*, *64*, 925–928.

Harper, R., Doorduyn, K., Reeves, B., et al. (1999). Evaluating the outcomes of low vision rehabilitation. *Ophthalmic and Physiological Optics*, *19*(1), 3–11. https://doi.org/10.1046/j.1475-1313.1999.00411.x.

Harris, M. J., Robins, D., Dieter, J. M., et al. (1985). Eccentric visual acuity in patients with macular disease. *Ophthalmology*, *92*, 1550–1553.

Hess, R. F. (1987). New and improved contrast sensitivity approaches to low vision. In G. C. Woo (Ed.), *Low vision principles and applications* (pp. 1–16). Springer-Verlag.

Hirnschall, N., Motaabbed, J. K., Dexl, A., et al. (2014). Evaluation of an electronic reading desk to measure reading acuity in pseudophakic patients. *Journal of Cataract and Refractive Surgery*, *40*(9), 1462–1468. https://doi.org/10.1016/j.jcrs.2013.12.021.

Ho, A., & Bilton, S. M. (1986). Low contrast charts effectively differentiate between types of blur. *American Journal of Optometry and Physiological Optics*, *63*, 202–208.

Hofeldt, A. J., & Weiss, M. J. (1998). Illuminated near card assessment of potential acuity in eyes with cataract.

Ophthalmology, *105*(8), 1531–1536. https://doi.org/10.1016/S0161-6420(98)98042-3.

Howell, E. R., & Hess, R. F. (1978). The functional area for summation to threshold for sinusoidal gratings. *Vision Research*, *18*, 369–374.

Hurst, M. A., & Douthwaite, W. A. (1993). Assessing vision behind cataract—A review of methods. *Optometry and Vision Science*, *70*, 903–913.

Kay, H. (1983). New method for assessing visual acuity with pictures. *British Journal of Ophthalmology*, *67*, 131–133.

Kessel, L., Andresen, J., Erngaard, D., et al (2016). Indication for cataract surgery. Do we have evidence of who will benefit from surgery? A systematic review and meta-analysis. *Acta Ophthalmologica*, *94*(1), 10–20. https://doi.org/10.1111/aos.12758.

Labiris, G., Panagiotopoulou, E., Chatzimichael, E., et al. (2020). Introduction of a digital near-vision reading test for normal and low vision adults: development and validation. *Eye and Vision*, *7*(1), 1–15. https://doi.org/10.1186/s40662-020-00216-0.

Legge, G. E. (1991). Glenn A. Fry Award Lecture 1990: three perspectives on low vision reading. *Optometry and Vision Science*, *68*, 763–769.

Legge, G. E., & Rubin, G. S. (1986). Contrast sensitivity function as a screening test: a critique. *American Journal of Optometry and Physiological Optics*, *63*, 265–270.

Legge, G. E., Ross, J. A., Isenberg, L. M., et al. (1992). Psychophysics of reading: clinical predictors of low vision reading speed. *Investigative Ophthalmology & Visual Science*, *33*, 677–687.

Lesmes, L. A., Lu, Z-L., Baek, J., et al. (2010). Bayesian adaptive estimation of the contrast sensitivity function: the quick CSF method. *Journal of Vision*, *10*(3), 1–21. https://doi.org/10.1167/10.3.17.

Logan, A. J., Gordon, G. E., & Loffler, G. (2020). The effect of age-related macular degeneration on components of face perception. *Investigative Ophthalmology & Visual Science*, *61*(6), 38.

Logan, A. J., Wilkinson, F., Wilson, H. R., et al. (2016). The Caledonian face test: a new test of face discrimination. *Vision Research*, *119*, 29–41. https://doi.org/10.1016/j.visres.2015.11.003.

Long, R. G., Reiser, J. J., & Hill, E. W. (1990). Mobility in individuals with moderate visual impairments. *Journal of Visual Impairment and Blindness*, *84*, 111–118.

Lotmar, W. (1980). Apparatus for the measurement of retinal visual acuity by Moiré fringes. *Investigative Ophthalmology & Visual Science*, *19*, 393–400.

Lovie-Kitchin, J. (2011). Reading with low vision: the impact of research on clinical management. *Clinical and Experimental Optometry*, *94*(2), 121–132.

Lovie-Kitchin, J. E., Bevan, J. D., & Hein, B. (2001). Reading performance in children with low vision. *Clinical and Experimental Optometry*, *84*(3), pp.148–154, John Wiley & Sons, Inc.

Lovie-Kitchin, J. E., Mainstone, J., Robinson, J., et al. (1990). What areas of the visual field are important for mobility in low vision patients? *Clinical Vision Sciences*, *5*, 249–263.

Lowe, J. B., & Drasdo, N. (1990). Efficiency in reading with closed-circuit television for low vision. *Ophthalmic and Physiological Optics*, *10*, 225–233.

MacKeben, M. (2008). Topographic mapping of residual vision by computer. *Journal of Visual Impairment and Blindness*, *102*(10), 649–655. https://doi.org/10.1177/0145482x0810201009.

Mackeben, M., & Colenbrander, A. (1992). How to stabilize gaze during vision tests in patients with maculopathies. *Investigative Ophthalmology & Visual Science*, *33*, 1415.

MacKeben, M., Nair, U. K. W., Walker, L. L., et al. (2015). Random word recognition chart helps scotoma assessment in low vision.

Optometry and Vision Science, 92(4), 421–428. https://doi.org/10.1097/OPX.0000000000000548.

Marron, J. A., & Bailey, I. L. (1982). Visual factors and orientation-mobility performance. *American Journal of Optometry and Physiological Optics, 59*, 413–426.

Mayer, D. L., & Dobson, V. (1982). Visual acuity development in infants and young children, as assessed by operant preferential looking. *Vision Research, 22*, 1141–1151.

McDonald, M. A. (1986). Assessment of visual acuity in toddlers. *Survey of Ophthalmology, 31*, 189–210.

McGraw, P. V., & Winn, B. (1995). Measurement of letter acuity in preschool children. *Ophthalmic and Physiological Optics, 15*, S11–S17.

Melki, S. A., Safar, A., Martin, J., et al. (1999). Potential acuity pinhole. *Ophthalmology, 106*(7), 1262–1267. https://doi.org/10.1016/s0161-6420(99)00706-x.

Minkowski, J. S., Palese, M., & Guyton, D. L. (1983). Potential acuity meter using a minute serial pinhole aperture. *Ophthalmology, 90*, 1360–1368.

Mollon, J. D., Astell, S., & Reffin, J. P. (1991). A minimalist test of colour vision. In B. Drum, J. D. Moreland, & A. Serra (Eds.), *Colour vision deficiencies X. Documenta Ophthalmologica Proceedings Series* (Vol. 54, pp. 59–67). Springer. doi:10.1007/978-94-011-3774-4_8.

Patel, P. J., Chen, F. K., Rubin, G. S., et al. (2008). Intersession repeatability of visual acuity scores in age-related macular degeneration. *Investigative Ophthalmology & Visual Science, 49*(10), 4347–4352. https://doi.org/10.1167/iovs.08-1935.

Patel, P. J., et al. (2011). Test-Retest variability of reading performance metrics using MNREAD in patients with age-related macular degeneration. *Investigative Ophthalmology & Visual Science, 52*(6), 3854–3859. https://doi.org/10.1167/iovs.10-6601.

Pelli, D. G., Robson, J. G., & Wilkins, A. J. (1988). The design of a new letter chart for measuring contrast sensitivity. *Clinical Vision Sciences, 2*, 187–199.

Pesudovs, K., Hazel, C. A., Doran, R. M. L., et al. (2004). The usefulness of Vistech and FACT contrast sensitivity charts for cataract and refractive surgery outcomes research. *British Journal of Ophthalmology, 88*(1), 11–16. https://doi.org/10.1136/bjo.88.1.11.

Pfäffli, O. A., Tamási, B., Hanson, J. V. M., et al. (2020). Colour vision testing in young children with reduced visual acuity. *Acta Ophthalmologica, 98*(1), e113–e120. https://doi.org/10.1111/aos.14219.

Radner, W. (2019). Standardization of reading charts: a review of recent developments. *Optometry and Vision Science, 96*(10), 768–779. https://doi.org/10.1097/OPX.0000000000001436.

Radner, W., & Diendorfer, G. (2014). English sentence optotypes for measuring reading acuity and speed—The English version of the Radner Reading Charts. *Graefe's Archive for Clinical and Experimental Ophthalmology, 252*(8), 1297–1303. https://doi.org/10.1007/s00417-014-2646-y.

Rayner, K. (1983). The perceptual span and eye movement control during reading. In K. Rayner (Ed.), *Eye movements in reading: perceptual and language processes* (pp. 97–102). Academic Press.

Reeves, B. (1991, 15th March). The Pelli-Robson Low Contrast Letter Chart. *Optician*, 18–27.

Reeves, B. C., Wood, J. M., & Hill, A. R. (1991). Vistech VCTS 6500 charts—Within and between session reliability. *Optometry and Vision Science, 68*, 728–737.

Regan, D. (1988). Low-contrast letter charts and sinewave grating tests in ophthalmological and neurological disorders. *Clinical Vision Sciences, 2*, 235–250.

Regan, D., & Neima, D. (1984). Low-contrast letter charts in early diabetic retinopathy, ocular hypertension, glaucoma and Parkinson's disease. *British Journal of Ophthalmology, 68*, 885–889.

Rumney, N. J. (1995). Using visual thresholds to establish low vision performance. *Ophthalmic and Physiological Optics, 15*, S18–S24.

Saunders, K. (2010). Testing visual acuity of young children: an evidence-based guide for optometrists. *Optometry in Practice, 11*(4), 161–168.

Schott, J. M., & Crutch, S. J. (2019). Posterior cortical atrophy. *CONTINUUM Lifelong Learning in Neurology, 25*(1), 52–75. https://doi.org/10.1212/CON.0000000000000696.

Schuchard, R. A. (1993). Validity and interpretation of Amsler grid reports. *Archives of Ophthalmology, 111*, 776–780.

Simunovic, M. P. (2016). Acquired color vision deficiency. *Survey of Ophthalmology, 61*(2), 132–155. https://doi.org/10.1016/j.survophthal.2015.11.004.

Sloan, L. L. (1980). Needs for precise measures of acuity: equipment to meet these needs. *Archives of Ophthalmology, 98*, 286–290.

Stifter, E., König, F., Lang, T., et al. (2004). Reliability of a standardized reading chart system: variance component analysis, test-retest and inter-chart reliability. *Graefe's Archive for Clinical and Experimental Ophthalmology, 242*(1), 31–39. https://doi.org/10.1007/s00417-003-0776-8.

Subhi, H., Latham, K., Myint, J., et al. (2017). Functional visual fields: relationship of visual field areas to self-reported function. *Ophthalmic & Physiological Optics, 37*(4), 399–408. https://doi.org/10.1111/opo.12362.

Subramanian, A., & Dickinson, C. (2006). Spatial localization in visual impairment. *Investigative Ophthalmology & Visual Science, 47*(1), 78–85. https://doi.org/10.1167/iovs.05-0137.

Swann, P. G., & Lovie-Kitchin, J. E. (1991). Age-related maculopathy II. The nature of the central field loss. *Ophthalmic and Physiological Optics, 11*, 59–70.

Tekavčič Pompe, M. (2020). Color vision testing in children. *Color Research and Application, 45*(5), 775–781. https://doi.org/10.1002/col.22513.

Teller, D. Y., McDonald, M., Preston, K., et al. (1986). Assessment of visual acuity in infants and children: The acuity card procedure. *Developmental Medicine and Child Neurology, 28*, 779–789.

Thayaparan, K., Crossland, M. D., & Rubin, G. S. (2007). Clinical assessment of two new contrast sensitivity charts. *British Journal of Ophthalmology, 91*(6), 749–752. https://doi.org/10.1136/bjo.2006.109280.

Trauzettel-Klosinski, S., Biermann, P., Hahn, G., et al. (2003). Assessment of parafoveal function in maculopathy: a comparison between the Macular Mapping Test and kinetic Manual Perimetry. *Graefe's Archives of Clinical Experimental Ophthalmology, 241*, 988–995.

Trauzettel-Klosinski, S., & Dietz, K. (2012). Standardized assessment of reading performance: the new International Reading Speed Texts IReST. *Investigative Ophthalmology & Visual Science, 53*(9), 5452–5461. https://doi.org/10.1167/iovs.11-8284.

Verbaker, J. H., & Johnston, A. W. (1986). Population norms for edge contrast sensitivity. *American Journal of Optometry and Physiological Optics, 63*, 724–732.

Vianya-Estopà, M., Douthwaite, W. A., Noble, B. A., et al. (2006). Capabilities of potential vision test measurements. Clinical evaluation in the presence of cataract or macular disease. *Journal of Cataract and Refractive Surgery, 32*(7), 1151–1160. https://doi.org/10.1016/j.jcrs.2006.01.111.

Vianya-Estopa, M., Douthwaite, W. A., Funnell, C. L., et al. (2009). Clinician versus potential acuity test predictions of visual outcome after cataract surgery. *Optometry, 80*(8), 447–453. https://doi.org/10.1016/j.optm.2008.11.011.

Wall, M., & May, D. R. (1987). Threshold Amsler Grid testing in maculopathies. *Ophthalmology, 94*, 1126–1133.

Watson, G. R., Wright, V., & De l'Aune, W. (1992). The efficacy of comprehension training and reading practice for print readers with macular loss. *Journal of Visual Impairment and Blindness, 86*, 37–43.

Whittaker, S. G., & Lovie-Kitchin, J. (1993). Visual requirements for reading. *Optometry and Vision Science, 70*, 54–65.

Whittaker, S. G., & Lovie-Kitchin, J. E. (1994). The assessment of contrast sensitivity and contrast reserve for reading rehabilitation. In A. C. Kooijman, P. L. Looijestijn, J. A. Welling, & G. J. van der Wildt (Eds.), *Low vision research and new developments in rehabilitation* (pp. 88–92). IOS Press.

Wood, J., Rubin, G. S., & Owsley, C. (2011). The role of vision in everyday activities. *Ophthalmic and Physiological Optics, 31*(3), 201–202. https://doi.org/10.1111/j.1475-1313. 2011.00842.x.

Woodhouse, J. M., Adoh, T. O., Oduwaiye, K. A. et al. (1992). New acuity test for toddlers. *Ophthalmic and Physiological Optics, 12*, 249–251.

Patient-Centred Outcome Measures

PATIENT-CENTRED OUTCOME MEASURES

These are also known as 'patient-reported outcome measures' and 'patient relevant outcome measures'. Patients are not only interested in improvements in clinical data (e.g. visual acuity), but rather in how treatments are going to affect their everyday functioning and quality of life (QoL) (Parrish, 1996; Mangione et al., 1999). Measures of patient-reported functioning are designed to capture these effects and have been growing in importance through many branches of healthcare.

The success of an operation or treatment was previously only measured by achievement of visual-impairment (VI) goals, in quantifiable measurements, but nowadays, self-reported visual function is very important to assess treatment outcomes (Ellwein et al., 1994). There is no perfect correlation between clinical measurements and patient perception of visual function. Visual-functioning assessment can detect impacts on performance that might not appear in a routine eye examination (Ellwein et al., 1994). However, several studies (Scott et al., 1994; Klein et al., 2001; Ghazi-Nouri et al., 2006) have found an association between scores of functional status, visual acuity and QoL. Lee et al. (1995), on the other hand, showed that measures of visual acuity, visual functioning, well-being, Amsler grid testing and retinopathy were independent of one another. In agreement with these findings, Steinberg et al. (1994) showed that measures of functional status provide information not covered by measures of visual acuity. In retinal detachment surgery, Okamoto et al. (2008) determined that in some cases, visual acuity was a bad predictor of QoL. Their findings demonstrated that even after what they considered a successful operation, with visual acuity almost back to normal, patients' scores of QoL were reduced.

QUALITY OF LIFE

Many studies have tried to define QoL (Galloway, 2005) and relate it to life satisfaction, well-being or happiness (Farquhar, 1995). QoL is a difficult term to define, as shown by the large number of papers in the literature trying to label and classify it. The World Health Organization (WHO, 1995) has defined QoL as a subjective perception of a person's situation in life. It has been described as a multidimensional concept, influenced by several factors (Camfield & Skevington, 2008). These factors include: mental and physical health; economic situation; education; friends and family. WHO (1995) terms these factors as domains and identifies: physical domain; psychological domain; level of independence; social relationships; environment; spirituality; religion; and personal beliefs.

Definitions and domains of QoL depend on the area of research and on the author. However, the majority of definitions are similar and, although using different terms, they refer to equivalent aspects, as observed in Table 4.1 (Galloway, 2005).

MEASURING 'VISION-RELATED QUALITY OF LIFE' IN ADULTS

Considering all the possible contributing factors, a decision has to be made as to which will be most relevant and meaningful to investigate. These measures of QoL often look at 'activity limitation' and sometimes 'adaptation to visual loss' and 'participation restriction'. However, the scope and definitions of each of these parameters does vary considerably between studies, and the terminology is not always used in accordance with International Classification of Functioning, Disability and Health (ICF) definitions. These studies usually use questionnaire or interview techniques to assess the

TABLE 4.1 Factors Influencing QoL According to Different Studies

AUTHOR				
Felce and Perry (1995)	Schalock (2000)	WHO QoL Definition (1993)	Hagerty et al. (2001)	Cummins (2000)
Field of Research				
Disability/Psychology		Health	Social Indicators	Disability
Six possible domains: 1. Physical well-being 2. Material well-being 3. Social well-being 4. Productive well-being 5. Emotional well-being 6. Rights or civic well-being	Eight core domains: 1. Physical well-being 2. Material well-being 3. Social well-being 4. Emotional well-being 5. Rights 6. Impersonal relations 7. Personal development 8. Self-determination	Six domains: 1. Physical 2. Environment 3. Social relationships 4. Psychological 5. Level of independence 6. Spiritual	Seven core domains: 1. Health 2. Material well-being 3. Feeling part of one's local community 4. Work and productive activity 5. Emotional well-being 6. Relationships with family and friends 7. Personal safety	Seven core domains: 1. Health 2. Material well-being 3. Community well-being 4. Work/productive activity 5. Emotional well-being 6. Social/family connections 7. Safety

QoL, Quality of life; *WHO,* World Health Organization.

perceived impact of the ophthalmic condition on physical (mobility, ambulation), psychosocial (alertness, communication, social interaction) and other (home management, sleep, hobbies) aspects of life. Wilkie et al. (2005) noted that very few questionnaires deal with participation restriction and devised the Keele Assessment of Participation to fill this gap.

In vision care, such questionnaires (often called 'instruments') were first used in relation to cataract surgery, both in deciding when to operate and in monitoring the improvement which the procedure brings. Bernth-Petersen (1981, 1982) was the first to suggest that a successful outcome for cataract surgery did not just mean a clear optical axis and a healthy eye as assessed by ophthalmoscopy but a patient who could function better as a result. Visual acuity is a useful measure to quantify VI, although other parameters such as peripheral vision, sensitivity to motion, contrast sensitivity or glare are important for a complete visual assessment (Kosnik et al., 1988; Sloane et al., 1992; Rubin et al., 1993). Even such a comprehensive assessment is limited as it cannot predict the visual functioning of patients in their daily activities, and their ability to perform everyday chores (Ellwein et al., 1994; Lee et al., 1995). It is well-accepted that visual acuity is not a good measure of when cataract operations should be performed and that the patient's 'satisfaction' with their vision is more significant. Considerable variation exists in the frequency of cataract operations in different geographical areas which have apparently similar populations, suggesting that different (probably highly subjective) criteria are being applied in these areas. The use of other visual tests, such as glare disability, will be discussed in Chapter 10, but the use of a 'functional status questionnaire' may offer another way of providing a quantitative description of function.

The general structure of questions (usually called 'items') on such tests is:

Does your vision cause you difficulty in doing tasks?

- *Yes*
  - *A little*
  - *A moderate amount*
  - *A great deal*
  - *Unable to do the task*
- *No*
  - *Not applicable-have never done this task*
  - *Reasons other than vision cause difficulty with task*

The question will be repeated for several tasks such as driving at night, reading a newspaper, watching television, or preparing food (Mangione et al., 1992; Steinberg et al., 1994).

Researchers who devise such questionnaires face some difficulty in providing evidence of their validity. Obviously some correlation with visual acuity would be expected, and it is greater for those tasks that you would expect to be visually demanding, such as reading in dim light (Rubin et al., 1994), than for a task like eating (Scott et al., 1994). The whole purpose of the questionnaires, however, is to overcome the apparent deficiency of visual acuity as a measure of functional status. Steinberg et al. (1994) reported a better correlation of functional status with the rather simplistic grading of patient 'satisfaction' (simply asking them if they were very satisfied, satisfied, dissatisfied or very dissatisfied): there was no correlation at all between visual acuity and satisfaction with vision! What is really required of course is to show that a visual improvement produces a proportional increase in functional status and QoL, and this has been reported for patients who have undergone cataract surgery (Brenner et al., 1993). As well as functional ability, QoL also embraces the emotional impact that poor vision has on the patient's perception of their well-being on such diverse scales as energy/

fatigue, social functioning and pain (Lee et al., 1993). In this extremely complex area, there may also be evidence of the corollary effect where patients with other health difficulties report greater problems with their vision than can be objectively measured (Wormald et al., 1993).

VI has an impact on QoL, with patient's feelings (e.g. hopelessness, depression) being similar to those caused by other chronic illnesses (Williams et al., 1998). Chia et al. (2004) determined that these effects are related to the severity of the VI and not to the eye condition. It has been accepted that when the vision decreases to the stage of low vision, the patient loses independence (Kupfer, 2000; Janiszewski et al., 2006). QoL has been related to dependency in activities of daily living (ADLs), suggesting that early detection and intervention might be crucial for a successful rehabilitation (Ivanoff et al., 2000).

Issues in Questionnaire Design

One of the problems that researchers encounter when they try to validate a questionnaire is the scoring (Massof & Rubin, 2001). The majority of questionnaires found in the literature use ordinal ranking data for each item (e.g. 1 to 5). However, sums of ordinal data, at face value, have no meaning, and individuals with the same score can represent very different characteristics. Then, various statistical models (Hambleton & Cook, 1977) can be used for validation purposes, such as the Rasch model (Andrich, 1978). The **Rasch model** helps to transform the raw data into a meaningful interval scale through logarithmic transformations and probabilistic equations (Bond & Fox, 2001). Rasch analysis (Fig. 4.1) does not assume that all items have the same level of difficulty and that all persons have the same ability but weights them accordingly (Bond & Fox, 2001; Court et al., 2007, 2010). Rasch analysis is a probabilistic model that helps to define the difficulty of an item independently of the population, and the ability of a person independently of the items resolved by this person (Bond & Fox, 2001).

Clinically, a measure of QoL is going to be useful if it is: reliable, valid and appropriate, responsive, interpretable, simple, quick to administer and complete, and easy to score (Aaronson et al., 1993; Thornicroft & Slade, 2000; Higginson & Carr, 2001).

Reliability refers to the consistency of a set of measurements or measuring instrument used to describe a given property or behaviour and has a number of aspects (Margolis et al., 2002). **Test-retest reliability** is the reproducibility of a given measure and refers to the degree to which scores stay the same over time, in a situation where no change is expected (Leidy et al., 1999). The participants should score similarly on the items between two assessments in a relatively short period of time (Margolis et al., 2002). Intraclass correlation coefficients (ICCs) should be higher than 0.60 over a 2-week period or less (Hays et al., 1998). Reliability does not imply validity; a measure can be reliable and not valid. Scores can be internally consistent and stable over time, and yet the instrument does not measure what it is supposed to determine.

Validity is the extent to which an instrument measures what it is supposed to be measuring (Leidy et al., 1999). Reliability is precision, whereas validity is accuracy (Cronbach, 1951). An instrument is said to have **content validity** if it covers all the aspects of a domain (e.g. social support: tangible, affectionate, instrumental, informational and positive social interaction) (Carmines & Zeller, 1979) and **face validity** if it seems to be measuring what it is supposed to measure: whether it 'looks like' is going to assess what it says, rather than it 'has been shown to work'. It refers to the degree to which a measure is sensitive to the participants' interests (Margolis et al., 2002).

According to de Boer et al. (2004), a questionnaire has good content validity when the authors design the items by examining the literature, as well as consulting patients and/or experts. They consider the consultation of patients a prerequisite, because the questions are about them or their feelings and how they perceive their problems. An initial (large) number of suggested questions should be reduced during the development process by removing those that are not applicable to a large section of the population; are too easy for the participants; ask about a different concept; or are redundant (with content covered by the rest of the questions).

Convergent (or concurrent) validity measures the degree to which an instrument correlates to other measures of the same or similar construct (the results of the measure are compared to the results of the gold standard obtained at approximately the same point in time) (Margolis et al., 2002). **Discriminant validity** is the capacity to differentiate between cases and controls or disease severity groups (Margolis et al., 2002). Cohen (1988) proposed that an r value of 0.10 was a low correlation, 0.30 was moderate, and 0.50 was a high correlation. **Construct validity** estimates how well a measure correlates with other indicators of similar related constructs (i.e. reflects the ability of an instrument to measure an abstract concept, or construct. There is not always a gold standard) (Margolis et al., 2002). Construct validity can be measured by the infit and outfit statistics (indices of measurement accuracy). **Infit** statistics detect unexpected patterns on responses to items (by individuals) that are targeted on them. **Outfit** statistics detect unexpected patterns on responses to items that are considered relatively easy or very hard for the individual.

Internal consistency is the extent to which all items measure the same construct and is tested using Cronbach's formula for coefficient alpha (Cronbach, 1951). Cronbach alpha should be higher than 0.70 for group comparisons and test-retest reliability (Leidy et al., 1999; Margolis et al., 2002).

When checking for subscales in the questionnaire, items that do not load (i.e. do not correlate with any other items measuring a similar construct) on any factor or that load in multiple factors should be eliminated. Cronbach alpha is a statistic commonly used to express this correlation (Cronbach, 1951) and should be between 0.70 and 0.90.

Margolis et al. (2002) also described the term **Responsiveness** as the extent to which the instrument can identify variations in individuals known to have a change in visual functioning. This will be particularly important if the instrument is to be used to assess the effect of a particular intervention. **Interpretability** is

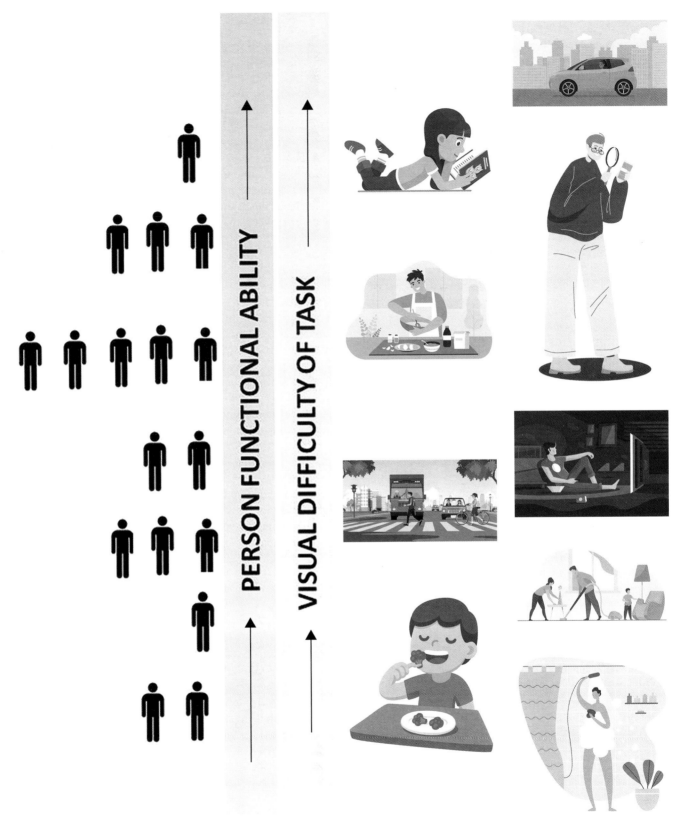

Fig. 4.1 A schematic representation of Rasch 'person-item' analysis of the results of a vision-related quality of life questionnaire. The questions/items are ranked by their visual difficulty, and the respondents/persons are ranked according to their functional ability. iStock.com/zuperia; iStock.com/IconicBestiary; iStock.com/Lyudinka; iStock.com/BRO Vector; iStock.com/jossnatu; iStock.com/intararit; iStock.com/SurfUpVector; iStock.com/Sudowoodo; iStock.com/Dmitrii Musku.

the ability to understand the scores on a measure (de Boer et al., 2004), and the degree to which it is possible to assign qualitative meaning to quantitative data (Lohr et al., 1996). For interpretability, mean scores and standard deviations should be given for the population on which the instrument was tested. **Respondent burden** (de Boer et al., 2004) is the demand imposed on the participants (i.e. usually mostly time, but also energy and emotional stress). Some participants may not complete the full questionnaire, and the proportion of missing values can be an indication of respondent burden.

A related issue which is particularly relevant to a visually impaired population is how the questionnaire will be delivered. The usual method is self-administration, often in written format. However, this can create difficulties for those with a VI or carry the risk that another person completes it on their behalf. In-person administration by the researcher or clinician can be time-consuming and lead to bias. Online completion and telephone interview with an independent person are possible alternatives that may be useful in some populations.

Questionnaires Designed for People With Visual Impairment

The Impact of Visual Impairment (IVI) questionnaire (Weih et al., 2002) was developed to assess the vision rehabilitation needs in the context of participation restriction and was supposed to be useful when measuring intervention outcomes.

According to de Boer et al. (2004), the IVI questionnaire is an instrument targeted at people with VI and it covers several dimensions of QoL, such as functional, social and psychological. The authors described a high content validity and reproducibility for this scale, whilst interpretability and respondent burden were considered to be average. Nevertheless, the IVI appears to address questions which relate to visual functioning of the patient and their limitation in their daily activities (e.g. reading labels and instructions in medicines) and patients' feelings (e.g. feeling embarrassed) and not just participation restriction aspects (e.g. 'I have taken part in social activities as and when I have wanted'). With such a wide-ranging content, it is difficult for a questionnaire to be responsive to simple rehabilitation strategies such as providing a magnifier.

The Low Vision Quality of Life (LVQOL) questionnaire aims to identify and quantify the impact of visual impairment on aspects like independence, mobility, time for oneself, and daily tasks (Wolffsohn & Cochrane, 2000). This questionnaire was developed using patients with a wide variety of conditions causing untreatable vision loss. The authors reviewed the literature in order to gather all the subjective questionnaires previously designed to measure QoL. The resulting items were combined, so no repetition occurred. The questions were then revised by a group of experts (optometrists, ophthalmologists, orthoptists, occupational therapists, welfare officers, audiologists and those with low vision), with items not relevant to the majority of persons with low vision excluded. The 74-item questionnaire was conducted on a random sample ($n = 150$ from the database of the Vision Australia Foundation) of subjects with low vision.

The LVQOL questionnaire is supposed to differentiate persons with low vision from those with 'normal' vision. For this purpose, the study included an age-matched and gender-matched control group of 70 subjects attending the optometric clinic (with minor eye conditions such as early cataracts, blepharitis, or dry eye). Internal consistency was calculated using the item-total correlation and Cronbach's α and reliability using the ICC. The authors determined that a homogeneous scale (internal consistency) was that which focused on the different aspects of the same attribute. Consequently, items should be moderately correlated to each other and to the total scale score. Furthermore, when the items are highly correlated, questions add little information (redundancy). However, when the correlations are very low, the questions refer to different attributes. Four questions were removed using this principle (Cronbach's α). The questionnaire was completed four times in a 4-week interval (short period for a potential change in patients' situation and long enough, so the participants do not remember their prior answers) to assess test-retest reliability. Those items that remained unchanged were selected. Using these methods, the scale was reduced to 25 items. The LVQOL questionnaire was confirmed to have high internal consistency (Cronbach's α = 0.88) and reliability (0.72). The questionnaire was designed to produce a summed score of the patients' QoL (between 0 and 125, with a higher score indicating better QoL).

Varimax rotation identified four principal factors (i.e. general vision, mobility and lighting issues; psychological adjustment; reading and fine work; and ADLs) in the LVQOL, each with internal consistency (Cronbach's α > 0.80). The questionnaire also appeared sensitive at differentiating people with low vision and those with normal sight. Less than 20% of the subjects with low vision scored 95 or higher in the questionnaire, compared with 65% in the control group. This scale is a suitable clinical tool to quantify the QoL of patients with low vision.

It takes 5 to 10 minutes to complete and it is easy to understand by the subjects. Furthermore, on the systematic review of QoL questionnaires conducted by de Boer et al. (2004), the LVQOL questionnaire (Wolffsohn & Cochrane, 2000) was considered to have high quality concerning psychometric aspects. Based on their research, the scale has good content validity (i.e. selection of items, item reduction, checking for subscales and internal consistency) and fair reproducibility and interpretability. The LVQOL was considered to be the gold standard at that time (de Boer et al., 2004) and therefore has been used in many studies (Van Nispen et al., 2011), when measuring QoL in people with low vision.

Another questionnaire specifically measuring visual functioning is the 48-item Veterans Affairs Low-Vision Visual Functioning Questionnaire (VA LV VFQ-48) (Stelmack et al., 2007). This instrument measures visual efficacy in terms of overall ability, mobility, visual information processing and visual motor skills (Stelmack et al., 2008). Theoretically, the questionnaire consists of 48 items (activities) that the subject has to categorise from not difficult to impossible to accomplish. But there are two further questions (is it difficult because of your vision?/how do you usually perform this activity?) that must be applied to every item of the questionnaire. Hence, the 48 items prove to be 144 questions, and as Stelmack and Massof (2007) observed takes around 35 minutes on the telephone. The short form of this questionnaire is only 20 items, again theoretically. In practice, these 20 items actually become 60 questions. The authors did not state how long the interview would last for this short form, but it would probably take about 15 minutes. The VA LV VFQ-48 scale is a very comprehensive tool to obtain accurate measures of the visual ability when time is not an issue: it has been designed to be sensitive to rehabilitation. The items were developed and chosen by a multidisciplinary team of clinicians and researchers as well as persons with vision loss. The items were calibrated with Rasch analysis to reflect their difficulty. The analysis includes standard errors of each estimate and reliability coefficients in order to calculate measurement precision. Test-retest reliability was assessed by readministering the questionnaire to 30 patients after 3 or 4 weeks (ICC = 0.98) (Stelmack et al., 2004). Stelmack et al. (2002) established the sensitivity and validity of the VA LV VFQ-48 as a measure of low-vision rehabilitation outcomes. In this study, the questionnaire was administered to 71 veterans (individuals with low vision and legally blind), before and 4 months after receiving rehabilitation. The results showed improved person measures postrehabilitation in legally blind patients. On the other hand, patients with less severe VI (near normal visual acuity) seemed to remain constant, before and after rehabilitation. The instrument appeared to be a sensitive measure for those patients with severe VI. As the VFQ has been Rasch analysed, it is possible to select only some of the items, and then the questionnaire responses can be scored using previously published algorithms (Stelmack & Massof, 2007). Based on this, a 15-item 'near vision' questionnaire was devised (NV-VFQ-15) by selecting appropriate items from the VFQ-48 questionnaire for a study which assessed the effectiveness of portable electronic vision enhancement systems (p-EVES) in addition to optical aids for patients seen in a hospital clinic (Taylor et al., 2017).

Massof et al. (2007) designed a visual function questionnaire (the Activity Inventory [AI]) which has the feature that each patient responds to an individually tailored set of questions. The questionnaire is divided into three objectives (daily living, social interactions and recreation), under which lie 50 goals and each goal (e.g. cooking) has a collection of tasks (e.g. reading a recipe). The patients have to rate the importance and difficulty of each goal as well as the difficulty of the tasks that serve these goals. The result of the patient's answers provides a functional history and the data needed to estimate the patient's visual ability. The reasoning for designing this questionnaire is interesting because it is true that when using a fixed-number-of-items questionnaire, some of the questions are not relevant to some patients (e.g. respondents are allowed to skip items based on responses to screening questions, or by permitting them to respond that the item is not applicable or that they do not do the activity described for reasons other than vision). The skipped answers lead to difficulty handling

these missing data in the final analysis, particularly when using conventional Likert-type scoring algorithms. Although Rasch analysis can overcome this problem, the authors argue that it would be even more reasonable to use a tailored questionnaire for each patient in addition to Rasch analysis.

The AI can be helpful in clinical practice to address goal-oriented components of the rehabilitation plan, as a tool to plan rehabilitation, evaluate patient progress and measure outcomes. The key is that it is possible to use this questionnaire to obtain specific information for a particular patient and plan and adapt the rehabilitation according to the patient's priorities and goals.

Other Vision-Related Questionnaires

There are other instruments described in the literature, such as the Visual Function Self-report (VF-14) (Steinberg et al., 1994), the Activities of Daily Vision Scale (Mangione et al., 1992), the Visual Activities Questionnaire (Sloane et al., 1992), the National Eye Institute Visual Function Questionnaire (NEI-VFQ) (Mangione et al., 2001), the Visual Disability Inventory (Newman & Houser, 1991), the Visual Disability Assessment (Pesudovs & Coster, 1998), the Michigan Commission for the Blind Functional Assessment Scale (Nieuwenhuijsen et al., 1991), and the Functional Assessment Self-Report Inventory (Szlyk et al., 1990).

Some questionnaires use a mixture of self-report, and of the clinician grading the performance of the individual whilst actually carrying out some of the tasks (e.g. Functional Low-Vision Observer Rated Assessment (FLORA; Geruschat et al., 2015) and the Melbourne Low Vision ADL Index (Haymes et al., 2001)).

However, some of the available instruments have been developed to evaluate medical treatments in clinical trials (e.g. the NEI-VFQ) or are disease-specific (e.g. MacDQoL (Mitchell & Bradley, 2004), the VF-14 (Steinberg et al., 1994), or the Daily Living Tasks Dependent on Vision (DLTV) (Hart et al., 1999)). A number of these questionnaires are time consuming (Carta et al., 1998) or have been designed for specific and likely treatable conditions (Desai et al., 1996; Okamoto et al., 2008) and not to address the overall impact of visual loss in a general low-vision population (Wolffsohn & Cochrane, 2000; Stelmack & Massof, 2007). The FLORA (Geruschat et al., 2015), for example, was developed to assess treatment or vision restoration in people with ultra-low vision, blinded with retinitis pigmentosa.

As noted earlier, the original NEI-VFQ was validated for an adult population with common eye diseases (Mangione et al., 2001) but not specifically for a low-vision population. This questionnaire, however, has been used widely (Broman et al., 2001) and for different age groups and degrees of visual loss (Klein et al., 2001). An abbreviated version was also developed and validated (the 7-item NEI-VFQ) for use in evaluating the Welsh Low Vision Service (Ryan et al., 2008).

Questionnaires may also be validated for a specific population (e.g. hospital sample) and then used on a different one (e.g. community settings or primary care practice) (Hilton et al., 2006). The LVQOL questionnaire was validated for self-administration, as well as in-person or telephone interviews and was specially designed for a low-vision population. Generalisation and robustness are more likely when the questionnaires have been validated for several populations and different forms of administration.

ADAPTATION TO VISION LOSS

As discussed previously, there is often a section (subscale) in a general VR-QOL questionnaire which assesses the responder's psychological state: their feelings and emotions (about their vision loss) and potential effects on well-being and relationships. These results should be kept separate from those related to practical activities and preferably dealt with in specific questionnaires.

The 'Adaptation to Vision Loss' (AVL) instruments (a 24-item and then a shortened 12-item version) were devised by Horowitz et al. (2007) for individuals with acquired vision loss. 'Adaptation' can be considered to be an acceptance of the condition (lack of denial), a willingness to explore rehabilitation strategies, and a healthy balance between independence and the acceptance of help (Horowitz & Reinhardt, 1998). Respondents have to give their level of agreement with statements such as 'Visually impaired persons cannot afford to talk back or argue with family and friends' and 'It is too hard for older people to learn new ways of doing things (that compensate for vision loss) if they become visually impaired'.

The design of the Vision Core Measure 1 (VCM-1) questionnaire began by asking a very wide range of visually impaired individuals, 'What are the main things that affect your quality of life as far as your eyesight is concerned?' which received many very varied answers. From a pool of over 200 questions, the authors selected 10 questions. Despite many of the items referring to specific tasks, such as shopping or reading, the final items are much more about the emotional reaction to the loss. Responders are asked, for example, 'How often have you worried about your eyesight getting worse?' or 'How often have you felt lonely or isolated because of your eyesight?'

The 19-item Acceptance and Self-Worth Adjustment Scale (AS-WAS) (Tabrett & Latham, 2010) was developed by using Rasch analysis of the 55-item Nottingham Adjustment Scale. It has questions on acceptance, self-efficacy, attitudes and self-esteem. Responders are asked to strongly agree or to strongly disagree with statements, some of which are phrased negatively and some positively. Examples are (in the self-esteem category) 'I am able to do things as well as other people' and (in the attitudes category) 'People with my sort of visual problem feel that they are worthless'.

MEASURING 'VISION-RELATED QUALITY OF LIFE' IN CHILDREN

Vision loss in early life has important psychological and functional implications (Day, 1997), and these affect QoL (Khadka et al., 2012; Rainey et al., 2016). Questionnaires to measure QoL are a popular tool because they are simple to use, inexpensive, quick, do not necessarily require attendance and can be applied to general population groups (Gothwal et al., 2003).

There are several questionnaires that have been used in different children populations. The LV Prasad-Functional Vision Questionnaire (LVP-FVQ) (Gothwal et al., 2003) was developed to assess the functional abilities of children with VI in India. The authors performed an extensive literature review in order to find a list of vision-related tasks performed by children with minimal or severe VI. They also conducted focus group discussions, including paediatric ophthalmologists, children with VI, parents of children with VI, and low-vision therapists, to understand the difficulties that these children encounter in their daily activities. The instrument consists of 19 items covering different domains, such as distance vision (six questions), near vision (six questions), colour vision (two questions) and visual field (five questions). There is an additional item, the 20th question, which asks the children to relate their vision to that of their friends. Rasch analysis showed higher reliability for item difficulty parameters (0.93) than for person ability (0.65). The LVP-FVQ confirms good criterion validity by its capacity to differentiate between those individuals with different visual abilities (e.g. 'seeing as well as' their normally sighted friends/ 'seeing a little worse' than their friends/ 'seeing much worse' than their friends). The LVP-FVQ is a valid and useful tool to measure functional vision performance in children with VI. This questionnaire was designed to use in children from 8 to 18 years old and more suited for low to middle-income countries, because of the tasks described.

The Cardiff Visual Ability Questionnaire for Children (CVAQC) (Khadka et al., 2010) is a 25-item instrument designed to evaluate the visual ability in children and young people between 5 and 18 years old with VI living in high income countries. The development methodology was similar to the LVP-FVQ, where focus group discussions, with children and young people with and without VI, were used to select the initial items. The questionnaire was piloted with children and young people ($n = 45$) with VI, and Rasch analysis was used to examine the response category function, as well as to facilitate selection of the final items. Validity and reliability were assessed on a group of visually impaired children ($n = 109$) using Rasch analysis and ICC. The results showed excellent person separation (2.28), high reliability (0.84), with the items well targeted to the subjects (-0.40 logit between item and person mean) and good temporal stability (ICC = 0.89). In other words, according to the statistical analysis, the children can be well differentiated into distinct groups given their abilities, and this differentiation is maintained across time—that is, if the test is administered on two different occasions, a longer test gap would not necessarily lead to a lower correlation.

The Children's Visual Function Questionnaire (CVFQ) (Felius et al., 2004) was designed for very young children (i.e. ≤7 years old) and based on proxy answers to determine parents' perceptions of treatment for the impairing conditions. This questionnaire was designed and developed in the United States.

The authors of the Impact of Visual Impairment on Children (IVI-C) questionnaire (Cochrane et al., 2008), used input, for the focus groups, from teachers, occupational therapists, orientation and mobility instructors, parents and children. However, the psychometric properties of the questionnaire were not described. This questionnaire was designed (in the United States) to be used in children between 8 and 18 years old to address the emotional and functional impact of their VI.

Another questionnaire developed in the UK is the Functional Vision Questionnaire for Children and Young People with Visual Impairment (FVQ_CYP) (Tadić et al., 2013). This questionnaire consists of 36 items and was designed for children between 10 and 15 years of age. The questionnaire was designed using focus groups and qualitative data was collected from semistructured interviews. The data collected were based on children's own perspectives of what it is like to live with VI. The items were pretested with 17 students with VI and piloted in 101 children with VI. The results were analysed with individual item response pattern, application of exploratory factor analysis, including parallel analysis and finally with Rasch analysis. According to the authors, this questionnaire is psychometrically robust, valid and reliable for the assessment of the self-perceived impact of VI on children and young people regarding the level of difficulty of performing vision-dependent activities. This questionnaire is expected to be a complementary measure to objective clinical assessments (e.g. visual acuity, contrast sensitivity, visual fields) and to other Patient Related Outcome Measures (PROMs), such as the Vision Quality of Life for Children and Young People (VQoL_CYP) questionnaire. The VQoL_CYP (Rahi et al., 2011) is a questionnaire to measure the emotional impact of vision loss in children and young people. This instrument was designed to understand the perceptions of the impact of living with a visual disability rather than focusing on the child's ability to perform tasks or activities that require vision (functional status). Sometimes, in the literature, the concepts of functional vision and vision-related QoL are used interchangeably. Here, the authors show the differences between these two concepts and state that these questionnaires (the FVQ_CYP and the VQoL_CYP) can complement each other, to understand how loss of vision affects children's ability to perform tasks which require vision (FVQ_CYP) and emotional status (i.e. psychosocial impact of vision loss) (VQoL_CYP). The VQoL_CYP is a 47-item scale designed for children between 10 and 15 years of age and it takes 15 to 20 minutes to administer.

SELECTING A QUESTIONNAIRE TO USE

With so many vision-related questionnaires available, it can be difficult to decide which instrument to use for a specific research or clinical question. The authors recommend reading scientific papers in the same area to determine which questionnaires have been shown to respond to the population of interest. Instruments which have been scaled using Rasch analysis, and those with accurate reliability statistics, are generally preferred. Data on demographics for the population in which the questionnaire was developed should also be considered, because validity, responsiveness and reproducibility will not necessarily be the same for all populations.

REFERENCES

Aaronson, N. K., Ahmedzai, S., Bergman, B., et al. (1993). The European Organization for Research and Treatment of Cancer QLQ-C30: a quality-of-life instrument for use in international clinical trials in oncology. *Journal of the National Cancer Institute, 85*(5), 365–376. https://doi.org/10.1093/jnci/85.5.365.

Andrich, D. (1978). A rating formulation for ordered response categories. *Psychometrika, 43*(4), 561–573.

Bernth-Petersen, P. (1981). Visual functioning in cataract patients. Methods of measuring and results. *Acta Ophthalmol, 59*, 198–205.

Bernth-Petersen, P. (1982). Outcome of cataract surgery. II. Visual functioning in aphakic patients. *Acta Ophthalmologica, 60*, 243–251.

Bond, T. G., & Fox, C. M. (2001). *Applying the Rasch model: fundamental measurement in the Human Sciences* (2nd ed.). Lawrence Erlbaum Associates Publishers.

Brenner, M. H., Curbow, B., Javitt, J. C., et al. (1993). Vision change and quality of life in the elderly: response to cataract surgery and treatment of other chronic conditions. *Archives of Ophthalmology, 111*, 680–685.

Broman, A. T., Munoz, B., West, S. K., et al. (2001). Psychometric properties of the 25-item NEI-VFQ in a Hispanic population: Proyecto VER. *Investigative Ophthalmology & Visual Science, 42*(3), 606–613.

Camfield, L., & Skevington, S. M. (2008). On subjective well-being and quality of life. *Journal of Health Psychology, 13*(6), 764–775.

Carmines, E. G., & Zeller, R. A. (1979). *Reliability and validity assessment.* Sage Publications.

Carta, A., Braccio, L., Belpoliti, M., et al. (1998). Self-assessment of the quality of vision: association of questionnaire score with objective clinical tests. *Current Eye Research, 17*(5), 506–512.

Chia, E., Wang, J. J., Rochtchina, E., et al. (2004). Impact of bilateral visual impairment on health-related quality of life: the Blue Mountains Eye Study. *Investigative Ophthalmology & Visual Science, 45*(1), 71–76.

Cochrane, G., Lamoureux, E., & Keeffe, J. (2008). Defining the content for a new quality of life questionnaire for students with low vision (The Impact of Vision Impairment on Children: IVI_C). *Ophthalmic Epidemiol, 15*, 114–120.

Cohen, J. (1988). *Statistical power analysis for the behavioral sciences* (2nd ed.). Lawrence Erlbaum Associates, Publishers.

Court, H., Greenland, K., & Margrain, T. H. (2007). Content development of the optometric patient anxiety scale. *Optometry and Vision Science, 84*(8), 730–744.

Court, H., Greenland, K., & Margrain, T. H. (2010). Measuring patient anxiety in primary care: Rasch analysis of the 6-item Spielberger State Anxiety Scale. *Value in Health, 13*(6), 813–819.

Cronbach, L. J. (1951). Coefficient alpha and the internal structure of tests. *Psychometrika, 16*(3), 297–334.

Cummins, R. A. (2000). Objective and subjective quality of life: an interactive model. *Social Indicators Research, 52,* 55–72.

Day, S. (1997). Normal and abnormal visual development. In D. Taylor (Ed.), *Paediatric Ophthalmology* (2nd ed., pp. 13–28). London: Blackwell Science.

de Boer, M. R., Moll, A. C., de Vet, H. C. W., et al. (2004). Psychometric properties of vision-related quality of life questionnaires: a systematic review. *Ophthalmic & Physiological Optics: The Journal of the British College of Ophthalmic Opticians (Optometrists), 24*(4), 257–273.

Desai, P., Reidy, A., Minassian, D. C., et al. (1996). Gains from cataract surgery: visual function and quality of life. *British Journal of Ophthalmology, 80*(10), 868–873. https://doi.org/10.1136/bjo.80.10.868.

Ellwein, L. B., Fletcher, A., Dominique Negrel, A., et al. (1994). Quality of life assessment in blindness prevention interventions. *International Ophthalmology, 18,* 263–268.

Farquhar, M. (1995). Definitions of quality of life: a taxonomy. *Journal of Advanced Nursing, 22*(3), 502–508.

Felce, D., & Perry, J. (1995). Quality of life: its definition and measurement. *Research in Developmental Disabilities, 16*(1), 51–74.

Felius, J. D. R. S., Berry, P., Salomao, S., et al. (2004). Development of an instrument to assess vision-related quality of life in young children. *American Journal of Ophthalmology, 138*(3), 362–372.

Galloway, S. (2005). Well-being and quality of life: measuring the benefits of culture and sport: a literature review and thinkpiece. Scottish Executive. *Social Research,* 4–97.

Geruschat, D. R., Flax, M., Tanna, N., et al. (2015). FLORA: Phase I development of a functional vision assessment for prosthetic vision users. *Clinical and Experimental Optometry, 98*(4), 342–347. https://doi.org/10.1111/cxo.12242.FLORA.

Ghazi-Nouri, S. M. S., Tranos, P. G., Rubin, G. S., et al. (2006). Visual function and quality of life following vitrectiomy and epiretinal membrane peel surgery. *British Journal of Ophthalmology, 90*(5), 559–562.

Gothwal, V. K., Lovie-Kitchin, J. E., & Nutheti, R. (2003). The development of the LV Prasad-Functional Vision Questionnaire: a measure of functional vision performance of visually impaired children. *Investigative Ophthalmology & Visual Science, 44*(9), 4131–4139. https://doi.org/10.1167/iovs.02-1238.

Hagerty, M. R., Cummins, R. A., Ferriss, A. L., et al. (2001). Quality of life indexes for national policy: review and agenda for research. *Social Indicators Research, 5,* 1–96.

Hambleton, R. K., & Cook, L. L. (1977). Latent trait models and their use in the analysis of educational test data source. *Journal of Educational Measurement, 14*(2), 75–96.

Hart, P. M., Chakravarthy, U., Stevenson, M. R., et al. (1999). A vision specific functional index for use in patients with age related macular degeneration. *British Journal of Ophthalmology, 83*(10), 1115–1120.

Haymes, S. A., Johnston, A. W., & Heyes, A. D. (2001). The development of the Melbourne Low-Vision ADL Index: a measure of vision disability. *Investigative Ophthalmology & Visual Science, 42,* 1215–1225.

Hays, R., Anderson, R., & Al, E. (1998). *Assessing reliability and validity of measurement in clinical trial.* Oxford University Press.

Higginson, I., & Carr, A. J. (2001). Using quality of life measures in the clinical setting. *British Medical Journal, 322*(7297), 1297–1300.

Hilton, T. M., Parker, G., McDonald, S., et al. (2006). A validation study of two brief measures of depression in the cardiac population: the DMI-10 and DMI-18. *Psychosomatics, 47*(2), 129–135. https://doi.org/10.1176/appi.psy.47.2.129.

Horowitz, A., & Reinhardt, J. (1998). Development of the adaptation to age-related vision loss scale. *Journal of Visual Impairment & Blindness, 92,* 30–41.

Horowitz, A., Reinhardt, J. P., & Raykov, T. (2007). Development and validation of a Short-Form Adaptation of the Age-Related Vision Loss Scale: The AVL12. *Journal of Visual Impairment and Blindness, 101*(3), 146–159.

Ivanoff, D. S., Sonn, U., Lundgren-Lindqvist, B., et al. (2000). Disability in daily life activities and visual impairment: a population study of 85-year-old people living at home. *Scandinavian Journal of Occupational Therapy, 7*(4), 148–155. https://doi.org/10.1080/110381200300008689.

Janiszewski, R., Heath-Watson, S. L., Semidey, A. Y., et al. (2006). The low visibility of low vision: increasing awareness through public health education. *Journal of Visual Impairment and Blindness, 100*(1_Suppl), 849–861. https://doi.org/10.1177/0145482x0610001s08.

Khadka, J., Ryan, B., Margrain, T. H., et al. (2010). Development of the 25-item Cardiff Visual Ability Questionnaire for Children (CVAQC). *British Journal of Ophthalmology, 94*(6), 730–735. https://doi.org/10.1136/bjo.2009.171181.

Khadka, J., Ryan, B., Margrain, T. h, et al. (2012). Listening to voices of children with a visual impairment: a focus group study. *The British Journal of Visual Impairment, 30*(3), 182–196. https://doi.org/10.1177/0264619612453105.

Klein, R., MOss, S., Klein, B., et al. (2001). The NEI-VFQ-25 in people with long-term type I diabetes mellitus: the Wisconsin Epidemiologic Study of Diabetic Retinopathy. *Archives of Ophthalmology, 119,* 733–740. https://doi.org/10.1097/00132578-200201000-00029.

Kosnik, W., Winslow, L., Kline, D., et al. (1988). Visual changes in daily life throughout adulthood. *Journal of Gerontology, 43*(3), 63–70.

Kupfer, C. (2000). The national eye institute's low vision education program: improving quality of life. *Ophthalmology, 107*(2), 229–230. https://doi.org/10.1016/s0161-6420(99)00094-9.

Lee, P. P., Hays, R., & Spritzer, K. (1993). The functional impact of blurred vision on health status. *Investigative Ophthalmology & Visual Science, 34,* 790.

Lee, P. P., Whitcup, S. M., Hays, R. D., et al. (1995). The relationship between visual acuity and functioning and well-being among diabetics. *Quality of Life Research, 4,* 319–323.

Leidy, N. K., Revicki, D. A., & Geneste, B. (1999). Recommendations for evaluating the validity of quality of life claims for labelling and promotion. *Value in Health, 2*(2), 113–127.

Lohr, K. N., Aaronson, N. K., & Al, E. (1996). Evaluating quality of life and health status instruments: development of scientific review criteria. *Clinical Therapeutics, 18*(2), 979–992.

Mangione, C. M., Phillips, R. S., Seddon, J. M., et al. (1992). Development of the 'Activities of Daily Vision Scale': a measure of visual functional status. *Medical Care, 30,* 1111–1126.

Mangione, C. M., Gutierrez, P. R., Lowe, G., et al. (1999). Influence of age-related maculopathy on visual functioning and health-related quality of life. *American Journal of Ophthalmology, 128*(1), 45–53. https://doi.org/10.1016/S0002-9394(99)00169-5.

Mangione, C. M., Lee, P. P., Gutierrez, P. R., et al. (2001). Development of the 25-item National Eye Institute visual function questionnaire. *Evidence-Based Eye Care, 119*, 1050–1059. https://doi.org/10.1097/00132578-200201000-00028.

Margolis, M. K., Coyne, K., & Al, E. (2002). Vision-specific instruments for the assessment of health-related quality of life and visual functioning. *Pharmacoeconomics, 20*(12), 791–812.

Massof, R. W., Ahmadian, L., Grover, L. L., et al. (2007). The activity inventory: an adaptive visual function questionnaire. *Optometry and Vision Science, 84*(8), 763–774. https://doi.org/10.1097/OPX.0b013e3181339efd.

Massof, R. W., & Rubin, G. S. (2001). Visual function assessment questionnaires. *Survey of ophthalmology, 45*(6), 531–548.

Mitchell, J., & Bradley, C. (2004). Design of an individualised measure of the impact of macular disease on quality of life (the MacDQoL). *Quality of Life Research, 13*(6), 1163–1175.

Newman, D. A., & Houser, B. P. (1991). Visual disability inventory: documenting functional impairment caused by cataract. *Journal of Cataract Refractive Surgery, 17*(2), 244–245.

Nieuwenhuijsen, E. R., Frey, W. D., & Al, E. (1991). Measuring small gains using the ICIDH severity of disability scale: assessment practice among older people who are blind. *International Disability Studies, 13*(2), 29–33.

Okamoto, F., Okamoto, Y., & Al, E. (2008). Vision-related quality of life and visual function after retinal detachment surgery. *American Journal of Ophthalmology, 146*(1), 85–90.

Parrish, R. K. (1996). Visual impairment, visual functioning, and quality of life assessment in patients with glaucoma. *Transactions of the American Ophthalmological Society, 94*, 919–1028.

Pesudovs, K., & Coster, D. J. (1998). An instrument for assessment of subjective visual disability in cataract patients. *British Journal of Ophthalmology, 82*(6), 617–624. https://doi.org/10.1136/bjo.82.6.617.

Rahi, J. S., Tadi, V., Keeley, S., et al. (2011). Capturing children and young people's perspectives to identify the content for a novel vision-related quality of life instrument. *Ophthalmology, 118*(5), 819–824. https://doi.org/10.1016/j.ophtha.2010.08.034.

Rainey, L., Elsman, E. B. M., van Nispen, R. M. A., et al. (2016, Oct). Comprehending the impact of low vision on the lives of children and adolescents: a qualitative approach. *Qual Life Res., 25*(10), 2633–2643. https://doi.org/10.1007/s11136-016-1292-8. Epub 2016 Apr 13.

Rubin, G. S., Adamsons, I. A., & Stark, W. J. (1993). Comparison of acuity, contrast sensitivity, and disability glare before and after cataract surgery. *Archives of Ophthalmology, 111*(1), 56–61.

Rubin, G. S., Bandeen Roche, K., Prasada-Rao, P., et al. (1994). Visual impairment and disability in older adults. *Optometry and Vision Science, 71*, 750–760.

Ryan, B., Court, H., & Margrain, T. H. (2008). Measuring low vision service outcomes: Rasch analysis of the 7 item NEIVFQ. *Optometry and Vision Science, 85*(2), 112–121.

Schalock, R. L. (2000). Three decades of quality of life. *Focus on Autism and Other Developmental Disabilities, 15*(2), 116–127.

Scott, I. U., Schein, O. D., West, S., et al. (1994). Functional status and quality of life measurement among ophthalmic patients. *Archives of Ophthalmology, 112*, 329–335.

Sloane, M., Ball, K., & Al, E. (1992). The visual activities questionnaire: developing an instrument for assessing problems in everyday visual tasks. *OSA Technical Digest Noninvasive Assessment of the Visual System, 1*, 26–29.

Steinberg, E. P., Tielsch, J. M., Schein, O. D., et al. (1994). The VF-14: an index of functional impairment in patients with cataract. *Archives of Ophthalmology, 112*, 630–638.

Stelmack, J. A., & Massof, R. W. (2007). Using the VA LV VFQ-48 and LV VFQ-20 in low vision rehabilitation. *Optometry and Vision Science, 84*, 705–709.

Stelmack, J. A., Tang, X. C., Reda, D. J., et al. (2008). Outcomes of the veterans affairs low vision intervention trial (LOVIT). *Archives of Ophthalmology, 126*(5), 608–617. https://doi.org/10.1097/IEB.0b013e31818913ca.

Stelmack, J. A., Szlyk, J., Stelmack, T., et al. (2002). Sensitivity of the VA LV VFQ-48 to change after low vision rehabilitation. *Investigative Ophthalmology & Visual Science, 43*(13), 3816.

Stelmack, J. A., Tang, X. C., & Al, E. (2004). Psychometric properties of the Veterans Affairs Low-Vision Visual Functioning Questionnaire. *Investigative Ophthalmology & Visual Science, 45*(11), 3919–3928. https://doi.org/10.1167/iovs.04-0208.

Stelmack, J. A., Tang, X. C., Reda, D. J., et al. (2007). The Veterans Affairs Low Vision Intervention Trial (LOVIT): design and methodology. *Clinical Trials, 4*(6), 650–660. https://doi.org/10.1177/1740774507085274.

Study protocol for the World Health Organization project to develop a Quality of Life assessment instrument (WHOQOL). (1993). *Quality of Life Research, 2*, 153–159.

Szlyk, J., Arditi, A., & Al, E. (1990). Self-report in functional assessment of low vision. *Journal of Visual Impairment and Blindness, 84*, 61–66.

Tabrett, D. R., & Latham, K. (2010). Derivation of the Acceptance and Self-Worth Adjustment Scale. *Optometry and Vision Science, 87*(11), 899–907.

Tadić, V., Cooper, A., Cumberland, P., et al. (2013). Development of the Functional Vision Questionnaire for children and young people with visual impairment: the FVQ-CYP. *Ophthalmology, 120*(12), 2725–2732. https://doi.org/10.1016/j.ophtha.2013.07.055.

Taylor, J. J., Bambrick, R., Brand, A., et al. (2017). Effectiveness of portable electronic magnifiers for near vision activities in low vision: a randomized crossover trial. *Ophthalmic and Physiological Optics, 37*, 370–384.

Thornicroft, G., & Slade, M. (2000). Are routine outcome measures feasible in mental health? *Quality in Health Care, 9*(2), 84.

Van Nispen, R. M. A., Knol, D. L., Langelaan, M., et al. (2011). Re-evaluating a vision-related quality of life questionnaire with item response theory (IRT) and differential item functioning (DIF) analyses. *BMC Medical Research Methodology, 11*. https://doi.org/10.1186/1471-2288-11-125.

Weih, L. M., Hassell, J. B., & Keeffe, J. (2002, April). Assessment of the impact of vision impairment. *Clinical and Epidemiologic Research, 43*(4).

WHO. (1995). WHOQOL: Measuring Quality of LIfe.

Wilkie, R., Peat, G., Thomas, E., et al. (2005). The Keele Assessment of Participation: a new instrument to measure participation restriction in population studies. Combined qualitative and quantitative examination of its psychometric properties. *Quality of Life Research, 14*(8), 1889–1899. https://doi.org/10.1007/s11136-005-4325-2.

Williams, R. A., Brody, B. L., Thomas, R. G., et al. (1998). The psychosocial impact of macular degeneration. *Archives of Ophthalmology, 116*(4), 514–520. https://doi.org/10.1001/archopht.116.4.514.

Wolffsohn, J. S., & Cochrane, A. L. (2000). Design of the Low Vision Quality-of-Life Questionnaire (LVQOL) and measuring the outcome of low-vision rehabilitation. *American Journal of Ophthalmology, 130*(6), 793–802.

Wormald, R. P. L., Wright, L. A., Popay, J., et al. (1993). Population-based study of the factors affecting visual function of visually disabled older people. *Investigative Ophthalmology & Visual Science, 34*, 788.

5

Magnification

POSSIBLE APPROACHES

If the low-vision patient cannot resolve the retinal image, despite the fact that it is optimally focussed onto the retina by their refractive correction, then it is necessary for it to be made larger. The intention is that the larger retinal image is sufficiently large for the patient to recognise, despite the ocular pathology impairing their visual performance.

From Fig. 5.1, it can be seen that the angles subtended at the nodal point of the eye by rays of light from both the object and the image are the same: that is, the ray of light from the top of the object passes straight through the nodal point without deviation, and forms the top of the image. Fig. 5.1A represents the situation before any magnifying device is introduced: it can be seen that the retinal image size is proportional to the angle subtended at the nodal point, and if there is to be an increase in the retinal image size, then this ray of light from the object must form a larger angle at the nodal point of the eye.

There are some important general points to be made concerning magnification as it relates to visual impairment (VI):

1. It is relative: it is the ratio comparing the situation before and after some change in the viewing environment, or perhaps with and without some optical or electronic appliance. Because magnification is relative, it cannot have a value of 0. Magnification may therefore be <1, in which case the retinal image is smaller, or it is >1, which is the situation required to improve acuity. (Note that the use of optical and electronic devices to minify images [magnification <1×], will be discussed in Chapter 12).

2. The apparent magnification achieved by an optical magnifier may not directly relate to the magnification formula.

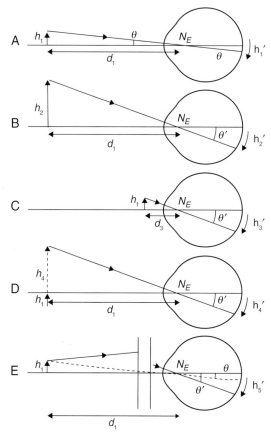

Fig. 5.1 A schematic representation of the retinal image size created by (A) an unmagnified object, in comparison to (B) to (E) which illustrate the four alternative ways to magnify the retina image: (B) increasing the object size; (C) decreasing the viewing distance; (D) transverse magnification and (E) angular magnification. d, object distance; h, object size; h', image size, N_E Nodal point of the eye; θ, angle subtended at nodal point by object; θ', angle subtended at nodal point by image.

For example, an observer looking through a magnifier lens might compare the image as seen outside and through the magnifier, but this is not the same as the change in retinal image size for the observer with and without the magnifier as expressed in the magnification formula. By contrast, for an electronic magnifier, the apparent magnification experienced by comparing the image outside and through the device relates well to the magnification formula.

3. The degree of magnification varies considerably for the different approaches to be described here: likely values range from 1.5× to 5× for simple strategies like changing object size and distance; 1.5× to 20× for optical devices; and 3× to 100× for electronic devices.

4. To put this degree of magnification into context, it can be compared to spectacle magnification. Spectacle magnification is the effect of plus and minus lenses used to correct ametropia: minus lenses make images smaller, whilst plus lenses make them bigger. This does affect retinal image size (the high myope in spectacles may have slightly poorer visual acuity (VA) than when wearing contact lenses) and also affects cosmetic appearance—the observer sees the spectacle wearer's eyes as smaller or larger. However, the amount of spectacle magnification is very small in comparison to magnifying devices—about 1% per dioptre. Putting this into terms of retinal image size increase, 4% spectacle magnification would be 1.04× magnification, for example: or to put it another way, 3× magnification would be 300%.

In mathematical terms:

$$\text{magnification (M)} = \frac{\text{new retinal image size}}{\text{original retinal image size}}$$

Fig. 5.1A shows the situation 'before' magnification, with the retinal image size proportional to θ, the angle subtended by the object at the nodal point of the eye (N_E). Figs. 5.1B to 5.1E show the situation 'after' the different forms of magnification have been used, with the magnified retinal image size proportional to the new angle θ' subtended at the nodal point of the eye.

Therefore,

$$\text{magnification} = \frac{\theta'}{\theta} \text{ which, for small angles,} \approx \frac{\tan\theta'}{\tan\theta}$$

There are four ways in which magnification can be achieved, which are summarised here and explored in detail in the forthcoming chapters.

Relative Size Magnification (Increasing Object Size)

This is illustrated schematically in Fig. 5.1B.

$$M = \frac{\tan\theta'}{\tan\theta} = \frac{h_2/d_1}{h_1/d_1} = \frac{h_2 \times d_1}{d_1 \times h_1}$$

$$M = \frac{h_2}{h_1} = \frac{\text{new object size}}{\text{original object size}}$$

The most common example of the use of this type of magnification is large print either commercially available (such as for books or music), in correspondence (such as a large print utility bill), locally printed (such as handouts for a student with VI in school) or on a screen (such as increasing font size to read messages on a smartphone). The magnification achieved can be determined very simply by a direct measurement of the size of the letter in the large print sample compared to an equivalent letter in a sample of the original text. In this case, we might not actually have the 'original' object to carry out the measurement, so it may be more accurate to say that the magnification is relative to a habitual or expected size for normal print. This form of magnification is usually limited to about 2.5× on paper because of physical limits to the size of book or page which can be obtained practically, but much larger amounts can be achieved on a screen (Fig. 5.2) (see Chapter 6). This form of magnification could also be used for a distance task: for example, obtaining a larger screen television. In this case, practicality (and cost) will limit the amount of magnification available.

Relative Distance Magnification (Decreasing Viewing Distance)

$$M = \frac{\tan\theta'}{\tan\theta} = \frac{h_1/d_3}{h_1/d_1} = \frac{h_1 \times d_1}{d_3 \times h_1}$$

$$M = \frac{d_1}{d_3} = \frac{\text{original object distance}}{\text{new object distance}}$$

One of the simplest ways to magnify is by decreasing the viewing distance (see Fig. 5.1C). A change in the viewing distance for watching television from 3 to 1 m would give 3× magnification, for example. The method is equally applicable to near vision, where moving the reading task from the typical 30 to 5 cm, for example, would give 6× magnification. The disadvantage now is that such a viewing distance will make a considerable accommodative (and convergence, if viewing is binocular) demand. Myopes can, and should be encouraged to, achieve a close viewing distance without excessive accommodation by removing their spectacles. For all other patients a way is needed to bring the object closer without any accommodative demand, and a simple plus lens can fulfil this requirement. If the object is placed at the focal point of the plus lens, the image is at optical infinity, and there is no demand on the accommodation.

In order to assign a magnification value to a particular plus lens, however, it must be compared to some standard 'before' value—by convention this is to +4.00 DS, provided either by a spectacle lens or by the patient's own accommodative effort. To

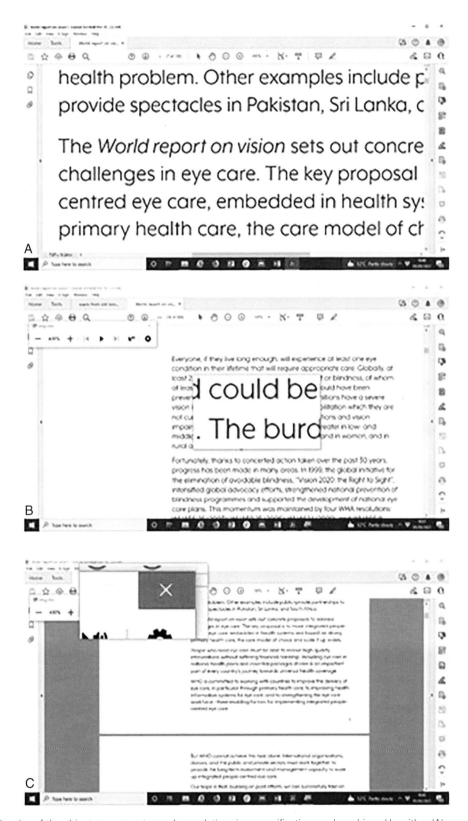

Fig. 5.2 Increasing the size of the object on screen to produce relative size magnification can be achieved by either (A) magnifying the document only using the Adobe software, or (B) magnifying a moving segment of the screen using 'Ease of Access' via the Windows Control Panel. The method in (A) does not affect the quality of the print display but that in (B) does; however, the moving magnifier also allows the toolbar and status bar to be magnified, as shown in (C).

be strictly accurate, of course, it is the focal lengths of the two lenses which are being compared: that is, the viewing distances allowed by each lens without requiring accommodation.

So the formula can be adjusted here to

$$M = \frac{\text{original object distance}}{\text{new object distance}}$$

$$= \frac{\text{focal length of} + 4.00DS \text{ lens}}{\text{focal length of magnifier lens}}$$

As power is the reciprocal of focal length, then for the example of a +40.00 DS lens,

$$M = \frac{\text{power of magnifier lens}}{+4.00} = \frac{+40.00}{+4.00} = 10x$$

Therefore, the magnification allowed by any plus lens is $M = F/4$ for an object at the focal point of the plus lens. It could also be expressed in terms of the 'original' and 'new' ('before' and 'after') viewing distances:

$$M = \frac{\text{focal length of} + 4.00DS \text{ lens}}{\text{focal length of magnifier lens}} = \frac{25cm}{2.5cm} = 10x$$

It must be emphasised that it is the viewing distance allowed by the lens which creates the magnification, hence plus lens magnification is an example of relative distance magnification (see Chapter 7).

Transverse (Real Image) Magnification

This is shown in Fig. 5.1D. This is typical of the situation with an electronic (video) system, where a magnified image of the object is created on a display screen. This real image is created in approximately the same location as the original object, and its size can actually be measured directly (with a millimetre scale) from the face of the magnifying device (Fig. 5.3). This is then compared to the size of the original object to determine

the magnification. A simple method is to use a millimetre scale as the object and use a second millimetre scale to measure its image (see Chapter 8).

$$M = \frac{\tan\theta'}{\tan\theta} = \frac{h_4/d_1}{h_1/d_1} = \frac{h_4 \times d_1}{d_1 \times h_1}$$

$$M = \frac{h_4}{h_1} = \frac{\text{size of real image}}{\text{size of original object}}$$

Angular (Telescopic) Magnification

In this case (see Fig. 5.1F.)

$$M = \frac{\tan\theta'}{\tan\theta}$$

$$= \frac{\text{angle subtended at eye by}\,(\text{telescope})\,\text{image}}{\text{angle subtended at eye by object}}$$

This is potentially a very versatile method of magnification, as it does not involve any change in the object or the viewing distance. Unfortunately, the optical system of the telescope presents considerable practical difficulties, which make it less widely used than might be expected from a simple consideration of this magnification formula. The magnification provided by the system makes an object seen through the telescope appear larger than the directly viewed object and a simultaneous comparison of the two retinal images allows the magnification to be estimated (Fig. 5.4).

If the patient was to view a distance acuity chart through a 4× telescope, the detail within the letters would be four times larger (or they may describe it as appearing four times closer). Thus, a letter which would be designated as 0.0 logMAR (6/6) would have the same angular subtense as one labelled 0.6

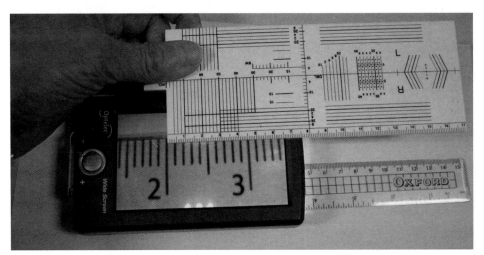

Fig. 5.3 To measure the transverse magnification produced by a portable electronic magnifier: the magnifier is used to display the image of a millimetre scale, and a second scale is used to measure the image size. In this case, an object size of 1 cm is magnified to an image size of 4.5 cm, giving 4.5× magnification.

TABLE 5.1 The Different Types of Magnification Strategy Available, the Effects on Viewing Distance and Field of View and the Task Distance for Which These Strategies Are Practical

Types of Magnification	Field of View	Working Space	Distance of Task
Increase size	No change	No change	N (I, D very limited)
Decrease distance	No change	Decreased	D, I or N
Decrease distance using plus lens	Decreased	Decreased	N
Transverse	Decreased	No change	N (I, D limited)
Angular (telescopic)	Decreased	No change	D, I or N

D, Distance; *I*, intermediate; *N*, near.

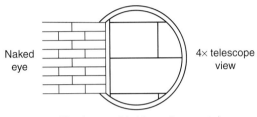

Fig. 5.4 The magnification provided by a distance telescope can be determined by direct comparison of the view obtained through the telescope and with the naked eye. If the object viewed has a repetitive structure (such as a brick wall), a quantitative estimate of telescope magnification can be made from the number of unmagnified bricks which are equivalent in height to one magnified brick.

logMAR (6/24) (i.e. 6/(6 × 4)) when seen directly. Put another way, an object which could just be resolved at 6 m could now be identified four times further away (at 24 m).

Of the many different types of magnification and magnifying device which are available, each falls into one of these four different categories. Each will be considered in more detail in the following chapters. Whilst it is not strictly necessary to understand the optics of all the devices in order to prescribe them, it is sensible to know as much as possible about the aids being used: it is then possible to determine exactly what '4×' means when written on the side of a magnifier, or whether a new design offers a worthwhile improvement on current designs.

Knowing the characteristics of the strategies available allows one to be selected to match the patient's requirements precisely. In addition to the differences in magnification available by the different methods, not all are equally suitable for all tasks. Table 5.1, which compares the different methods, shows, for example, that plus lens magnifiers are only suitable for near tasks, whereas telescopes can potentially be used at all distances (see Chapter 9).

COMBINING MAGNIFICATION

Different types of magnification can be used in combination with each other, and the total magnification created is the product of the two (or more) individual values. Consider the example of a patient trying to read print with a letter size of 5 mm directly from the page, without magnification, at a distance of 40 cm. The patient then views the same print magnified to a size of 50 mm on the screen of an electronic magnifier, at a distance of 20 cm. This patient is using two types of magnification, and combining 'transverse' magnification (M_1) with 'relative distance' magnification (M_2), so taking each in turn:

$$M_1 = \frac{\text{size of real image}}{\text{size of original object}} = \frac{50 \text{ mm}}{5 \text{ mm}} = 10\text{x}$$

$$M_2 = \frac{\text{original object distance}}{\text{new object distance}} = \frac{40 \text{ cm}}{20 \text{ cm}} = 2\text{x}$$

The combined magnification is

$$M_{\text{TOTAL}} = M_1 \times M_2 = 10 \times 2 = 20\text{x}$$

So the retinal image of the letters viewed on the screen from the closer distance is 20× the size of the original image of the letters viewed direct from further away.

6

Relative Size Magnification: Increasing the Object Size

LARGE PRINT

Increasing the size of the object is most commonly put into practice in the form of 'large print', when it may be used alone, or in addition to another form of magnification such as a hand-held plus lens.

The size of print used varies between sources, but is approximately 18- to 24-point. Print of 16-point size may be called 'enlarged' and 'giant' print is 24-point or greater. As well as the increase in size of approximately 1.5× to 2.5× provided by large print in comparison to 'standard' print (which is typically 10- or 12-point), the typeface, letter spacing, and line length and spacing, may all differ. These features, along with the colour of the text and background, and the print contrast, could be changed in order to increase legibility. There is no standard for large print, and publishers seem to select print characteristics for aesthetic reasons, so not all large print books will be read equally easily by a particular individual.

There is an extensive research literature on the topic of typeface legibility in reading (Bigelow, 2019), including some studies of readers who are visually impaired. One very noticeable characteristic of a font is whether it is proportionally spaced, (a thin letter like l takes up less space than a wide letter like m) or fixed-width (monospaced: all letters take up the same space). Nowadays most fonts are the former, although the latter makes it easier to estimate word length (important when planning eye movements for reading) and may be better for those with central vision loss who may experience more crowding (Chung, 2014). Kerning can also be added to software fonts. This is an increase in the spacing between certain letter pairs to avoid confusion: so, for example, cl is not mistaken for d, or nn is not read as m.

Sans-serif fonts are thought to be easier to read than seriffed letters, and feature in texts aimed at those with learning disabilities. The Tiresias and the American Printing House for the Blind fonts (APHont) for visually impaired readers also use that rationale. Gary Rubin and colleagues found that people with low vision read Tiresias more quickly than three other fonts (Helvetica, Foundry Form Sans and Time New Roman), but that this was because at each font size, Tiresias is slightly larger than the other fonts (Rubin et al., 2006). When x-height was equalised, there was no difference in reading speed between these typefaces by people with low vision. Xiong et al. (2018) tested two other specially designed fonts—Eido and Maxular—against Courier, Helvetica and Times Roman (Fig. 6.1) (Xiong et al., 2018). They found that Courier allowed those with macular degeneration to read text with a significantly smaller x-height (i.e. better reading acuity), but Courier (and the other fonts with wider spacing) led to slightly lower reading speed.

People with macular disease read more quickly and with fewer errors when line spacing and word spacing are increased (Blackmore-Wright et al., 2013) although this effect is quite small and is suggested only for those with very slow reading speed (Calabrèse et al., 2010). Increased spacing on printed text requires considerably more paper and is not always practical to implement.

Large Print Books and Other Publications

Previously only produced by specialist publishers, large print books are now also in the catalogues of mainstream publishers, and available from online suppliers. They are also commonly available through local public libraries, although the range of titles available varies considerably. A number of religious publishers produce large print versions of the Bible, and devotional literature for a number of denominations is available. Technically, there is no limitation to how printed material could be formatted, but there are extensive copyright restrictions, which limit the ability to modify or distribute a published work.

A 'Big Print' TV and radio guide is available from Royal National Institute of Blind People (RNIB) on subscription. Both RNIB and the Partially Sighted Society sell crossword

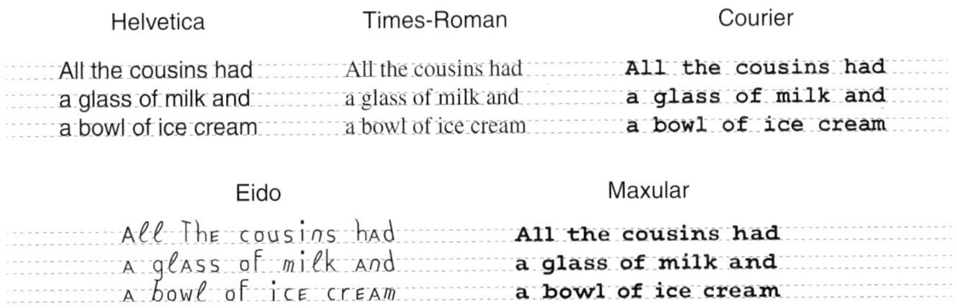

	Helvetica	Times-Roman	Courier

All the cousins had
a glass of milk and
a bowl of ice cream

All the cousins had
a glass of milk and
a bowl of ice cream

All the cousins had
a glass of milk and
a bowl of ice cream

Eido

Maxular

All The cousins had
A glass of milk And
A bowl of ice cream

All the cousins had
a glass of milk and
a bowl of ice cream

Fig. 6.1 Samples of five different fonts used to display the same sentence, matched for x-height (the *dashed lines* are included to confirm this). Eido and Maxular fonts were specifically developed for readers with macular degeneration. From Xiong, Y. Z., Lorsung, E. A., Mansfield, J. S., Bigelow, C., & Legge, G. E. (2018). Fonts designed for macular degeneration: Impact on reading. Investigative Ophthalmology and Visual Science, 59(10), 4182–4189. https://doi.org/10.1167/iovs.18-24334.

and puzzle books, diaries and calendars in their online shops; RNIB also offer recipe books. CustomEyes produces about 4000 children's titles (both educational and fiction) as books with a user-selected format (Guide Dogs, n.d.). The typeface, weight (bold or normal), font size, line spacing, paper colour and binding (e.g. spiral, so the pages lie flat) can all be customised. Specialist centres such as the Joseph Clarke Service in London can produce books in specific formats, although it may take some time for these books to be made. It will often be easier for students to obtain books electronically and to read them on a tablet computer or e-reader. Alternatively, the RNIB library provides textbooks in electronic formats which can be printed out in the font, colour and spacing chosen by the person with low vision.

Other Large Print Documents

It is a requirement of the *Equality Act 2010* that service providers do not treat the users of their services less favourably because of their disability. Providers are required to make reasonable adjustments, and one very simple option which is offered is the provision of large print information (other accessible formats are also usually offered such as Braille or audio). Banks, utility companies and local councils, should therefore, on request, provide any correspondence or information leaflets in the preferred format.

From July 2016, the *Health and Social Care Act 2012* required that organisations providing NHS health and adult social care must follow the Accessible Information Standard. This requires that individuals with a disability or sensory loss are asked if they have any information or communication needs, and how those needs should be met. They must then receive information in a format they can access, and large print would be an important option. Accessing information about their medication, and reading pharmacy labels, are acknowledged concerns of patients with visual impairment (Latham et al., 2011; Leat et al., 2016). These issues should be addressed by the Accessibility Standard, but there was poor awareness of its existence amongst patients (NHS, 2017) and of the needs of visually impaired patients amongst pharmacists (Barnett et al., 2017). Patients should therefore be encouraged to be proactive if they are experiencing problems managing their medications, or indeed in receiving any health information

in an inaccessible format. The RNIB have published a 'toolkit' giving guidance on how to proceed (Royal National Institute of Blind People (RNIB), n.d.a).

There are a number of commercial transcription services which specialise in producing documents in Braille, and a number of them are also equipped to provide large print. There is obviously some expense and delay inherent in having items produced this way. Large print material can, however, be produced by enlargement on a photocopier, and this could be suggested to a patient for, for example, a favourite knitting pattern or recipe. Local public libraries and high-street stationery shops often have such equipment, and charges should be modest. If copying is done repeatedly to increase print size still further, the print contrast will diminish rapidly. It should be noted that smaller font sizes have proportionally greater letter spacing, so text magnified by photocopying (or indeed by viewing it through any magnifying device) will have greater spacing than when printing the document using a larger font size.

Large print music is available which is produced in a slightly different format to standard musical scores. If the standard score is simply enlarged overall, then the spacing between notes becomes excessive, and there is increased risk of the reader losing the line. Modified Stave Notation (MSN) is used, where the symbols are enlarged (and can be repositioned and/or explained by words), and redundant spaces are eliminated: typically any text is 24-point bold. Music notation software, available in the form of an app, has made the production of MSN much easier, and users can customise and store their preferred layout.

Advantages and Disadvantages of Large Print as a Rehabilitation Strategy

Using large print as a method of magnification has the following advantages and disadvantages:

Advantages

1. The patient's habitual reading posture can still be used; the object is viewed binocularly at a 'normal' reading distance.
2. No special instruction or training in use is required, whereas this would be necessary to benefit fully from the use of an optical aid.

3. There is no unusual cosmetic appearance, nor any of the restrictions apparent with optical aids (such as aberrations, or a reduced field-of-view). Some school students may, however, be sensitive to being seen by peers with very large-scale worksheets or examination papers when they have requested large print.

4. No eye examination or professional advice is required: the patient can take the initiative and try the method out for themselves.

Disadvantages

1. In the case of a printed book, as the print size has increased, the book itself must also increase proportionately in physical size. This can make it difficult to handle, and to carry home from the library! In some very thick books (such as the Bible), the publishers may use very thin paper to moderate the size of the book, and this can be difficult to read because of shadows partially seen through from the reverse of the page.

2. As most books are in portrait format, enlarged print can mean very few words per line, which can make navigating around the page more challenging: the reader has to make more return sweep eye movements from the end of one line to the beginning of the next line.

3. There is often only a standard, limited amount of magnification available, rarely exceeding 2×. Nonetheless, the RNIB survey (Bruce et al., 1991) found that 58% of blind and 75% of partially sighted individuals could comfortably read a print sample of bold 16-point type, thus suggesting that this strategy may be more widely applicable than previously thought.

4. Only a limited range of book titles is available (probably <1% of the titles available in print), with the publishers concentrating on fiction likely to appeal to a wide readership. There are almost no technical or reference books, although some dictionaries are available. When diagrams or tables are enlarged, the captions may remain in a smaller font. There are also relatively few children's fiction books, particularly for those in their teens.

5. If enlarged print is prepared by photocopying, the print contrast and quality will suffer and pictures will usually be black-and-white. All material must be organised and prepared well in advance (which may be a disadvantage for vocational or educational use).

There is some controversy about whether children should invariably be encouraged to use large print, rather than using 'normal' print and gaining magnification with an optical device. There are further criticisms in using large print in the educational setting: it does not provide the child with a means of access to general print sources outside school, and it does not remove the need for other aids to cope with magnification needs for intermediate and distant tasks (e.g. art and craft work, or mobility). Corn and Ryser (1989) found that children using optical aids and normal print continued to show an increase in reading speed and ability throughout their school career, whereas the performance of those who used large print appeared to plateau. Koenig et al. (1992)

describe an objective procedure for determining a child's reading performance under these different circumstances to decide which method is 'best': in general, however, large print did not increase reading speed, accuracy or the working distance. McLeish (2007), however, suggests that optical aids provide a slower reading speed for children, and that in fast-moving interactive classroom sessions, the large print option will prove much more practical (McLeish, 2007). For adult readers, Lovie-Kitchin and Whittaker (1998) found no difference between reading performance using relative size or relative distance magnification.

E-BOOKS

Electronic books, or e-books, are publications which are made available digitally and which can be accessed via reading from the screen of a computer or smartphone or from a dedicated e-reader (Fig. 6.2).

Usually the e-readers do not use a standard LCD screen, but a so-called 'electronic ink' display which consists of microcapsules which, depending on the charge applied to them, can appear black or white. Whilst this display maintains its contrast under any lighting conditions (unlike an LCD), it is also a relatively low contrast display (~60% Michelson contrast) (Crossland et al., 2010). This may make it unsuitable for those users with poor contrast sensitivity, as the contrast reserve (see Chapter 3) will be too low to support high fluent reading, although newer screens may offer higher contrast.

E-books are popular (with normally sighted individuals as well) for the convenience of downloading titles online, and being able to 'carry' many titles within a lightweight handheld device. For users with visual impairment, they give the additional benefit of being able to modify the way the text is displayed (although different devices will have a different range of options): depending on the specific device used, there may also be a text-to-speech audio, or Braille display, option. However, some of the accessibility options only apply once the book is 'opened', and are not available on the entry screen.

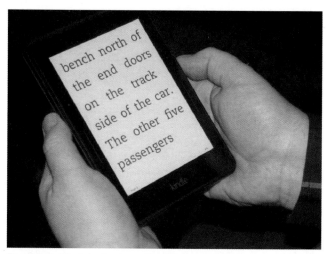

Fig. 6.2 A 'Kindle' e-book reader with the text displayed at the maximum size.

Technical books are well-suited to the format because the text can be searched for keywords. Despite the fact that they have only existed for a comparatively short time, the mainstream popularity of e-books means there are many more titles available than there are in physical large print books.

Unfortunately, e-books do not all use the same electronic file systems, and so an e-book designed for one e-reader will not work on a different e-reader. E-books can be purchased online, and are available to borrow free of charge through local public libraries (through the Libby or Overdrive apps). Project Gutenberg and Standard Ebooks are both organisations which make e-books available free of charge, but these are restricted to those which are not covered by copyright restrictions, so tend to be older 'classics'.

Magazines, periodicals and newspapers are also available in equivalent formats for reading electronically.

Gill et al. (2013) compared the reading performance using e-readers and printed text of equal size for individuals with macular degeneration and varied levels of near vision. Individuals preferred the large print because of its simplicity. However, the iPad allowed slightly faster reading speed (which the authors attributed to increased contrast of the display), whilst reading using the Sony e-reader was slower, which was attributed to the restricted display size (likely to be a particular issue with larger text sizes).

As electronic devices usually weigh less than a large print book, it is easier for the person to hold it close, providing some relative distance magnification.

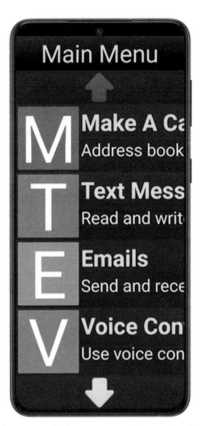

Fig. 6.3 The large text display on a smartphone using Synapptic software. Synapptic Ltd.

LARGE TEXT IN EVERYDAY USAGE

A Dymo labelling machine can produce labels with letters up to 24-point size. Landline or mobile phones with clear numerals and/or extra-large keypads are available from commercial suppliers or the RNIB (Fig. 6.3).

Easy-to-see large-numeral clocks, watches and calculators are available from the RNIB. RNIB also sell a remote control with large clearly marked buttons, which can be used to replace an existing one which has markings which are too small to see: however, the user will need to use their existing remote to programme the new device initially. Examination of the wide range of household appliances which are generally available will show that the control panels are very variable and idiosyncratic in the size and contrast of the labelling that they use. An individual with visual impairment might want to add the requirement for large, high contrast labelling of the controls (and a large print instruction book) to the list of their requirements when purchasing an oven or washing machine. There are some appliances designed specifically for the visually impaired user, but they are likely to place more emphasis on providing audio descriptions of control functions.

LARGE TEXT ON THE COMPUTER

As computer monitors have got larger, more people with visual impairment can manage with a 'standard' display,

especially if text size can be selected within the programme and the viewing distance can be reduced to allow relative distance magnification to be used as well (e.g. a desktop monitor stand with a flexible arm). It is important that the individual has a refractive correction that is appropriate, especially if unusual viewing distances are used. Large-character computer keyboards (or stick-on enlarged numerals to adapt a standard computer keyboard) are available to make the characters easier to see (and usually also come in reverse contrast and black-on-yellow combinations). If electronic documents can be edited, these can be printed in any size or layout required.

With regard to the information on screen, there are many accessibility options which allow the user to customise the appearance of the display, one of which is increasing text size. The RNIB (n.d.b) and AbilityNet (n.d.) give detailed guidance on how to implement this: the latter also offers assistance with suggested adaptations for motor, hearing and cognitive difficulties. In brief, in Windows, via the 'Ease of Access' settings, you can magnify just the text, or magnify the screen as well. The screen magnification also comes with the option to magnify the whole screen (which can make navigation more difficult because of the difficulty of locating the required section of the text), or part of the screen as a horizontal section scrolling down the screen, or the so-called 'magnifier' view which just magnifies the area around the cursor and displays it within an outlined oblong. Many other display colour and contrast changes are possible (in addition to screen reading options) and the mouse cursor can be enlarged and made higher contrast.

On Apple computers, these settings are changed through the accessibility section of the system preferences. Apple have advisors in their high-street stores who can guide users through the available settings. Working through accessibility options on any computer can be daunting to users who are not very comfortable with technology. Often a friend or relative can help and several charities for visual impairment have technology helplines. Alternatively, users may be able to seek in-person advice from local Digital Inclusion Officers employed by local societies or Social Services.

If these accessibility changes are insufficient, there are a number of software programs which will enhance the display (e.g. ZoomText [n.d.] and Dolphin [n.d.]). The commercially available systems may not be compatible with older devices, or with some types of software, but the manufacturers may provide free trials which allow a test to be made.

REFERENCES

AbilityNet. (n.d.). My Computer My Way. Retrieved February 3, 2022, from https://mcmw.abilitynet.org.uk/impairment/vision.

Barnett, N., El Bushra, A., Huddy, H., et al. (2017). How to support patients with sight loss in pharmacy. *Pharmaceutical Journal, 299*(7904), 1–11. https://doi.org/10.1211/PJ.2017.20203346.

Bigelow, C. (2019). Typeface features and legibility research. *Vision Research, 165*, 162–172. https://doi.org/10.1016/j.visres.2019.05.003.

Blackmore-Wright, S., Georgeson, M. A., & Anderson, S. J. (2013). Enhanced text spacing improves reading performance in individuals with macular disease. *PLoS ONE, 8*(11), e80325. https://doi.org/10.1371/journal.pone.0080325.

Bruce, I., McKennell, A., & Walker, E. (1991). Blind and partially sighted adults in Britain: The RNIB Survey Volume 1. HMSO.

Calabrèse, A., Bernard, J. B., Hoffart, L., et al. (2010). Small effect of interline spacing on maximal reading speed in low-vision patients with central field loss irrespective of scotoma size. *Investigative Ophthalmology & Visual Science, 51*(2), 1247–1254. https://doi.org/10.1167/iovs.09-3682.

Chung, S. T. L. (2014). Size or spacing: Which limits letter recognition in people with age-related macular degeneration? *Vision Research, 101*, 167–176. https://doi.org/10.1016/j.visres.2014.06.015.

Corn, A., & Ryser, G. (1989). Access to print for students with low vision. *Journal of Visual Impairment & Blindness, 83*, 340–349.

Crossland, M. D., Macedo, A. F., & Rubin, G. S. (2010). Electronic books as low vision aids. *British Journal of Ophthalmology, 94*(8), 1109. https://doi.org/10.1136/bjo.2009.170167.

Dolphin. (n.d.). SuperNova. Retrieved January 3, 2022, from https://yourdolphin.com/en-gb/products/individuals/supernova-magnifier-screen-reader.

Gill, K., Mao, A., Powell, A. M., & Sheidow, T. (2013). Digital reader vs print media: The role of digital technology in reading accuracy in age-related macular degeneration. *Eye, 27*(5), 639–643. https://doi.org/10.1038/eye.2013.14.

Guide Dogs. (n.d.). CustomEyes books. Retrieved January 3, 2022, from https://www.guidedogs.org.uk/getting-support/help-for-children-and-families/living-independently/customeyes-books/#.WeBcfztrzIU.

Koenig, A. J., Layton, C. A., & Ross, D. B. (1992). The relative effectiveness of reading in large print and with low vision devices for students with low vision. *Journal of Visual Impairment & Blindness, 86*, 48–53.

Latham, K., Waller, S., & Schaitel, J. (2011). Do best practice guidelines improve the legibility of pharmacy labels for the visually impaired? *Ophthalmic and Physiological Optics, 31*(3), 275–282. https://doi.org/10.1111/j.1475-1313.2010.00816.x.

Leat, S. J., Krishnamoorthy, A., Carbonara, A., et al. (2016). Improving the legibility of prescription medication labels for older adults and adults with visual impairment. *Canadian Pharmacists Journal, 149*(3), 174–184. https://doi.org/10.1177/1715163516641432.

Lovie-Kitchin, J., & Whittaker, S. (1998). Relative-size magnification versus relative-distance magnification: Effect on the reading performance of adults with normal and low vision. *Journal of Visual Impairment and Blindness, 92*(7), 433–446. https://doi.org/10.1177/0145482x9809200704.

McLeish, E. (2007). A study of the effect of letter spacing on the reading speed of young readers with low vision. *The British Journal of Visual Impairment, 25*(2), 133–143. https://doi.org/10.1177/0264619607075995.

NHS England. (2017). *Accessible Information Standard: Post-implementation review-report (1–22).* https://www.england.nhs.uk/accessibleinfo.

Royal National Institute of Blind People (RNIB). (n.d.a). *Accessible health information.* https://www.rnib.org.uk/campaigning/current-campaigns/accessible-information/accessible-health-information.

RNIB. (n.d.b). *Desktop accessibility.* Retrieved January 3, 2022, from https://www.rnib.org.uk/sight-loss-advice/technology-and-useful-products/technology-resource-hub-latest-facts-tips-and-guides/desktop-accessibility.

Rubin, G. S., Feely, M., Perera, S., et al. (2006). The effect of font and line width on reading speed in people with mild to moderate vision loss. *Ophthalmic & Physiological Optics, 26*(6), 545–554. https://doi.org/10.1111/j.1475-1313.2006.00409.x.

Xiong, Y. Z., Lorsung, E. A., Mansfield, J. S., et al. (2018). Fonts designed for macular degeneration: Impact on reading. *Investigative Ophthalmology & Visual Science, 59*(10), 4182–4189. https://doi.org/10.1167/iovs.18-24334.

ZoomText. (n.d.). *Zoomtext magnifier/reader.* Retrieved January 3, 2022, from https://www.freedomscientific.com/products/software/zoomtext/.

7

Relative Distance Magnification: Decreasing the Viewing Distance

THE OPTICAL PRINCIPLES OF PLUS-LENS MAGNIFIERS

The plus lens used as a magnifying aid is creating an increased retinal image size by allowing an object to be held close to the eye without requiring the accommodative effort that would usually be expected from viewing at this distance. (The individual with active accommodation can be thought of as having this magnifier inside their eye.) Optimum positioning is achieved by placing the object at the anterior focal point of the positive convex lens, so that parallel light leaves the lens, the virtual image is at infinity, and the patient's accommodation can be relaxed (Fig. 7.1A). It can be seen that the ray of light from the top of the object will pass through the optical centre of the positive lens, making an angle θ' with the optical axis. As all the rays of light leaving the lens are parallel to each other, they all make this same angle with the optical axis, including the ray which passes through the nodal point of the eye. Although the magnifier-to-object distance must be held constant and equal to the (short) focal length of the plus-lens, the magnifier-to-eye distance can be increased without affecting θ' and so the magnification remains the same (Fig. 7.1B).

In this way it is possible to use a plus-lens magnifier close to the eye, or remote from it: it can be spectacle-mounted, hand-held or on a stand, depending on the visual task requirements of the patient. Spectacle-mounted plus-lenses are occasionally called 'microscopic' lenses from the obsolete term 'simple microscope' applied to such systems. The confusing term 'loupe' may also be applied to magnifying plus lenses. This is variously defined as a hand-held plus lens held remote from the eye (Linksz, 1955), a low-power spectacle-mounted binocular correction, and, in British Standard (BS) 3521, as either a magnifier of power 5× or higher, or a low-powered binocular magnifier (BS 3521, 1991). Both these terms should be abandoned to avoid misinterpretation.

A Problem in Defining Magnification

The plus lens creates magnification by allowing the patient to adopt a closer viewing distance, and so

$$M = \frac{\text{original object distance}}{\text{new object distance}}$$

where the 'new object distance' will be the focal length of the plus lens. The 'original object distance'—the distance at which objects were habitually held—will be individual for each patient, but in order to allow the convenient labelling of magnifiers, some standard value must be adopted. Traditionally this is taken to be 25 cm, and if this viewing distance were to be used by the patient, they would require 4.00 DS of

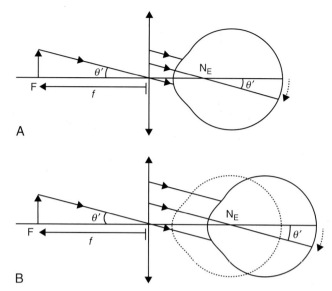

A

B

Fig. 7.1 (A) The use of a plus lens as a magnifier when held close to the eye, and with the object positioned at the anterior focal point (F) of the lens so that parallel light enters the eye. (B) The same plus lens used with an increased eye-to-magnifier distance, showing that the retinal image size remains unchanged. θ', Angular subtense; N_E, nodal point of the eye; f, focal length.

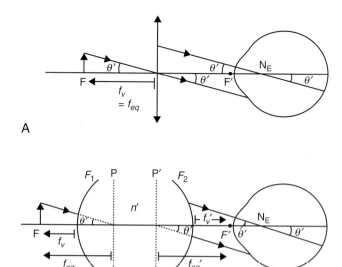

A

B

Fig. 7.2 The angular subtense (θ') at the nodal point of the eye (N_E) of an object placed at the anterior focal point (F) of a thin (A) and a thick (B) plus lens. The thick lens is in air, so the nodal points (N, N') coincide with the principal points (P, P'). The front (f_v) and back (f_v') vertex focal lengths are measured from the respective lens surfaces, and the equivalent focal lengths (f_{eq}, f_{eq}') are measured from the principal points. Comparison of (A) and (B) shows that it is the angle subtended at the nodal points of the thick lens system which determines its magnification.

accommodation or a +4.00 DS reading addition, or some combination of the two.

Thus the formula is restated as

$$M = \frac{\text{focal length of +4.00 DS lens or accommodation}}{\text{focal length of magnifier lens}}$$

$$= \frac{\text{power of magnifier lens}}{+4.00} = \frac{F}{4}$$

This formula causes some controversy, because the assumed 'standard' viewing distance of 25 cm may bear no relation to the actual reading distance that the patient has been using, and the reading addition in their prescription may not be +4.00 DS. This has led to suggestions that all plus-lens magnifiers should simply be labelled with the measured power, and then the prescriber could calculate the magnification provided in each individual case. It would be possible to devise a formula unique to the particular patient concerned: if a presbyopic patient habitually read at 40 cm with a +2.50 addition (i.e. with the object at the focal point of the lens), then their own magnification formula would be

$$M = \frac{\text{focal length of +2.50 DS ens}(40\,\text{cm})}{\text{focal length of magnifier lens}}$$

$$= \frac{\text{power of magnifier lens}}{+2.50} = \frac{F}{2.5}$$

To take another example, if a young child usually accommodated to read at a distance of 33 cm, this would require 3 DS of accommodation and his magnification formula would be $M = F/3$. These formulae would then describe, for these individual cases, exactly how much larger the retinal image

would be when using the magnifier as compared to the habitual reading situation.

Specifying Magnifier Power

A further difficulty exists, however, even in specifying the refractive power of these positive convex lenses: should the value of F in the magnification formula be front vertex power, back vertex power, or equivalent power? For a thin lens, these are all equal, but for a thick lens (Fig. 7.2):

Back vertex power

$$F_v' = \frac{1}{f_v'} = \frac{F_1 + F_2 - \left(\dfrac{t}{n'}\right)F_1F_2}{1 - \left(\dfrac{t}{n'}\right)F_1} = \frac{F_{eq}}{1 - \left(\dfrac{t}{n'}\right)F_1}$$

Front vertex power

$$F_v = \frac{1}{f_v} = \frac{F_1 + F_2 - \left(\dfrac{t}{n'}\right)F_1F_2}{1 - \left(\dfrac{t}{n'}\right)F_2} = \frac{F_{eq}}{1 - \left(\dfrac{t}{n'}\right)F_2}$$

where F_1 is the front surface power, F_2 is the back surface power, F_{eq} is the equivalent power, t is the lens centre thickness, and n' is the refractive index of the lens material. Both these power values can be determined using a focimeter, by placing the respective surface (vertex) of the lens against the lens rest of the instrument. It can be seen by comparing Figs. 7.2A and B, however, that it is equivalent power which is the relevant measure. As noted earlier, the retinal image size is determined by the angle subtended at the nodal point of the eye by the parallel beam of rays leaving the magnifier lens. This angle is that made by the ray entering the lens from the top of the object, which passes undeviated through the lens, and which makes an angle θ' at the optical centre of the thin lens or at the nodal point (principal point) of the thick lens. Thus, for a thick lens, the angle θ is inversely proportional to the equivalent focal length, and thus depends on the equivalent power.

For a plus-lens therefore the magnification formula is more accurately stated as:

$$M = \frac{\text{magnifier equivalent power}}{4} = \frac{F_{eq}}{4}$$

Labelling of plus-lens magnifiers by the manufacturer with this value of F_{eq} would allow the clinician to devise a measure of magnification that was more appropriate to the individual patient circumstances. Despite this, it is often not available, and if a power value is given it may well be that of back vertex power. It can be seen from Fig. 7.2B that the vertex focal lengths are often shorter than the equivalent focal length, so the corresponding power is higher: this may suggest a better patient performance with the magnifier than will be borne out in practice.

Equivalent power

$$F_{eq} = \frac{1}{f_{eq}} = F_1 + F_2 - \left(\frac{t}{n'}\right)F_1F_2$$

and this cannot be measured using a focimeter, although if the magnifier lens is plano-convex with $F_2 = 0$, the first principal plane coincides with the front surface of the lens, $f_{eq} = f_v$, and so the equivalent power (F_{eq}) is equal to the front vertex power (F_v). For other lens forms, there are two methods by which equivalent power can be measured relatively easily in practice.

Measuring Equivalent Power

Method 1—Suitable for Large-Diameter Single-Lens Systems

The formula below is used to determine equivalent power

$$F_{eq} = F_1 + F_2 - \left(\frac{t}{n'}\right)F_1F_2$$

with direct measurement of the unknown parameters.

A lens measure placed centrally on the surface is used to determine F_1 and F_2, but the lens measure will be calibrated for crown glass ($n' = 1.523$) so the readings must be compensated for this by multiplying the measured surface powers by the factor $(n' - 1)/(1.523 - 1)$ where n' is the refractive index of the magnifier lens. Thickness callipers can be used to measure t (which must be converted into metres for the calculation), and n' is available from reference sources.

This method, although straightforward, is only suitable for certain magnifiers. The magnifying system must be a single-lens system with only two surfaces (so that the overall power derives only from the combination of these), and it must be possible to place a lens measure across each surface: in some cases the lens diameter is smaller than the separation of the pointed feet on the lens measure, or a large plastic rim/housing around the lens prevents the lens measure from touching the lens surface. If the lens is aspheric, the surface power will be decreasing from centre to edge. If the lens diameter is large compared to the distance between the legs of the lens measure, this will not lead to much inaccuracy: however, for lower diameter lenses with surfaces above 10 DS, the power will be underestimated.

Method 2—Applicable to Any Plus-Lens System

This method can be used to measure a single- or multi-lens system, and can be performed on lenses of any diameter (Bailey, 1981a).

Fig. 7.3A shows the thick lens magnifier with parallel light from an infinitely distant object now being brought to a focus at the anterior focal point. The reciprocal of f_{eq}' would give equivalent power, but this cannot be measured accurately because the principal plane cannot be located. The image height h' can be measured, however, and power determined indirectly. To do this, the object must be moved closer than infinity (Fig. 7.3B). The angle subtended by the object at the first principal point is the same as the angle subtended by the image at the second principal point, and so in the image space

$$\tan\theta = \frac{-h'}{l'}$$

and in the object space

$$\tan\theta = \frac{h}{-l}$$

where h is the object size, l the object distance, and l' the image distance.

Equating these gives

$$\frac{-h'}{l'} = \frac{h}{-l}$$

So

$$l' = \frac{h'l}{h}$$

If the object distance l is assumed to be close to infinity, then the image distance l' approximates to the equivalent focal length f_{eq}' and

$$f_{eq}' = \frac{h'l}{h}$$

so

$$F_{eq} = \frac{h}{h'l} \qquad \text{Eq. (7.1)}$$

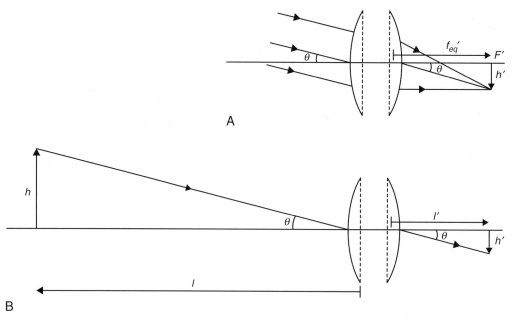

A

B

Fig. 7.3 (A) Shows the magnifier, with parallel light from an infinitely distant object forming an image of height h' at the posterior focal point, which is a distance f_{eq}' from the principal plane. (B) Shows the optical system for the practical determination of F_{eq}'. The object of height h is a distance l from the principal plane of the lens. The image of height h' is formed at a distance l' from the principal plane, but if l is large, $l' = f_{eq}'$. F' is the focal point.

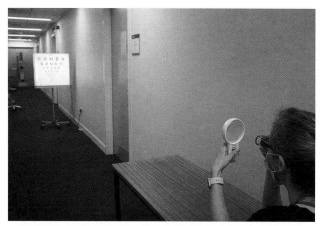

Fig. 7.4 The observer taking a measurement of the image formed by the plus lens magnifier, using a magnifier with measuring scale attached held close to their eye. The illuminated test chart acts as a distant object.

If all the measurements are taken in metres, F_{eq} is in dioptres. An illuminated Snellen letter chart makes a suitable object, with the height of the illuminated panel (or an individual letter on it) being measured to determine the object size h. The object distance (l) should be as large as possible so that the inaccuracy in locating the principal plane of the magnifier is insignificant: either 3 or 4 m should be possible in the average consulting room. The observer should be about 20 cm from the securely held plus-lens, viewing the (blurred) object through the plus-lens with a small measuring magnifier held up to the eye (Fig. 7.4).

The observer then approaches the plus lens until the (inverted) image is clearly in focus and superimposed on the

millimetre scale of the magnifier. The image size (h') should then be measured as accurately as possible, and all the values obtained (in metres) substituted into Eq. (7.1) to determine the equivalent power. To minimize percentage error, the object should be chosen so that the image size is approximately 5 mm.

Practical Considerations

Working Space and Working Distance

All plus-lens magnifiers placed in the spectacle plane produce magnification by allowing the patient to bring the object closer to the eye than the patient's available accommodation will allow. As long as parallel light leaves the magnifying system, however, the system-to-eye distance can be varied without affecting the magnification, and the *working distance* from eye to object can be large. Under these circumstances, it is the magnifier-to-object distance—the *working space*—that must be restricted, and which determines the magnification achieved. Hand-held and stand-mounted magnifiers are obviously designed to take advantage of the variable magnifier-to-eye distance, but it is also exploited by some spectacle-mounted devices where the back vertex distance is extreme (Fig. 7.5)

Despite this increase in the working distance, however, the working space remains limited—at its largest, this cannot be greater than the anterior focal length of the system. Herein lies one of the major limitations of all plus-lens magnifiers: they range in power up to +80.00 DS, when the working space drops as low as 12.5 mm. There are some tasks where this is feasible (e.g. reading for short periods), although psychologically difficult because it is so conspicuous and unusual. It may also

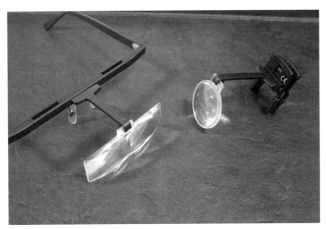

Fig. 7.5 Spectacle-mounted plus lenses, designed with an extended back vertex distance in order to increase working distance.

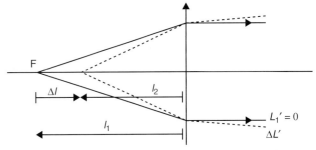

Fig. 7.6 With the object at the focal point F, a distance l_1 from the magnifier, the vergence of light leaving the lens is $L_1' = 0$. When the object moves a short distance Δl closer to the lens, the vergence changes by $\Delta L'$. The new object distance is l_2. If $\Delta L'$ is the minimum change detectable by the observer, then the depth-of-field is $2 \times \Delta l$ (since the object can move towards or away from the lens).

be very tiring to maintain the working space and difficult to illuminate the task area where the magnifier or patient overshadows it: the use of auxiliary reading stands and built-in illumination may need to be considered. For other tasks, such a restricted working space is impossibly small (e.g. writing, knitting or playing music) and in such cases alternative methods of magnification may need to be sought.

Depth-of-Field

Positioning of the object of interest at the anterior focal point of the magnifier (or in fact at any designated position) is critical, and movement of the object away from this plane will cause the vergence of light, leaving the magnifier to alter. Assuming that the eye's accommodative state remains unchanged, this will cause the previous retinal point focus to become a blur circle. The range of magnifier-to-object separations over which the object (or the magnifier) can be moved without the patient noticing any change in image clarity is termed the depth-of-field. This depth-of-field will differ for different patients using the same magnifier, as the size of the retinal blur circle depends on the pupil size, and patients will differ in their ability to detect blur. Nonetheless, it has long been recognised that depth-of-field is very small in plus-lens magnifiers, and this is in fact one of the justifications for using a stand-mounted magnifier. Short 'distance posts' could be fitted to the temporal front of a spectacle frame containing high-plus lenses to allow the maintenance of the correct working space, or a length of string of the correct working distance could be attached to the frame as a reminder of where to hold the task.

Fig. 7.6 illustrates the situation of an object placed a distance l_1 from a plus-lens magnifier (in this case, the object is at the focal point and l_1 is equal to the focal length of the magnifier). The object can move to a distance of l_2 from the lens before the patient notices that the image is blurred, so the linear depth-of-field is Δl for movement of an object towards the lens (and of course, the object could also move an equivalent distance away from the lens).

By simple geometry,

$$-l_1 = -l_2 + \Delta l$$

$$\Delta l = l_2 - l_1 = \frac{1}{L_2} - \frac{1}{L_1}$$

Considering the refraction of light by the magnifier,

$$L_2' = L_2 + F_M \quad \text{so} \quad L_2 = L_2' - F_M$$

And

$$L_1' = L_1 + F_M \quad \text{so} \quad L_1 = L_1' - F_M$$

Therefore:

$$\Delta l = \frac{1}{L_2' - F_M} - \frac{1}{L_1' - F_M} \qquad \text{Eq. (7.2)}$$

To take an example, consider a magnifier of power $F_M = +4.00$ DS, with the object at the focal point ($L_1' = 0$). Assume that a ± 0.50 DS change in vergence is the minimum that could be detected by a patient, so L_2' (the depth-of-focus) is ± 0.50 DS. If $L_2' = -0.50$ DS (for the case in which the object moves towards the lens), substituting into Eq. (7.2) gives

$$\Delta l = \frac{1}{-0.50 - 4.00} - \frac{1}{0 - 4.00}$$

$$= -0.222 - (-0.25) = +0.028 \text{ m} = +28 \text{ mm}$$

If $L_2' = +0.50$ DS (the object moves away from the lens),

$$\Delta l = \frac{1}{+0.50 - 4.00} - \frac{1}{0 - 4.00}$$

$$= -0.285 - (-0.25) = -0.035 \text{ m} = -35 \text{ mm}$$

This gives a total depth-of-field of 63 mm for a +4.00 DS ($M = 1\times$) magnifier. If we wish to investigate how the depth-of-field alters as the magnifier power changes, the previous method is rather lengthy, and a more direct method is preferable (Bennett & Rabbetts, 1984). As shown in Fig. 7.6, with the object distance equal to the focal length of the magnifier, the rays of light (shown as solid lines) which leave the magnifier are parallel ($L' = 0$, image at infinity). As the object moves a small distance Δl closer to the magnifier, the vergence of the rays of light (now shown by dashed lines) leaving the lens changes by a small amount $\Delta L'$. When this change $\Delta L'$ reaches a certain detectable value (which will be different for each patient), the image seen by the patient becomes blurred.

In terms of vergences, the refraction by the lens can be expressed as:

$$L' = L + F$$

So

$$L = L' - F$$

And

$$l = \frac{1}{L' + F} \qquad \text{Eq. (7.3)}$$

To find the effect of a change in l by a small amount Δl, the corresponding small change $\Delta L'$ in L' can be found by differentiating Eq. (7.3):

$$\Delta l = \frac{((L' - F) \times 0) - (1 \times 1)\Delta L'}{(L' - F)^2}$$

$$\Delta l = \frac{-\Delta L'}{(L' - F)^2}$$

The change in L' is occurring about the position where $L' = 0$, so the formula becomes:

$$\Delta l = \frac{-\Delta L'}{F^2}$$

or, in words,
maximum tolerable change in object position (in metres) is equal to

$$\frac{-(\text{minimum noticeable change in vergence (DS)})}{(\text{lens power})^2}$$

In the low-vision context, devices are more often labelled with the magnification rather than the power, and

$$M = \frac{\text{lens power}}{4}$$

So lens power = $4 \times M$
Therefore:

$$\Delta l = \frac{-\Delta L'}{(4M)^2}$$

Now the change in object position here is in metres, although this is likely to be a very small number. Changing the formula so that Δl is measured in millimetres gives:

$$\Delta l = \frac{-1000 \times \Delta L'}{16 \times M^2} = \frac{-62.5 \times \Delta L'}{M^2}$$

This gives the tolerable change in object position moving towards the lens (Δl positive, as $\Delta L'$ negative), but of course the object can also move away with a corresponding decrease in L' ($\Delta L'$ positive and Δl negative). This means that the full tolerable range of possible object positions (the depth-of-field) is:

$$\text{total depth} - \text{of} - \text{field(mm)}$$
$$= \frac{125 \times \text{minimum noticeable change in vergence}}{\text{magnification}^2}$$

For the example already given earlier, where $M = 1$, it can be seen that:

$$\text{total depth} - \text{of} - \text{field (mm)} = \frac{125 \times 0.5}{1^2} = 62.5 \text{ mm}$$

which matches well to the value of 63 mm calculated by the alternative method given earlier. By comparison, if the magnifier power is now increased, for example, to +20.00 DS, and $M = 5\times$,

$$\text{total depth} - \text{of} - \text{field (mm)} = \frac{125 \times 0.5}{5^2} = 2.5 \text{ mm}$$

Thus, whilst the depth-of-field is large for the low-powered magnifier, the entire permissible range of movement within which the object will be seen clearly through the +20.00 DS magnifier is only 2.5 mm, which illustrates one of the practical difficulties encountered in using such devices. Of course, the visually impaired patient may not be so sensitive to blurring of the image and may be able to tolerate more movement. Equally, a patient with active accommodation may be able to alter their accommodative effort to aid in focussing the image. It is also apparent that a change in object position can be useful to create a change in the vergence of light leaving the magnifier lens, which will compensate for uncorrected spherical ametropia.

Field-of-View

The field-of-view of a magnifying lens is defined as the angle subtended by the lens periphery at the image of the eye's entrance pupil.

Considering Fig. 7.7, the entrance pupil is at E, a distance a behind the lens, with its image at E' with an image distance a'.

Refraction of light by the magnifier (F_M) gives, in terms of vergences:

$$A = A' + F_M$$

or

$$\frac{1}{a'} = \frac{1}{a} - F_M$$

so

$$a' = \frac{a}{1 - aF_M} \qquad \text{Eq. (7.4)}$$

$$\tan \phi = \frac{D}{2a'} \quad \text{and substituting from Eq. (7.4)}$$

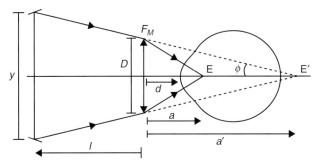

Fig. 7.7 The linear field-of-view y of magnifying lens of power F_M which has diameter D. ϕ is the angular semi-field-of-view. E is the entrance pupil of the eye, and E' its image, formed a distance a' from F_M. l is the magnifier-to-object distance, d is the magnifier-to-eye distance and a is the distance from the magnifier to E, which is approximately equal to $d + 3$ mm.

$$\tan \phi = \frac{D(1 - aF_M)}{2a} \qquad \text{Eq. (7.5)}$$

This gives the angular semi-field-of-view ϕ of the plus lens, but in purely practical terms, it is more useful to know the linear dimension y of the field-of-view, as this can be more easily related to a task (e.g. the width of a column of newsprint). From Fig. 7.7:

$$\tan \phi = \frac{y}{2(a' - l)} = \frac{y}{2\left[\dfrac{a}{(1 - aF_M)} - l\right]}$$

$$= \frac{y(1 - aF_M)}{2(a - l + laF_M)} \qquad \text{Eq. (7.6)}$$

Equating Eqs. (7.5) and (7.6):

$$\frac{D(1 - aF_M)}{2a} = \frac{y(1 - aF_M)}{2(a - l + laF_M)}$$

So total linear extent of field-of-view:

$$y = \frac{D(a - l + laF_M)}{a} \qquad \text{Eq. (7.7)}$$

sometimes written as

$$y = D\left[1 - \frac{l}{a} + \frac{l}{f'_M}\right] \qquad \text{Eq. (7.8)}$$

Eqs. (7.7) and (7.8) are general expressions applicable in any circumstances, but Eq. (7.7) can be considerably simplified by considering the situation where the magnifier is used with the object at the anterior focal point so that $l = -f'_M$ and

$$y = \frac{D(a - (-f'_M) + (-f'_M aF_M))}{a}, \text{ so}$$

$$y = \frac{D}{aF_M} \qquad \text{Eq. (7.9)}$$

In fact, for all practical purposes, in low-vision work, these formulae are equally valid if the substitution $a = d$ is made, so Eq. (7.9) becomes

$$y = \frac{D}{dF_M}$$

where D is magnifier diameter, F_M is the equivalent power of the magnifier, and d is the distance of the magnifier from the corneal vertex. All of these formulae can be applied to spectacle, hand-held or stand-mounted plus-lens magnifiers.

Thus the field-of-view which the patient obtains with a magnifier depends on the following:

1. The magnifier-to-eye distance. Halving this, for example, will double the field-of-view, and whenever possible, the patient should be encouraged to hold the magnifier close to the eye. This is illustrated in Fig. 7.9 which shows the dramatic increase in the field-of-view when the magnifier is spectacle-mounted. This parameter is the most powerful influence on the area which can be viewed through the lens.
2. The lens diameter. When the patient is bothered by the limited field-of-view, complaining that only a few letters are visible through the magnifier, this is the parameter which the patient feels should be changed. It must be explained that there are practical limitations of weight, manufacturing capability and peripheral aberrations which limit lens diameter, although using the optimum lens form may allow increased diameter whilst maintaining image quality.
3. The power of the lens. As lens power increases, the field-of-view decreases, in addition to the secondary effect that more powerful lenses are usually smaller in size. This is one of the reasons for the practice in low-vision work of giving the minimum magnification which allows the patient to perform the task. It can be seen from Fig. 7.8, however, that lens power is of less significance than the magnifier-to-eye distance: for example, the field-of-view of an 8× magnifier at 10 cm from the eye is greater than that of a 4× magnifier with a 25 cm magnifier-to-eye distance.

To maximise field-of-view then, the patient must be encouraged to hold the magnifier as close to the eye as possible (i.e. as close as the particular task allows). As already pointed out, changes in this magnifier-to-eye distance do not alter the magnification, but in fact, the patient may often feel that magnification is actually greater with the longer magnifier-to-eye distance. The reason for this is illustrated in Fig. 7.9.

On the right-hand side, the real situation shows the decreasing angular subtense of the magnifier lens, with the word seen within the aperture remaining the same size but gradually taking up more of the field-of-view: the field-of-view has decreased whilst magnification has stayed constant. It may be perceived by the patient, however, as the situation on the left-hand side of Fig. 7.9: it appears as if the subtense of the magnifier itself (i.e. the field-of-view) remains constant, so as the word being seen fills more of the available field-of-view, it must be increasing in size.

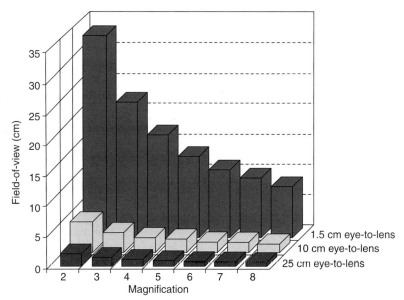

Fig. 7.8 The field-of-view (in centimetres) for plus-lens magnifiers of 2× to 8× magnification positioned in the spectacle plane (1.5 cm from eye), and at 10 and 25 cm from the eye. A lens diameter of 40 mm is assumed in each case.

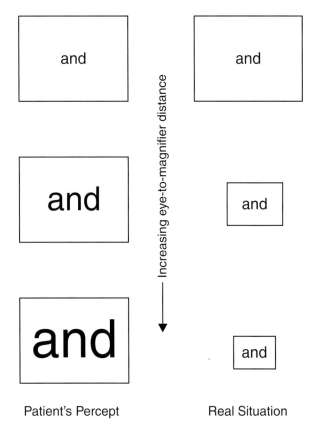

Patient's Percept   Real Situation

Fig. 7.9 The effect of increasing eye-to-magnifier distance on magnification and field-of-view. The 'real situation' is that magnification remains constant (note the size of the word 'and') whilst field-of-view decreases, but the 'patient's percept' is often of a constant field-of-view with increasing magnification.

Lens Forms for Minimum Aberration

Whether lenses are to be used to correct ametropia or as magnifying aids, there is obviously a desire to minimise the aberrations which will affect the quality of the image created by the lens, and presumably the patient's visual performance. There is little experimental evidence, however, to support the assumption that the lens form which gives the clearest image will give the best performance: it is certainly possible that the visual system of the visually impaired patient is not capable of detecting imperfections in the image, and would be less affected by them than a normally sighted subject would be. Nonetheless, magnifier lenses are designed to be optimal for the normal visual system.

The aberrations which can be identified for a lens can be divided into *chromatic* and *monochromatic*. The monochromatic aberrations are further subdivided into *spherical aberration, coma, oblique astigmatism, field curvature and distortion*. Whilst they are separated in this way for descriptive purposes, all the aberrations would actually be present simultaneously in the image to some extent. Fig. 7.10 shows a grid pattern which can be used to visualise each of these aberrations, and each is best seen using a large-diameter (~70 mm) plano-convex or meniscus lens of approximately +8.00 DS.

Chromatic aberration describes the greater power of the lens for blue light than red, due to its higher refractive index for these wavelengths. The greater the refractive index difference shown by the lens material between the extremes of the spectrum, the greater this power difference and the *dispersion* shown by the lens. It is desirable to minimise dispersion, and this quality is usually represented by a high value of the reciprocal of dispersion—*constringence*. Once the lens material is selected, there is little that can be done to reduce chromatic aberration with a single lens. It can be eliminated with an achromatic lens system: this would typically be a doublet combining a positive and a negative lens, each made of a different material. The refractive powers of the two lenses sum to give the required effect, whilst the chromatic dispersion of one is cancelled by the other. To visualise transverse chromatic aberration, place the grid target at about 30 cm from

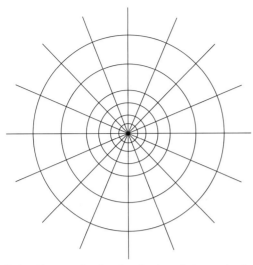

Fig. 7.10 A grid target for the visualisation of chromatic aberration, oblique astigmatism and field curvature. Modified with permission from Jalie, M. (1995). The design of low vision aids. In C. Dickinson (Ed.), The Ophthalmic Lens Year Book 1995 (pp. 14–30). WB Saunders.

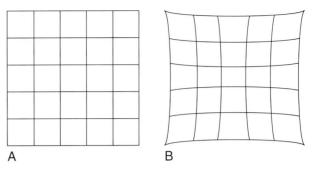

Fig. 7.11 (A) A regular square grid, which shows pincushion distortion when viewed through a powerful plus lens, and appears as in (B). Reproduced with permission from Jalie, M. (1995). The design of low vision aids. In C. Dickinson (Ed.), The Ophthalmic Lens Year Book 1995 (pp. 14–30). WB Saunders.

the eye, and the plus-lens flat on top of it with the geometrical centre of the lens over the centre point on the grid. Then bring the lens slowly off the page until the outer circle on the grid becomes slightly blurred, and at that point, its black outline will be edged with blue on the inner side and yellow on the outer edge. The effect is more noticeable on the circles seen through the edge of the lens, because the prismatic effect (deviation) is greater through these outer zones: transverse chromatic aberration is the difference in the prismatic effect of the lens for the extremes of the spectrum. The coloured fringes are only seen with high-contrast, black-white targets, due to the different image size created by rays of different wavelength. With low-contrast targets, this difference in image size simply creates a blurred edge to the image, reducing its sharpness and clarity: in normal viewing conditions, therefore, the effect of chromatic aberration is simply to blur images seen through the lens periphery rather than create coloured fringes.

Of the monochromatic aberrations, spherical aberration and coma are clinically insignificant for spectacle-mounted lenses until very high powers are reached (>+48.00 DS, 12× magnification). This is because these aberrations are apparent in the image when rays from the periphery of the lens are refracted to a different focus to those passing through a point closer to the optical centre. When the lens is worn close to the eye, the eye's pupil acts as the aperture stop and the limited-diameter bundle of rays entering the eye has passed through a restricted area of the lens, within which the power should vary very little. In hand-held or stand-mounted magnifiers, by contrast, the longer eye-to-magnifier distance means that the eye pupil no longer forms the aperture stop of the system: rays of light entering the entire magnifier aperture can enter the eye simultaneously, and so spherical aberration and coma can adversely affect the image. The problem increases with the aperture of the lens, so one possible solution is simply to decrease magnifier diameter; the use of aspheric surfaces can also effectively reduce spherical aberration, as can the use of a doublet or triplet lens system.

The main aberrations to be considered in magnifier lenses, however, are oblique astigmatism, field curvature and distortion. Placing the plus-lens over the grid in Fig. 7.10 as before, it should be moved gradually off the page, and it will be seen that the outer rings of the grid pattern go blurred before the inner rings. This indicates that the image distance decreases progressively for correspondingly more peripheral rays, creating a curved image plane—the so-called field curvature. Examining the blurring ring at one point, however, it will be seen that the radiating spokes on the grid are still clear, whilst the concentric circle has blurred: the lens is showing oblique astigmatism for rays passing off-axis through the lens. Placing the plus-lens over the square grid in Fig. 7.11A, and drawing the lens slowly off the page produces an image as in Fig. 7.11B, where the shape of the image shows pincushion distortion.

These same aberrations are also problematic when plus lenses are used to correct a hypermetropic refractive error, and oblique astigmatism and field curvature are controlled (and a 'best form' lens produced) by careful combination of back and front surface powers. The lens wearer adapts to the distortion in the image because of their awareness of the true nature of their environment, and this does not usually need to be considered. In magnifier lenses, there is no such compensation for spatial distortion, and this becomes an important influence on image quality unless lens form is adjusted accordingly. A more significant difference, however, is the fact that ametropic corrections are optimised for viewing an object at distance (infinity) or at a 'normal' near working distance (about 33 cm), whereas the magnifier will be used with the object at the anterior focal point (or even closer). Unfortunately, even taking this into account, no single lens form can eliminate all of the aberrations simultaneously, and the lens designer must decide which aberration will most significantly affect image quality and arrive at the best compromise design. This was attempted in the 'Stigmagna' range of lenses which correct for oblique astigmatism and distortion (Bennett, 1975) and in the calculations of Lederer (1955) which attempt to minimise field curvature as well.

As lens power increases beyond +20.00 DS (5× magnification), careful choice of spherical surfaces is no longer sufficient to produce adequate image quality, and aspheric surfaces must be used. In contrast to a spherical surface where the radius of curvature remains constant across the entire diameter, aspheric surfaces flatten (the radius of curvature increases) towards the periphery. The degree of flattening increases as the surface chosen changes from elliptical to paraboloid and is greatest for a hyperboloid form. By careful manipulation of the spherical back surface power, and the particular aspheric form used for the front surface, oblique astigmatism and distortion can both be made negligible. The 'Hyperocular' lens form for magnifiers (Bennett, 1975) is one such design where in lower powers (4× to 5×), an ellipsoid front surface is used, but for higher powers (8× to 12×), the degree of flattening must be greater and a hyperboloid surface is needed (Jalie, 1995). In order to determine whether a particular plus-lens surface is spherical or aspheric in form, a lens measure can be placed perpendicular to, and centrally on, the surface. Keeping the lens measure perpendicular to the surface, it should now be moved towards the periphery of the lens, and the reading noted: a progressive decrease in the power will occur on the flattening aspheric surface, whereas the reading will remain constant on a spherical surface.

Table 7.1 illustrates the range of lens forms which can be used to minimise the aberrations of spectacle-mounted magnifiers. Whilst lower-powered plus lenses which use spherical surfaces are often meniscus in form with a concave back surface, those above approximately +17.00 DS and those which use aspheric surfaces are usually bi-convex. It is usual in a spectacle-mounted lens to have the most convex surface away from the eye (as it would be if used for correcting refractive error) but when the lens is used away from the eye in a hand-held or stand-mounted form, this position should be reversed and the most convex surface held towards the eye to minimise aberrations. In fact, the 'change-over' between these two positions occurs when the eye-to-magnifier distance is equal to the focal length of the lens.

The same adjustment of the lens forms with increasing lens power will be required in hand-held and stand magnifiers, although in this case, the aberrations are likely to become more severe at lower powers. This is because the pupil of the eye no longer forms the aperture stop of the system, with the consequence that rays of light passing through the whole lens aperture are present in the final image. This causes greater problems with spherical aberration, and aspheric surfaces are often employed in low-powered hand and stand magnifiers as the flattening of the lens surface and the consequent fall-off in power help to counteract this. Thus, a lens of a particular power can be made in larger diameter, whilst still retaining acceptable image quality, if aspheric surfaces are used. Even so, the increased eye-to-magnifier distance increases aberrations to such a degree that the use of compound systems may also become necessary at lower powers.

Lens Forms for Minimum Thickness

The design of the Fresnel lens (and prism) is such that the refracting effect of the optical surfaces is retained (the appropriate curvature for the lens, or the correct angle for the prism), but the bulk of the material in between is removed. This is shown schematically in Fig. 7.12.

This makes it possible to have very thin and lightweight lenses with either very large diameter (Fig. 7.13) or very high power, or both, and they could be used in hand-held or spectacle-mounted form. Although these seem to be an attractive option, visual performance with them is often very poor. The reduction in image contrast caused by scattering of light is particularly problematic to those with poor contrast sensitivity, and in spectacle form, the wearer may be aware of a regular pattern of reflections from the facets.

Diffractive optical elements represent another potentially attractive alternative to conventional lens forms, especially in high plus powers, because the optical element is thin and does not vary in thickness as the power increases. Conventional lenses use refraction of light at curved surfaces to bend light to the required focal point: in white light, this bending effect is greater for short wavelengths, leading to chromatic aberration. Diffraction occurs as light passes through a thin slit: if a diffraction grating is used which has several slits, generating overlapping beams of light, then a pattern of maxima and minima of brightness is created by constructive and destructive interference, respectively. If the 'slits' in the opaque medium are circular, and with appropriate spacing,

Approximate Power Range (DS)	Lens Form
Up to +8.00/+10.00 DS (2× to 2.5×)	'Standard' prescription best form, spherical surfaces, meniscus
+8.00 to +16.00 (2× to 4×)	Lenticular (restricted aperture), spherical surfaces, meniscus
+10.00 to +24.00 (2.5× to 6×)	Stigmagna or Lederer 'special' spectacle magnifier form, spherical surfaces, meniscus in low power, plano-convex and bi-convex in higher powers
+16.00 to +48.00 (4× to 12×)	Hyperocular, aspheric front surface (ellipsoid lower powers, hyperboloid in higher powers), biconvex
+40.00 to +80.00 (10× to 20×)	Achromatic doublet or triplet lens system

TABLE 7.1   The Range of Lens Forms Which Can Be Used to Optimise the Image Quality When Using Spectacle-Mounted Plus-Lens Magnifiers of Various Powers

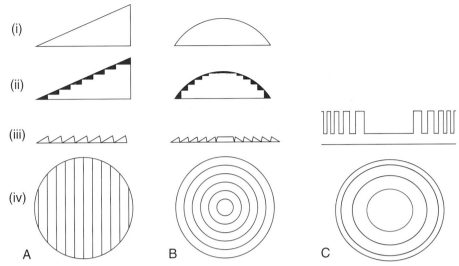

Fig. 7.12 A schematic diagram showing the design of a Fresnel prism (A) and lens (B). *(i)* shows the full-aperture element in section, and in *(ii)*, the *shaded areas* show the important areas of the element which give its refractive power. In *(iii)* the section of the Fresnel element is shown which contains the refracting elements, but the bulk of the lens material has been removed. In *(iv)* the front view is shown. For comparison, a diffractive lens (a phase reversal zone plate) is shown in (C). *(iii)* shows the section (not to same scale) and *(iv)* the front view.

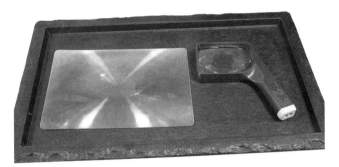

Fig. 7.13 A Fresnel sheet magnifier shown in comparison to a conventional lens design of similar power.

then the maximum occurs at a focal point, and the action is similar to a refractive lens. Such an element is called a 'zone plate'—or sometimes a Fresnel zone plate, which is not to be confused with a Fresnel lens. The disadvantage is the loss of the light caused by having the opaque zones, so a 'phase reversal zone plate' is used, where the previously opaque sections are replaced by a transparent zone of increased thickness to slow the light wave passing through it and change its phase such that it also constructively interferes at the focal point. So the appearance of such a diffractive optical element is a transparent thin lens with concentric circular zones with minimally different thickness: different focal lengths (powers) are created by changing the width and spacing of these thicker zones (see Fig. 7.12C). This design appears to have been implemented in the Eschenbach 'noves' range of half-eye spectacles. Shorter wavelengths are diffracted less than longer ones, so the chromatic aberration is in the opposite direction to that created by refractive lenses. For this reason, a hybrid optical element composed of both a refractive and a diffractive component may represent an even better option.

Combining Plus-Lens Magnifiers With Accommodation or Reading Additions

It has been assumed that the object is to be placed at the focal point of the plus-lens magnifier, and thus parallel rays of light leave the lens and the image is at infinity. This allows the user to obtain a clearly focused retinal image whilst wearing the distance refractive correction, and with the accommodation relaxed. It is likely, however, that the patient may not intuitively use the magnifier in this way. It would be natural for the pre-presbyopic patient to converge and accommodate for the physically near location of the object, and if the presbyopic patient uses a hand-held or stand-mounted magnifier for reading, they may well expect to wear their reading spectacles. In order to now create a focused retinal image, the rays of light must be divergent when leaving the magnifier lens, and the converging effect of the reading addition or the accommodation will bring the rays to parallel. This will require the lens-to-object distance to be decreased, so the object will be closer to the lens than the focal point (Fig. 7.14).

In either situation, the magnifying system is no longer the single plus-lens magnifier: it is now a combined system of two spaced elements, one being the positive magnifier and the other being the positive accommodation or reading addition. Very little inaccuracy is introduced by the approximation, which is illustrated in Fig. 7.15. Accommodation is taken to be represented by a thin positive lens placed at the corneal vertex, and thus the combined system of the convex magnifier (F_M) and the accommodation (F_A) produces the image at infinity. If the patient uses a reading addition, this is represented as a thin positive lens (of power F_A) placed at any required distance from the eye. In fact, because parallel light leaves this second element, it can be positioned at any distance from the eye—the vertex distance of the reading

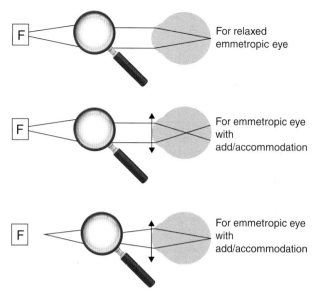

For relaxed
emmetropic eye

For emmetropic eye
with
add/accommodation

For emmetropic eye
with
add/accommodation

Fig. 7.14 (*Upper*) The user obtains a clear retinal image whilst wearing their distance refractive correction, and with accommodation relaxed. (*Middle*) The patient accommodates or uses a reading add so the retinal image is no longer focused. (*Lower*) The lens-to-object distance is decreased, so the object will be closer to the lens than the focal point (F), light is now divergent when leaving the magnifier lens, and the retinal image is in focus.

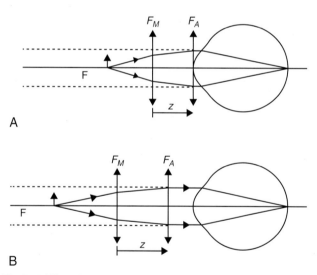

Fig. 7.15 When the object is placed closer to the magnifier (F_M) than the anterior focal point (F), divergent light leaves the magnifier lens and either (A) accommodation (represented as a thin lens F_A placed at the corneal vertex) or (B) a reading addition F_A is required to produce a clear retinal image. The combined two-element system with separation z between the two components creates a virtual image at infinity in each case.

spectacles will not affect the magnification. The magnification produced by this combined system obviously depends on its equivalent power, and this is given by:

$$F_{eq} = F_M + F_A - zF_MF_A$$

where $z = $ the separation of the two elements in the system—either the distance of the magnifier (F_M) from the cornea in the case where accommodation provides the second component

(F_A) in the system, or the distance of the magnifier from the reading spectacles (F_A). This value of equivalent power can then be used to calculate the magnification:

$$M = \frac{F_{eq}}{4}$$

Fig. 7.16 summarises the effect on F_{eq} (y-axis) of using a magnifier in combination with another plus lens (F_A on the x-axis). If $F_A = 0$, then F_{eq} is equal to F_M, regardless of the distance of the magnifier from the eye (z, expressed here in terms of multiples of f_M, the focal length of the magnifier). Fig. 7.16 shows how the value of F_{eq} (in terms of F_M, the magnifier power) changes for different values of separation (z) and F_A.

It can be seen that where z is small (equal to zero or, more realistically, $0.2f_M$) (and the magnifier is close to the spectacle plane), there is an increase in the combined power over that expected when using the magnifier with the object at the focal point. When the two components are separated by a distance equal to the focal length of the magnifier lens ($z = f_M$) the magnification is not affected by the power of the reading addition and $F_{eq} = F_M$, regardless of the value of F_A.

It is when the separation z becomes greater than the focal length of the magnifier that the combined power of the system begins to decrease dramatically in proportion to that separation. The effects can be extreme: to take an example (reading from the graph), a +40.00 DS ($F_M = +40$) magnifier combined with 4.00 DS ($F_A = +4.00$) of accommodation gives an equivalent system power of +44.00 DS if the two components are touching, but only +20.00 DS ($F_{eq} = F_M - 20 = +40 - 20$) if they are separated by 15 cm ($z = 15$ cm $= 6f_M$). Therefore, if a magnifier is positioned away from the eye/spectacle plane, the magnifier-to-object distance should be maximised to ensure there is no/little accommodation, and the presbyope should wear their distance correction.

Minimum magnification occurs when $z = f_A$ (the focal length of F_A). This is when the magnifier is in contact with the object (Fig. 7.17) and does not contribute to the system power ($F_{eq} = F_A$).

Previously, Eq. (7.9) was derived which allows the linear field of view through a magnifier to be derived, when the object is at the focal point of the magnifier. In this two-component system, this is no longer the case, so this equation cannot be used. However, the object is at the focal point of the combined system (with power F_{eq}), so the equation can be amended to:

$$y = \frac{D}{aF_{eq}}$$

The patient may notice that the field of view is larger, for example, when using their reading spectacles compared to using their distance spectacles, but this is only because of the decrease in F_{eq} in the former case.

Trade Magnification

The magnification of a plus-lens is derived by comparing the viewing distance it allows (i.e. its focal length), to that

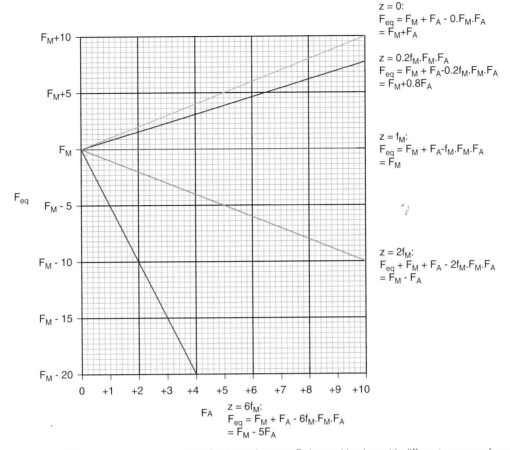

Fig. 7.16 The equivalent power (F_{eq}) achieved by using a magnifier lens of power F_M in combination with different powers of accommodation/reading addition (F_A), for different separations (z) of the two components. F_{eq} is expressed as a function of F_M, and z is expressed as a function of f_M' (the focal length of the magnifier). $z = 0$ is the situation where the two components are in contact.

achieved with a +4.00 DS lens, or 4.00 DS of accommodation. It has been argued that the effect of this reading addition should continue to be taken into account, and the effect of the magnifier lens added to it, rather than replacing it. Thus, the magnification obtained with a magnifier and the +4.00 DS addition would be compared with the effect of the +4.00 DS addition alone. If the magnifier is used in conjunction with a +4.00 DS addition, the magnification of the two-component system is:

$$M = \frac{F_{eq}}{4}$$

where

$$F_{eq} = F_M + F_A - zF_M F_A$$

F_M is the magnifier power, F_A is the reading addition (+4.00 DS in this case) and z is the separation of the two components. If it is assumed that the magnifier is held in the spectacle plane, touching the addition lens, so $z = 0$, then

$$F_{eq} = F_M + (+4.00) - (0 \times F_M \times (+4.00)) = F_m + 4$$

and

$$M = \frac{F_M + 4}{4}$$

or

$$M = \frac{F_M}{4} + 1$$

This formula is that for 'trade magnification', and is sometimes used by manufacturers in labelling their magnifiers. Bennett (1982), rather more descriptively, called it 'iso-accommodative' magnification. Although it is in common usage, it is not very realistic as there is no reason to assume that the patient always has a +4.00 reading addition (or equivalent accommodation), and it is not likely that the magnifier will be held in contact with the spectacles.

HAND-HELD MAGNIFIERS

The principle of all plus-lens magnifiers is identical: the magnification remains constant regardless of the eye-to-magnifier distance, providing that the object is placed at the anterior focal point. This gives the option of taking the plus lens and placing it in a mounting, perhaps with a handle, and holding it away from the eye. There are literally hundreds of different designs of hand magnifier to choose from, and they are available from many different sources: they are often designed primarily for hobbies such

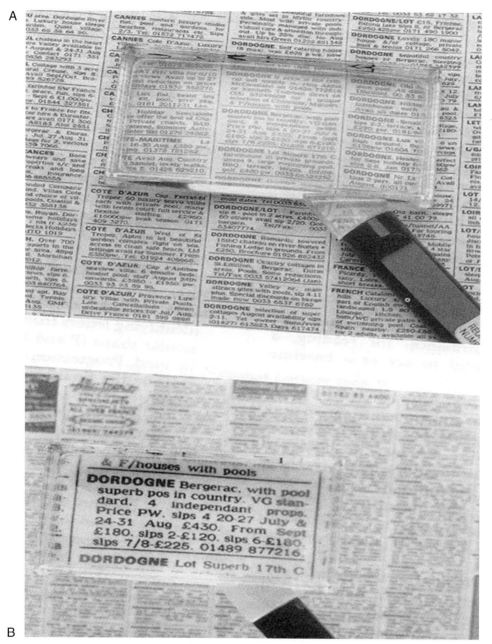

Fig. 7.17 (A) The magnifier flat on the page gives no magnification, and it must be slowly raised to where the object is close to the focal point (B), when magnification is optimal.

as stamp-collecting or needlework rather than for visually impaired patients.

Advantages and Disadvantages
Advantages

1. Convenient and most suitable for short-term 'spot' or 'survival' reading (see section on 'Visual Requirements for Reading' in Chapter 3) such as price tags whilst shopping, or looking up a telephone number, rather than a longer-duration task such as reading a novel.
2. The magnifier-to-eye distance can be extended without affecting magnification, providing the magnifier-to-object distance is kept constant and equal to the focal length of the magnifier. This can be useful when it would not be safe to approach the task too closely (perhaps setting dials and gauges on an oven), or if the patient rejects the unusual close working distance associated with spectacle-mounted lenses.
3. Can have internal illumination if necessary, which is useful out of the home where lighting is unpredictable; and is strongly recommended for a patient with log contrast sensitivity <1.00. Having the light source below the lens also limits annoying reflections from the lens surfaces.
4. Psychologically acceptable to the patient because they are freely available devices often used by those with no visual impairment.

5. Often very familiar to the patient who has obtained and used one of these aids before reaching the stage of seeking professional advice.

6. Usually compact, lightweight and portable. Some are heavy due to the use of glass lenses, which do have greater surface hardness. Plastic lenses are preferred to reduce the weight, especially if the rim around the lens forms a flange which protects the curved lens surface from being scratched by any surface on which it is placed.

7. With the exception of the large diameter (and therefore low-powered) aspheric lenses, these magnifiers are usually inexpensive.

Disadvantages

1. Even though a long eye-to-magnifier distance can be used, this is associated with a limited field-of-view. This may make it practically necessary to hold the lens close to the eye and can cause the patient to ultimately reject the device in favour of a spectacle-mounted lens.

2. Must have suitable and comfortable hand-grip. Some are specific to right- or left-handed grip, but if interchangeable, there must be some way for the patient to distinguish which is the correct orientation: the more convex surface should be placed towards the eye.

3. May prove unsatisfactory if obtained (often by family or friends on behalf of the patient) and used without instruction by a naive presbyopic patient. The natural reaction will be to buy the largest available lens, which will inevitably be of low power: it will be assumed that spectacles with a reading addition should be worn, and the magnifier will usually be positioned at the habitual reading distance (~30 cm). This will create a two-component magnifying system, with a large separation between the reading addition and the magnifier lens, thus producing low equivalent power and magnification.

Types Available

Table 7.2 summarises the characteristics of the hand-held magnifiers currently available (see Figs. 7.18 to 7.20). The division into three different power categories is arbitrary and is done simply for comparative purposes. The large diameter of the low-powered devices makes them very difficult to hold close to the eye, but the field-of-view is acceptable even with a long eye-to-magnifier distance (a value of 25 cm is chosen as an example). It can be seen that the field-of-view of the high-powered magnifiers is very small, and this means that the lens cannot be held away from the eye and must be used close to the distance spectacles.

STAND-MOUNTED MAGNIFIERS

The importance of placing the object at the focal point of the plus-lens magnifier has already been discussed. This positioning is critical, with slight alterations in object distance producing large changes in the vergence of light leaving the magnifier, usually creating a noticeably blurred image for the patient. Casual inspection of the view through the magnifier illustrates this very limited depth-of-field, but a possible solution to the problem of maintaining the precise magnifier-to-object distance is to place the magnifier lens on a stand to fix that position. This is the principle of the stand magnifier, of which there are several distinct categories:

1. Fixed focus
2. Variable focus
   a. High-powered
   b. Low-powered

Fixed-Focus

Although the stand allows the object to be placed at a fixed position relative to the magnifier lens, fixed-focus stand magnifiers are in fact typically designed so that the magnifier-to-object distance is *less* than the anterior focal length of the lens. This means that light is divergent when leaving the magnifier, and thus the image is not at infinity but at some finite distance from the eye. The patient must therefore accommodate to neutralise the divergence (i.e. accommodate for the apparent distance of the image) or, if presbyopic, wear a reading addition appropriate to that image distance. In either case, the combination of the accommodation or reading addition (F_A

TABLE 7.2	**A Summary of the Types of Hand-Held Magnifiers Currently Available**		
Characteristics	**Low-Powered (Fig. 7.18)**	**Medium-Powered (Fig. 7.19)**	**High-Powered (Fig. 7.20)**
Power/magnification range	<+16.00 DS (4×)	From +16.00 to +32.00 DS (4× to 8×)	>+32.00 DS (8×)
Lens form and diameter	Spherical up to 75 mm Aspheric up to 100 mm	Aspheric up to 50 mm Spherical up to 25 mm	Doublet/triplet lens systems up to 20 mm
Typical linear field-of-view	40 mm with 25 cm eye-to-magnifier distance	10 mm with 25 cm eye-to-magnifier distance; 150 mm with magnifier close to spectacle plane	25 mm with magnifier close to spectacle plane
Other features	Large single lens, often with surrounding flange to protect from scratching; may have internal illumination; potential for binocular viewing through lens	As low-powered, or folding design	Typically folding 'pocket' lenses

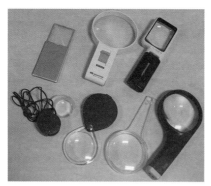

Fig. 7.18 A selection of low-powered hand magnifiers, both illuminated and nonilluminated, of various designs.

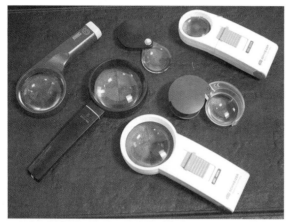

Fig. 7.19 A selection of medium-powered hand magnifiers, both illuminated and nonilluminated, of various designs.

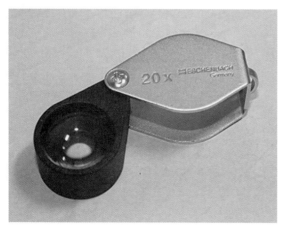

Fig. 7.20 A high-powered hand magnifier of typical folding style, with a multiple lens system.

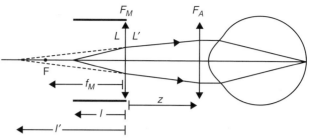

Fig. 7.21 The use of a fixed-focus stand magnifier with the object plane (at the base of the stand) in front of the anterior focal point (F) of the magnifying lens (F_M). The magnifier-to-object distance (l) is less than the magnifier focal length (f_M) requiring a reading addition (F_A) in the system, so parallel light enters the eye and a clear retinal image is formed. z is the lens separation; l and L are object distance and object vergence; l' and L' are image distance and image vergence.

Consider an example of a stand magnifier with a +20.00 DS lens, and a stand height of 4 cm (shorter than the focal length of 5 cm). The value of F_M is therefore +20.00 DS and the object distance l (see Fig. 7.21) is −0.04 m. L is the vergence of light reaching the magnifier, and L' is that leaving the magnifier. Therefore

$$L = \frac{1}{l} = \frac{1}{-0.04} = -25.00 \text{ DS}$$

$$L' = L + F_M = -25.00 + (+20.00) = -5.00 \text{ DS}$$

$$l' = \text{image distance} = \frac{1}{-5.00} = -0.20\text{m} = -20 \text{ cm}$$

If the patient's eye is directly behind the magnifier ($z = 0$), the initial image created by the magnifier alone is 20 cm from the eye, and accommodation or a reading addition of +5.00 DS will be required to view at 20 cm (or, to put it another way, to neutralise the divergence of light from that point). If the magnifier-to-eye separation increases, however, and $z = 20$ cm, for example, the initial image would now be 40 cm from the eye ($z + l' = (-20) + (-20) = -40$ cm), and this will require accommodation or a reading addition of +2.50 DS to neutralise the divergence and focus the image clearly on the retina. If the patient happened to be wearing a +6.00 DS reading addition, they would never see the object clearly, regardless of the magnifier-to-eye separation: the reading addition is stronger than is required to neutralise the divergence. In this case, the light entering the eye is converging and focuses in front of the retina.

Thus, the presbyope needs a reading addition (or the pre-presbyope needs to accommodate) in order to use a fixed-focus stand magnifier, but the degree of accommodation required depends on the design of the magnifier (how much shorter the stand height is than the focal length) and the distance of the magnifier lens from the eye. The equivalent power and magnification is now that of a two-component

in Fig. 7.21) and the magnifier lens (F_M) creates a two-component magnifying system where the final image is at infinity, and parallel light enters the eye. As the object is no longer at the anterior focal point of the magnifier lens, the magnification of the system is not constant, but varies with the power of F_A and the separation of F_A and F_M, which is z.

system. Considering the two examples already quoted above:

In the first case,

$$F_M = +20.00, F_A = +5.00, z = 0$$

$$F_{eq} = F_M + F_A - zF_MF_A$$

$$F_{eq} = +20.00 + (+5.00) - (0 \times (+20.00) \times (+5.00))$$
$$= +25.00$$

So

$$M = \frac{F_{eq}}{4} = \frac{+25.00}{4} = 6.25\times$$

But, in the second case,

$$F_M = +20.00, + F_A = +2.50, z = 20 \text{ cm} = 0.20 \text{ m}$$

$$F_{eq} = F_M + F_A - zF_MF_A$$

$$F_{eq} = +20.00 + (+2.50) - (0.2 \times (+20.00) \times (+2.50))$$
$$= +12.50$$

so

$$M = \frac{F_{eq}}{4} = \frac{+12.50}{4} = 3.1\times$$

As the magnifier lens itself had a power of +20.00 DS, it might have been expected to have a magnification of 5× ($M = F_{eq}/4$). However, as demonstrated previously, in a two-component system consisting of a reading addition (or accommodation) and a magnifier lens, the higher the reading add, and the closer the reading add and the magnifier lens are to each other, the higher the magnification will be. The reading add cannot be greater in magnitude than the divergence of light leaving the magnifier lens, however, or a clear retinal image cannot be formed. If the patient finds that the print is difficult to read and blurred, regardless of its size, this suggests that the reading add is not optimal (or their accommodative effort is inappropriate). If the patient reports that lifting the magnifier stand off the page improves their vision, this suggests an insufficient reading add—by moving the magnifier off the page the focal point is being placed nearer to the object, and reducing the divergence of light leaving the magnifier. If this process makes vision worse, it suggests that the reading add is already too high, and decreasing the divergence is making this worse. It is possible to optimise the reading addition

on a trial-and-error basis by adding trial lenses in ±0.50 DS steps to the patient's reading correction whilst the magnifier is in use in the habitual (or intended) working position.

The position of the image created by the stand magnifier, and the way in which the magnifier is positioned, will thus dramatically affect the magnification obtained. This is rarely taken into account by the manufacturers when labelling stand magnifiers. In addition, there is no 'standard' reading addition or accommodative effort: manufacturers vary in the object position selected, and often vary within a particular range of magnifiers of different powers. A very quick check can be performed by the practitioner viewing some reading material through the magnifier which is held close to the eye: if the print remains clear when a +4.00 DS trial lens is added over the magnifier lens, it shows that the light is indeed divergent when leaving the magnifier, and the presbyopic patient will need a reading correction. In general, the lower the dioptric power of the magnifier lens, the greater the divergence of light leaving the lens—up to −10.00 DS in some cases—whereas very high-powered magnifiers often have the object plane almost coincident with the anterior focal point, resulting in light being almost parallel as it leaves the lens. There appear to be a number of practical reasons why this should be so. Firstly, a low-powered stand magnifier will have a long focal length, and this would require a physically large stand if the object were to be at the focal point. Typically, the stand height is shortened to a more practical size, resulting in a considerable divergence of light leaving the lens. Considering the case where this is −10.00 DS, the image will be positioned 10 cm behind the lens: if the patient held the magnifier up to their eye, they would need a +10.00 DS reading add, or 10.00 DS of accommodation. As this lens is of low-power, however, it will also have a relatively large diameter, and thus the patient can achieve an acceptable field-of-view whilst holding the magnifier at a 'normal' reading distance. Consider, for example, the lens being placed 30 cm from the eye; the image will now be 40 cm from the eye and will require a +2.50 DS reading add (or 2.50 DS accommodation) to see it clearly. It must be realised, of course, that this large separation of the magnifier and the reading addition in the two-component magnifying system will create a low equivalent power, and hence low magnification: nonetheless, it is more practical, because the patient is more likely to already possess a pair of reading spectacles with a +2.50 addition, rather than a +10.00 DS addition which would need to be specially prescribed. On the contrary, a high-powered stand magnifier would not give sufficient field-of-view if used away from the eye, and it will usually be positioned almost touching the spectacles. If the divergence of light leaving this magnifier is much smaller (perhaps −2.50 DS), the image will be 40 cm behind the magnifier lens, and 40 cm from the eye. This will require a +2.50 reading addition, or 2.50 DS of accommodation, to clearly see the image, which, once again, is within the range where the patient may be expected to have such a correction already (Sloan & Jablonski, 1959). A genuine difficulty can arise with these high-powered stand magnifiers, however, when the patient's reading correction is in the form of bifocal lenses.

When the magnifier is held very close to the spectacles, the patient's natural gaze is straight ahead, through the *distance* portion of the lens, and downwards gaze through the reading segment can be difficult to achieve. In such a case, a special pair of full-aperture reading spectacles may be required: alternatively, one of the stand magnifiers which has a stand height equal to the focal length could be selected. This, of course, has parallel light leaving the magnifier lens.

Determining the Emergent Vergence

Fixed focus stand magnifiers are typically made so that the stand height is less than the focal length of the magnifier lens, such that light is divergent as it leaves the magnifier lens. The precise 'emergent vergence' can easily be determined in practice (Bailey, 1981b). With the magnifier in normal use with an object level with the base of the stand, the divergent rays leaving the lens can be made parallel using a plus lens. This auxiliary plus lens introduced as close as possible to the magnifier (Fig. 7.22A) neutralises this divergence and measures its value. An observer placing their eye some distance behind this lens would find the maximum plus-lens power which still allowed the object to be seen clearly. This would be the lens which neutralised the full amount of divergence of the emerging rays, and the rays of light entering the observer's eye would then be parallel. In the case of a relaxed, unaccommodating observer, these rays would be clearly focused on the retina. It is, however, extremely difficult to reach this endpoint because the observer often accommodates due to the close proximity of the object, thus underestimating the divergence of the rays. The difficulty in determining the point at which the emergent rays are exactly parallel can be overcome by using one of two alternative methods.

Method 1—Viewing Through a Distance Telescope. When viewing through a telescope, the observer is much more sensitive to defocus. The arrangement used is shown in Fig. 7.22B, where the observer selects the most positive lens power which still allows a clear image of the object under the magnifier lens. This time, however, a telescope is introduced close to the observer's eye and the object is viewed through this. This telescope must be focused for a very long working distance (>10 m if possible) before beginning. This means that the telescope is focused for parallel light, so the image created by the magnifier and the additional plus lens will only be seen clearly if the light emerging from the combination is parallel, and the additional lens is making the divergent rays parallel. If a plus lens in the ray path makes the image clearer, but not optimally clear, it is helpful to know whether the power of the plus lens needs to be increased or decreased. If the lens is lifted away from the magnifier, and the image focus improves, then the power should be increased: if the image blur worsens, the power should be decreased.

Method 2—Reversing the Ray Path. The passage of light through the lens combination can be reversed, and a distant object could act as a source of parallel rays of light which are converged by the auxiliary lens and magnifier to form an image at the base of the stand (Fig. 7.22C). The auxiliary lens which forms the clearest image is that which neutralises the emergent vergence. In practical terms, a piece of translucent tape is placed across the bottom of the stand magnifier to be tested, to form a screen on which to view an image. Using a distant illuminated object (such as a test chart) in a darkened room, the image of this object formed by the magnifier can be seen on the translucent tape screen (Fig. 7.23).

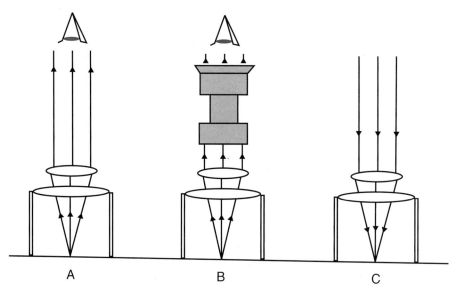

Fig. 7.22 (A) The observer views through the stand magnifier combined with a plus lens of the maximum power which still allows a clear view of the object. This combination will create parallel rays of light leaving the lens, so will be seen clearly if viewed by an emmetropic observer with relaxed accommodation. In (B), the observer views through a telescope focused for infinity to ensure that the image created by the lens/magnifier combination will only be clear if the emergent rays are exactly parallel. In (C), the direction of the light path is reversed, with the same lens/magnifier combination producing an image of an infinitely distant object in the plane of the magnifier base.

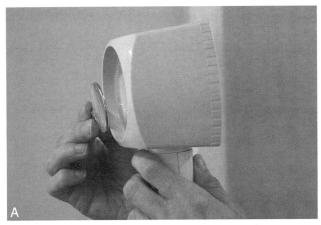

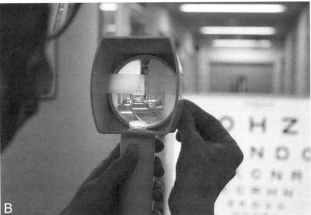

Fig. 7.23 (A) Introducing a plus lens of the correct power to (B) form an image of a distance test chart on the translucent tape attached to the base of the fixed-focus stand magnifier.

This image will usually be blurred initially, because it is not being formed at the same position as the screen. Various plus lenses can now be introduced in front of the magnifier lens, touching its surface. This lens is changed until the one which produces the clearest image is determined: this is the power of the lens which neutralises the emergent divergence. As earlier, the effect of changing the auxiliary lens position can be used to determine any change of power required: if increasing the separation from the magnifier lens improves image clarity, the power should be increased. For maximum sensitivity, when optimum focus is approached, observation of the image through a band magnifier will allow it to be examined more carefully.

Variable Focus

These come in two distinct types: high-powered and low-powered.

High-Powered (F_{eq} >+40.00 DS)

These are small diameter, compound or aspheric lens systems designed to be used monocularly in the spectacle plane. Their characteristic feature is the facility to alter the stand height, or to move the lens vertically to change its distance from the object plane. In this way, the vergence of light leaving the magnifier lens can be altered: for example, the divergence could be increased so that a larger reading addition

could be used in combination with the magnifier to increase the equivalent power (and hence magnification) of the two-component system, or to allow a myope to remove their spectacles and still experience a focused image. Alternatively, the stand height could even be made greater than the focal length of the magnifier lens to create convergent emergent rays, which may allow a hypermetrope to use the magnifier without the need for their usual distance refractive correction: the advantage of this would be to allow the lens to be placed even closer to the eye so maximising the field-of-view.

Low-Powered (F_{eq} <+10.00 DS)

These are usually large diameter lenses, often with spherical surfaces, held on an adjustable or flexible stand, or suspended around the neck on a cord. The position of the object plane can be freely selected by the patient, so they can be used like a hand-held magnifier with the object placed at the focal point of the magnifier lens and the distance refractive correction in place (and in fact, this will give greater magnification than using the magnifier at a long distance from the reading addition). The fact that the lens is supported leaves the patient's hands free and avoids fatigue, and these lenses are most frequently used by the patient wishing to write or do handicrafts. Illumination may be incorporated, or the magnifier lens can actually be attached to the housing of a lamp (Fig. 7.24).

Advantages and Disadvantages

Despite the distinctive differences between the various types, stand-mounted magnifiers share the following features:

Advantages

1. Accurate working distance is easily maintained, and this is particularly useful when the patient has hand tremor or weakness. It is especially beneficial in high-powered lenses where depth-of-field is restricted.
2. Support of the magnifier lens (especially for low-powered designs where the working space is larger) may leave the hands free to perform a manipulative task such as writing, DIY or handicrafts.
3. As the stand is likely to obstruct ambient light falling on the task, these magnifiers are most commonly available with built-in illumination, which avoids the need to arrange separate task lighting.
4. Some people find the larger handle of most stand magnifiers easier to grip than smaller hand magnifiers.

Disadvantages

1. The patient may require a special pair of reading spectacles to neutralise the emergent divergence from the magnifier lens in a fixed-focus design. The required reading addition depends on magnifier design and magnifier-to-eye distance, so it is not easily applicable to changes in position for different visual tasks, or any change in magnifier which may be required if the patient's vision changes. Great care must be taken when providing 'reading' spectacles of this type: despite careful explanation to the contrary, the patient often expects the spectacles alone to be sufficient for reading (or

an improvement on their current lenses), and alternative terminology, such as 'magnifier spectacles' or 'special spectacles' may be preferable in describing this correction.

2. Stand design and construction are critical to the success of the device. A firm and robust stand completely surrounding the lens is best for accurate location of the lens but prevents access to the working plane for manipulative tasks, and unless such a stand is transparent, internal illumination is essential, and the magnifier cannot be used if the batteries fail. The bottom of the stand should not be visible to the patient as they look through the lens, or it will further restrict the limited field-of-view.

3. The stand (and the power supply in the case of an internally illuminated design) may make the magnifier heavy and unwieldy to carry around.

4. In some designs, the stand surrounding the lens makes it impossible to read words near the spine of a tightly bound book.

5. The magnifier cannot be used on a non-flat surface, such as a tin of food or a bottle of medicine.

6. It is often difficult to write under a stand magnifier, although it is possible with some larger (lower power) stand magnifiers.

Types Available

Low-powered fixed-focus stand magnifiers allow a sufficient field-of-view to be positioned away from the eye and so typically have a high value of emergent vergence: even though the image is formed only a short distance behind the lens, it is still remote from the eye and so does not demand excessive accommodation or reading addition. The lens in such magnifiers may be cylindrical to give magnification in the vertical meridian only (Table 7.3, Figs. 7.24 to 7.26).

SPECTACLE-MOUNTED OR HEAD-MOUNTED PLUS LENSES

Not to be confused with spectacle-mounted telescopes, this method involves placing the magnifying plus lenses close to the patient's eye (in, or close to, the spectacle plane), which gives the potential for the optimum field of view, and binocular viewing. As with other plus-lens systems, the object is positioned at the focal point of the lens, such that parallel rays of light leave the lens and the patient's accommodation is relaxed. Prescribing of spectacle-mounted plus-lenses does not actually require any special equipment in the practice. The patient can be tested using standard trial-case lenses, in an appropriately centred trial frame, and then the required spectacles could be ordered from the prescription house. Trial lenses are labelled with back vertex power, and for magnification we are concerned with equivalent power. However, reduced aperture trial lenses have a plano-convex form (flat front surface), so equivalent power is equal to back vertex power. If using full-aperture trial lenses (which can be beneficial if the patient has an unusual head or eye position), these are usually made in equiconvex form for higher plus powers. Therefore, a pragmatic assumption is that the F_{eq} is approximately +0.50 less than the F'_v for every +10 DS of power: for example, if you want to achieve F_{eq} = +16.00, use full-aperture trial lenses to the labelled power of +16.75.

Binocular Versus Monocular Correction

Hand-held and stand-mounted magnifiers can rarely be used binocularly, as the (typically) small diameter lenses must be used close to one eye in order to increase the field-of-view.

TABLE 7.3	**A Summary of the Types of Stand-Mounted Magnifiers Currently Available**			
Characteristics	**FIXED-FOCUS**		**VARIABLE-FOCUS**	
	Low-Powered (Fig. 7.25)	**Medium-/High-Powered (Fig. 7.26)**	**Low-Powered (Fig. 7.24)**	**High-Powered**
Power/magnification range	<+16.00 DS (4×)	From +16.00 DS to +80.00 DS (4 to 20×)	<+10.00 DS (2.5×)	>+40.00 DS (10×)
Typical emergent vergence	Up to −10.00 DS	Zero to −4.00 DS	Variable	Variable
Lens form and diameter	Spherical up to 75 mm Aspheric up to 100 mm	Aspheric up to 50 mm Doublet lenses up to 20 mm	Spherical up to 100 mm Aspheric up to 150 mm	Aspheric up to 30 mm
Typical linear field-of-view	40 mm with 25 cm eye-to-magnifier distance	100 mm with magnifier close to spectacle plane	100 mm with 25 cm eye-to-magnifier distance	30 mm with magnifier close to spectacle plane
Other features	Stand design must allow illumination of, and access to, object plane	Commonly internally illuminated	May be worn suspended around the neck; many originally designed for industrial situations, so are robust but expensive	Very few examples of this type of magnifier are produced

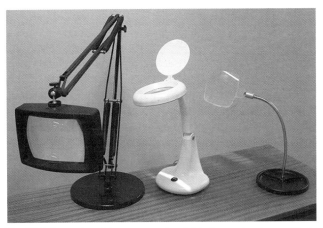

Fig. 7.24 Examples of low-powered variable focus stand magnifiers.

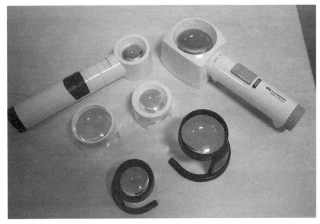

Fig. 7.26 Various medium- and high-powered (4× to 20×) stand magnifiers, showing both illuminated and non-illuminated designs.

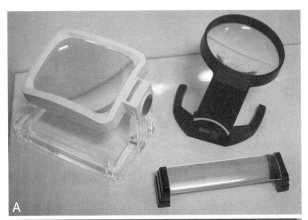

A

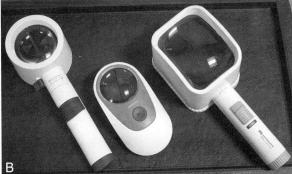

B

Fig. 7.25 A selection of (A) non-illuminated, and (B) illuminated, low-powered (<4×) fixed-focus stand magnifiers.

They could only be considered for binocular viewing if the lens is of large aperture (and therefore of low power and low magnification) and held at a long eye-to-magnifier distance. If the monocular fields are to overlap, it is also necessary that the lens be placed on the user's midline and this means that each eye views obliquely through the lens and thus experiences greater aberrations than if the lens is directly in front of one eye, whose visual axis coincides with the optical axis of the lens. Binocular viewing through a magnifying plus lens can, however, be achieved in some cases by placing the lenses in the spectacle plane. It is often desirable to use binocular viewing because it has the following advantages (Fonda, 1970):

1. Larger total field-of-view.
2. Improved acuity.
3. 'Normal' appearance.
4. Patient's psychological preference for using both eyes.
5. An occluder can be provided to change to monocular viewing with either eye if binocular viewing later becomes impractical/impossible.
6. For a patient with patchy vision loss, the functional field in one eye could theoretically compensate for the missing areas in the other eye.

Binocular correction would, however, be contra-indicated if there was:

1. No evidence of binocularity. The patient could be tested for intact binocular perception using a Bagolini lens, a Mallett fixation disparity test (in which the patient viewing through polarising filters sees the target letters O X O with both eyes, but two adjacent bars are each seen by only one eye), or a Worth four-dot test (the patient views through goggles containing one red and one green lens, and must have binocular vision in order to correctly report the presence of each of the white, green and red target lights). In each case, the test must be placed at the distance at which the patient is intending to read, and the intended plus-lens correction must be worn. If these tests were not available, a simple bar-reading test could be used. In the latter, a pen or thin bar is placed on the midline, midway between the patient's eyes and the reading matter. It acts as an occluder for each eye in turn, obscuring the view of each eye for different words along a line. Uninterrupted reading of the text suggests that both eyes are viewing simultaneously, with one eye compensating for the missing view of the fellow eye.
2. A large discrepancy in the monocular acuities measured. If the difference is a factor of two or more, there is unlikely to be any visual advantage in binocular correction, and monocular correction of the better eye will usually be more appropriate.

In either case (1) or (2), whilst binocular vision does not help the patient visually, it may still be used because it is cosmetically or psychologically preferred. In other situations, such as (3) and (4) below, the binocular vision may actually be worse, and restricting the patient to monocular viewing is essential. (This is not usually a problem with hand or stand magnifiers, as the patient can adjust the lens position to optimise use by the better eye).

3. A central or paracentral scotoma or distortion in a previously dominant eye. The patient can find this impossible to suppress, and binocular vision is poor: the distorted vision in the worse (dominant) eye may rival the clear image seen by the better (non-dominant) eye. The poorer dominant eye may need to be occluded, and correction confined to the better eye. The degree of occlusion required will vary between patients: sometimes a blurring lens or a frosted occluder will suffice, but on other occasions it proves necessary to use an opaque black cover or even an occlusive contact lens.

4. Too large a convergence demand created by the close working distance, causing discomfort or diplopia. The angle through which each eye must rotate is ϕ in Fig. 7.27:

$$\tan \phi = \frac{\frac{(PD)}{2}}{ws + u}$$

where PD is the distance between the centres of rotation of the eyes ($R_R R_L$) and is equal to the interpupillary distance of the patient; ws is the working space, which is the distance from the magnifying lens to the object, and this will

typically be equal to the focal length of the lens; and u is the distance from the spectacle plane to the centre of rotation of the eyes (for a lens positioned in the conventional spectacle plane, this is usually assumed to be 27 mm; consisting of a vertex distance of 12 mm, and a distance from the cornea to the centre of rotation of 15 mm).

To convert to prism dioptres from degrees, the tangent of the angle is multiplied by 100, so the total convergence demand for both eyes together is

$$convergence = \frac{100\,PD}{ws + u}$$

This can be shown to be 1Δ base-out for every millimetre of interpupillary distance, to view an object at a distance of 10 cm from the centre of rotation of the eye. Because the lenses are high-powered positive lenses, the amount of base-out prism to be overcome will be increased still further if the lenses are not sufficiently decentred inwards.

Determining the Correct Centration

To determine the required centration for binocular correction in conventional reading spectacles, the near centration distance (NCD) would usually be measured directly using a millimetre rule or a pupillometer whilst the patient was converging to view an object at their required working distance. This technique is not usually applicable to the very short working distances to be considered here, so the required NCD should be calculated or estimated by a 'rule-of-thumb'.

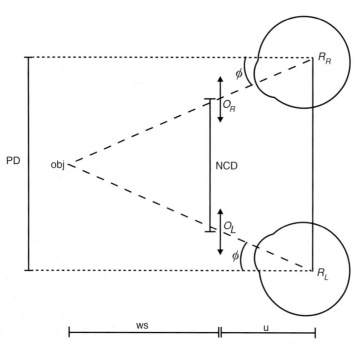

Fig. 7.27 Binocular viewing of an object (*obj*) through spectacle-mounted plus lenses, positioned a distance *u* from the centres of rotation of the eyes (R_R and R_L), showing the required optical centre distance (*NCD*) for a small working space (*ws*). Each eye must rotate through an angle of ϕ, to view the object binocularly. The distance $R_R R_L$ is equal to the interpupillary distance (*PD*). O_R and O_L are the optical centre of the right and left lenses.

Calculation

Fig. 7.27 illustrates schematically the binocular fixation at near with the eyes rotated about their respective centres-of-rotation R_R and R_L, so that the visual axes converge on the object (obj). The object is usually at the focal point of the plus lenses, so the working space (*ws*) (magnifier-to-object distance) is equal to the focal length f_M. The optical centres of the plus lenses have been decentred inwards and $O_R O_L$ is the required NCD—the optical centre distance which will give no prismatic effect.

By similar triangles

$$\frac{R_R R_L}{O_R O_L} = \frac{PD}{NCD} = \frac{ws + u}{ws}$$

So

$$NCD = \frac{ws \times PD}{ws + u}$$

If the correction was in bifocal form, the segments would need to be inset so that the horizontal distance between the geometrical centres of the two segments was equal to NCD. In this case

$$inset \text{ for each lens} = \frac{PD - NCD}{2}$$

It is important to remember that this near centration must also be used with the lenses in the trial frame when testing the patient, as well as in the final completed spectacles. Example:

What is the required NCD for an emmetropic patient with PD = 66 mm who is to have a reading addition of +10.00 made up as single-vision lenses? $F_M = +10.00$, so *ws* (which is equal to $f_M = 1/F_M = 0.1$ m) = 100 mm: assume that $u = 27$ mm)

$$NCD = \frac{ws \times PD}{ws + u}$$

$$NCD = \frac{100 \times 66}{(100 + 27)} = 52 \, mm$$

Clinical 'rules-of-thumb'

As the previous method requires a calculator, various simply applied rules have been suggested which should only require some mental arithmetic. These methods actually calculate the required total decentration for near, which is in fact the difference between the PD and the NCD. As can be seen by working through the same example for each, they do not produce precisely the same result, but each is within the limits of clinically acceptable tolerance:

1. Bailey's method
   Total decentration for near = PD − NCD

   $$= (1.5 \times \text{working space in dioptres}) + (1 \, mm \text{ if } PD > 65 mm)$$

   For the previous example, working space = 10.00 DS and PD = 66 mm
   so

   $$PD - NCD = (1.5 \times 10) + 1 = 16 \, mm$$

   $$66 - NCD = 16, \text{ so } NCD = 50 \, mm$$

2. Lebensohn's rule

   $$\text{total decentration for near} = PD - NCD$$

   $$= \frac{PD \text{ in mm}}{(ws \text{ in inches} + 1)}$$

   Again considering the same example, working space is 10 cm which is 4 in, so

   $$PD - NCD = \frac{66}{(4 + 1)} = 13.2$$

   $$66 - NCD = 13.2 \text{ so } NCD \approx 53 \, mm$$

   These methods each aim to provide accurate centration for lenses so that unwanted base-out prismatic effect can be avoided. Nonetheless, the convergence demand is still extreme, and Fonda (1957) recommends extra decentration inwards (a smaller NCD) to give the patient a base-in prismatic effect in near viewing.

3. Fonda's recommendation
   Total decentration for near = PD − NCD = (2 × working space in dioptres)
   In the example already given where working space is 10.00 DS and PD = 66 mm,

   $$PD - NCD = 2 \times 10 = 20$$

   $$66 - NCD = 20, \text{ so } NCD = 46 mm$$

   These extremes of inwards decentration may not be possible to achieve practically in some cases. The size of the uncut lens may be insufficient or, particularly in the case of lenticular lenses of limited aperture, or small bifocal segments, the fields-of-view may no longer be maximally coincident. In order to maximise the field-of-view through the lens aperture, the patient's visual axis should pass through the *geometrical* centre of the aperture when the eyes are converging to the required object distance. If the decentration is too large to be practical, working base-in prism on each lens is a possible solution: Fonda suggests 1Δ per dioptre of working space.

Even if Fonda's recommendation is followed, the convergence demand remains high, and Bailey (1979) has suggested the following assessment of the likelihood of achieving comfortable binocular single vision with the various addition powers:

+6.00—easy

+8.00—difficult

+10.00—risky

+12.00—highly unlikely

Some manufacturers have produced binocular spectacle-mounted aids with a longer-than-normal back vertex distance (see Fig. 7.5). This increases the working distance (eye-to-object distance) and therefore reduces convergence demand. Care must be taken, however, because the visual axes pass through the plus lens more nasally and thus more base-out prism is induced.

In the examples quoted previously, it has been assumed that the patient is an emmetrope with relaxed accommodation: in this case the object will be seen clearly when placed at the anterior focal point of the plus lens and parallel light leaves the lens. In this case, ws is equal to f_M. It is possible, however, that the pre-presbyopic patient will accommodate and create a more powerful plus-lens system: for practical purposes it can be assumed that the total power of the two-component system is simply the sum of the accommodation and the magnifier power, with the object being held at the focal point of this combined system. In this case the patient's working space will be correspondingly reduced, and their convergence (and therefore the required decentration of the lenses) increased.

There is also an influence of uncorrected ametropia on the magnification and working space achieved. If, for example, an uncorrected 4.00 DS myope uses a +8.00 DS spectacle lens, this will have the magnifying effect of a +12.00 DS lens. It is as if the myope was wearing −4.00 DS (to correct their myopia), plus +12.00 DS as a magnifying lens, and in total this gives +8.00 DS. The magnifying component being of power +12.00 DS, however, means that it will provide 3× magnification ($M = F_{eq}/4 = +12.00/4$) and the working space will be 8.3 cm ($ws = f_M = 1/F_M = 1/+12.00 = 8.3$ cm). The uncorrected 4.00 DS hypermetrope using the same +8.00 DS magnifying lens, however, only has the magnifying effect of a +4.00 DS lens: +4.00 DS of the plus lens power has been 'used up' to correct the ametropia. The +8.00 DS total power is effectively made up of +4.00 DS (to correct the hypermetropia), and +4.00 DS as a magnifying lens, and in total this gives +8.00 DS. The magnifying component being of power +4.00 DS, however, means that it will only provide 1× magnification ($M = F_{eq}/4 = +4.00/4$) and the working space will be 25 cm ($ws = f_M = 1/F_M = 1/+4.00 = 25$ cm). These influences on working space must be considered when deciding on the optical centre distance to be used in a binocular correction.

Advantages and Disadvantages

Advantages

1. The patient has both hands free to hold, or to carry out, the particular task.
2. The field-of-view is maximal as the lens is as close as possible to the eye. It has been suggested that field-of-view is a major factor in achieving a fast reading speed (Mancil & Nowakowski, 1986).
3. The spectacle frame can be fitted with distance posts or some similar device to ensure the task material is correctly positioned.
4. There is a similar cosmetic appearance to conventional spectacles, particularly in low to moderate powers.

Disadvantages

1. Obviously the system cannot be worn binocularly for walking around (although bifocal, half-eye and clip-on/flip-up forms of these lenses are all available), and even the blurred vision experienced when simply looking up from the visual task may make the patient feel disorientated or nauseous.
2. Account must be taken of the patient's ametropia, as discussed previously, with less magnification being experienced by the hypermetrope wearing a given lens, than by an emmetrope with the same magnifier. Conversely, the myope obtains an effective increase in magnification. For an astigmatic patient, it can be difficult to obtain the special high-powered lenses required with cylindrical correction incorporated, but typically cylinder powers of less than 2.00 DC do not influence the patient's acuity.
3. Often quite expensive, unless in clip-on form.
4. The short working space makes task illumination difficult, although small LED light sources are available which can clip on to the side of the spectacle frame and produce very high illuminance direct on the task (Fig. 7.28) which may become an advantage of this form of magnification. This is not a concern for viewing illuminated tasks such as tablet computers or a smartphone. The working space may be too restricted for the performance of some manipulative tasks.

Types Available

As noted previously, the performance of the patient with a spectacle-mounted plus lens can be tested using standard trial-case lenses, in an appropriately centred trial frame, and then the required spectacles could be ordered from the prescription house (see point [5] below). This does not, however, allow the patient to see the cosmetic result of the finished spectacles or to try the device at home to judge its effectiveness, and the lenses will be expensive. It is better, if possible, to begin with a device (such as those in points [1] to [3] below) which are extremely useful to loan to a patient for trial at home before deciding whether to proceed with a permanent correction, although many patients continue to use them on an extended basis.

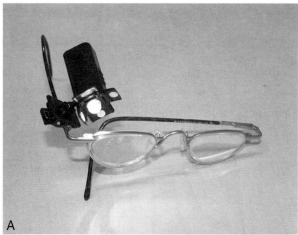

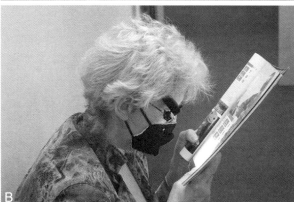

Fig. 7.28 (A) An LED light can be clipped onto the side of the frame of a spectacle-mounted magnifier to produce extremely high illumination directly on the task. (B) The device in use.

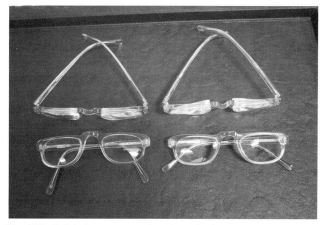

Fig. 7.29 Coil half-eye spectacles. The paired +10.00 lenses on the right have greater base-in prism than the +6.00 lenses on the left.

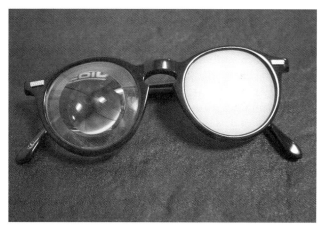

Fig. 7.30 An example of a hyperocular lens.

In giving examples of the products of particular manufacturers, the magnification or power ratings which they use will be quoted, in order that the products can be identified: the equivalent power should be verified experimentally as required.

There are many ways in which spectacle-mounted plus-lenses can be provided, and these are available from a number of different manufacturers, whose websites give extensive information about their individual products.

1. Ready-glazed in standard frame or mount

a. Paired lenses (with base-in prisms)

Various manufacturers produce a fixed range of powers, equal for right and left eyes, which incorporate standard amounts of base-in prism in order to reduce the convergence demand. Minor degrees of cylindrical refractive error, or slight anisometropia, are not usually a contraindication to this choice of correction. A limited range of frame styles and sizes are available from a number of suppliers (Coil; Mattingley; Multilens), including metal and plastic frames; full-aperture and half-eye; and small sizes (kids or 'quarter-eye'). A typical range of powers would be +4.00 DS/6Δ (1×); +6.00 DS/8Δ (1.5×); +8.00 DS/10Δ (2×); +10.00 DS/12Δ (2.5×); +12.00 DS/14Δ (3×) and +14.00 DS/16Δ (3.5×) (Fig. 7.29). The exact prismatic effect experienced will depend on the wearer's interpupillary distance. Eschenbach use a standard mount with adjustable nosepads and a lens attachment which gives a long vertex distance (see Fig. 7.5). The interchangeable lenses are clipped in and can be easily changed: although labelled as 2×, 2.5× and 3×, they actually measure +2.50 DS, +4.75 DS and +7.50 DS, respectively (and each incorporates base-in prism).

b. Monocular corrections

Coil produces a range of Hyperocular aspheric lenses glazed to a standard frame (Fig. 7.30). As the powers available are 4× to 12× (and these lenses are labelled with the equivalent powers), binocular viewing is not possible, so no prism or decentration is required: the other lens aperture contains a plano lens. These frames are available with a lens fitted in front of both eyes: these are NOT binocular corrections but are useful for the practitioner to use when trialling with patients because a requirement for either a right or left eye correction can be met with a single pair.

2. Added over patient's own spectacles

These are most commonly in a clip-on/fitover design, for use on an intermittent basis, but others are more permanent. The clip-on type is also ideal for loan to the patient to try at home, especially in the case of moderate to high cylindrical or spherical ametropia.

Monocular

a. Coil Magniclip monocular clip-on/flip-up. The manufacturer rates these as 2.5×, 3.5× and 4.75×, but these are 'trade magnification', the lenses being labelled +6.00 DS, +10.00 DS and +15.00 DS, respectively. There is also a chavasse lens available to occlude the uncorrected eye. If placed over a steeply curved or deep spectacle lens, the clip-on may lie at an oblique angle and the patient may not be able to view through it.

b. Eschenbach clip-on with extended vertex distance attachment, 4× and 7× (Fig. 7.5, right).

c. A more permanent addition to the patient's existing (distance or near) correction can be provided by the stick-on Eschenbach uniVISION segments. These are extremely thin and lightweight 22 mm diameter 'segments' with equivalent powers from +6.00 to +40.00. The lens can be temporarily positioned (as for a bifocal segment) for checking and then is 'permanently' stuck in position. Although it cannot be routinely taken on and off, it can be moved to the patient's new pair of spectacles, or replaced if a new power is needed. A similar effect, although optically this would be considerably inferior, could be achieved with a stick-on Fresnel bifocal segment, or a full-sized Fresnel lens which had been cut down to the required segment shape and size, and then attached to the conventional single-vision prescription.

Binocular

d. Eschenbach 2×, 2.5×, 3×: these are the same lenses as used in (1a) above, again with the extended vertex distance mount, but this time with a clip to attach across the bridge of the patient's own frame.

e. Multilens Sight Optimiser: these lenses, on a mount, which fits over existing spectacles, offer only a small addition (from +1.00 to +3.00), so would need to be combined with near spectacles to provide magnification.

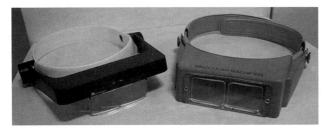

Fig. 7.31 Headband magnifiers.

3. Aids adapted from occupational use

a. Headband magnifiers are used mainly for industrial inspection use and are only usually available up to approximately +10.00 DS (2.5×) because they are invariably binocular. Some designs have an auxiliary lens which can be added for monocular viewing (Fig. 7.31). They are very poor cosmetically and are often clumsy and heavy.

b. A watchmaker's eyeglass (available from 2× to 8× magnification) is held in the orbit by muscular pressure.

c. Jeweller's loupes [sic], can be single or double lenses, up to +32.00 DS (8×), flips out of the way when not in use.

d. Ary loupe [sic], up to 5×. This attachment is not interchangeable between right and left lenses, and it is difficult to fit on large frames.

4. Exchangeable lenses in a carrier mounting

If high-powered lenses are limited in diameter, then this reduces weight and thickness. These can be placed into a standard mounting which is inserted into a plano carrier, which itself is edged to fit into the chosen spectacle frame. The effect is similar to that of a lenticular lens. The advantage is that the central optical element can consist of more than one lens (to better manage aberrations) and can be changed if required (e.g. if the patient requires additional magnification). This is the basis of the Multilens A2, and Aplanat, lenses, where two plano convex lenses are combined with curved surfaces facing to create an aplanatic system with equivalent powers (for the A2) from +10.00 (2.5×) to +52.00 (13×). An additional lens to correct refractive error can also be added into the mounting.

5. Edged lenses glazed into frame

A wide variety of lenses are available which can be glazed to the patient's preferred spectacle frame. In the UK, it would be possible to use an NHS Spectacle Voucher to contribute to the cost of such an appliance. Unless otherwise stated, powers quoted are back vertex power.

Single Vision

a. 'Conventional' glass or plastic prescription lenses: best form (meniscus) spherical lenses will offer adequate image quality up to approximately +10.00 DS, then lenticular and aspheric designs are better optically. It is important to remember that the aberration control in these lenses is designed for the correction of ametropia at long viewing distances, so image quality will not be optimal for the very short viewing distances adopted in low-vision aids. Similarly the advantage of blended aspherics (e.g. Essilor Omega and Rodenstock Perfastar) is predominantly in eliminating the ring scotoma to aid mobility, and so these are not beneficial for near vision. High-index lenses will offer a better cosmetic appearance (and perhaps higher power availability) but a poorer image quality due to the increased dispersion (reduced V-value/Abbe number).

Full-aperture lenses are available up to approximately +15.00, depending on index. Lenticulars are available up to +48.00, although the aperture reduces as the lens power increases. The use of digital (free-form) surfacing increases the range of lenticular designs which could be utilised: for example, a lens could be lenticular and aspheric on both surfaces (Chadwick Optical).

b. Specific magnifier lens forms using spherical surfaces: Stigmagna or Lederer designs in powers from +10.00 DS to +24.00 DS do calculate the optimum form for the very short working distance to be used. These lenses are not commercially available, but they could be worked to order.

c. Other specific magnifier lens forms: examples are the Hyperocular with an aspheric front surface and 34 mm aperture in equivalent powers from +16.00 DS (4×) to +48.00 DS (12×); and the Designs for Vision Full Diameter Microscope range which are doublet lenses with an aperture from 27 to 36 mm and powers from 2× to 20×.

d. Stick-on, flexible, plastic Fresnel lenses are available in powers up to +16.00 DS, which could be attached to a plano-/low-powered lens. Although they offer a potentially useful temporary or trial correction, they create very poor image contrast which may cause the patient to reject the spectacles.

Bifocals—Surfaced Lenses

e. Watchmakers spot segment (15 mm diameter) with add +10.50 to +25.00. This is designed to be fitted monocularly with the segment in the upper portion of one lens.

f. Glass lens with flat-top 25 mm diameter segment cemented to back surface: addition up to +16.00 DS (4×) (Zeiss).

g. Plastic solid downcurve 22/25/28 mm diameter segment with addition up to between +10.00 DS and +20.00 DS (depending on segment diameter).

h. Plastic flat-top 25 or 35 mm diameter segment with addition up to +8.00 DS (although this does depend on the distance prescription).

Bifocals—Made to Order From Single-Vision Components

Any single vision lens can theoretically be used as one of the lens components, so the range of powers available will be better than for catalogue lenses: any limitation will be due to the technical challenges of combining the two component lenses into a single entity. The earliest bifocal lens—the (Franklin) split bifocal—is made by cutting the top half from a lens with the distance prescription, and the bottom half from a lens with the near prescription. The straight-line bifocal lens is formed when these two components are held together in a frame: technically this is much easier to achieve with a metal frame.

The other alternatives are to cement the smaller addition lens onto the full size distance lens, or to insert the addition lens into an aperture of appropriate size drilled into the main lens (Norville 'Presto' (Fig. 7.32) or Multilens 'MLOptio'; Chadwick Optical).

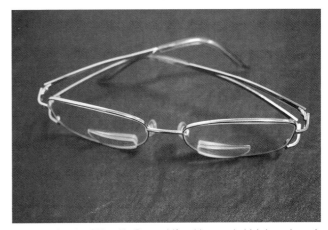

Fig. 7.32 A pair of Norville Presto bifocal lenses (which have base in prism in the segments).

Procedure for Dispensing a High-Plus Spectacle Magnifier

Frame Choice

The frame chosen should be a full-rimmed metal or plastic frame, of small to moderate size, and rounded lens shape. Ideally the patient's interpupillary distance (PD) should be only slightly less (2 to 4 mm) than the frame boxed centre distance (minimal decentration), and with the pupils only slightly above the horizontal centre line in straight-ahead gaze. If the lens to be used is made up of more than one component, it will usually be necessary to make sure the whole of the high-powered zone will fit within the aperture. If choosing a half-eye frame, a very shallow oblong shape is not suitable because of the extreme edge thickness created at the upper and lower rims.

Binocular or Monocular

If magnification to be provided is ≤3×, and the acuity difference between the two eyes is ≤2× (0.3 log units), then binocular correction can be considered. If a monocular correction is chosen, then it is also necessary to select a suitable lens to be placed in front of the uncorrected eye. This could be a (balance) lens of the same power, to match the cosmetic appearance, or a low power or plano lens (and perhaps single vision rather than bifocal) to keep the cost down (and perhaps allow the patient to look up and use that eye for distance). If the patient has severe vision loss in a previously dominant eye, this can be difficult for them to ignore and the eye may need to be occluded. A frosted lens, or even an opaque occluder can be ordered. Alternatively, a stick-on Bangerter foil would be better cosmetically and may be discarded later as the patient adapts to monocular viewing.

Material and Lens Type

As noted previously, the extreme add will give very blurred vision when the wearer looks up from the near task. This can make the patient feel disorientated or nauseous, so a bifocal option (or a half-eye) may be a good option. A bifocal intended for this purpose would probably still only be worn during the near task, rather than constantly. If this is the case, the segment could be fitted 2 to 3 mm higher than usual. A bifocal is an excellent cosmetic option, as the high-powered segment does not significantly affect overall lens thickness/weight/appearance. To experience the cosmetic advantage for yourself, compare the thickness of a full-aperture and reduced aperture trial lens of equal (high plus) power. There is a restriction on the availability of different segment sizes, especially for very high adds. The limited diameter obviously restricts the field of view, but this is mitigated by the short eye-to-lens distance. The field of view ($y = D/aF_{eq}$) can be calculated for the diameter of the bifocal segment, to decide whether this is too restrictive: in fact, a 20 mm diameter segment allows a field of view of 33 cm with a +4.00 add, although this does reduce to 6 cm with a +20.00.

From a cosmetic point of view, high index lens materials and aspheric form will give the thinnest, lightest lens with minimum spectacle magnification: the latter is not significant visually but may be so cosmetically.

Horizontal Centration

This depends on whether a binocular or monocular correction is to be dispensed. If monocular, the lens can be centred to match the monocular distance PD (no convergence is required). If binocular, then it is necessary to decide whether to fit to accurate NCD or to use extra decentration/inset to aid convergence: a large D-segment can often be inset by up to 10 to 12 mm if required. If the required amount of decentration/inset is not achievable, then working base-in prism on a single vision lens is straightforward. A bifocal lens (when the prism is for near only), would require a special lens type (e.g. Presto, Franklin split, cemented). However, the extra thickness at the base of the prism (thickness difference g) will also be considerably less in the small bifocal segment than in the full aperture lens. The formula for thickness difference is

$$g = \frac{P \times D}{100(n-1)}$$

where P is the worked prism, D is the lens diameter, and n is the refractive index. Taking an example, for CR39 lenses ($n = 1.5$ approximately), a 20 mm segment with 6Δ prism would have a thickness difference of 2.4 mm, whereas, for a full aperture lens of 50 mm diameter, the corresponding value would be 6 mm.

Vertical Centration

In single vision lenses, the ideal situation is for the wearer to view along the optical axis of the lens. If the frame has been fitted with some degree of pantoscopic tilt (almost inevitable to optimize the cosmetic appearance and prevent the lens being too far from the wearer's face), then this is achieved by moving the optical centres downwards. This involves determining the lens position directly in line with the pupil centres

in distance vision and then decentring the lenses downwards by 0.5 mm for each 1° of pantoscopic tilt (Jalie, 2007). In reality, this tends to place the optical centres close to the default position on the horizontal centre line, as the pantoscopic angle is usually close to 10°, and the pupil centres are typically 5 mm above the horizontal centre line. If this is not the case, and vertical decentration becomes extreme, then the effect on lens thickness may be problematic (and perhaps a different frame should be chosen).

Vertex Distance

When dispensing high-powered lenses to correct ametropia, it is critical that vertex distance is measured, and the prescription compensated for any differences in vertex distance between the trial lens and the chosen spectacle frame. This is not required for near corrections, because the working distance is not usually rigidly fixed: any discrepancy in power can be overcome by the wearer adjusting their working distance slightly.

Required Power to Order

Some high-powered spectacle lenses are specifically designed as magnifiers and so may be specified by their equivalent power or magnification (e.g. the Hyperocular range). However, 'standard' prescription lenses are ordered in terms of power, rather than magnification. Further, this is back vertex power, rather than equivalent power. If the required magnification to order has been determined by testing the patient using reduced aperture trial lenses, then this will be an accurate value for F_{eq}: although these lenses are marked with their F'_v, the front surface is plano, so $F_{eq} = F'_v$.

If it is necessary to find the correct back vertex power to order, then consider the formula

$$F'_V = \frac{F_{eq}}{\left[1 - \frac{t}{n'}F_1\right]}$$

It is difficult to account for this exactly, because the front surface curvature and thickness for the finished lenses is unknown, but it is clear from the formula that the back vertex power will need to be greater than the equivalent power. The discrepancy will increase as the power of the lens increases, and will be greater for lenses which are thicker, have a larger diameter (because of the effect this has on thickness), and have more steeply curved front surfaces. In view of the fact that two important variables (F_1 and t) are unknown at the time of ordering the spectacles, any power adjustment (to a higher ordered value) will need to be on a pragmatic basis and is typically of the order of 1.00–2.00 DS in the relevant power range.

INTRAOCULAR LENSES

Intraocular lenses (IOLs) have the potential to provide magnifying power in a way which is always available to the patient (unlike, for example, a hand magnifier) and does not create an unusual cosmetic appearance (as a spectacle aid would do). Routine cataract surgery uses monofocal lenses, but multifocal lenses are available, and these could be made with higher adds by putting the add on both surfaces. Borkenstein and Borkenstein (2020) report the LENTIS MAX LS-313 MF 80 IOL, which has a +8.00 add (reported equivalent to a +6.00 in the spectacle plane), being used successfully in individuals with macular degeneration.

An alternative is the Scharioth macular lens (SML) which is an add-on IOL for a patient who is already pseudophakic, or who will be simultaneously fitted with a conventional monofocal IOL. The lens is fitted monocularly to the better eye and is placed in the ciliary sulcus, which is the space between the posterior iris and anterior ciliary body. This IOL has no refractive effect in the lens periphery, but a central 1.5-mm zone with +10.00 power, which is claimed to provide 2× magnification at a 15 cm viewing distance. For any lens which allows simultaneous vision through different optical zones, the image which is defocused on the retina has the effect of reducing the retinal image contrast of the focused image. This will be partially avoided by the pupil constriction which occurs when fixating at near (part of the near triad), meaning very little of the light is passing through the peripheral zone of the lens, but it could be a consideration for individuals with already poor contrast sensitivity. A patient with similar acuity in both eyes may require occlusion of the nonimplanted eye to avoid confusion.

Scharioth (2015) reported that patients had much better acuity postoperatively with the SML, than they did preoperatively when reading at 15 cm with a +6.00 spectacle add, and he attributed this to the better image quality of the IOL. However, Srinivasan et al. (2019) suggests the results under these two conditions are very similar, if lighting and viewing distance are well controlled.

None of these lenses have been tested in randomised controlled trials.

One particular monofocal IOL (Eyemax mono) has been designed specifically for patients with macular degeneration, with an aspheric surface which aims to provide good image quality across an enlarged visual field (up to 10° from the fovea) (Qureshi et al., 2018; Robbie et al., 2018). It is suggested that this would be more beneficial than standard IOLs if the individual uses eccentric viewing and fixates with a nonfoveal area. Rather than targeting emmetropia as the final refractive error, it can be planned that the individual is left moderately hypermetropic and so get additional spectacle magnification from their correcting lenses. There is some disagreement about the extent of magnification available: Robbie et al. (2018) suggest a +2.00 to +3.50 correction provides between 10% and 20% (1.1× to 1.2×), whereas Qureshi et al. (2018) calculated a 9% increase (1.09×) for a +2.70 spectacle power. Alternatively, planning for postoperative myopia would allow the uncorrected patient to be focused for a close working distance and experience relative distance magnification. This should certainly be discussed with patients who were myopic prior to their cataract.

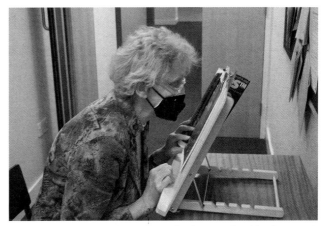

Fig. 7.33 Using a reading stand to maintain a comfortable close working distance.

OPTIMISING THE USE OF MAGNIFIERS

Reading Stands

The necessity of using a fixed (and usually small) magnifier-to-object distance has already been discussed. This typically makes the reading posture very different to that to which the patient has been accustomed previously. In addition, it can be most uncomfortable to maintain such a posture for a prolonged period, and the low-vision patient may well complain of neck ache and/or aching arms. In these cases, a reading stand or raised desk-top can be helpful, as it provides a firm working surface with variable tilt on which to support the visual task. The required working space can then be maintained without undue effort. Reading stands can be home-made, and are also commercially available (Fig. 7.33). In addition to the models designed for low-vision work, or intended for use by patients with other physical limitations, there are also office copy-holders or tilting tables which can be adapted: over-the-bed tables may often be provided with a tilting top. School children may benefit from a sloping desk.

In deciding which model to buy, the following points should be considered:

- What weight will it need to hold? Some copy-holders are not robust enough to hold more than a few sheets of paper, nor could they support the weight of the patient writing on them.
- Does the patient need a device to hold the book or magazine open at the page? If to be used for single sheets, is a line marker which can slide down the page required? Would such a guide-rail be a useful rest for a stand magnifier? Some stands with a magnetised work surface can have a magnetic page holder which slides down the page acting as a line guide.
- Does it need to be portable and adjustable to be used in different locations and for different tasks?
- Will it be free-standing on a table-top (does it need a weighty base?) or clamped? The latter might be required, for example, when reading music whilst playing an instrument.

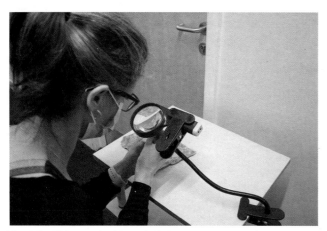

Fig. 7.34 Using a double-ended clamp to create a variable focus stand magnifier from a hand magnifier.

When the patient is reading with a magnifier and their field of view is restricted (either due to the magnifier diameter, or to their visual characteristics) the use of scrolled text or steady eye strategy (see Chapter 13) is often beneficial: keeping the head and eyes still and moving the task. This ensures that the patient's visual axis is parallel to the optical axis of the magnifier lens, and it also maintains the correct focal distance. This will not be possible if a reading stand is used, because the reading material must be held by the patient. In this case, the use of a clipboard or a sheet of thick card or hardboard should be considered in order to keep the object supported. It is almost impossible to use a stand magnifier properly for reading a newspaper or single sheet of paper, like a letter, without such a device. Many patients are very reluctant to make what they consider to be unnecessary and elaborate preparations to optimise reading conditions. Every opportunity must be taken to convince the patient that if the working conditions and the lighting are poor, the performance of their magnifier will be disappointing and inadequate.

Double-Ended clamp

Various methods exist to convert a hand magnifier into a stand magnifier, which is useful, for example, where a stand is required for writing, but a hand magnifier could be more easily carried for reading prices when out shopping. Fold-away legs, or a separate support into which the magnifier can be placed, are possible options. The clamp is a further option, consisting of a flexible rod with a clamp at each end—one can be used to hold the magnifier, and the other to attach to a table or shelf to leave the hands free, and create a variable focus stand magnifier (Fig. 7.34).

REFERENCES

Bailey, I. L. (1979). Centering high-addition spectacle lenses. *Optometric Monthly, 70,* 523–527.

Bailey, I. L. (1981a). Verifying near vision magnifiers—Part 2. *Optometric Monthly, 72*(2), 34–38.

Bailey, I. L. (1981b). Locating the image in stand magnifiers. *Optometric Monthly, 72*(6), 22–24.

Bennett, A. G. (1975). Igard hyperoculars: their origins and development. *Ophthalmic Optician, 15,* 1151–1154.

Bennett, A. G. (1982). Spectacle magnification and loupe magnification. *Optician, 183*(4740), 16–18, 36.

Bennett, A. G., & Rabbetts, R. B. (1984). *Clinical visual optics* (pp. 304–305). Butterworths.

Borkenstein, A. F., & Borkenstein, E. M. (2020). Four years of observation to evaluate autonomy and quality of life after implantation of a high-add intraocular lens in age-related macular degeneration patients. *Case Reports in Ophthalmology, 11*(2), 448–456. https://doi.org/10.1159/000508914.

BS 3521. (1991). *Terms relating to ophthalmic optics and spectacle frames part 1. Glossary of terms relating to ophthalmic lenses.* British Standards Institute.

Fonda, G. (1957). Binocular correction for low vision: rationale for rule of thumb for decentration. *American Journal of Ophthalmology, 45,* 23–27.

Fonda, G. (1970). Binocular reading additions for low vision. Report of 120 cases. *Arch Ophthalmol, 83,* 294–299.

Jalie, M. (1995). The design of low vision aids. In C. Dickinson (Ed.), *The ophthalmic lens year book 1995* (pp. 14–30). W.B. Saunders Company Ltd.

Jalie, M. (2007). *Ophthamic lenses and dispensing* (3rd ed.). Butterworth-Heinemann.

Lederer, J. (1955). A new development in aids for subnormal vision. *British Journal of Physiological Optics, 12,* 184–187.

Linksz, A. (1955). Optical principles of loupe magnification. *American Journal of Ophthalmology, 40,* 831–840.

Mancil, G. L., & Nowakowski, R. (1986). Evaluation of reading speed with four low vision aids. *American Journal of Optometry and Physiological Optics, 63,* 708–713.

Qureshi, M. A., Robbie, S. J., Hengerer, F. H., et al. (2018). Consecutive case series of 244 age-related macular degeneration patients undergoing implantation with an extended macular vision IOL. *European Journal of Ophthalmology, 28*(2), 198–203. https://doi.org/10.5301/ejo.5001052.

Robbie, S. J., Tabernero, J., Artal, P., et al. (2018). Initial clinical results with a novel monofocal-type intraocular lens for extended macular vision in patients with macular degeneration. *Journal of Refractive Surgery, 34*(11), 718–725. https://doi.org/10.3928/1081597X-20180831-01.

Scharioth, G. B. (2015). New add-on intraocular lens for patients with age-related macular degeneration. *Journal of Cataract and Refractive Surgery, 41*(8), 1559–1563. https://doi.org/10.1016/j.jcrs.2015.07.018.

Sloan, L. L., & Jablonski, M. D. (1959). Reading aids for the partially blind: classification and measurement of more than 200 devices. *Archives of Ophthalmology, 62,* 465–484.

Srinivasan, S., Scharioth, G., Riehl, A., et al. (2019). Implantation of Scharioth macula lens in patients with age-related macular degeneration: results of a prospective European multicentre clinical trial. *BMJ Open Ophthalmology, 4*(1), e000322. https://doi.org/10.1136/bmjophth-2019-000322.

Transverse Magnification

ELECTRONIC VISION ENHANCEMENT SYSTEMS

Optical magnifying systems are limited practically to a maximum magnification of about 20×. If using a plus-lens, this would require a +80.00DS lens with a working space of only 1.25 cm (equal to the anterior focal length of the lens). Such a high-powered system would also have considerable aberrations and be severely restricted in field-of-view. Transverse or 'real-image' magnification is available up to extremely high levels and does not require a change in the working space from the patient's preferred or habitual position.

The most efficient way to provide real image magnification is electronically, using a video camera to create a magnified image on a screen. The patient can be the same distance from the image on the screen as from the original object, so the existing refractive correction will be equally appropriate. Such a Closed-Circuit Television (CCTV) system was first proposed in 1959 (Potts et al., 1959), but much credit for the development from prototype to commercial production model must go to Sam Genensky, a mathematician with visual impairment who worked at the Rand Corporation (Genensky, 1969; Genensky et al. 1978). These systems are usually used for near or intermediate tasks, with the image presented on a screen close to the patient, although the camera can be pointed at a distant object, for example, a lecture screen or whiteboard. Flat panel LCD screens were incorporated into CCTVs in the early 2000s, making them smaller and lighter, and portable electronic video magnifiers have been used for about 20 years.

Since the early 1990s, researchers have attempted to develop wearable or head-mounted electronic magnifiers, such as the Low Vision Enhancement System (LVES) designed in conjunction with NASA (Massof & Rickman, 1992), although it is only since the availability of smaller lightweight screens that these have been used more widely (Deemer et al., 2018).

As electronic magnifiers have become more diverse, and to avoid confusion with security cameras, Peterson and colleagues suggested the more appropriate term Electronic Vision Enhancement Systems (EVES) is used for all electronic systems which use image manipulation such as magnification and contrast enhancement (Peterson et al., 2003).

Magnification and Field-of-View

The magnification of EVES is expressed as a direct increase in the linear size of a feature as measured on the display screen, compared to that of the original object:

$$M = \frac{\text{linear size of image on screen}}{\text{linear size of original object}}$$

There is no theoretical limit to the magnification which an electronic system can provide: up to 70× or even more is not unusual. In the early days of EVES, this extremely high magnification was emphasised, and it was suggested that patients who could not be helped with optical aids would be able to read with an electronic system. Nowadays, it is more common for the devices to be used by patients who use optical aids for some tasks, but revert to EVES when a long working space is needed, or longer duration tasks must be performed.

It may take some time for patients to become familiar with EVES (Ehrlich, 1987), and their ability to use it can increase with practice (Goodrich et al., 1977; Burggraaff et al., 2012). Desktop and portable EVES (p-EVES) seem to allow faster reading than optical magnifiers (Goodrich & Kirby, 2001;

Peterson et al., 2003), although this improvement is not seen with wearable systems (Culham et al., 2004; Wittich et al., 2018a; Crossland et al., 2019).

All EVES require a certain degree of manipulative skill, as indeed do optical aids, but in addition, the patient with limited sight must be able to distinguish all the controls: if these are all located on the same panel, they should be of different shapes or have tactile markings. When reading, text must be manipulated below the camera in a predictable and regular fashion. For desktop systems, this is usually achieved by using an X-Y platform to move the material in the X (left-right to read along the line and then return to the beginning) or Y (towards-away to move to the beginning of the next line) planes without any oblique movement. These platforms often have stops and adjustable resistance to movement to prevent overshoot of the area of interest. It is technically possible, though rare, to have semi-automatic hand or foot-operated push-button control of the platform movement or to have text presented digitally one line, or one word, at a time.

Field-of-View

If the field-of-view is defined as the area of the task (e.g. the number of words of text) visible at a given time, then this will not be influenced by the monitor-to-eye distance. The number of characters seen simultaneously on the screen depends on the magnification and the screen size. Increasing the screen size will obviously increase the field-of-view, but will give a heavier, bulkier system which may be difficult to transport or house. Patients are generally advised to use the minimum magnification possible, which will maximise the available information on the screen: given a free choice, they will usually select much higher magnification than used in optical magnification, even though this must restrict the field-of-view. Patients can also produce additional magnification by using a very close viewing distance. People with low vision habitually obtain magnification using a combination of reduced viewing distance and increased print size, with the latter being the primary method for most people (Granquist et al., 2018).

Encouraging the patient to get closer to the screen to maximise this 'relative distance magnification' whilst using the minimum real image magnification on the screen, will optimise the field-of-view. For example, the same retinal image size will be produced by viewing a screen with 10× magnification at 40 cm, as by viewing a screen with 5× magnification from 20 cm. In the second case, however, twice as many letters will be seen simultaneously.

Contrary to intuitive impressions, there is experimental evidence that reading can be very fast with a field-of-view of only 4 characters (Legge et al., 1997; Cheong et al., 2008) but in these cases the text was being automatically scanned. When the patient has to perform their own 'page-navigation', optimal performance may require 15 characters or more (Lovie-Kitchin & Woo, 1988; Lowe & Drasdo, 1990).

Advantages and Disadvantages

These can be summarised as follows.

Advantages

1. The use of zoom lenses permits a rapid change of magnification without altering focus. This allows the use of low magnification for overall assessment of the task before higher magnification is selected for examination of detail; for example, scanning newspaper headlines before zooming in on the text of an article.
2. When compared to optical aids, EVES usually increase reading speed, reduce the number of errors made when reading and can be used for longer durations without fatigue (Goodrich & Kirby, 2001; Burggraaff et al., 2012).
3. The systems typically have magnification adjustable over a wide range, so the patient can use it for a wide variety of tasks, and can continue to use it if their vision changes.
4. EVES might be psychologically more acceptable than optical aids, particularly in a school or work environment where screens are on every desk.
5. Binocular viewing of the screen from a 'normal' working distance is usually possible, so there are fewer restrictions on posture or convergence.
6. Many patients with severe field restrictions and reduced visual acuity can read more efficiently with EVES than with the same magnification produced by an optical aid. This appears to be because they can fixate on a single area of the screen and use the X-Y platform to scan the image through this area. In contrast, when using an optical aid they appear to use refixation saccades and miss out lines or words. Although this 'steady eye strategy' can be taught with optical aids, it is more difficult to learn (see section 'Central Field Loss' in Chapter 13).
7. Most EVES allow contrast reversal—electronic alteration of the polarity of the image on the screen, to transform black-on-white text to a white-on-black image. This is particularly useful for patients with media opacities because the average intensity of the image is considerably reduced, and thus light scatter within the eye is decreased.
8. EVES provide a higher contrast image than optical systems. This particularly benefits patients with poor contrast sensitivity for whom the optical aid provides insufficient 'contrast reserve' (see section 'Visual Requirements for Reading' in Chapter 3). Some systems allow a wide choice of background and text colour combination. There does not appear to be a systematic strategy to the selection of these, but some users claim to find them beneficial.
9. Desktop EVES may be useful for people with other comorbidities, such as those with tremor who find it difficult to hold optical aids steady.
10. Text can be underlined on the screen, and electronic windows can be created to blank out unwanted areas of the image.
11. Some EVES allow split screen presentation to enable two different tasks to be viewed simultaneously. This could be used, for example, for distance and near, such as taking notes from a whiteboard.

Disadvantages

1. In comparison to optical aids, these systems are usually bulkier and more obtrusive.
2. Those less familiar with technology may require more practice with EVES than with optical aids to become proficient in their use (Goodrich et al., 1977), although formal training is usually not required (Burggraaff et al., 2012).
3. EVES are usually more expensive to buy than optical magnifiers, and may not be funded by low vision clinics.
4. They may be difficult to repair in the case of malfunction.
5. There is some persistence of the image on the display, causing 'smearing' of the image as it moves across the screen. This can be worse with white-on-black images than with black-on-white and can limit the maximum reading speed attainable.
6. EVES are often provided 'off-the-shelf' without a full low-vision assessment. They do need to be prescribed like any other aid to ensure that they are suitable, and to be backed-up by optical aids for the tasks for which EVES are unsuitable. In some cases, a patient may purchase an EVES without realising a simpler and cheaper optical aid can perform the task just as well.
7. The depth-of-field is limited, and scanning across the page of a thick book can cause the image to go out of focus. The autofocus on some systems can take about a second to adjust to different object distances.
8. Viewing quickly moving images on EVES, particularly on wearable systems, can induce nausea and dizziness (Crossland et al., 2019).
9. At very high levels of magnification, pixels may be visible on the screen, limiting image quality.
10. EVES typically take longer to turn on and setup than optical magnifiers, and portable and wearable systems are often limited by short battery life.
11. Some systems have standard component or control positions that are not suited to a left-handed user.

CLASSIFICATION

The term 'electronic vision enhancement system' applies to a wide range of devices, which can be classified by object distance, portability, power source and other parameters (Table 8.1; Fig. 8.1). Broadly, these systems can be grouped into those that are desktop-based; those that are easily portable; and those which are worn, such as head-mounted devices.

Desktop EVES

Desktop EVES consist of a camera, a processor and a screen (Fig. 8.1, *left*). Modern systems typically incorporate a camera mounted underneath the screen, pointing down towards the x,y table on which text is placed. A large working space is available under the camera, which makes it suitable for use in hobbies or handicrafts—for example, building models or repairing domestic appliances. The patient must learn to look at the magnified view of their hands performing the task on the screen, rather than directly: this becomes more difficult as the screen is positioned further away from the task area.

Diagonal screen size is typically 12 to 24 in (30–60 cm), and magnification can be increased to about 75×. Controls for

TABLE 8.1 Classification of EVES Devices Currently Available

Object Distance	Portability	Power Supply	Camera	Display	Field of View	Image Magnification Type	Image Magnification Range	Image Manipulation
Distance	Fixed location	Mains	Independent	Standard TV	Small/restricted	Fixed	Low (≈2×–3×)	Contrast reversal
Intermediate	Transportable	Rechargeable	Rotatable	Standard monitor/laptop	Large	Steps	High (≈10×)	Colour change
Near	Handheld		Mouse-style	Head mounted		Continuous	Extreme (≈100×)	Image capture/freeze frame
Variable	Wearable		Incorporated opposite display	Incorporated				Line windowing/marking
			Incorporated in-line	Electronic reader				Mirror reversal
								Text reformatting
								Adding fixation marker
								Contrast enhancement
								Edge enhancement
								Stabilisation

EVES, Electronic vision enhancement systems.
From Dickinson, C., Hernández Trillo, A. H., & Gridley, A. (2017). Electronic vision enhancement for low vision. *Optometry in Practice, 18*(2), 93–102.

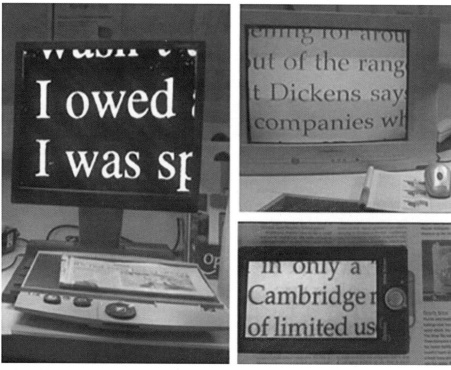

Fig. 8.1 Reading a magazine with various electronic vision enhancement systems. *(Left)* Desktop electronic vision enhancement systems (EVES). *(Top right)* Television magnifier. *(Bottom right)* Portable EVES (p-EVES).

magnification level and image manipulation are usually placed beneath the screen or in front of the x,y table. More advanced systems include optical character recognition, text-to-speech and other sensory substitution options (see Chapter 15).

Although usually designed for use in one location, smaller desktop EVES may fold up for transportation. Transportable magnifiers usually have a screen of about 10 to 16 in (around 25–40 cm).

Some desktop and transportable EVES can also be used for distance viewing, using a different camera or by rotating the camera to point at a distant object. These were used widely in schools and colleges, although an electronic system to relay the whiteboard image on to a tablet computer or laptop is now more common. They are sometimes used for intermediate tasks such as DIY or applying makeup (and for this purpose may allow a 'reversed' image, as would be seen looking in a mirror).

Television and Mouse-Based Magnifiers

A cheaper option is for patients to use an electronic system with their existing television screen or computer monitor. In these devices, the camera is mounted in a handheld unit which looks like a computer mouse, connected to the screen by a cable. Magnification is typically fixed or variable between a few levels and will be dependent on the size of the screen used. These may have some simple image manipulation modes. It can be difficult to trace a line of text with these systems, and holding the camera straight can be hard for some users. However, they were the first genuinely 'cheap' electronic magnifiers, typically costing less than one-tenth the price of desktop EVES.

Portable EVES

In the last 20 years, dozens of portable electronic vision enhancement systems have become available. p-EVES incorporate a camera, light source, processor and screen in a single handheld device. Screen size varies between about 2 in and about 8 in (5–20 cm), although the point at which a p-EVES device becomes a transportable device is not well defined. p-EVES usually weigh less than 500 g and have a battery life of up to 5 hours. They have a more modest magnification range than desktop EVES, generally having a maximum level of about 10×, which may be stepped or on a continuous zoom function. They generally offer reversed contrast and may provide some other colour options, although this will typically be more restricted than on a full-featured desktop system. Manipulation of a p-EVES requires practice to learn to follow lines of text and return to pick up the next line. The action required, however, is not that different to scanning an optical magnifier across text, and most patients master the skill relatively easily: placing a strip of wood across the page and pushing the camera against it whilst moving across the page may be useful in the early stages. Some systems have a stand into which the camera can be clipped to convert it to 'conventional' operation if portability is not required.

Unlike desktop EVES, portable systems do not improve reading speed when compared to optical aids (Taylor et al., 2017), although they do improve near visual acuity. In Taylor's study, people could read for longer with p-EVES than with optical devices, but optical low vision aids (LVAs) were used more frequently and for more tasks (Taylor et al., 2017). The limited screen size and reduced field of view is likely to be the major factor in reducing reading ability with portable devices: it is not physically possible to magnify text to the very high levels possible on a large-screen desktop EVES.

Wearable and Head-Mounted EVES

As cameras, screens, batteries and processors have got smaller and lighter, wearable EVES have become a more acceptable form of LVA for some patients. The principle of these systems is similar to desktop or p-EVES, although the camera is generally optimised for distance viewing. Wearable EVES comprise a camera mounted on a pair of spectacles, which also include an LCD or organic light-emitting diode (OLED) screen to display the magnified or manipulated image (Fig. 8.2). The battery may be included on the spectacles or connected by a cable. Magnification of up to 25× is available and is typically adjusted using a wired or wireless remote control. Some systems also have a minification mode for people with restricted visual fields. Image processing options may include reversed contrast, edge enhancement and adjustable brightness. The first commercially available head-mounted system—the LVES, introduced in 1994—weighed nearly a kilogram; but modern equivalents are nearly 10 times lighter (Deemer et al., 2018).

Head-mounted EVES improve visual acuity and contrast sensitivity (Wittich et al., 2018a; Crossland et al., 2019), and may improve some aspects of vision-related quality of life. However, current devices are limited by their weight and cosmetic appearance; about half of those who were asked to wear a similar system in public for a study said they felt self-conscious (Golubova et al., 2021). Some wearable EVES artificially restrict the visual field, and walking when observing a magnified view has negative effects on balance, eye movements and the vestibulo-ocular reflex (Massof & Rickman, 1992). Technical solutions for this are possible, although they will require almost instant image processing (Deemer et al., 2018).

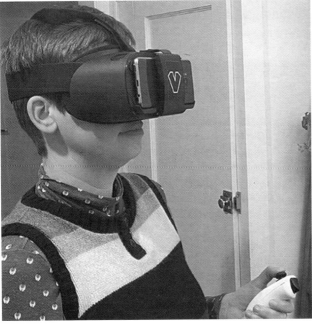

Fig. 8.2 A wearable electronic vision enhancement systems (EVES) in use (SightPlus™ by GiveVision Birmingham, UK).

In one study only about half of people who tried a wearable device thought they would help them, and 20% experienced side-effects including nausea, dizziness and headache (Crossland et al., 2019). The authors are only familiar with a small number of patients who use current head-mounted EVES, and they are generally used for specific tasks such as playing video games, going to the theatre, or for some work meetings.

CONSUMER DEVICES

Smartphones and tablet computers usually have bright screens, high-resolution cameras and an LED torch, so can be used as a simple electronic vision enhancement system. Many patients use their phone's camera to zoom in to a scene, particularly for spot reading tasks or for quick viewing of a distant object such as a street name or train departure board (Crossland et al., 2014). Dozens of magnification apps are available, which may offer more advanced options such as contrast reversal, image stabilisation and freeze frame modes. Typically these apps are used for less than 3 minutes at a time (Luo, 2020) and reading ability is comparable to p-EVES for spot tasks (Wittich et al., 2018b). For prolonged reading, a stand can be added to a tablet computer to create a rudimentary desktop electronic vision enhancement system.

FINANCING THE PURCHASE OF EVES IN THE UK

In the UK, optical LVAs are provided through the Hospital Eye Service (HES) on permanent loan, and the patient makes no contribution towards the cost. Optical devices are also available privately, but costs are relatively modest, with most plus-lens magnifiers costing less than £60 and telescopic systems up to about £350. In contrast, electronic devices range from about £100 for a television magnifier to almost £10,000 for the most expensive head-mounted EVES. In Wales, some p-EVES are funded through the Welsh Low Vision Service, but we are not aware of National Health Service (NHS) funding for EVES in other nations of the United Kingdom.[1]

School students may receive funding for EVES through their school or local authority, following a technology assessment by their Specialist Teacher for Visual Impairment. Students may not be allowed to take these devices home for homework and leisure, but the VICTA charity will provide grants to purchase EVES for home use (see Appendix 1). Students in higher education can obtain a Disabled Students Allowance, which includes an element for equipment, and this could well be used to purchase an EVES. The Access to Work scheme will fund some or all of the cost of assistive technology, including EVES, following a workplace assessment. This scheme is available to those who are employed, looking for work, or who are self-employed, including those on fixed-term or part-time contracts.

---

[1] Two of the authors met with a Secretary of State in the Department of Health to make the case that p-EVES should be funded by the NHS but were unsuccessful in changing policy.

Some national and local sight loss charities will fund the purchase of EVES such as Blind Veterans UK and VICTA (see Appendix 1), as might local branches of groups such as the Lions Club, the Round Table, and the Rotary Club. Some larger libraries have desktop EVES available for shared use.

People who are registered as severely sight impaired (SSI) and buy themselves an electronic vision enhancement system may use the saving made on their bind person's personal tax allowance to pay for the device. EVES are zero-rated for VAT, although patients may need to fill in a form declaring that they are registered as sight impaired or SSI to obtain this exemption.

Some suppliers of EVES offer an extended trial period before committing to purchasing the device, and others have a subscription scheme, where a device is provided for a monthly fee rather than being bought outright. Finally, second-hand EVES can sometimes be found: the Macular Society magazine is a good place to find advertisements.

BAR AND FLAT-FIELD MAGNIFIERS

Although these magnifiers are very different from electronic systems, they also provide transverse magnification. They are single solid lenses of hemicylindrical (bar; magnifying only in the vertical meridian) or hemispherical (flat-field; magnifying the image overall) form, designed to be placed directly onto the object—usually the page of a book (Fig. 8.3). For purely practical reasons, the lower lens surface may be held about 1 mm away from the task by a flange around the lens, to protect the lens from scratching. These may be called 'paperweight', 'dome', or 'Visolett' magnifiers. Despite the fact that these magnifiers are plus lenses, their magnifying properties are derived from lateral magnification of the object, rather than from the change in viewing distance which other plus-lens magnifiers allow (Fonda, 1976).

From elementary optical principles magnification of the system is given by

$$M = \frac{image\ size}{object\ size} = \frac{h'}{h} = \frac{L}{L'}$$

but $L' = F_2 + L$

so $M = \dfrac{L}{(F_2 + L)}$

Since $F_2 = \dfrac{(n' - n)}{r}$ and $L = \dfrac{n}{l}$

$$M = \frac{\dfrac{n}{l}}{\left[\dfrac{(n' - n)}{r} + \dfrac{n}{l}\right]}$$

$$= \frac{nr}{l(n' - n) + nr}$$

For this magnifier $l = t$ (thickness) and $n' = 1$ (air), so

$$M = \frac{nr}{t(1 - n) + nr}$$

To assess the effect of thickness on magnification, t can be expressed as a function of r (radius of curvature).

If $t = r/2$,

$$M = \frac{2n}{n + 1}$$

When the magnifier is exactly hemispherical with the thickness equal to the radius of curvature ($t = r$),

$$M = n$$

A theoretical maximum size (although not practically achievable) occurs if the magnifier is spherical, and $t = 2r$, giving

$$M = \frac{n}{2 - n}$$

Thus the thicker the magnifier in relation to its radius of curvature, the higher will be its magnification: this is unlikely to exceed 3× in practice. It can be seen (see Fig. 8.3) that, regardless of magnifier thickness, the image is formed very close to the original object, so magnification has not been created by a reduction in the viewing distance (as with other plus lenses). There is no advantage in decreasing the eye-to-magnifier distance to increase the field-of-view: the number of words seen through the magnifier will only be affected by the lens diameter. Magnification is increased by lifting the magnifier a few millimetres from the page (Fonda, 1976).

Advantages and Disadvantages
Advantages
1. As the image is formed close to the patient's normal reading distance, this demands no change in habitual reading posture. Binocular viewing of the image is possible, and any reading addition already prescribed will still be appropriate.
2. A useful additional feature of these magnifiers is their light-gathering property, whereby the illumination of the working plane viewed through the magnifier is increased relative to the surrounding area in the presence of diffuse background illumination (see Fig. 8.3). There are few reflections from the lens surface, although occasionally a single bright task light may need to be repositioned.
3. As the magnifier rests on the page, the focus of the image is unaffected by hand tremor. The patient does not need to hold the lens, and can simply push it along the lines of text, making it useful for those with grip problems.
4. The periphery of the lens suffers none of the aberrations usually associated with optical systems, the image having equal clarity across its full width.

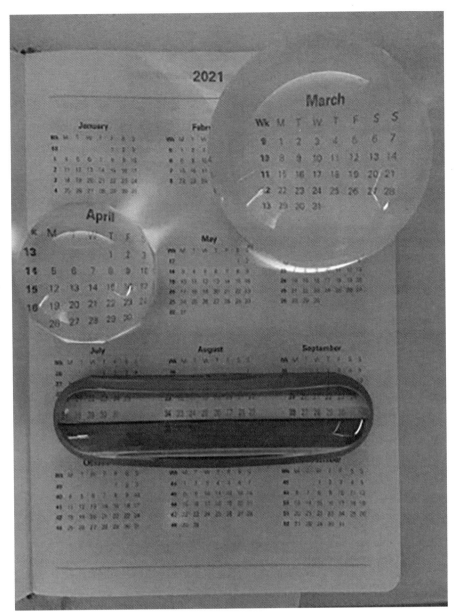

Fig. 8.3 Flat-field and bar magnifiers. *(Top left)* COIL Bright magnifier (40 mm diameter). *(Top right)* 65-mm diameter dome magnifier. *(Bottom)* COIL VTM bar magnifier with guide line. Note that magnification is not affected by flat-field diameter, and the reflection of room lights on the lens surface.

5. It can be used in conjunction with a spectacle-mounted system to double (nearly) the magnification, whilst leaving the working space unchanged. This would be particularly appropriate for the patient wearing a binocular spectacle correction in which any increase in the power of the lens would create too great a convergence demand.

6. Some bar and flat-field magnifiers have a guide-line to help follow a line of text. Additionally, some have a slightly opaque region away from the centre of the lens, acting as a typoscope (see Fig. 8.3, *bottom*).

Disadvantages

1. These lenses are often large (up to 90 mm diameter) and can be heavy, particularly when made of glass. Plastic versions are lighter but prone to scratching. Smaller versions, which are lighter and more convenient to carry, have a correspondingly small field-of-view. The field-of-view is not increased by holding the magnifier closer to the eye.

2. They are only suitable for reading on a firm, flat surface. A newspaper, for example, would need to be placed on a board, and they cannot be used for reading a curved surface, such as the ingredients list on a can of beans.

3. The curved surface of the lens can be prone to reflections (see Fig. 8.3).

4. Bar magnifiers only magnify in one dimension (vertically), creating some image shape distortion.

REFERENCES

Burggraaff, M. C., van Nispen, R. M. A., Hoeben, F. P., et al. (2012). Randomized controlled trial on the effects of training in the use of closed-circuit television on reading performance. *Investigative Ophthalmology & Visual Science, 53*(4), 2142–2150.

Cheong, A. M. Y., Legge, G. E., Lawrence, M. G., et al. (2008). Relationship between visual span and reading performance in age-related macular degeneration. *Vision Research, 48*(4), 577–588.

Crossland, M. D., Silva, R. S., & Macedo, A. F. (2014). Smartphone, tablet computer and e-reader use by people with vision impairment. *Ophthalmic & Physiological Optics, 34*(5), 552–557.

Crossland, M. D., Starke, S. D., Imielski, P., et al. (2019). Benefit of an electronic head-mounted low vision aid. *Ophthalmic and Physiological Optics, 39*(6), 422–431.

Culham, L. E., Chabra, A., & Rubin, G. S. (2004). Clinical performance of electronic, head-mounted, low-vision devices. *Ophthalmic & Physiological Optics, 24*(4), 281–290.

Deemer, A. D., Bradley, C. K., Ross, N. C., et al. (2018). Low vision enhancement with head-mounted video display systems: Are we there yet? *Optometry and Vision Science, 95*(9), 694–703.

Ehrlich, D. (1987). A comparative study in the use of closed-circuit television reading machines and optical aids by patients with retinitis pigmentosa and maculopathy. *Ophthalmic and Physiological Optics, 7*(3), 293–302.

Fonda, G. (1976). Visolett magnifier: Evaluation and optics. *Archives of Ophthalmology, 94*(9), 1614–1615.

Genensky, S. M., Petersen, H. E., Clewett, R. W., et al. (1978). A second-generation interactive classroom television system for the partially sighted. *Optometry and Vision Science, 55*(9), 615–626.

Genensky, S. M. (1969). Some comments on a closed circuit TV system for the visually handicapped. *Optometry and Vision Science, 46*(7), 519–524.

Golubova, E., Starke, S. D., Crossland, M. D., et al. (2021). Design considerations for the ideal low vision aid: Insights from de-brief interviews following a real-world recording study. *Ophthalmic and Physiological Optics, 41*(2), 266–280.

Goodrich, G. L., & Kirby, J. (2001). A comparison of patient reading performance and preference: Optical devices, handheld CCTV (Innoventions Magni-Cam), or stand-mounted CCTV (Optelec Clearview or TSI Genie). *Optometry, 72*(8), 519–528.

Goodrich, G. L., Mehr, E. B., Quillman, R. D., et al. (1977). Training and practice effects in performance with low-vision aids: A preliminary study. *Optometry and Vision Science, 54*(5), 312–318.

Granquist, C., Wu, Y. H., Gage, R., et al. (2018). How people with low vision achieve magnification in digital reading. *Optometry and Vision Science, 95*(9), 711–719.

Legge, G. E., Ahn, S. J., Klitz, T. S., et al. (1997). Psychophysics of reading—XVI. The visual span in normal and low vision. *Vision Research, 37*(14), 1999–2010.

Lovie-Kitchin, J. E., & Woo, G. C. (1988). Effect of magnification and field of view on reading speed using a CCTV. *Ophthalmic and Physiological Optics, 8*(2), 139–145.

Lowe, J. B., & Drasdo, N. (1990). Efficiency in reading with closed-circuit television for low vision. *Ophthalmic and Physiological Optics, 10*(3), 225–233.

Luo, G. (2020). How 16,000 people used a smartphone magnifier app in their daily lives. *Clinical and Experimental Optometry, 103*(6), 847–852.

Massof, R. W., & Rickman, D. L. (1992). Obstacles encountered in the development of the low vision enhancement system. *Optometry and Vision Science, 69*(1), 32–41.

Peterson, R. C., Wolffsohn, J. S., Rubinstein, M., et al. (2003). Benefits of electronic vision enhancement systems (EVES) for the visually impaired. *American Journal of Ophthalmology, 136*(6), 1129–1135.

Potts, A. M., Volk, D., & West, S. S. (1959). A television reader as a subnormal vision aid. *American Journal of Ophthalmology, 47*, 580–581.

Taylor, J. J., Bambrick, R., Brand, A., et al. (2017). Effectiveness of portable electronic and optical magnifiers for near vision activities in low vision: A randomised crossover trial. *Ophthalmic and Physiological Optics, 37*(4), 370–384.

Wittich, W., Lorenzini, M. C., Markowitz, S. N., et al. (2018a). The effect of a head-mounted low vision device on visual function. *Optometry and Vision Science, 95*(9), 774–784.

Wittich, W., Jarry, J., Morrice, E., et al. (2018b). Effectiveness of the Apple iPad as a spot-reading magnifier. *Optometry and Vision Science, 95*(9), 704–710.

9

Angular Magnification

OUTLINE

THE OPTICAL PRINCIPLES OF TELESCOPES

The principle of angular magnification is to use an optical system to change the angle formed at the nodal point of the eye by the rays of light from the object. Telescopes are a very effective way of producing this angular magnification, which occurs without changing the object or the viewing distance. The patient can achieve an enlarged retinal image whilst staying at their chosen distance from the task, whether this is at distance (street signs, bus numbers, whiteboard), intermediate (TV, music, playing cards, game console) or near (writing, handicrafts). The disadvantage is the very restricted field-of-view (FOV) allowed by such devices, and they can rarely be used whilst the patient is mobile (although some special designs for this purpose are described in the section on 'Telescopes for Mobility'). Even if the patient is stationary, telescopes are often used to view moving objects (e.g. watching sport) which is challenging because of the FOV, and magnification of the object's apparent speed.

Telescopes in low-vision work are often required to focus on objects closer than infinity, and they can be modified to correct for the wearer's refractive error. Their optical principles, however, are those of *afocal* systems, where parallel rays of light enter the telescope from an infinitely distant object, and parallel rays leaving the telescope form a final image at infinity. The two types of telescope used in low-vision work are illustrated simply in Fig. 9.1A, the astronomical (Keplerian), and Fig. 9.1B, the Galilean telescope. In the astronomical telescope, a ray from the bottom of the object forms the top of the image, and thus the image is inverted (and also laterally reversed). This is obviously unsuitable for low-vision work, so a reflecting system (a combination of prisms or mirrors) is always included

to reorient the image. The more correct name for such a telescope is 'terrestrial', but 'astronomical' has become accepted in the low vision field. In the astronomical telescope, the convex objective lens F_O forms an image of the distant object (focuses the incident parallel light) at F'_O, the second focal point of this lens. The distance between the image and the objective lens is obviously the second focal length, f_O. Light then diverges from this focus and is refracted by the convergent eyepiece lens F_E. If this lens is positioned so that its first focal point F_E coincides exactly with F'_O and the image, then parallel light will emerge from the system. For the Galilean telescope, the eyepiece lens F_E is negative and is positioned so that its first focal point is coincident with F'_O: rays of light converging towards F'_O are intercepted before focusing and emerge parallel from the system. The ray of light which left the top of the object emerges at the top of the image: the image is erect and no additional components are required to make practical use of the system.

The reflecting system which the astronomical telescope requires to produce an erect image is usually a prism system which takes advantage of total internal reflection. A typical example is illustrated in Fig. 9.2, where the use of two right-angled (Porro) prisms is illustrated. This also illustrates how the use of prisms allows the optical path length between the objective and eyepiece lenses to be 'folded', thus reducing the overall length of the telescope. The separation of the two lenses $t = f_O + f_E$, and as these second focal lengths are both positive in the astronomical telescope, this will be longer than the Galilean telescope of equivalent magnification (where f_E is negative): folding of the light path as described above may be able to reduce the difference in physical size between the finished telescopes.

Fig. 9.3 illustrates the extra-axial rays from an infinitely distant object which shows how the angular magnification is produced by the telescopes: there is an increase in the angle made by the rays with the optical axis after passing through the telescope.

$$\text{Magnification}(M) = \frac{\text{angle subtended at eye by image}}{\text{angle subtended at eye by object}}$$

$$= \frac{\theta'}{\theta}$$

since the object would subtend an angle θ at the eye without the telescope.

From the shaded triangles in Fig. 9.3:

a. Astronomical

$$\theta = \frac{-h'}{f'_O}$$

and

$$-\theta' = \frac{h'}{f'_E}$$

So

$$\theta' = \frac{h'}{f'_E}$$

b. Galilean

$$\theta = \frac{-h'}{-f_O} = \frac{-h'}{f'_O}$$

and

$$\theta' = \frac{-h'}{-f'_E} = \frac{h'}{f'_E}$$

Thus for either afocal telescope,

$$M = \frac{\theta'}{\theta} = \frac{h'}{f'_E}\frac{-f'_O}{h'} = \frac{-f'_O}{f'_E}$$

or

$$M = \frac{-F_E}{F_O}$$

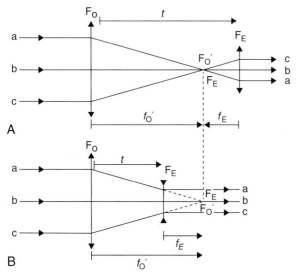

Fig. 9.1 A schematic representation of the optical system of (A) an astronomical and (B) a Galilean telescope. In the astronomical telescope, the top-most ray 'a' entering the telescope becomes the lowest ray of the exiting bundle, so the image is inverted. In the Galilean telescope, the order of the rays is the same on entering and exiting, so the image is erect. See text for explanation of variables.

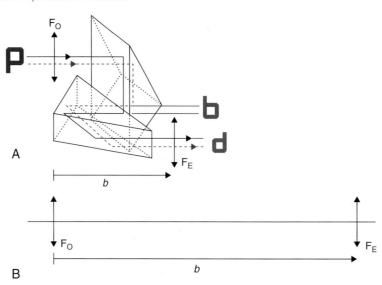

Fig. 9.2 The use of two right-angled (Porro) prisms as an example of the way in which the image in an astronomical telescope can be laterally and vertically inverted. The prisms also allow the light path to be 'folded' to the reduced distance *b* shown in (A). The full path length between the objective (F_O) and eyepiece (F_E) lenses is shown in (B).

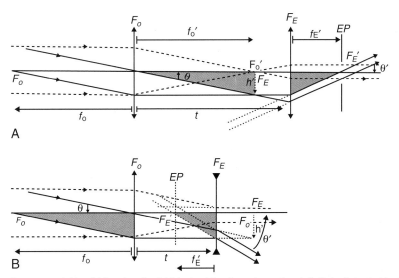

Fig. 9.3 The path of rays from the extra-axial (*solid lines*) and axial (*dashed lines*) portions of an infinitely distant object through (A) an astronomical and (B) a Galilean afocal telescope. In each case the objective lens (F_O) and the eyepiece lens (F_E) are a distance t apart and are assumed to be thin. The object subtends an angle θ at F_O and the image subtends an angle θ' at the eye. h' is the size of the primary image formed by F_O. The position of the exit pupil (*EP*) is also shown.

As both component lenses are positive in the astronomical telescope, the resultant magnification value is negative, showing that the image is inverted and that an erecting system is required: magnification for the Galilean telescope is positive indicating an erect image. In both systems, to obtain magnification values numerically greater than one requires that the eyepiece lens must be the more powerful. In purely practical terms, the powers of both components should be high, so the corresponding focal lengths will be short and the overall length of the telescope minimised. The use of more powerful lenses will inevitably cause aberrations to affect the final image quality. Thus, in high-magnification astronomical systems (up to 14× is available) the eyepiece and objective lenses each consist of up to four components to minimise aberrations. This large number of air/glass interfaces (added to those of the erecting system) inevitably causes a loss of image brightness, even with antireflection-coated lenses. By contrast, Galilean systems are not generally available beyond 3.5× distance magnification due to the poor image quality associated with the higher powers. This means that the objective and eyepiece lenses are generally of lower power than in the astronomical designs, and in the interest of producing compact and lightweight aids, each component may be reduced to a single aspheric lens.

Focal Telescopes

The telescopic systems used in low-vision work are therefore basically afocal, and the formula derived for their magnification ($M = -F_E/F_O$) is only applicable when they are used in that way. However, telescopes are rarely used by emmetropic eyes to view infinitely distant objects: in normal circumstances, ametropic eyes viewing objects at less remote distances need to be considered. When the telescopes are used in this way, the magnification will be changed, but it is possible to calculate the extent to which this occurs.

The 'Vergence Amplification' Effect

It will be realised by anyone using a telescope that it needs to be refocused for each different object distance and that the observer's own accommodation cannot be used to create clear retinal images of near objects. The reason for this is that the amount of accommodation required for viewing objects at a finite distance through the telescope is greatly in excess of the expected value. The incident vergence has in fact been 'amplified' by its passage through the telescope. Freid (1977) derived a precise formula for the actual emergent vergence:

$$U' = \frac{M^2U}{(1 - tMU)}$$

where U' is the emergent vergence as it leaves the telescope eyepiece; U is the actual incident vergence at the telescope objective; M is the magnification of the telescope (positive for Galilean, negative for astronomical) and t is the optical path length of the telescope.

An approximate formula has become commonly used:

$$U' = M^2U$$

In words, this becomes:

$$\text{emergent vergence} = (\text{magnification})^2 \times \text{incident vergence}$$

or in terms of its effect on the patient:

$$\text{actual accommodation required} = (\text{magnification})^2 \times \text{expected accommodation}$$

In fact, this approximate formula is only accurate for a limited range of conditions, but it does illustrate the general problem that patients rarely possess the amount of accommodation required for even modest viewing distances. For example, a 3× telescope used for viewing at 1 m may require approximately 9.00 DS of accommodation rather than the expected 1.00 DS.

Compensating for Ametropia

There are three ways in which either astronomical or Galilean telescopes could be adapted to compensate for spherical ametropia:
1. Adding the full refractive correction to the eyepiece
2. Adding a partial refractive correction to the objective
3. Changing the telescope length

Considering the practicalities of each of these methods in turn:

Adding the Full Refractive Correction to the Eyepiece. This is a very simple strategy. In practice, it is realised by the patient holding the telescope up against their spectacles; or the telescope being clipped over the spectacles; or a small auxiliary lens being attached behind the eyepiece lens of the telescope. The magnification of the telescope is unchanged, because the telescope is still afocal: parallel light leaves the telescope and it is only then that its vergence is changed before entering the eye. The method allows both spherical and cylindrical refractive errors to be corrected.

Adding a Partial Refractive Correction to the Objective. It is theoretically possible to place a partial correction in front of the objective lens, to slightly alter the vergence of light entering the telescope. This vergence would then be amplified by its passage through the telescope, to the extent that the vergence of light leaving the telescope would be appropriate to correct the refractive error. This method is never used practically because the degree of correction required, and its influence on the magnification, are difficult to calculate, and it offers no practical advantage.

Changing the Telescope Length. The uncorrected myope could shorten the telescope by the amount required to make the previously parallel light leaving the afocal telescope into light which is divergent to the correct extent to correct the refractive error and be clearly focused on the retina. The hypermetrope would lengthen the telescope to create a convergent emergent beam. This is a useful practical strategy in cases of low (in Galilean telescopes) to moderate/high (in astronomical telescopes) degrees of ametropia. Cylindrical ametropia cannot be corrected in this way, but it has been suggested that uncorrected astigmatism up to 2.00 DC does not influence acuity. Larger spherical ametropias may also create problems because of physical restrictions in the change of telescope length that the housing of the telescope lenses will permit. The telescope is clearly no longer afocal, but a method of calculating the change in magnification can easily be determined by using an example:

Consider a Galilean telescope consisting of an eyepiece lens $F_E = -50.00$ DS and an objective lens $F_O = +20.00$ DS. The magnification, if the telescope is operating as an afocal telescope, is $M = -F_E/F_O = -(-50.00)/+20.00 = +2.5×$. Fig. 9.4A shows the relative position of the lenses, separated

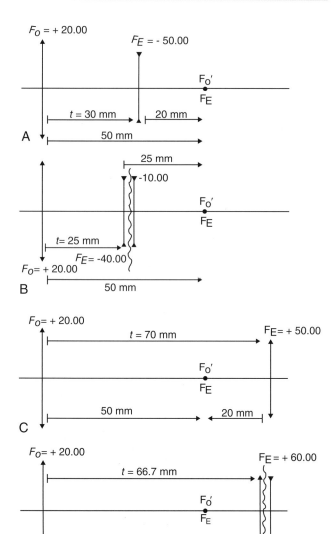

Fig. 9.4 (A) A diagram showing the distances (t) between the component lenses (F_O and F_E) in a 2.5× Galilean telescope, focussed for infinity (afocal). (B) shows the same telescope focussed for use by an uncorrected −10.00 DS myope. (C) shows the equivalent component lens positions for a 2.5× astronomical telescope, focused for infinity. (D) shows the astronomical telescope focussed for use by an uncorrected −10.00 DS myope. F_O' and F_E are the focal points of the objective and eyepiece lenses respectively.

by the algebraic sum of their focal lengths: $t = f_O + f_E = 50$ mm $+ (-20$ mm$) = 30$ mm.

If a −10.00 DS myope were to use the telescope, and the ametropia were corrected by a spectacle correction placed behind the eyepiece, no focusing of the telescope (i.e. no change in length) would be required, and the magnification would remain at 2.5×. If the uncorrected −10.00 DS myope is now to look through the telescope, refocusing would be required. The situation can be thought of as shown in Fig. 9.4B. Consider the −50.00 DS eyepiece to be made of two components, a −10.00 DS element which is being 'borrowed' to correct the ametropia, and a −40.00 DS element which is the eyepiece of an afocal telescope. In order to make the 'new' Galilean telescope afocal, the length of the telescope must be altered to $t = f_O + f_E = 50 + (-25)$ mm $= 25$ mm, so it is shortened by 5 mm in the focusing process. In addition, the magnification changes: the effective eyepiece power is now $F_E = -40.00$ DS (the original -50.00 DS $- (-10.00$ DS)) which has been used to correct the ametropia. Magnification $M = -F_E/F_O = -(-40.00)/+20.00 = +2.0\times$. Therefore, the myope obtains *less* magnification by using the telescope in this way.

If the telescope were an astronomical one of equivalent power, but with a positive eyepiece this time, the analogous calculations can be made (Figs. 9.4C and D):

Assume that the eyepiece lens $F_E = +50.00$ DS and the objective lens $F_O = +20.00$ DS. The magnification, if the telescope is operating as an afocal telescope, is

$$M = -\frac{F_E}{F_O} = -\frac{+50.00}{+20.00} = -2.5\times$$

If the ametropia were corrected by a spectacle correction placed behind the eyepiece, no focusing of the telescope (i.e. no change in length) would be required, and the magnification would remain at 2.5×. This is exactly analogous to the situation when using the Galilean telescope. Fig. 9.4C shows the relative position of the lenses, separated by the algebraic sum of their focal lengths: $t = f_O + f_E = 50 + 20$ mm $= 70$ mm. Consider the +50.00 DS eyepiece to be made of two components, a -10.00 DS element which is being 'borrowed' to correct the ametropia, and a +60.00 DS element which is the eyepiece of an afocal telescope. In order to make the 'new' astronomical telescope afocal, the length of the telescope must be altered to $t = f_O + f_E = 50 + 16.7$ mm $= 66.7$ mm, so it is shortened by 3.3 mm in the focusing process. In addition, the magnification changes: the effective eyepiece power is now $F_E = +60.00$ DS (the original +50.00 DS $- (-10.00$ DS) which has been used to correct the ametropia). Magnification $M = -F_E/F_O = -(+60.00)/+20.00 = -3.0\times$. Therefore, the myope gets *more* magnification by using the telescope in this way, rather than placing the telescope over their spectacle lens. The equivalent argument applied to the hypermetropic wearer shows that this patient would get *more* magnification if using the Galilean telescope and lengthening it to correct the ametropia, but *less* magnification if using the astronomical telescope. The effects in the astronomical and Galilean telescopes are opposite because it is the apparent power of the eyepiece lens which is changing, and this is of opposite sign in the two instruments.

Of course, the effects on magnification were quite dramatic in the example given, because the degree of ametropia to be corrected was large—more limited effects will be experienced with low refractive errors. There are also occasions when the choice presented here is not available for practical reasons—the patient may, for example, be a contact lens wearer who cannot remove the correction just to use the telescope intermittently. As is clear from the diagrams in Fig. 9.4, the length changes required seem practical, and they are even less if the eyepiece lens is of higher power. However, as suggested previously, Galilean telescopes are often not manufactured to have an extensive focusing ability. The typical range of ametropia compensated may be ±3.00 DS, compared to ±15.00 DS or more in an astronomical system.

Intermediate and Near Viewing

As discussed earlier, the telescope user will not be able to accommodate to view at these distances. In an analogous manner to the way in which ametropic correction is provided, there are three ways in which the afocal telescope can be adapted to intermediate or near viewing:

1. Adding full correction for the viewing distance to the objective
2. Adding increased correction for the viewing distance to the eyepiece
3. Focusing the telescope by changing (increasing) the telescope length

Considering the practicalities of each of these methods in turn:

Adding Full Correction for the Viewing Distance to the Objective. This is the simplest practical solution, because the power of the correcting lens, the working space, and the 'new' magnification of the system are all easily determined. If, for example, the patient wishes to view a near object at a distance of 50 cm, the light entering the telescope would be divergent (vergence = -2.00 DS), and the telescope would no longer be afocal. Addition of a +2.00 DS lens in front of the objective lens would neutralise this divergence: parallel light would now enter the telescope, which would once again be afocal. This positive lens power can be incorporated into the objective lens or can be clipped over the objective as a *reading cap*. The use of a reading cap is the more versatile option, as the cap can be removed or changed so that the telescope can be used for a variety of purposes. This modified system is often called a *telemicroscope* (Fig. 9.5).

The magnification of the system is the product of that provided by its individual components, so

total magnification = afocal telescope magnification
× plus-lens reading cap
magnification

$$M_{TOTAL} = M_{TEL} \times \frac{F_{RC}}{4}$$

Such a formula can also be used to calculate the plus-lens reading cap which will be required to produce a particular total magnification. For example, if the patient required

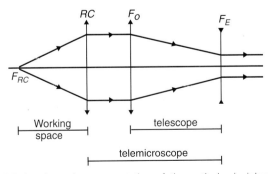

Fig. 9.5 A schematic representation of the optical principles of a telemicroscope—a telescope with full correction for the near viewing distance added over the objective lens (F_O) as a reading cap (*RC*). The object is placed at the anterior focal point (F_{RC}) of RC, so parallel light enters the (still afocal) telescope (Galilean in this case). F_E is the telescope eyepiece lens.

6× magnification at near, and the telemicroscope was to be formed using a 2× telescope as its base, then

$$M_{TOTAL} = M_{TEL} \times \frac{F_{RC}}{4}$$

And substituting gives

$$6 = 2 \times \frac{F_{RC}}{4}$$

$$\frac{F_{RC}}{4} = 3,$$

so

$$F_{RC} = +12.00 \text{ DS}$$

The working space is not affected by the afocal telescope, so (as for any plus-lens system) it is simply the anterior focal length of the plus lens:

$$f_{RC} = \frac{1}{F_{RC}} = \frac{1}{+12.00} = +0.0833 \text{ m} = 8.33 \text{ cm}$$

It is now possible to see the advantage of such a system over that which uses a plus-lens alone. To continue with the same example, if 6× magnification was to be produced using only a plus lens, then

$$M = \frac{F_{eq}}{4}$$

So $F_{eq} = 4 \times M = 4 \times 6 = +24.00 \text{ DS}$

The working space is the anterior focal length of the plus lens, so

$$f_{eq} = \frac{1}{F_{eq}} = \frac{1}{+24.00} = +0.0417 \text{ m} = 4.17 \text{ cm}$$

So using the telescopic system has allowed the working space to be increased by 2×; that is, by a factor equal to the magnification of the telescope used. If a 3× telescope had been used to form the basis of the system, the working space would have been increased by 3×.

This can be stated mathematically as:

$$f_{RC} = M_{TEL} \times f_{eq}$$

where f_{RC} is the anterior focal length of the near telescope (i.e. the anterior focal length of the reading cap), MTEL is the telescope magnification, and f_{eq} is the anterior focal length of the plus-lens of equal magnification.

Whilst the working space of a plus-lens is fixed once a particular level of magnification has been chosen, the near telescopic system could be any one of a number of combinations of afocal telescope and reading cap. Taking the example of 2.5× magnification, the plus-lens which would provide this would have power +10.00 DS, and a working space of 10 cm

$(F_{eq} = 4M, f_{eq} = 1/F_{eq})$. A variety of near telescopes (telemicroscopes) could give the same magnification:

A 1.5× afocal telescope with a +6.75 DS reading cap, working space ~15 cm

A 2.0× afocal telescope with a +5.00 DS reading cap, working space 20 cm

A 4.0× afocal telescope with a +2.50 DS reading cap, working space 40 cm

The anterior focal length of an unknown system, and hence the working space of a near telescope, can be determined by measurement of its front vertex power (the reciprocal of this distance) using a focimeter. Despite the increased working space, there are situations where it is so small that it has no clinical advantage. For example, even if the working space is 2× larger with a telescope than with a plus lens, this will not be useful in functional terms if the increase is only from 2 cm to 4 cm: it has been suggested that the increase must be at least 5 cm to be practically worthwhile. In fact if the full working distance is considered, measured from the eye to the task, this includes the length of the magnifying system, as well as the working space. As the telescopic system is longer than a plus-lens, this will further increase the advantage of such a device (Fig. 9.6).

As well as the obvious advantage of increased space in which to perform manipulative tasks, or more comfortable working postures, the more remote position of the task renders binocular viewing easier to achieve. Whereas binocular magnification is almost impossible beyond 2.5× with a plus-lens system (F_{eq} = +10.00 DS, working space = f_{eq} = 10 cm), telescopic systems are commercially available up to 5× magnification. Binocular magnification at near is not without its problems, however, because a way must be found to accurately convergence the two telescope tubes to match the convergence of the patient's visual axes. This requires a way of compensating for the interpupillary distance of the patient, and the particular working distance employed.

Adding Increased Correction for the Viewing Distance to the Eyepiece. If the afocal telescope is used to view a near or intermediate object, the divergent light from the object which enters the telescope objective will have its vergence amplified by passage through the telescope. Thus, it would require a much stronger plus-lens placed over the eyepiece in order to make the light parallel than would be required if positioned over the objective. The power of such a lens, and the resultant magnification of the 'new' system, are difficult to calculate unless the system parameters are known in detail, and the high power of the lens makes the method practically unprofitable. It may be worth considering if the patient already possesses a very high-power reading addition in spectacle-mounted form to provide near magnification, but the final effect on magnification and working space would be unpredictable.

Focusing the Telescope by Changing (Increasing) the Telescope Length. Changing the length of the telescope by increasing the separation of the objective and eyepiece is a practical and often-used method of adapting the afocal telescope for finite working distances. The only limit is in the physical restriction on practical tube lengths allowed by the

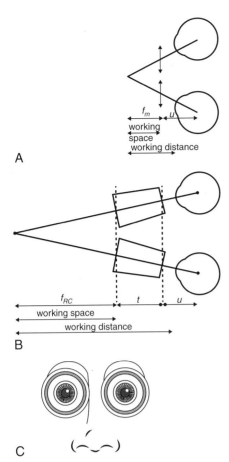

A

B

C

Fig. 9.6 A comparison of the degree of convergence required for near vision in (A) plus-lens and (B) telescopic systems of equivalent magnification. *u* is the distance of the magnifier from the eye's centre of rotation: working space in (A) is the focal length of the plus lens magnifier (f_M) but in (B) it is the anterior focal length of the reading cap (f_{RC}). In the latter case, the working distance is also increased by the length of the telescope (*t*). The telescope tubes must be correctly centred for the patient's pupillary distance and correctly angled for the convergence of the visual axes. This position is achieved when the view of the patient's eyes from directly in front appears as in (C).

particular device, with astronomical telescopes in general allowing a greater range of focus than Galilean devices. A consideration of some examples will show why this is the case. The effect of focussing for intermediate or near distances by changing the telescope length can be found in an analogous way to that used when considering the effects of correcting for ametropia by changing the telescope length. In the case of correcting for ametropia, this was considered as 'borrowing' some of the power of the eyepiece to do this, whereas when focusing for near objects, this will instead borrow some of the *objective* lens power. The aim is the same: it is necessary to be able to consider the system as an afocal telescope, as the optical characteristics of such a device are well-known.

Consider two 3× telescopes, one Galilean and one astronomical, which have component lenses of equivalent powers, as illustrated in Table 9.1.

Now consider focusing each telescope on an object at a distance of 20 cm in front of the objective lens. The vergence of light reaching the objective lens would be −5.00 DS, which would require a power of +5.00 DS to neutralise

it. As described previously, the use of a separate reading cap to neutralise this divergence is shown, but this +5.00 DS of power could also be provided by 'borrowing' it from F_O. This will create a 'new' afocal telescope with a lower objective lens power, and the 'focussing' will have been accomplished by increasing the separation of F_E and F_O.

The telescopes can now be thought of as having a 'virtual' reading cap of +5.00, over the objective lens of an afocal telescope whose objective lens power $F'_O = +10.00$, giving the original power of +15.00 (+10.00 + (+5.00)). The characteristics of these 'virtual' telescopes are then shown in Table 9.1.

As the change to the telescope is affecting the *objective* lens, which has the same sign in each case, it is not surprising that it affects both Galilean and astronomical telescopes in the same way. The length of both the telescopes is increased by the same amount, and this is substantial (33 mm in this example). However, the magnification is also greater, and it is therefore more beneficial in these terms (when it is possible) to focus the telescope for close distances by increasing its length rather than adding separate supplementary reading caps onto the fixed-focus distance telescope. Magnification can actually increase quite dramatically, as consideration of the formula makes clear: if

$$M = \frac{-F'_E}{F'_O}$$

then as positive power is being borrowed from the objective, it is effectively decreasing in power, so magnification increases. This is most beneficial in a telescope with lower-powered components, because the *percentage* change in F'_O is larger. This method cannot always be used, however, because it requires changes in the telescope length, and these rapidly increase beyond the range of practical instrument tube lengths especially when the component lenses are of low power. Astronomical telescopes offer more scope for focusing at close distances, because the component lenses used are typically more powerful than those in the Galilean systems: a necessary consequence of producing short enough telescopes whilst at the same time achieving magnifications up to 10× or 12×. In terms of magnification, then, it is always better to be able to refocus the telescope to compensate for intermediate and near distances rather than add auxiliary reading caps. However, this will noticeably reduce the FOV, and in this respect, the use of a reading cap is advantageous. A further reason to use a reading cap is to avoid the increase in length, which can make the device unwieldy, especially if it is to be spectacle mounted.

The Ocutech Vision Enhancement System (VES) design of astronomical telescope is particularly suited to spectacle mounting and can also be focused for near without changing the physical size of the device. This telescope was developed by Greene et al. (Greene et al., 1991), in which the optical components are parallel to the front of the spectacle frame, instead of extending out from the carrier lens (Fig. 9.7, *bottom left*). This makes the telescope relatively inconspicuous and means that the weight is balanced on both sides of the

TABLE 9.1   A Step-by-Step Calculation of Magnification for Example Telescopes Focussed for Near Viewing Using Two Alternative Methods: Adding a Reading Cap and Increasing the Length

	Galilean	Astronomical
Afocal telescope components	$F_E = -45.00$ $f'_E = -22\,mm$ $F_O = +15.00$ $f'_O = -67\,mm$ $t = f'_E + f'_O = (-22) + 67 = 45\,mm$ $M_{TEL} = -(-45)/+15 = 3\times$	$F_E = +45.00$ $f'_E = 22\,mm$ $F_O = +15.00$ $f'_O = 67\,mm$ $t = f'_E + f'_O = 22 + 67 = 89\,mm$ $M_{TEL} = -45/15 = -3\times$
Add separate reading cap to focus for 20 cm (+5.00 required)	$M_{TOTAL} = M_{TEL} \times M_{RC} = M_{TEL} \times (F_{RC}/4) = 3 \times (5/4) = 3 \times 1.25 = 3.75\times$ **(no change in length of telescope)**	
Refocus telescope for 20 cm	'Borrow' +5.00 DS from objective; 'new' telescope has $F_O = +15.00 - (+5.00) = +10.00$	
Telescope focussed for near	$F_E = -45.00$ $f'_E = -22\,mm$ $F_O = +10.00$ $f'_O = 100\,mm$ $t = F'_E + f'_O = (-22) + 100 = 78\,mm$ $M_{TEL} = -(-45)/+10 = 4.5\times$	$F_E = +45.00$ $f'_F = 22\,mm$ $F_O = +10.00$ $f'_O = 100\,mm$ $t = F'_E + f'_O = 22 + 100 = 122\,mm$ $M_{TEL} = -45/10 = -4.5\times$
Borrow power from objective to focus for near	$M_{TOTAL} = M_{TEL} \times M_{RC} = M_{TEL} \times (F_{RC}/4) = 4.5 \times (5/4) = 4.5 \times 1.25 = 5.6\times$ **(increased overall magnification, but increased length)**	

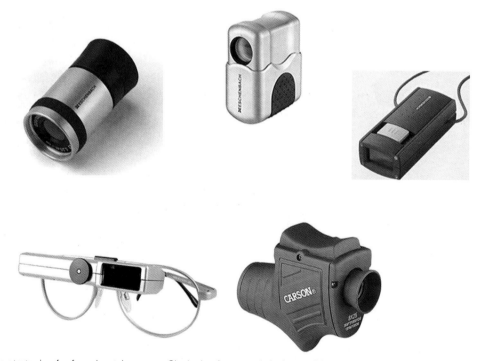

Fig. 9.7 The various strategies for focusing telescopes. Clockwise from *top left*: the traditional method of rotating the objective end of the telescope tube; fixed focus with no adjustment; slide focus (silver button moves sideways); rocking focus (on *top*); rotating knob in centre front (this telescope is also available in autofocus design).

spectacle frame, even though the device is monocular. It can be positioned so that the eyepiece is in front of the better eye. Some users find it confusing that the objective lens is in front of the opposite eye to the eyepiece: for example, the world as seen from the right side is projected into the left eye. This is particularly noticeable when the telescope is being used in near vision. The lens movements required for focusing are also internal to the system and not apparent to the user. Manual focusing is achieved using a small centrally placed ring, but the design also lends itself to the addition of an autofocus capability (Greene et al., 1992). Autofocus systems typically use an infra-red pulse from an LED which is directed towards the object at which the telescope is pointed. It is partially reflected by this target and falls on a Position Sensitive Detector on the telescope mounting. The system is completed by a signal processing circuit which computes the distance to the target. There must then be a motorised system which can alter the lens separation and, in the case of a binocular device, alter the angle between the right- and left-eye telescopes to take account of convergence. To date, only a monocular device is available commercially for low vision (Ocutech Falcon: https://ocutech.com/ves-falcon-autofocus-bioptic/).

As well as the optical consequences of focusing a telescope, there are the practical implications of how well the user can carry this out. Sometimes it may only be possible to use a fixed focus (or autofocus) design; other focusing strategies are used in different devices which may be simpler than the traditional method of rotating the objective end of the tube (see Fig. 9.7).

PRACTICAL CONSIDERATIONS

A number of optical parameters, such as FOV, aberrations, depth-of-field and binocular viewing have already been discussed in relation to plus-lens magnifiers, and it is now useful to compare the performance of telescopic systems.

It is immediately obvious to anyone who has looked through a telescope that the FOV is severely restricted. This may mean that only a portion of the task is visible at any one time, and the patient must scan across the area to gain a complete view. The limiting aperture in a telescope is assumed to be the edge of the objective lens, and this forms the entrance pupil of the system. Any ray from the object which enters the telescope through the entrance pupil will leave it through the exit pupil (EP), which is the image of the edge of the objective lens as seen from the eyepiece side of the system. It can be seen from Fig. 9.1 that for both telescope designs, the exiting bundle of rays has a much smaller diameter than the incident bundle. In fact, the diameter of the exiting bundle, and hence the EP size, can be determined from

$$EP\ diameter = \frac{objective\ lens\ diameter}{magnification\ of\ telescope}$$

The location of the EP in each telescope is shown in Fig. 9.3.

The EP of the astronomical telescope is beyond the eyepiece lens, but for the Galilean system, it is internal to the system. This feature allows the telescope type to be easily distinguished. The telescope is held at a distance of approximately 20 cm, with the eyepiece towards the observer and the objective lens pointing towards a plain light-coloured wall. A bright circle of light can be seen in the centre of the eyepiece lens—this is the EP. As the observer holds the telescope still and moves their head from side to side, the EP will also appear to move (Fig. 9.8).

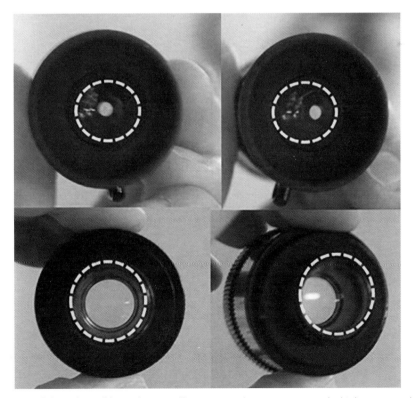

Fig. 9.8 The apparent movement of the exit pupil in a telescope. The *top row* shows an astronomical telescope, and the *bottom row*, a Galilean telescope. A *dashed line* indicates the edge of the eyepiece lens. The viewer begins by viewing along the axis of the telescope (*left images*) and the exit pupil (*light circle*) appears centrally placed in the eyepiece lens. If the viewer now moves their head to the left, the exit pupil may move to the opposite side of the eyepiece (an AGAINST movement as seen for an astronomical telescope [*upper image*]) or to the same side of the eyepiece (a WITH movement which is characteristic of a Galilean telescope [*lower image*]).

If the observer moves their head to the left and the EP also moves to the left (a 'WITH' movement) the EP is within the telescope which is therefore Galilean. If the movement of the EP is to the right (an 'AGAINST' movement), the EP is in the space between the observer and the eyepiece and the telescope is ASTRONOMICAL (remember A for Against and Astronomical!). This method can always be used to identify an unknown telescope, but it should not be assumed that looking at the eyepiece lens is a reliable indicator of telescope type. The rear surface of the eyepiece that can be seen will not necessarily be concave in a Galilean telescope and convex in an astronomical telescope, because the eyepiece may be a compound system of several lenses (in an attempt to minimise aberrations). Further clear evidence of astronomical design is when the telescope lenses do not share a common optical axis—that is, the light changes direction on passing through the telescope (see Fig. 9.7, *bottom row*). This is possible through appropriate positioning of the reflecting system which is needed to make the image erect in an astronomical telescope.

Field-of-View

A telescope gives the maximum FOV if the objective lens is as large as possible, but the eyepiece lens can be relatively much smaller, and will not influence FOV unless it is so small that it cuts off the peripheral exiting rays. Manufacturers often give information about objective lens diameter, but in any case it is easily measured with a millimetre rule. A telescope may be labelled '4 × 12' or a pair of binoculars '8 × 24': in each case the first number is the magnification, and the second is the objective lens diameter in millimetres. In these examples, the EP would be 3 mm in diameter in both cases. To gain the maximum FOV when using the telescope, the patient's pupil should be placed as close as possible to the EP of the telescope, and should match it in size exactly. This may be difficult to achieve, especially in the Galilean telescope where the EP is virtual, and inside the system (see Fig. 9.3B): the FOV will be noticeably larger with an astronomical compared to Galilean design of the same magnification. As the eye moves further away from the EP, the axial rays will still be imaged on the retina, but off-axis ray bundles from the periphery of the object will 'miss' the eye pupil and the FOV will be less than the theoretical value. Even if it means losing some of the imaging rays, it is often better that the exit bundle of rays is comfortably larger than the patient's eye pupil (or that the patient's pupil is not too close to the EP). If the patient's pupil and EP are exactly matched in size, any movement of the telescope causes part of the patient's FOV to become dark as one part of the pupil has no rays entering. The larger EP will allow the same image to be seen even if there is slight misalignment or tremor.

Although the theoretical calculation of FOV for distance tasks can be useful in comparative terms, the restrictions described earlier mean that a practical measurement of the FOV actually achieved in use is more useful. Fig. 9.9 shows examples of the linear FOV obtained at different viewing distances for a typical angular field of 10°.

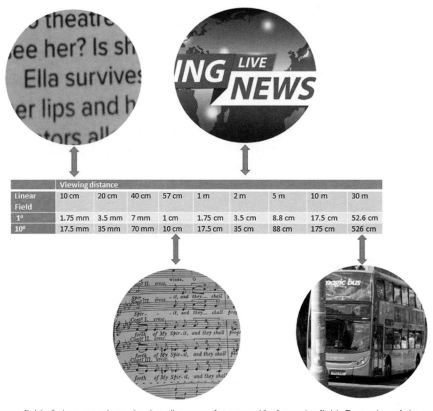

Linear Field	Viewing distance								
	10 cm	20 cm	40 cm	57 cm	1 m	2 m	5 m	10 m	30 m
1°	1.75 mm	3.5 mm	7 mm	1 cm	1.75 cm	3.5 cm	8.8 cm	17.5 cm	52.6 cm
10°	17.5 mm	35 mm	70 mm	10 cm	17.5 cm	35 cm	88 cm	175 cm	526 cm

Fig. 9.9 The linear telescope field-of-view at various viewing distances for every 1° of angular field. Examples of the actual linear field obtained viewing through a typical astronomical telescope with 10° angular field are shown: the page of a book at 10 cm; a sheet of music at 57 cm; a TV screen at 2 m; and a bus at 30 m.

The FOV increases in direct proportion to the viewing distance, but attempting to maximise the FOV by getting further away will obviously reduce the overall magnification because of the effect of relative distance magnification. For example, the patient who sits watching TV at 1 m without a telescope will have the same retinal image size as when using a 3× telescope at 3 m, but the FOV in the latter case will be much more restricted, and the patient will have to contend with holding or wearing a heavy and uncomfortable optical appliance. It would only be worthwhile suggesting the use of a telescope in these circumstances if the patient could not sit at 1 m from the TV (perhaps in the large lounge of a residential home), or if they could use the telescope and sit at 1 m as well. In this case, the patient would benefit both from relative distance magnification and angular magnification, and the retinal image would be much larger, but the FOV available would be very limited.

The most useful comparison of the FOV is that of telescopes for near viewing, with plus-lens magnifiers of equivalent magnification. The formula for plus lenses was derived in Chapter 7, where total linear of FOV was found to be given by

$$y = D\left[1 - \frac{l}{a} + \frac{l}{f'_M}\right]$$ Eq. (9.1)

This could be simplified by considering the situation where the magnifier is used with the object at the anterior focal point so that $l = -f'_M$ and

$$y = \frac{D}{aF_M}$$ Eq. (9.2)

To derive the corresponding formulae for a telescope, the limiting aperture is now the objective lens of the telescope.

In Fig. 9.10 it can be seen that the objective lens power of this near telescope is now $(F_O + F_{RC})$—the power of the objective lens of the afocal distance telescope plus the power of the reading cap which is required to adapt the telescope to focus for a near working distance. Fig. 9.10 shows the linear FOV (y) of the telescope, and by comparison with Fig. 7.7, it can be seen that the objective lens has an equivalent effect to

the magnifier lens F_M. In Fig. 9.10, it is seen that the objective lens acting alone would form an image at E', a distance $(p' + t)$ from the objective lens. This distance is equivalent to the distance a in Fig. 7.7, where the plus-lens F_M forms its image at E. In the case of the telescope, the eyepiece lens F_E then diverges the rays which would have been focussed at E' and focuses them at E, the eye's entrance pupil, which is a distance p behind the eyepiece lens.

Eq. (9.1) can be applied to the telescope by substituting

$$a = (p' + t)$$

where t is the length of the telescope ($= f'_O + f'_E$) and p' is the distance from the eyepiece F_E to the image of the entrance pupil which it forms.

Applying a simple vergence formula to the telescope eyepiece F_E:

$$P = (P' + F_E)$$

and in terms of distances, this becomes

$$\frac{1}{p} = \frac{1}{p'} + F_E$$

and

$$p' = \frac{p}{1 - pF_E}$$

So Eq. (9.1) becomes:

$$y = D\left[1 - \frac{l}{(p' + t)} + l(F_o + F_{RC})\right]$$ Eq. (9.3)

where $p' = \frac{p}{1 - pF_E}$, p is the distance from the telescope eyepiece to the eye's entrance pupil, l is the object distance, F_O and F_E are the powers of the objective and eyepiece lenses of the telescope, and F_{RC} is the power of the reading cap.

In the same way that Eq. (9.2) represents a simplified equation for FOV of a plus-lens, we can simplify the corresponding Eq. (9.3) as it applies to a telescope. If the object is placed in the conventional position, at the anterior focal point of the

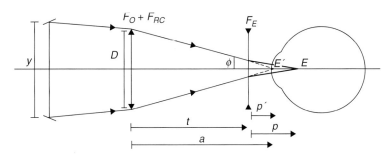

Fig. 9.10 The linear field-of-view y of a near (Galilean) telescope consisting of eyepiece lens of power F_E and an objective lens of power ($F_O + F_{RC}$) which has diameter D. The separation of the telescope lenses is t. ϕ is the angular semi-field-of-view. E is the entrance pupil of the eye, and E' its image, formed a distance p' from F_E. p is the distance between F_E and E, and a is the distance between the objective lens and E'.

reading cap lens, then the object distance will be equal to the focal length of the reading cap:

$$l = -f_{RC}$$

and substituting this into Eq. (9.3) gives:

$$y = D\left[1 - \frac{-f_{RC}}{(p'+t)} - f_{RC}\left(F_O + F_{RC}\right)\right]$$

$$y = D\left[1 + \frac{1}{F_{RC}(p'+t)} - \frac{F_O}{F_{RC}} - \left(f_{RC}F_{RC}\right)\right]$$

$$y = D\left[1 + \frac{1}{F_{RC}(p'+t)} - \frac{F_O}{F_{RC}} - 1\right]$$

$$y = \frac{D}{F_{RC}}\left[\frac{1}{(p'+t)} - F_O\right] \qquad \text{Eq. (9.4)}$$

where, as before

$$p' = \frac{p}{1 - pF_E}$$

These FOV formulae are only strictly valid for thin lenses. Whilst this can never be strictly true of plus-lenses or Galilean telescopes, the formulae do give reasonable approximations. They cannot be used, however, for astronomical telescopes, because of their more complex optical design.

Eq. (9.4) is now in a useful form for comparison, and by analogy with the case of a plus-lens magnifier, it can be seen that the FOV will increase as the diameter of the objective lens increases, and as the power of the reading cap decreases.

The term $\left|\frac{1}{(p'+t)} - F_O\right|$ depends on the parameters of the particular telescope and is a constant if the telescope is kept at the same distance from the eye. It can be shown that it decreases as the telescope magnification decreases but varies only slightly as the telescope component lenses are changed.

Applying the corresponding formulae to near-vision telescopes and plus-lenses of equal magnification shows that the FOV advantage of the plus-lens systems is considerable, although the telemicroscopes allow a much greater working space: the object must be positioned at the anterior focal point of the plus-lens, but at the focal point of the reading cap for the telescopic system. Fig. 9.11 shows the relationship between magnification, FOV and working space for three different systems; a plus-lens, a telemicroscope based on a 2× telescope and a telemicroscope made up of a 3× telescope with a reading cap. It is clear that whilst careful choice of telemicroscope components can significantly change the working space, it can do little to improve the FOV, which will always be dramatically better with a plus-lens. Whilst the working space with a near telescope improves (in this

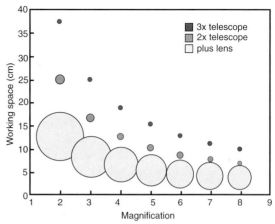

Fig. 9.11 The working space (in centimetres) of plus lens and telemicroscope systems of various magnifications. The horizontal extent of each symbol indicates the approximate relative linear field-of-view of the system. The *largest symbol* represents a linear field-of-view of over 33 cm, compared to the *smallest* which is only 1 cm. The plus lens is of 40 mm diameter and is 15 mm from the eye's entrance pupil. The telescope is mounted in the same position. The 2× telescope has component lenses $F_E = -30.00$, $F_O = +15.00$ and has diameter 30 mm. In the 3× telescope, F_E is increased to −45.00.

example) by a factor of 2× or 3× (depending on whether the system is based on a 2× or 3× telescope) compared to a plus-lens of the same magnification, the FOV decreases by a much greater extent—a factor of approximately 5.5×, and 7.5×, respectively.

Depth-of-Field

The depth-of-field is the maximum distance that the object can be moved around the optimal position before the patient notices image blurring, and it is the change in the vergence of light which this object movement produces which is detected by the patient. The minimum detectable amount will vary between patients, depending on their pupil diameter and sensitivity to blur, but a permissible change in vergence of ±0.50 DS would seem to be useful for comparison. For a plus-lens magnifier, the change in vergence of light leaving the magnifying system (emergent vergence) is the same as that entering (incident vergence). For a telescopic system, however, the incident vergence alteration is amplified by passage through the system. This means that the change in the incident vergence which can occur before it is noticeable by the patient is less than it would be in a plus-lens system. As noted earlier, an approximate formula for vergence amplification by the telescope is:

$$\text{emergent vergence} = (\text{magnification})^2 \times \text{incident vergence}$$

This means that, taking the example of a 2.5× telescope:

$$\text{emergent vergence} = 2.5^2 \times \text{incident vergence}$$
$$= 6.25 \times \text{incident vergence}$$

TABLE 9.2 The Depth-of-Field Experienced by the User of a 2.5× Telemicroscope Magnifier Whose Tolerance to Blur is ±0.50 DS

			Incident Vergence at Magnifier	Object Distance	
2.5× telescope with +4.00 reading cap	Correctly Positioned With Object at Focal Point of Reading Cap, Zero Vergence at Eye		−4.00	−25 cm	
	Change in Vergence at Eye	Change in Vergence Entering Magnifier			Acceptable Range of Object Distances (Depth-of-Field)
	+0.50	+0.08	−3.92	−25.5 cm	25.5–24.5 cm = 1 cm
	−0.50	−0.08	−4.08	−24.5 cm	

If the allowable emergent vergence is taken as ±0.50 DS, the equation can be rearranged to find the range of incident vergences which are allowable:

$$\text{incident vergence} = \frac{\text{emergent vergence}}{6.25}$$

$$= \frac{\pm 0.50}{6.25} = \pm 0.08\,DS$$

The effect of this on the depth-of-field in a telescopic system can be found by considering an example of a telescope focused for near vision by a reading cap. Suppose a magnifier consists of a 2.5× Galilean afocal telescope with a +4.00 reading cap to focus the system for 25 cm (the anterior focal point of the +4.00 reading cap). Table 9.2 illustrates the results, showing that the change in object position from 0.5 cm in front of the focal point to 0.5 cm behind, induces the maximum tolerable change in vergence of light entering the telescope (±0.08 DS), which having undergone vergence amplification is, in fact, a change of vergence of ±0.50 DS entering the eye.

For comparison, consider the example of a plus-lens being used to create the same overall magnification: $M = 2.5\times$, $F_{eq} = 4M = +10$ DS. The optimum object position for the nonaccommodating emmetrope is at the anterior focal point, 10 cm in front of the plus lens, and this is obviously much closer to the system than if the magnification was created solely by a telescopic system. It was shown in section 'Depth-of-Field' in Chapter 7 that for a plus-lens magnifier, the full tolerable range of possible object positions (the depth-of-field) is

$$\text{total depth-of-field (mm)}$$

$$= \frac{125 \times \text{minimum noticeable change in vergence}}{\text{magnification}^2}$$

which in this case, assuming a tolerance to defocus of ±0.50 DS, gives

$$\text{total depth-of-field} = \frac{125 \times 0.50}{2.5^2} = 10\,mm$$

As can be seen from this example, the depth-of-field is actually the same *linear* distance for the two types of device,

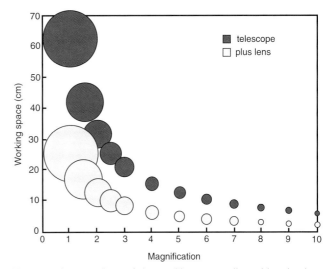

Fig. 9.12 A comparison of the working space allowed by plus lens (*light grey symbol*) and telescopic (*dark grey symbol*) systems with overall magnification from 1 × to 10×. The near telescope is based on a 2.5× distance afocal telescope, and different total magnification is created using appropriate reading caps. The horizontal extent of each symbol in each case indicates the approximate relative range of distances at which clear vision is possible—that is, the depth-of-field. The *largest symbol* represents a total depth-of-field of over 6 cm, compared to the *smallest* which is less than 1 mm.

and in fact Smith (1979) and Spitzberg and Qi (1994) have shown that this formula is equally applicable to telescopic magnifying systems. To summarise, therefore, the depth-of-field depends only on the magnification, rather than the design of the particular system but equivalent magnification in the two types of device is associated with very different working space: these are illustrated by Fig. 9.12. If we compare the same magnification in the two devices, then the acceptable range of object distances, around the optimum position, is the same. Nonetheless, patients often report that the telescope appears more restrictive: this may be because the depth-of-field is lower as a percentage of the working space, and aberrations cause portions of the field to blur and become patchy more quickly than the calculated values suggest. Other features which should be noted from Fig. 9.12 are that both types of devices obviously have decreasing depth-of-field as the magnification increases and that the depth-of-field is extremely short for all high-powered devices.

Compensating for Ametropia

The phenomenon of depth-of-field could actually be reconsidered in a positive way: it is actually a change in object position away from the focal point which causes a change in the emergent vergence from parallel light to divergent or convergent. This change in object position could therefore be used to provide the required refractive correction in spherical ametropia—for example, by moving the object *closer* than the focal point, the uncorrected myope could cause the rays leaving the magnifier to be sufficiently divergent to produce a clear retinal image. The greater the change in the object position, the greater the change in vergence which would occur. To determine the extent of this object movement, the depth-of-field equation needs to be stated in a slightly different way, especially as the movement must be in one specific direction from the focal point: *towards* the magnifier to correct myopia, and *away* to create the convergent emergent beam to be in focus for the uncorrected hypermetrope:

$$\text{object movement from focal point (mm)}$$

$$= \frac{-62.5 \times \text{required refractive correction}}{\text{magnification}^2}$$

Example 1. An uncorrected myope is not wearing their distance correction of −2.00 DS and uses a +10.00 DS plus-lens magnifier. The expected object position for the emmetropic user would be at the anterior focal point of the lens, $f_{eq} = -1/F_{eq} = -100$ mm (10 cm). The magnification of the system is 2.5× ($M = F_{eq}/4$), so

$$\text{object movement from focal point (mm)}$$

$$= \frac{-62.5 \times (-2.00)}{2.5^2} = +20 \text{ mm}$$

New object position = −100.00 + 20.00 = −80.00 mm: the myope has brought the object 20 mm closer to the lens, to a reduced working space of 80 mm (8 cm) to compensate for their uncorrected refractive error and produce a clear retinal image. In fact, the same result could have been obtained by considering the uncorrected −2.00 DS myope as being like an emmetrope wearing an additional +2.00 DS lens. Thus, the overall lens power experienced is +12.00 DS (+10.00 + (+2.00)) and the required object position is at the focal point of this lens, $f_{eq} = -1/F_{eq} = -1/+12.00 = -80$ mm (8 cm).

Example 2. An uncorrected hypermetrope with a refractive error of +10.00 DS uses a 2× telescope with a +8.00 DS reading cap. Overall magnification for near, M, is

$$M_{TOTAL} = M_{TEL} \times \frac{F_{RC}}{4}$$

so

$$M_{TOTAL} = 2 \times \frac{8}{4} = 4\times$$

and the expected object position for the emmetropic observer is at the focal point of the reading cap

$$f_{RC} = \frac{1}{F_{RC}} = -125 \text{ mm (12.5 cm)}$$

$$\text{object movement from focal point (mm)}$$

$$= \frac{-62.5 \times \text{required refractive correction}}{\text{magnification}^2}$$

$$\frac{-62.5 \times (+10.00)}{4^2} = -39.06 \text{ mm}$$

New object position = −125.00 − 39.06 = −164.06 mm: the hypermetrope has moved the object 39.06 mm further from the telescopic system and actually needs to have an increased working space of 164.06 mm (16.4 cm) to produce a clear retinal image.

Thus, it is possible to change the object position, and hence the working space, to compensate for uncorrected spherical ametropias. Obviously the larger errors require more extreme adjustments to the working space, and this may on occasions make the system practically impossible to use. If such were the case, consideration would have to be given to placing the refractive correction behind the eyepiece (e.g. clipping or holding the telescope over the spectacles): in this case, the magnifying system performs as it would for an emmetropic observer.

Binocularity and Convergence Demand

For distance viewing, there is no reason why Galilean or astronomical telescopes of any magnification could not be used binocularly if required. Such systems are readily available on standard spectacle-frames, or special mountings: more difficult, but not impossible, to align are two individual monocular telescopes attached to the patient's own refractive correction.

The main limitation in the higher powers is simply the weight of the spectacle-mounted systems, and so the astronomical binocular systems of 6× and higher are more often hand-held (Fig. 9.13).

For near viewing, it seems initially that telescopic systems will have considerable advantage over spectacle-mounted plus lenses. For an equal magnification, the telescopic system will require the patient to converge to an object position which is much further away. For the plus lens, the distance from the eye's centre of rotation to the object plane is:

$$u + f_M$$

where u is the distance from the spectacle plane to the centre of rotation, and f_M is the anterior focal length of the magnifier (see Fig. 9.6A). In comparison, the equivalent distance for the telescope is:

$$u + t + f_{RC}$$

where u is the distance from the spectacle plane to the centre of rotation, t is the length of the telescope, and f_{RC} is the

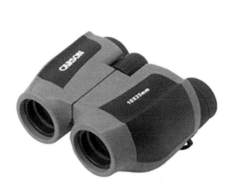
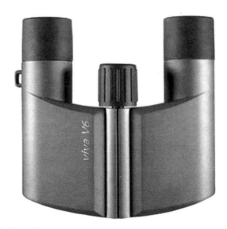

Fig. 9.13 Typical hand-held binocular astronomical telescopes, with only limited focusing range.

anterior focal length of the reading cap (see Fig. 9.6B). This more remote object plane lessens the convergence demand. In the plus lens system, there is also the risk of base-out prism being introduced by inadequate inward decentration of the lenses, making the required convergence even greater. Near vision telescopes which allow binocular magnification up to 5× are available commercially: this compares to approximately 2.5× as the limit of binocular magnification for near with plus-lens systems.

However, it will be appreciated that for longer or larger aperture telescopes, fitted to a patient with small interpupillary distance (PD), the required angling of the tubes may not be physically possible. It is also apparent that the degree of angling and PD adjustment needs to be very precise, and the frame or mount must have facilities to accomplish this. In order to check the centration of a binocular telescope, the observer places their right eye on the patient's midline at the required viewing distance, and the patient focuses the system optimally for this distance. The observer now views each of the patient's eyes with their right eye, looking through the telescope tubes. Every circular aperture of each telescope tube should appear concentric with each other, and with the patient's pupil (see Fig. 9.6C). If the viewing distance decreases, for example, the eyes will converge and the angle between the visual axes will increase. It will therefore be necessary for the angle between the two telescope tubes to change in a similar way, but it is uncommon that a practical system has sufficient adjustment to take account of the wide range of viewing distances possible with a focusing telescope and/or a large selection of reading cap powers. Consequently, most systems are likely to be one of two options: they either have variable focus in a monocular system, or fixed focus (or a limited variation in focus) in a binocular system. Another third theoretical strategy is to fit the telescopes with their optical axes parallel and to incorporate prism into the reading caps to make the reading fields coincident.

When Should Telescopes Be Recommended?

Some low vision clinics prescribe very few telescopic magnifiers: this may be partly due to the high cost, or perhaps

to previous experiences with patients discontinuing use (Crossland & Silver, 2005). However, in other clinics they form a high proportion of the aids provided, and it is clear that they do offer an important strategy in situations where other devices may not be appropriate (Table 9.3). Watson et al. (1997) asked patients to identify all the tasks they carried out with each device they had received. As can be seen, telescopes were rarely used for near activities, such as reading and writing, but were the only practical optical aid for travelling and watching TV. They can therefore serve a very useful rehabilitation function for many patients. The following guidelines are useful to follow in deciding whether this is going to be successful for the patient (Ocutech, n.d.).

For distance tasks outdoors:

1. Although the practitioner may be aiming for a target acuity of 6/6 or 6/9, if the visual acuity (VA) achieved is less than 6/15 it is unlikely to be useful functionally. Consider, however, that performance in the consulting room can be limited by the loss of light occurring by reflection from multiple optical interfaces within the device. VA may actually be much better outdoors where the ambient light level is higher, especially for high-powered astronomical telescopes (>6×).

2. The patient's poor contrast sensitivity may limit their ability to appreciate more detail within the image, even if it is larger. Asking the patient to report on facial expressions seen across the room through the telescope can form a test of the potential improvement for low contrast objects.

3. The dominance of the better eye should preferably be well-established if a monocular device is suggested: the patient should spontaneously choose their better eye and be able to position the telescope correctly, when given the device. If not, then careful training/adaptation will be required.

Whilst a distance telescope, especially if bioptic, may be used for a variety of tasks, for near/intermediate tasks, it is likely that the telescope is very specific to that one task (e.g. painting or music). Again there are some important guidelines to consider:

1. The patient should be questioned carefully to identify the exact working distance/viewing conditions required (and

TABLE 9.3   **The Percentage of Each Type of Magnifier Used for the Activities Listed**

| | Plus Lens Magnifiers | | Video Magnifiers | Telescopes | |
| | Hand/Stand | Spec-Mounted | | Hand-Held | Spec-Mounted |
Activities	*N* = 273	*N* = 114	*N* = 70	*N* = 146	*N* = 130
Reading	82	58	97	1	2
Writing	18	28	76		
Typing	4	13	16	1	1
Travel				73	21
Watching TV				1	68
Identifying faces				23	27
Repairing	20	40	34	1	
Cooking	20	19	29	1	
Lawn and garden	6	6	1	56	33
Grooming and health care		13	14	1	1

Some devices were used for more than one task, so the column totals are greater than 100%.
Modified from Watson, G. R., de l'Aune, W., Stelmack, J., Maino, J., & Long,. S. (1997). National survey of the impact of low vision device use among veterans. *Optometry and Vision Science, 74*(5), 249–259.

whether these could be changed). The restricted FOV (and the inability to see 'around' the device, unless bioptic) must be explained to the patient. The possibility of other alternative strategies to allow access to the tasks should be explored.

2. The patient should preferably be familiar already with optical magnifiers and their limitations, and have shown good visual performance, and good handling ability, with them.

For all types of telescope, the patient must be fully aware of the appearance of the finished device and be happy to use this in public.

MEASURING TELESCOPE MAGNIFICATION

Distance Telescopes

Telescopes are often marked with their magnification, but the methods described here may be used to check the rating given, to determine magnification of the patient's own telescope which has lost its label, or to verify a custom-made device. There are several available methods, but they are all suitable for use in the practice setting as they do not require any specialist apparatus.

Method 1—Direct Comparison

This method simply estimates the size ratio of the magnified view to the apparent size of the object without the telescope. Most people with binocular vision find it easier and more accurate to simultaneously compare the magnified view in one eye with the nonmagnified view in the other, by using the first eye to view through the telescope and the second eye to view the object directly. Looking at a regular periodic pattern, Fig. 5.4 shows the percept obtained, and the observer simply has to judge, for example, how the height of an 'unmagnified'

brick corresponds to the height of one 'magnified' brick. Sometimes, with high degrees of magnification, it is difficult to make this judgement because of hand-shake, or because the magnified brick is too large to be contained within the limited FOV available. In this case, the telescope can be reversed, with the objective held nearest to the observer's eye, and the degree of minification of the image determined.

Method 2—Using the Exit Pupil

The EP of the telescope is the aperture through which all the rays leaving the system emerge. The EP is the image of the objective lens as seen from the eyepiece side of the telescope. The telescope is held, with its eyepiece towards the observer, about 20 cm from the observer's eye, and pointed towards a blank white wall: the observer can then see a bright circle within the boundary of the eyepiece, and this is the EP.

$$\text{EP diameter} = \frac{\text{diameter of objective lens}}{\text{magnification}}$$

As the EP (and hence the exiting bundle of rays) is so small, the eyepiece lens in any telescope is typically also much smaller than the objective.

Rearrangement of this formula shows how the magnification of the telescope can be found:

$$\text{magnification} = \frac{\text{diameter of objective lens (mm)}}{\text{exit pupil diameter (mm)}}$$

To take an accurate measurement of EP size, the telescope is firmly clamped horizontally. Viewing from the eyepiece side of the instrument, a millimetre scale is positioned as close as possible to the EP, and its size measured (Fig. 9.14).

In the astronomical telescope, this is relatively straightforward because the EP is behind the eyepiece, but the Galilean

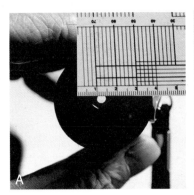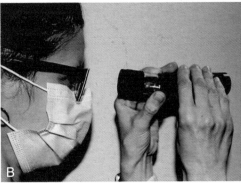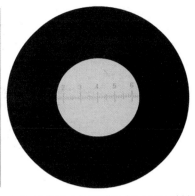

Fig. 9.14 (A) Holding the telescope away from the eye and pointing it towards a bright field allows the bright exit pupil to be seen within the eyepiece aperture: introducing a millimetre scale allows this to be measured. (B) To measure the exit pupil more accurately, the observer views through a measuring magnifier held behind the telescope eyepiece (*left*) so that the exit pupil focusses on the millimetre scale. (*right*) The view of the observer, showing the bright exit pupil and the measurement scale.

telescope EP is inside the system and the scale simply has to be placed as close to the eyepiece as possible. To increase the accuracy of measurement (to nearest 0.1 mm), the EP can be imaged on the scale of a measuring magnifier, which is held such that the EP is clearly imaged (see Fig. 9.14B). The objective diameter can easily be measured directly with a millimetre scale, but it is often written on the telescope as part of the specification—for example, an 8×30 telescope has a magnification of 8× and an objective diameter of 30 mm.

Although these two methods have acceptable precision for clinical purposes, the following method is more accurate. It makes use of the so-called 'vergence amplification' effect in which the incident vergence at the objective lens is relatively modest, but this is increased by passing through the telescope, and the emergent vergence leaving the eyepiece is much greater.

Method 3—Using the Focimeter

This method (Bailey, 1979a) is not suitable for checking astronomical telescopes because:
1. They are usually too long to fit onto the lens rest of the focimeter.
2. The internal prism system often allows 'folding' of the light path so that the true telescope length cannot be measured.
3. The higher power of the component lenses leads to the use of compound systems, so it is difficult to determine the position of their principal planes.

If an *afocal* telescope was placed on a focimeter with its eyepiece against the lens rest, the back vertex power should be *zero* (by definition) (if a finite power was measured, this would represent the distance refractive correction incorporated in the telescope for the benefit of the ametropic user). Freid's (1977) formula for actual emergent vergence

$$U' = \frac{M^2 U}{1 - tMU}$$

(where U' is the emergent vergence, U the incident vergence, t the telescope length and M the telescope magnification) shows that any change in vergence on the 'objective side' of the telescope is followed by a correspondingly greater change

on the 'eyepiece side'. Therefore, if a lens of power U is placed against the objective, the vergence of light emerging from the objective will need to be altered by a corresponding amount in order to maintain clarity of the focimeter target. To create this change in vergence on the objective side will require a larger change in vergence on the eyepiece side: this will be U', and it will actually be the new back vertex power of the telescope, measured on the focimeter. By rearrangement of Freid's formula, these changes in vergence can be used to determine magnification from Eq. (9.5) below:

$$M = \frac{-tU'}{2} \pm \sqrt{\left(\frac{tU'}{2}\right)^2 + \frac{U'}{U}} \qquad \text{Eq. (9.5)}$$

If measured values are substituted into the formula, two possible answers will be obtained, one positive and the other negative: the former applies if the telescope is Galilean and the latter if astronomical. Table 9.4 provides a look-up for the results of these calculations.

Practical Procedure
1. Looking at a far distant target (>10 m), focus the telescope as accurately as possible.
2. Place the telescope in the focimeter with the eyepiece against the lens rest, and the objective pointing towards you. Measure the back vertex power. This reading will be called BVP$_1$: if the telescope is genuinely afocal this should of course be zero, but the method can still be used even if the telescope incorporates a refractive correction. *Example: BVP$_1$ is recorded as −0.50.*
3. Now place a +1.00 DS trial-case lens up against the surface of the objective lens. The focimeter target will now blur and should be refocused. The power reading corresponding to this clear image should be taken, and this is BVP$_2$. *Example: With the +1.00 trial lens in place, BVP$_2$ is recorded as +2.50.*
4. The change in 'incident' vergence—the vergence on the objective side of the telescope—was the +1.00 DS from the added trial-case lens, so $U = +1.00$. The change in

TABLE 9.4 Determining the Magnification of Galilean Telescopes by Measuring Telescope Length and the Amount of Change in Back Vertex Power (BVP) That Results From Adding a +1.00 DS Lens in Front of the Objective

	Telescope Length (mm)			
Change in BVP	10	20	30	40
1.00	1.00	0.99	0.99	0.98
1.50	1.22	1.21	1.20	1.20
2.00	1.40	1.39	1.38	1.37
2.50	1.57	1.56	1.54	1.53
3.00	1.72	1.70	1.69	1.67
3.50	1.85	1.84	1.82	1.80
4.00	1.98	1.96	1.94	1.92
4.50	2.10	2.08	2.05	2.03
5.00	2.21	2.19	2.16	2.14
5.50	2.32	2.29	2.26	2.24
6.00	2.42	2.39	2.36	2.33
6.50	2.52	2.49	2.45	2.42
7.00	2.61	2.58	2.54	2.51
7.50	2.70	2.66	2.63	2.59
8.00	2.79	2.75	2.71	2.67
8.50	2.87	2.83	2.79	2.75
9.00	2.96	2.91	2.87	2.83
9.50	3.04	2.99	2.94	2.90
10.00	3.11	3.06	3.02	2.97
10.50	3.19	3.14	3.09	3.04
11.00	3.26	3.21	3.16	3.10
11.50	3.33	3.28	3.22	3.17
12.00	3.40	3.35	3.29	3.23

'emergent' vergence—the vergence on the eyepiece side of the telescope is now calculated from $(BVP_2 - BVP_1)$ and this is equal to U'.

Example: $U' = BVP_2 - BVP_1 = +2.50 - (-0.50) = +3.00$

5. Measure the length of the telescope (in m); this is t.

   Example: $t = 20$ mm or 0.02 m

6. Look up the magnification in Table 9.4, and find $M = 1.70\times$

As can be seen from Table 9.4, a small inaccuracy in measuring t will have an insignificant effect on the results, and it is only inaccurate focimeter readings which could be sources of error. A potential influence on accuracy (whose significance cannot be reduced) is that the measurement of emergent vergence should be made from the second principal plane of the system. The focimeter measures this vergence from the back surface of the eyepiece and if the principal plane is a significant distance from this, it will lead to errors.

Near Telescopes

An afocal telescope can be modified practically for near-vision use by increasing the separation of the objective and eyepiece lenses, or by adding a plus-lens reading cap to create a telemicroscope. Either of these systems can be thought of as a distance afocal telescope, with an additional plus-lens incorporated into (or added over) the objective lens in order to provide focussing for the close working distance. This additional plus-lens (whether real or apparent) makes the divergent light from the near object parallel and so the object must obviously be placed at its anterior focal point. Such a system can be thought of as being composed of two components, the telescope and a plus lens, and the total magnification is equal to the product of the telescope magnification and the reading cap magnification (calculated in the same way as any plus lens):

$$M_{TOTAL} = M_{TEL} \times \frac{F_{RC}}{4}$$

For a near telescope, then, the crucial parameters to measure are its magnification and anterior focal length (f_{RC}): the latter is the working space for which the patient will be focused. The latter is measured quite easily: the anterior focal length is just the reciprocal of the front vertex power measured by focimeter, which is also F_{RC} in the previous formula.

Having measured the front vertex power, this can be neutralised by using a trial-case lens of equal power and opposite sign and placing it in contact with the telescope objective lens. As the effect of the reading cap has now been eliminated, the power of the distance telescope can be found using the focimeter, as described in the previous section (Bailey, 1978b). As noted earlier, this method of measuring telescope power with a focimeter is only suitable for Galilean systems, and this is equally true of this method for near-vision telescopes.

Practical Procedure

1. Place the near-vision telescope with its objective lens against the lens rest of the focimeter, and read the front vertex power. This is the power of the reading cap, and the reciprocal—its focal length—is the working space which this telescope will allow the patient to use.

   Example: The front vertex power of a Galilean telescope is found to be +6.00, which means the working space is equal to the front vertex focal length which is 16.7 cm.

2. Take a lens of opposite sign but equal power from the trial case. Turn the telescope round so that it now has its objective surface pointing towards you and you are now able to measure back vertex power. Place the 'neutralising lens' over the objective and take a reading of back vertex power—BVP_1—which should be close to zero if the telescope is genuinely afocal.

   Example: A −6.00 lens is held against the objective, and BVP_1 is recorded as −0.25.

3. Now change the neutralising lens to one with an extra +1.00 DS power, and measure the back vertex power again: this is BVP_2.

Example: The neutralising lens is changed to −5.00 (−6.00 + (+1.00)) and BVP$_2$ is now recorded as +3.25.

4. The change in 'incident' vergence—the vergence on the objective side of the telescope—was the +1.00 DS from the changed neutralising lens, so $U = +1.00$. The change in 'emergent' vergence—the vergence on the eyepiece side of the telescope—is now calculated from $(BVF_2 − BVF_1)$ and this is equal to U'.
   Example: $U' = BVP_2 − BVP_1 = +3.25 − (−0.25) = +3.50$

5. Measure the length of the telescope (in m); this is t.
   Example: t = 25 mm or 0.025 m

6. This can be determined from Table 9.4 by extrapolation. In this case, the magnification of the telescope is 1.83×.

7. This is the (afocal distance) telescope magnification, but it is now necessary to also consider the effect of the additional plus-lens reading cap and calculate total magnification.

$$M_{TOTAL} = M_{TEL} \times \frac{F_{RC}}{4}$$

Example: The power of the reading cap F_{RC} has already been determined as +6.00, so substituting values into the formula,

$$M_{TOTAL} = 1.83 \times \frac{6}{4} = 1.83 \times 1.5 = 2.75\times$$

TYPES AVAILABLE

Astronomical telescopes are available from many different sources: this includes shops supplying bird-watching and photographic equipment, as well as specialist low-vision aid companies. Spectacle-mounted binocular distance Galilean telescopes are often sold as 'sports glasses' or for going to the theatre; spectacle-mounted binocular near astronomical telescopes are used by surgeons and dentists in their work. Many of the hand-held telescopes are very similar in design and construction and are just marketed under different names from the different suppliers. Many devices are very versatile and can be used in several different ways (Fig. 9.15), depending on the patient's requirements (Table 9.5; Figs. 9.16 and 9.17).

The design of Galilean telescopes can be broadly divided into the categories shown in Table 9.6 (Fig. 9.18).

TELESCOPES FOR MOBILITY

Of the telescopes described so far, all have been intended for sedentary or 'spotting' tasks: the FOV of all those described has been insufficient for even limited mobility. Yet obviously a device which can magnify at long distances would be useful if it could be mounted before the eye and used when mobile. There are several ways in which attempts have been made to achieve this goal.

Bioptic Systems

Bioptic is a general term used to describe a system in which two different retinal images (typically magnified and non-magnified) are presented to the patient at the same time. As applied to telescopes, it refers to a system where the refractive correction forms a carrier lens, and a compact telescope is mounted in the upper part of this (Korb, 1970) (see Fig. 9.7, *bottom left*). When the wearer is looking straight ahead, the telescope is positioned with the lower edge at the top of the pupil, and the telescope is tilted about 10 degrees

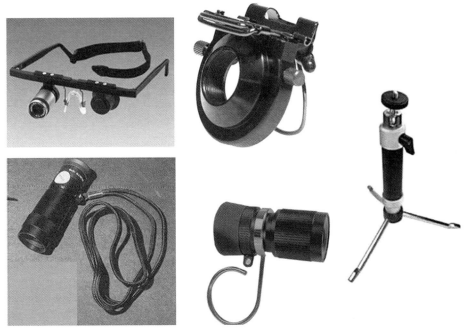

Fig. 9.15 Several different ways in which a telescope can be used, depending on patient requirements and preferences. Clockwise from *top left*: permanent mounting on carrier frame (with optional headband); clip-on/flip-up mount; table-top tripod; finger-ring for one-handed focusing; neck-cord.

TABLE 9.5	**The Characteristics of Currently Available Astronomical Telescopes**		
Characteristics	**Astronomical**		
	Monocular (Fig. 9.16)	**Binocular**	
		Distance	**Near**
Magnification range	2.75× – 14×	4× – 10×	4× – 8×
Focussing distance	Infinity to ~20 cm; or fixed focus for infinity	Infinity to ~2 m	Fixed focus
Mounting available (see Fig. 9.15)	Finger-ring Neck/wrist cord Clip-on/flip-up or fixed frame-mounted (up to 6×) Table-top tripod-mounted (8× and over)	Hand-held Table-top tripod-mounted (Rare) spec-mounted	Spec-mounted
Features	Can have reading caps (including additional plus lens to make very high-powered stand magnifier ~30× (Fig. 9.17)	Limited adjustment for PD	Working distance varies, depending on design and magnification Mounted on or through prescription lenses

PD, Interpupillary distance.

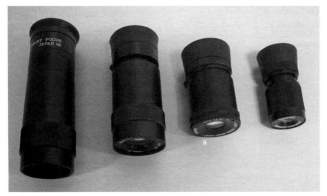

Fig. 9.16 A range of monocular astronomical telescopes, with magnification (from *left* to *right*) 8×; 6×; 4×; 2.75×.

upwards. To view through the telescope, the wearer drops their head slightly, so the telescope is now horizontal and its optical axis aligns with the wearer's visual axis. This allows 'normal' viewing through the spectacle lens, with the magnified view available as required during distance vision on lowering the chin down. Several manufacturers offer the same range of telescopes to be fitted either in a bioptic or a 'full-aperture' position (i.e. positioned for use when viewing in the primary position). Bioptic devices are frequently used to help the patient achieve independent travel, which is a very important goal for many. The majority of states in the United States, and some European countries, allow driving using bioptic devices, although the licence may be restricted (Barron, 1991). There is evidence that with careful fitting (Bailey, 1979b) and an intensive and structured training programme (Park et al., 1993; Kooijman et al., 2009), the success rate (Feinbloom, 1977) and safety record (Kelleher, 1979) achieved are good. Their potential safety is questioned by some clinicians, however, as the bioptic is only a spotting

aid, designed for occasional use (Fonda, 1974): for over 98% of the time, the driver is in an unaided visually impaired state (Wang et al., 2020). The device is used in the same way as a normally sighted driver uses a rear-view mirror, with occasional glances (median duration: 1.4 seconds, Wang et al., 2020) to obtain extra information about the road ahead. Although both magnified and unmagnified fields can be viewed simultaneously if the device is monocular, the telescope housing creates a considerable ring scotoma around the magnified zone. In addition, the dissimilar simultaneous views create rivalry which also limits hazard detection (Doherty et al., 2015).

Contact Lens Telescopes

The fields-of-view of both Galilean and astronomical telescopes are very small, due to the distance of the objective lens from the eye. Feinbloom (1940) and Dittmer (1939) both proposed making a telescope in contact lens form to improve on this. A more realistic system (and the type of system which would now be called a contact lens telescope) uses a negative contact lens as the eyepiece and a positive spectacle lens as the objective of a Galilean telescope (Bettman & McNair, 1939), with the length of the telescope being equal to the separation of the lenses (the vertex distance of the spectacles). This system is of particular interest in the UK because it would appear to be the only magnifying appliance which would be permissible for driving (Silver & Woodward, 1978). The FOV of the telescope is determined by the diameter, power and position of the spectacle lens and is equivalent to that of the highly hypermetropic spectacle wearer. Due to the prismatic effect of the lens edge, there is a ring scotoma following the shape of the lens periphery: this can be avoided by the use of a blended aspheric lens (e.g. Essilor Omega or Rodenstock Perfastar), where the power gradually decreases to zero at the lens edge beyond a useful diameter of approximately 45 mm. Even when the contact lens power, spectacle lens power

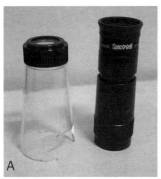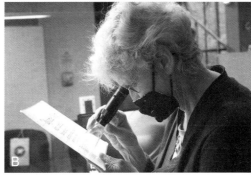

Fig. 9.17 (A) A high-powered focusing astronomical telescope, and a reading cap which attaches to the objective. (B) The assembled device which is a very high magnification device (>25×), but which gives an extended working distance.

TABLE 9.6 The Characteristics of Currently Available Galilean Telescopes (Fig. 9.18)

Characteristics	Fixed Focus/Limited Focussing Ability		Fixed Focus with Caps	Fixed Focus for Near
	Distance	Near		
Magnification range	1.2× – 4×	1.5× – 4×	[a]1.6× – 20×	1.6× – 4.5×
Binocular (B) or monocular (M)	B or M	B or M	M or B (B may be achieved by prism in reading cap)	B or M
Viewing distance (Distance (D); Intermediate (I); Near (N))	D to I (≈60 cm)	N (40 cm) to very near (<10 cm)	D, I and N if appropriate caps available	N
Mounting available	Clip-on, hand-held, spec-mounted[b] (including bioptic)	Spec-mounted[b]	Spec-mounted (including bioptic)	Spec-mounted
Examples	Eschenbach MaxTV Eschenbach Binocular Distance Telescopes TechOptics	Eschenbach MaxDetail COIL Near Telescope	Zeiss Telescopic Spectacles Designs for Vision Full Diameter Multilens Vidi	Designs for Vision Reading Telescope Multilens CombiShort

[a]Some manufacturers give the total magnification available, although others label by the distance magnification and list cap powers/working distances separately. If high magnification is produced by using a high-powered reading cap, working space will be very limited.
[b]If in a standard mount for binocular viewing, there may be limited/no interpupillary distance (PD) or height adjustment.

and vertex distance are maximised, the magnification limit is only 1.8× to 2.0× (Byer, 1986; Lewis, 1986): it is unlikely to exceed this even in a hypermetrope in whom the uncorrected ametropia increases the effective power of the eyepiece (Fig. 9.19)—the uncorrected +10.00 DS hypermetrope wearing a −30.00 DS contact lens would have an 'effective eyepiece power' of −40.00 DS.

It can be seen that the longer the vertex distance, the greater the magnification which can be achieved, but it is difficult to go beyond 25 mm, even if a spectacle frame is hand-made to have an inset bridge (Fig. 9.20). Although unusual custom-made mountings can be devised, it must be remembered that as the positive spectacle lens (which is the telescope objective lens) gets further from the eye, the FOV decreases such that the system no longer has any advantage over a conventional telescope. The patient may have difficulty inserting the contact lenses, as once they are in place the vision is extremely poor until the spectacles are worn. This is obviously not a system which can be discarded or adopted rapidly. The restricted magnification of contact lens systems

led Jose and Browning (1983) to develop a bioptic telescope for use in front of the spectacle objective lens of a contact lens telescope. This can achieve a magnification of 3.2× but reduces FOV considerably.

As the magnification of the contact lens telescope is limited, it would be most useful in a patient with only a modest loss of acuity, and patients with (idiopathic) infantile nystagmus are ideal candidates. Although the magnified view of their moving eyes can be rather disconcerting to the casual observer, people with nystagmus may see better with contact lenses as they move with the eye (so long as they have stable orientation). It has also been suggested that this optical system could be creating stabilisation of the retinal image (Drasdo, 1965; Drasdo & Sabell, 1979). (These issues are discussed in more detail in Chapter 14.)

People with infantile nystagmus almost never perceive apparent object motion (oscillopsia) in the environment despite the constant retinal image motion. Remarkably, whatever compensation mechanism these patients have continues to function despite the increased retinal image motion produced by the

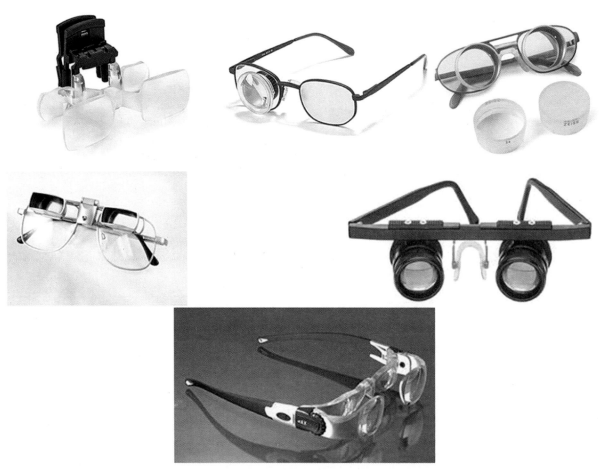

Fig. 9.18 Examples of spectacle-mounted Galilean telescopes. Clockwise from *top left*: clip-on distance telescope (fixed focus; fixed centration); fixed focus near monocular telescope; binocular telescope with reading caps; near telescope (note the convergence of the tubes) (limited focus; and variable centration); distance telescope (limited focus; fixed centration); bioptic (fixed focus for distance).

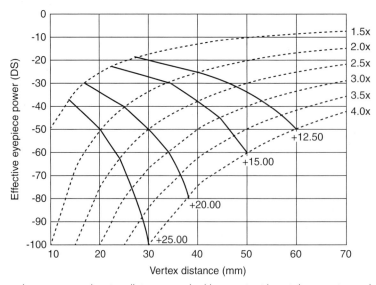

Fig. 9.19 The combination of eyepiece power and vertex distance required in a contact lens telescope to produce magnifications from 1.5× to 4×, which are represented by the *dashed lines*. Appropriate spectacle lens (telescope objective) powers to achieve a particular magnification are shown by the *solid lines*. It can be seen that high magnification requires an extremely powerful contact lens eyepiece and/or a large vertex distance.

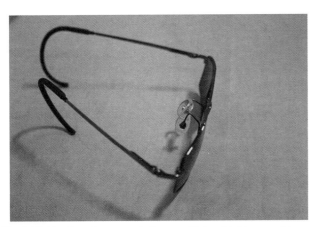

Fig. 9.20 Hand-made spectacle frame with inset bridge used to create a large vertex distance.

magnification. Nonetheless, the patient should be questioned carefully about the presence of oscillopsia when viewing through a hand-held telescope before proceeding with contact lens fitting, as on rare occasions, an individual with nystagmus viewing through a telescope does experience disabling oscillopsia.

It is important to create a stable but physiologically acceptable contact lens fit, as any lens movement will induce a corresponding but magnified image motion, and scleral (Ludlam, 1960; Drasdo & Sabell, 1979) rigid corneal (Silver & Woodward, 1978) and hydrogel (Lewis, 1986) lenses have all been recommended as suitable: the latter is recommended if the required power can be obtained. Due to vergence amplification, it will be impossible for the patient to accommodate for intermediate and near distances through the telescope, and they will require a reading addition (although the patient initiating a small increase in the vertex distance of this high-powered spectacle lens, when required, may provide sufficient additional power in practice). This can be incorporated into the high-plus spectacle lens which is the telescope objective, and the lens power to be added is that which has a focal length equal to the patient's required working distance. Optically, this behaves as a 'reading cap', and it can be fitted in single-vision or bifocal form. A further variation involves the use of a Fresnel spectacle lens to achieve high power combined with low weight (Gerstman & Levene, 1974). Filderman (1959) has suggested using a lenticular form of both the spectacle lens and contact lens so that the central portion of each is of high power, with the periphery of the contact lens containing the ametropic correction and the spectacle carrier portion being afocal. In this way, the magnified and unmagnified images are present simultaneously.

Practical Procedure

It is likely that a team approach with multidisciplinary expertise in low vision, contact lens fitting and spectacle frame dispensing will be needed to perform this procedure.

1. Refract the patient and determine the spectacle correction. Carry out keratometry and an assessment of suitability for contact lens wear.
2. With the spectacle prescription in place, demonstrate a hand-held telescope with approximately 2× magnification

to the patient. Measure the improvement in acuity, and (in the presence of nystagmus) question the patient about possible oscillopsia.
3. Unless there are contra-indications to its use, select a soft contact lens of power approximately −25.00 DS to −35.00 DS as a trial lens. When settled in the eye, place a trial frame in position with the longest possible back vertex distance and over-refract with plus trial lenses. Measure the vertex distance and the acuity improvement. Using Fig. 9.19, confirm that the acuity improvement is in approximate agreement with the magnification expected.
4. Alter the contact lens if required to obtain a different power, or to improve the physical fit: this may need to be ordered, and require another visit by the patient. Repeat stage (3) with this new lens in place.
5. Fit a spectacle frame with the largest possible vertex distance. Measure this value and, if necessary, compensate the spectacle prescription obtained in (3) to be correct for this distance. If possible choose a frame with adjustable pads so that minor changes in vertex distance can be achieved when the system is collected, and with curl sides to ensure a stable fit. Select a suitable positive lens form: a blended aspheric will eliminate the ring scotoma normally experienced by the wearers of high-plus lenses.
6. When the patient collects the completed spectacles and optimum contact lens, demonstrate the reduced FOV and poor near vision. When the patient has adapted to the system, perform an over-refraction for the habitual near viewing distance to determine the required reading correction. It is worth delaying prescription of near spectacles, because the wearer may prefer to obtain extra power by a slight increase in the vertex distance of their 'distance' spectacles.

Intraocular Lens Telescopes

To create a Galilean telescope using a high-minus intraocular lens (IOL) in conjunction with a high-plus spectacle lens is a logical progression from the contact-lens telescope, and as the two lenses are further apart, the magnification can be higher. Koester and Donn (1984) fitted patients with macular degeneration and cataract (subsequently removed), obtaining magnification in the range 2× to 4×. Garnier and Colonna De Lega (1992) created an approximately 3× Galilean telescope by using an IOL of power −50.00 DS and a spectacle lens of approximately +30.00 DS. They found that whilst the vision was improved to at least the level obtained with a conventional 3× magnifier preoperatively in all 50 patients treated, 44% were not satisfied with the result because the improvement was not sufficient for their needs. This suggests that very careful patient screening is required before embarking on these procedures. Temel et al. (1993) report their results of a similar study, but an unusual aspect of the report is their recommendation of monocular correction so that the patient can voluntarily swap between magnified and unmagnified viewing. They give no details of whether the patient covers one eye or suppresses the unwanted image, or whether both images are seen simultaneously as in a monovision contact lens correction. Other suggested designs have included an IOL with both the conventional positive power, and a supplementary negative power zone. A recent study has suggested much more modest 'minus' powers, in the form of an IOL which is less positive than that required to result in emmetropia (Iizuka et al., 2007). Of course, before the advent of IOLs, all cataract surgery rendered the patient aphakic, and these patients all experienced the telescope created by the 'minus eye' and the high plus spectacle lens, creating around 25% (1.25×) magnification.

From a cosmetic perspective, a better alternative would be to place the entire optical system within the eye. Beyond considerations of the optical device itself, this raises a number of concerns:

1. The device is larger than a conventional IOL, so surgery is more invasive (larger incision), and there is a risk of the front surface of the device touching the posterior cornea, and further compromising the integrity of the corneal endothelium.

2. If all the light entering the eye is imaged through the telescope, the FOV will be limited. This may require the device to be fitted monocularly to allow peripheral vision by the unoperated eye: this disparity between the two monocular views will require considerable familiarisation and adaptation by the patient.

3. The actual device itself is only part of what is happening to the patient. The existing natural lens, with possible opacity, will be removed; any residual hypermetropic refraction will be corrected with spectacles that create spectacle magnification; and the patient is trained to make the best use of their residual vision. The latter may be particularly significant, as studies have reported improvement in the non-operated eyes (e.g. Dag et al., 2019; Hudson et al., 2006). Without clinical trials which control for these variables, it is difficult to unequivocally identify the contribution of the device (Colenbrander et al., 2008).

4. These devices require considerably more surgical skill (and time) than is required to implant a conventional IOL.

5. If the patient requires monitoring or treatment of a progressive retinal disease, visualising the fundus is challenging through these IOLs.

6. There is a risk of the device blocking the passage of aqueous into the anterior chamber, or through the drainage angle, with a possibility of a transient or permanent rise in intraocular pressure. For this reason, a prophylactic peripheral iridotomy or iridectomy is sometimes performed.

7. Some devices are unsuitable for individuals who are already pseudophakic.

8. If the patient does not tolerate the system, further surgery is required to explant the device.

The most common systems have been based on a Galilean design, so separation of the lenses is critical. The IOL-Vip (Intraocular Lens for Visually Impaired People) consisted of a −64 DS IOL to form the eyepiece placed in the capsular bag, and a +53 DS IOL as the objective, placed in the anterior chamber. Although it only provided a theoretical 1.3× magnification

(with 80-degree FOV), the acuity gains reported by Orzalesi et al. (2007) were markedly in excess of that, leading to the reservations expressed by many experts about the reason for the improvement (Colenbrander et al., 2008). In particular, some patients had significant cataract removed, and a high degree of residual hypermetropia (subsequently corrected by high-plus spectacle lenses) was often found, due to the lenses not being as far apart as optical theory required. The IOL-Vip Revolution device relies less on the judgement of the surgeon to position the lenses. In this case, both lenses are placed in the capsular bag, with a ring of acrylic material positioned between the two lenses to hold them in the correct position (Dag et al., 2019). The iol-AMD again used a similar lens combination, but each lens has angled haptic supports to hold the lenses at the required separation (Hengerer et al., 2015). For all these systems, fitting can be either monocular or binocular. However, in each design (and particularly the iol-AMD), it is suggested that the component lenses should have prism incorporated, or be laterally displaced, to create prismatic effect, to attempt to move the image onto a better functioning area of the retina (see section 'Prism Relocation' in Chapter 13). If this is implemented, it is likely that binocular vision will create diplopia.

The IMT (Implantable Miniature Telescope) has the whole telescope (with either 2.2× or 3× magnification available) within a rigid housing 4.4 mm long, which sits in the capsular bag and protrudes through the pupil. This telescope is intended to be fitted monocularly, so one eye sees a magnified view, whilst the other unoperated eye provides peripheral vision. This is because the telescope only provides a 20° to 24° (depending on magnification) FOV (Hudson et al., 2006). Patients require substantial training before and after the surgery, to help them adapt to using the two eyes in different ways. The device is focussed at around 3 m, with the option to prescribe distance and/or near spectacles to optimise vision.

An alternative telescope design is the basis of the Lipshitz Mirror Implant (LMI) device. This uses a Cassegrain telescope based on mirrors, which has a magnification of 2.5× (Agarwal et al., 2008). As implemented in an IOL design, it is possible to have the central area of the lens (2.8 mm in diameter) containing the mirror elements, providing magnification, but a peripheral zone which allows an unobstructed peripheral view. Nonetheless, this is fitted monocularly, and the patient will still have to adapt to the conflicting images from the two eyes. Some patients are disturbed by reflections and glare from the mirrors: interestingly, Agarwal et al. (2008) report this as an issue when the patients are driving, illustrating that this is one of very few magnifying aids that might be acceptable for that purpose. The Orilens is a similar device designed for patients who are already pseudophakic.

The effectiveness of these intraocular devices has only been reported in observational studies, although some of these have been large. Gupta et al. (2018) have pointed out the poor quality of the evidence in the absence of randomised controlled trials. However, the results with the different devices are critically compared in two reviews (Dunbar & Dhawahir-Scala, 2018;

Grzybowski et al., 2020). Unfortunately, measurement of visual improvements has often been based solely on letter acuity (e.g. Hudson et al., 2006): this is especially problematic as a measure of near vision, for which word acuity and reading speed are more appropriate outcomes. Assessing a patient in advance of surgery, using an external telescope of equivalent magnification, should give a reasonable indication of expected VA. Careful counselling (regarding loss of binocularity, potential simultaneous vision of conflicting images and the need for adaptation/training) is also an important part of preparing the patient for the procedure.

REFERENCES

Agarwal, A., Lipshitz, I., Jacob, S., et al. (2008). Mirror telescopic intraocular lens for age-related macular degeneration. Design and preliminary clinical results of the Lipshitz macular implant. *Journal of Cataract and Refractive Surgery, 34*(1), 87–94. https://doi.org/10.1016/j.jcrs.2007.08.031.

Bailey, I. L. (1978). New method for determining the magnifying power of telescopes. *American Journal of Optometry and Physiological Optics, 55,* 203–207.

Bailey, I. L. (1979a). A lensometer method for checking telescopes. *Optometric Monthly, 70,* 216–219.

Bailey, I. L. (1979b). A scientific angle on bioptic telescopes. *Optometric Monthly, 70,* 462–466.

Barron, C. (1991). Bioptic telescopic spectacles for motor vehicle driving. *Journal of the American Optometric Association, 62,* 37–41.

Bettman, J. W., & McNair, G. S. (1939). A contact-lens telescopic system. *American Journal of Ophthalmology, 22,* 27–33.

Byer, A. (1986). Magnification limitations of a contact lens telescope. *American Journal of Optometry and Physiological Optics, 63,* 71–75.

Colenbrander, A., Fletcher, D. C., Berlin, A. J., et al. (2008). Letter to the editor: rehabilitation and intraocular telescopes. *Ophthalmology, 115*(8), 1437–1438.

Crossland, M. D., & Silver, J. H. (2005). Thirty years in an urban low vision clinic: changes in prescribing habits of low vision practitioners. *Optometry and Vision Science, 82*(7), 617–622. https://doi.org/10.1097/01.opx.0000171336.40273.3f.

Dag, M. Y., Afrashi, F., Nalcaci, S., et al. (2019). The efficacy of "IOL-Vip Revolution" telescopic intraocular lens in age-related macular degeneration cases with senile cataract. *European Journal of Ophthalmology, 29*(6), 615–620. https://doi.org/10.1177/1120672118803831.

Dittmer, A.F. (1939). US Patent 2,164,801.

Doherty, A. L., Peli, E., & Luo, G. (2015). Hazard detection with a monocular bioptic telescope. *Ophthalmic and Physiological Optics, 35*(5), 530–539. https://doi.org/10.1111/opo.12232.

Drasdo, N. (1965). An experimental and clinical system for producing retinal image constraint under quasi-normal viewing conditions. *American Journal of Optometry and Archives of American Academy of Optometry, 42,* 748–756.

Drasdo, N., & Sabell, A. G. (1979). A supplementary note on contact lens telescopes. *Ophthalmic Optician, (January 20th),* 36.

Dunbar, H. M. P., & Dhawahir-Scala, F. E. (2018). A discussion of commercially available intra-ocular telescopic implants for patients with age-related macular degeneration. *Ophthalmology and Therapy, 7*(1), 33–48. https://doi.org/10.1007/s40123-018-0129-7.

Feinbloom, W. (1940). US Patent 2,198,868.

Feinbloom, W. (1977). Driving with bioptic telescopic spectacles (BTS). *American Journal of Optometry and Physiological Optics, 54,* 35–42.

Filderman, I. P. (1959). The Telecon lens for the partially sighted. *American Journal of Optometry and Archives of American Academy of Optometry, 36,* 135–136.

Fonda, G. (1974). Bioptic telescopic spectacles for driving a motor vehicle. *Archives of Ophthalmology, 92,* 348–349.

Freid, A. N. (1977). Telescopes, light vergence and accommodation. *American Journal of Optometry and Physiological Optics, 54,* 365–373.

Garnier, B., & Colonna De Lega, X. (1992). Low-vision aid using a high-minus intraocular lens. *Applied Optics, 31,* 3632–3636.

Gerstman, D. R., & Levene, J. R. (1974). Galilean telescopic system for the partially sighted. *British Journal of Ophthalmology, 58,* 761–765.

Greene, H. A., Beadles, R., & Pekar, J. (1992). Challenges in applying autofocus technology to low vision telescopes. *Optometry and Vision Science, 69,* 25–31.

Greene, H. A., Pekar, J., Brilliant, R., et al. (1991). The Ocutech Vision Enhancing System: utilization and preference study. *Journal of the American Optometric Association, 62,* 19–26.

Grzybowski, A., Wang, J., Mao, F., et al. (2020). Intraocular vision-improving devices in age-related macular degeneration. *Annals of Translational Medicine, 8*(22), 1549. https://doi.org/10.21037/atm-20-5851.

Gupta, A., Lam, J., Custis, P., et al. (2018). Implantable miniature telescope (IMT) for vision loss due to end-stage age-related macular degeneration. *Cochrane Database of Systematic Reviews, 30*(5), 5. https://doi.org/10.1002/14651858.CD011140.pub2.

Hengerer, F. H., Artal, P., Kohnen, T., et al. (2015). Initial clinical results of a new telescopic IOL implanted in patients with dry age- related macular degeneration. *Journal of Refractive Surgery, 31*(3), 158–162. https://doi.org/10.3928/1081597X-20150220-03.

Hudson, H. L., Lane, S. S., Heier, J. S., et al. (2006). Implantable miniature telescope for the treatment of visual acuity loss resulting from end-stage age-related macular degeneration: 1-Year results. *Ophthalmology, 113*(11), 1987–2001. https://doi.org/10.1016/j.ophtha.2006.07.010.

Iizuka, M., Gorfinkel, J., Mandelcorn, M., et al. (2007). Modified cataract surgery with telescopic magnification for patients with age-related macular degeneration. *Canadian Journal of Ophthalmology, 42*(6), 854–859. https://doi.org/10.3129/I07-152.

Jose, R., & Browning, R. (1983). Designing a bioptic-contact lens telescopic system. *American Journal of Optometry and Physiological Optics, 60,* 74–79.

Kelleher, D. K. (1979). Driving with low vision. *Journal of Visual Impairment and Blindness, 73,* 345–350.

Koester, C. J., & Donn, A. (1984). Ocular telephoto system for patients with macular degeneration. *Journal of the Optical Society of America, 1,* 1268.

Kooijman, A. C., Melis-dankers, B. J. M., Peli, E., et al. (2009). The introduction of bioptic driving in The Netherlands. *NIH Public Access, 10*(1), 1–9.

Korb, D. R. (1970). Preparing the visually handicapped person for motor vehicle operation. *American Journal of Optometry and Archives of American Academy of Optometry, 47,* 619–628.

Lewis, H. T. (1986). Parameters of contact lens-spectacle telescopic systems and considerations in prescribing. *American Journal of Optometry and Physiological Optics, 63,* 387–391.

Ludlam, W. M. (1960). Clinical experience with the contact lens telescope. *American Journal of Optometry and Archives of American Academy of Optometry, 37,* 363–372.

Ocutech. (n.d.). *Bioptic telescope prescribing protocol.* Retrieved January 4, 2022, from https://ocutech.com/wp-content/uploads/2021/documents/Ocutech. Prescribing Protocol .pdf

Orzalesi, N., Pierrottet, C.O., Zenoni, S., et al. (2007). The IOL-Vip System: a double intraocular lens implant for visual rehabilitation of patients with macular disease. Ophthalmology, 114, 860–865.

Park, W. L., Unatin, J., & Hebert, A. (1993). A driving program for the visually impaired. *Journal of the American Optometric Association, 64,* 54–59.

Silver, J. H., & Woodward, E. G. (1978). Driving with a visual disability—A case report. *Ophthalmic Optician,* (28th October), 794–795.

Smith, G. (1979). Variation of image vergence with change in object distance for telescopes: the general case. *American Journal of Optometry and Physiological Optics, 56,* 696–703.

Spitzberg, L. A., & Qi, M. (1994). Depth of field of plus lenses and reading telescopes. *Optometry and Vision Science, 71,* 115–119.

Temel, A., Bavbek, T., & Kanpolat, A. (1993). Clinical application of contact lens telescopes. *International Journal of Rehabilitation Research, 16,* 148–150.

Wang, S., Moharrer, M., Baliutaviciute, V., et al. (2020). Bioptic telescope use in naturalistic driving by people with visual impairment. *Translational Vision Science and Technology, 9*(4), 1–11. https://doi.org/10.1167/tvst.9.4.11.

Watson, G. R., de l'Aune, W., Stelmack, J., et al. (1997). National survey of the impact of low vision device use among veterans. *Optometry and Vision Science Official Publication of the American Academy of Optometry, 74*(5), 249–259. https://doi.org/10.1097/00006324-199705000-00019.

10

Contrast and Glare

IMPROVING VISIBILITY OF THE RETINAL IMAGE

Into this category come a wide range of very simple strategies which are designed to aid vision, but do not affect the vergence or direction of rays of light entering the eye. They do not increase the size or improve the focus of the retinal image, but rather improve the visibility of the image in other ways. In addition to making an object easier to see, it is often possible to add a tactile back-up to give extra help in recognition—for example, one may put a coloured mark on a light switch to make it easier to see, but also make the mark raised above the surface so that it can be easily felt. 'Hi-marks' is a fluorescent orange substance like toothpaste which is squeezed from a tube to make coloured, tactile markings which set to a hard lump; 'Bump-ons' are self-adhesive plastic dots which are clearly visible and easily felt when used as markers (Figs. 10.1 and 10.2), and there are many other examples. Improving object visibility often involves increasing the contrast of the retinal image, and these strategies will be equally effective regardless of the cause of the visual impairment. For those patients with media opacities, however, the ability to detect low-contrast objects may be particularly impaired in the presence of high ambient illumination when there may be scattering of light within the eye, reducing the contrast of the retinal image. This can be tackled by removing any possible sources of scattered light, thus maximising the contrast of the retinal image: these methods will be considered later in the section 'Possible Approaches to Glare Reduction'.

Luminance contrast

Michelson contrast is equal to

$$\frac{L_{max} - L_{min}}{L_{max} + L_{min}}$$

where L_{max} is the luminance of the brightest and L_{min} the luminance of the dimmest areas within the image. In the case of a black object on a white background, or a white object on a black background, contrast can approach 100%. Many low-vision patients have very poor sensitivity to low-contrast targets, and if the contrast is insufficient, then improving the lighting or magnifying the image may not help. If, for example, the patient has difficulty in seeing the edge of a sheet of white paper against a pale desk-top when writing, then there is insufficient contrast between it and the background because the two surfaces have almost equal luminance. The simple solution of providing a darker surface or edge (a sheet of black paper covering the desktop or surrounding a light switch) will make the border of the sheet or the switch visible, even if vision is poor (Figs. 10.3A and B).

It has been suggested that electronic enhancement of video images could be performed in order to improve the contrast (and hence visibility) of images presented on a TV screen.

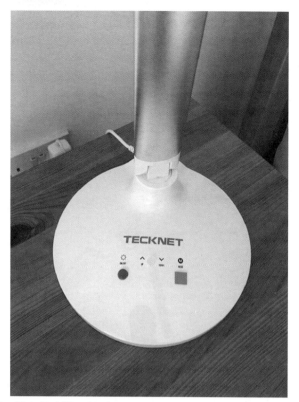

Fig. 10.1 An LED table lamp with different types of 'bump-ons' to increase visibility.

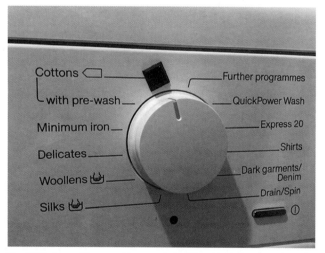

Fig. 10.2 A washing machine control with a black 'bump-on' on the most used programme to increase visibility.

This might apply to television programmes, films or videos, or might extend to image enhancement for text and images presented on an electronic vision enhancement system (EVES). Peli and coworkers found improved performance of visually impaired patients for recognition of faces, expressions, and other details on still photographs (Peli et al., 1991) and video films (Peli et al., 1994). This group did not find any improvement in reading performance for text which had been enhanced in this way: this is in marked contrast to the results of Lawton (1989) who reported dramatic increases in reading speed. This technique is incorporated on several new wearable EVESs although data have not been published on how many people use these modes.

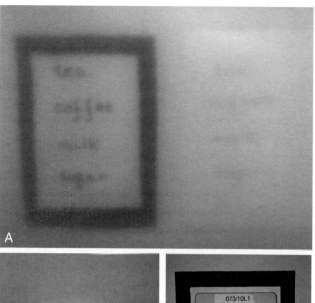

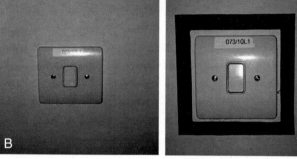

Fig. 10.3 (A) The edge of a piece of white paper is more easily seen if placed on a dark background, and higher contrast letters are achieved with fibre-tip pens *(left)* when compared to ball-point pen or pencil *(right)*. These techniques considerably enhance visibility even in the presence of blur. (B) Light-switch contrast aid to make the switch more visibile (Henshaws).

Chromatic (colour) contrast

It is possible to have chromatic contrast within an image in addition to, or instead of, luminance contrast. In fact, it is possible for someone with good colour vision to be able to distinguish an object from a background of equal luminance, if the two are of different colours—such as a green object against a red background. There are some ocular pathologies in which colour perception would be impaired to the extent that such an object would be invisible, whereas luminance contrast is always a potent source of visual information. This might suggest that black-and-white should be the only colour combination used, but in many cases extra information can be provided by maximising both luminance and chromatic contrast (Sicurella, 1977).

There have been several studies looking at preferred colour combinations in a variety of contexts. Jacobs (1990) looked at reading performance with various colour combinations for text displayed on a screen and found that whilst there were strong subjective preferences, there was no combination which led to improved performance. Legge and Rubin (1986) measured reading rate for different coloured letters against a black background and found very little variation in performance. In a study by Silver et al. (1995) of the preferred colours for the screen display of a bank self-service cash dispenser, there was a marked preference for white-on-black in most older subjects: in the group of cataract patients, white-on-blue was slightly more popular but this is likely to offer almost as much contrast when one considers the attenuation of the blue background luminance by the yellowed crystalline lens. For reading text, then, it appears that maximising luminance contrast is the only way to optimise performance, although patients may subjectively prefer to introduce colour contrast as well: this may be beneficial providing that high luminance contrast is maintained.

Wurm et al. (1993) investigated the hypothesis that colour would improve object recognition for the blurred images seen by low-vision patients even more than it would for those with good vision (as with good vision, additional shape and texture information can be seen, which might render colour redundant). After carefully controlling for luminance contrast in the images, they found that colour did improve the speed and accuracy of naming familiar objects (food items): this led them to suggest that colour contrast is a useful practical strategy to use when the patient has to perform a *recognition* task.

Optimising both luminance and colour contrast would appear to offer the best practical approach. In considering which colours to select, it is worth remembering that the normal visual system is much more sensitive to wavelengths from mid-spectrum—the peak of photopic sensitivity being at 555 nm (yellow)—with less sensitivity to the spectral extremes. Even if there is no specific colour vision defect associated with the visual impairment, one would expect the patient to lose the ability to detect the red and blue wavelengths as sensitivity overall diminishes (Knoblauch & Arditi, 1994). It is also likely that the ability to discriminate between similar hues of equal luminance will become impaired: patients often report a difficulty in distinguishing between black and blue, or between white and yellow (Fig. 10.4). To maximise luminance contrast needs a bright object and a dark background, or vice versa, and chromatic contrast requires selection of colours widely separated in the spectrum. If choosing a colour from mid-spectrum and one from a spectral extreme, it makes sense to have that from the extreme at low-luminance, with the brighter one chosen from mid-spectrum. If the choice is reversed, it is possible that the patient's loss of sensitivity will tend to equalise the apparent brightness of each. Thus, a 'good' combination would be bright yellow and dark blue, but bright red and dark green would be a poor choice. Other poor choices would be those hues close together in the spectrum (such as green and turquoise) or pastel shades where hue is indistinct (such as yellow and grey): in these cases, detection would be especially difficult if the two were of equal brightness.

There are many suggestions for putting such strategies (along with many other helpful adaptations) into practice for everyday tasks:

https://www.rnib.org.uk/sight-loss-advice/reading-home-and-leisure/your-home/practical-adaptations

https://www.henshaws.org.uk/knowledge-village/henshaws-life-hacks/

Using Luminance Contrast

1. Writing with a fine felt-tip or fibre-tip pen produces higher-contrast letters, which are more visible than those written with ball-point pen, even when the two are the same size. It is also possible to have lined paper with lines which are thicker and darker than 'normal'. Various writing frames can also be used which provide the patient with a dark marker along which to write, thus keeping the words in straight lines: this might be done, for example, by moving a dark elastic line marker progressively down the page (Fig. 10.5), or having a cover over the page which

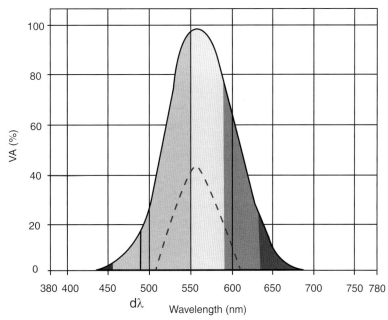

Fig. 10.4 Sensitivity of normal eye peaks in mid-spectrum (green, i.e. *550 nm*), decreased sensitivity at extremes of spectrum (blue, i.e. *450–495 nm* and red, i.e. *620–750 nm*). Patients are likely to lose sensitivity equally throughout the spectrum. Light from ends of the spectrum will therefore produce very little reponse. *Blue* and *red* objects may just seem 'dark'. *VA,* Visual acuity.

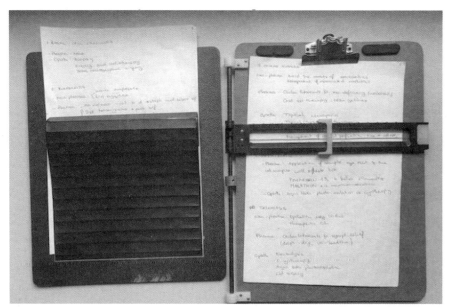

Fig. 10.5 Writing frames.

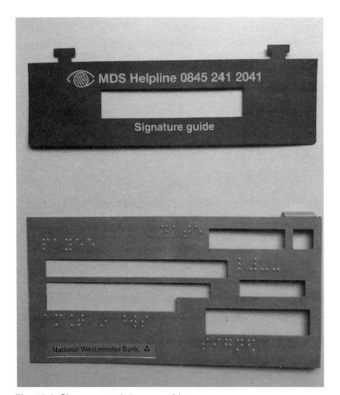

Fig. 10.6 Signature and cheque guide.

is folded down section-by-section to reveal each new line in turn. There are also envelope and cheque guides and signature guides (Fig. 10.6): each is in essence a dark card with sections cut out to reveal the spaces on the page beneath into which the patient must write.

2. A staircase should be evenly lit to avoid shadows from the vertical risers.

3. A white napkin or handkerchief on a dark table-top helps the patient to locate dark objects placed there, such as a purse or spectacle case.

4. Tools can be carried around the house or garden in a large white bucket. This stops them from being lost, or forming a hazard when left lying on the ground, and the bucket will be noticed easily against the background.

5. Decor should include pale carpets and walls (matt) to reflect the available light, and to contrast with dark furniture. If the furnishing fabric is striped, then the stripes will orient in different directions on the horizontal and vertical planes and will define the direction of each.

6. Dark contrasting door knobs will be more easily seen on a light surface and may stop the patient from bumping into the door. Shiny door knobs are most effective on a dark door.

7. Vegetables should be peeled or chopped against a light work surface, whereas pastry should be rolled out on a dark board. Sponge cake mixture should be made in a dark-coloured bowl, but chocolate cake mixed in a light container!

8. Pale crockery will be seen best against a dark tablecloth or, if using a white tablecloth, choose crockery with a dark edge band.

9. Kitchens are often uniformly pale in colour, providing no contrast against which to view light objects. A sheet of black paper against the wall forms a useful background for pouring pale liquids.

10. If making tea/coffee in white cups, the tea/coffee should be poured in before the milk because milk will not be seen (Fig. 10.7).

Using Chromatic Contrast

The selection of appropriate coloured backgrounds is often a very individualised choice. If there is a particular task to be performed, this should be tried against different backgrounds provided by coloured sheets of paper to see which is best. A 'good' combination should also provide significant luminance contrast. In some of these examples, colour is also used for

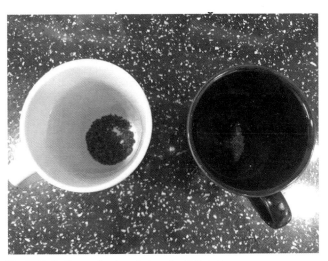

Fig. 10.7 Coffee grains in a dark and a light cup.

'coding' and identifying particular objects. This will only be possible if the patient retains useful colour perception.

1. Glass tumblers are available which have coloured plastic holders to make them easy to see. A clear glass container is almost invisible against a white tablecloth.
2. Food should be arranged on a plate of contrasting colour, such as carrots on a white plate, or fish on a blue plate. Green vegetables placed between fish and mashed potatoes on the plate will aid in the location of each.
3. The handles of garden tools could be painted bright yellow to make them easy to locate.
4. Brightly coloured straps around suitcases can be used for identification.
5. A standard lamp with a pale shade will not contrast with the wall, and may be knocked into, but a brightly coloured wall hanging behind it will make it clearly visible.
6. Coloured electrical sockets and/or plugs can be used. The colour contrast makes each easier to see, and can be used for identification (e.g. red for kettle, blue for microwave).
7. Old felt-tip pens can be used as markers for seedlings in the garden.
8. Toothpaste and shaving cream should be bought in different coloured tubes, and dangerous substances like bleach or white spirit in a distinctively coloured bottle so that these are not mistaken.
9. Grab rails on the sides of the bath can be wound with fluorescent tape.
10. Crockery could be selected from nonmatching sets: the shape of cups, milk jugs and sugar bowls is often similar, so choose the latter two from sets of different colour, preferably with a different shape.
11. Kitchen utensils should not be from a matched set, but deliberately chosen to differ in design: the can opener with a red handle, potato peeler with a yellow handle, etc. If utensils are all the same colour, different coloured tape can be wound around the handles.
12. Plastic freezer bags are available with different coloured stripes, and these can also be used for coding—green for vegetables, red for meat, blue for fish, etc.
13. Tablecloths should be selected which contrast with the crockery, placemats and serving bowls.
14. Low vision aids (LVAs) should have different colour tape attached so they stand out against a table or shelf: something which manufacturers often overlook.

GLARE

Illumination is often extremely valuable for vision enhancement, but there are occasions when it must be carefully controlled, due to the symptoms of glare described by the patient. 'Glare' is a word which is used very informally by many clinicians and patients; however, it covers a range of difference experiences, and it is not clear that everyone is applying the term in the same way. Glare phenomena are experienced by everyone, but patients with visual impairment face some specific/additional challenges. Careful investigation and questioning are required to determine the exact nature of the problem.

Definitions

Photophobia is acquired as a result of pathology affecting the trigeminal (ophthalmic division) axon reflex (Lebensohn, 1934, 1951). Stimulation of the trigeminal sensory nerve endings of the cornea by keratitis, for example, causes reflex vasodilation in the iris. This leads to miosis and a painful response to further light-induced miosis. It is this pain, accompanied by blepharospasm and tearing, which is characteristic of true photophobia: symptoms are alleviated by mydriasis, pending treatment of the underlying condition. In contrast, dazzling or glare is a sense of excessive brightness within the visual field which can create discomfort (discomfort glare) or impair visual performance (disability glare) (Waiss & Cohen, 1992). It must be emphasised that glare and photophobia are completely different phenomena: mydriasis might reduce the photophobia experienced by the patient with anterior segment disease, and yet the dilated pupil may increase the glare experienced (Lebensohn, 1934).

Discomfort glare occurs physiologically (and transiently) in normal vision when a person is suddenly subjected to a much higher level of luminance than that to which they have adapted. The discomfort can be long-lasting if the visual environment requires a difference in adaptation level between adjacent areas of the visual field. For example, the recommendations for workplaces (BS EN 12464: 2011) (European Committee for Standardization, 2011) suggest that for a task illuminance of 750 lx, the immediate surround (<50 cm) of the task should be at least 500 lx, and the background (3 m) at least 160 lx. The amount of discomfort glare created by a discrete light source within the visual field can be predicted to be proportional to the brightness of the source and its angular subtense at the eye, and inversely proportional to its distance from the visual axis and the brightness of the background. However, such a formula tells us nothing about the subjective perception of the glare phenomenon. This glare does not affect vision and may just be annoying, or it may cause the individual to screw up their eyes or avert their gaze. In pathological conditions, discomfort glare occurs when the eye is constantly subjected to levels of illumination which are higher than those to which it can adapt. Sometimes it is easy to see why this would be the case, with conditions such as albinism or aniridia (where the light reaching the retina will be considerably greater than normal) or rod monochromatism (where only the low-light scotopic rod photoreceptor system is operational). Many other conditions (such as refractive error, glaucoma, optic atrophy and retinitis pigmentosa) have been associated with discomfort glare, although in these cases the mechanism of the visual symptoms is not so obvious. There are various subjective scales with which a patient could be asked to rate the amount of glare they experience (Allan et al., 2019): the simplest is a four-point scale of *imperceptible, noticeable, disturbing, intolerable*. The LUMIZ 100 (Montés-Micó et al., 2020) consists of a headset which the patient holds over their eyes, and this allows the amount of light required to reach the individual's discomfort threshold to be accurately measured. It is not yet clear how such a device will be used in clinical practice.

Disability glare may occur at the same time as discomfort glare, but is distinguished by the change in retinal image contrast, and hence reduction in vision, which it creates.

By definition,

$$contrast = \frac{L_{max} - L_{min}}{L_{max} + L_{min}}$$

and in the case of a black object (L_{min} = 0.0) on a white background (L_{max} = 1.0), or a white object on a black background, contrast can approach 100%:

$$contrast = \frac{1.0 - 0.0}{1.0 + 0.0} = 1.0 \ (or \ 100\%)$$

A glare source will add a constant luminance to both the light and dark areas of the high contrast image (e.g. 0.25) so that the contrast reduces. L_{min} = 0.25, and L_{max} = 1.25, so

$$contrast = \frac{1.25 - 0.25}{1.25 + 0.025} = 0.67 \ (or \ 67\%)$$

The high contrast object simply appears faded or washed out to the observer, but a low contrast target may disappear completely.

EFFECT OF GLARE ON VISION

The loss of sensitivity for low-contrast targets in patients with media opacities may be particularly apparent in the presence of high ambient illumination (an extremely bright white background, or a separate glare source), as this will increase the amount of scattering (due to fine particles along the light path) within the eye. This is termed 'disability glare'. Another type of disability glare occurs when an extraneous light source falls onto the object of interest and reduces the contrast of the object, thereby leading to poor contrast in the image. An example of this might be light from a window falling onto a computer screen or a lamp reflecting from a glossy magazine. This is completely independent of any ocular effect, so

it is often distinguished by being referred to as 'veiling glare' (Fig. 10.8).

Scatter occurs to a small extent even in normal eyes, and instead of the retinal image being perceived against a dark background, it creates a certain background illumination, which reduces the visibility of the target. This has led to the concept of 'equivalent luminance', and the scattered light from a glare source can be matched in luminance to a real light source. This can be achieved with a technique called 'flicker photometry', which has been developed into a commercial instrument (C-Quant straylight meter, Oculus Optikgeräte, GmbH, Wetzlar, Germany) (Franssen et al., 2006). In flicker photometry, two different lights are alternated very quickly, and if the lights are of different luminance, flicker is easily perceived. As the lights are adjusted to equal luminance, the flicker ceases, and in the C-Quant, the patient can therefore match the equivalent luminance of the scattered light within their eye, to a standard source.

Of more direct interest within a low vision assessment, is the assessment of visual performance in the presence of glare (rather than the glare itself). This is particularly true because the classic optical sources of scatter within the eye (corneal and lenticular opacities) do not easily explain the disability glare in eyes with other ocular diseases. There could be scatter

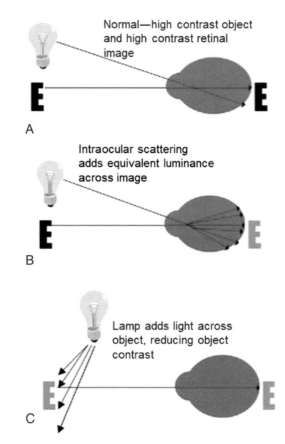

Fig. 10.8 A schematic representation of discomfort and disability glare. (A) The peripheral light source has no effect on the retinal image (visual performance), but if bright, it could create discomfort glare. (B) The scatter of light by a lens opacity creates disability glare because of the reduced retinal image contrast. (C). Inappropriate illumination on the visual target leads to a reduction in object contrast, and a form of disability glare known as veiling glare.

from the retina, especially if there was extensive scarring, or through the iris and sclera in albinism (Kruijt et al., 2011) but many cases would be difficult to explain.

Clinical testing methods have included simple but uncontrolled procedures such as placing the test chart against a window (Junker, 1976), shining a pen-torch or reading lamp towards the eyes (Maltzman et al. 1988), or comparing outdoor acuity facing towards and away from the sun (Neumann et al., 1988a). Expensive purpose-built instruments which deliver a controlled glare source are also available (Neumann et al., 1988b), and these may use focal 'point' sources of light, or (more commonly) an extended light background. For example, the Miller-Nadler test uses a back-projector to present Landolt rings of variable contrast against a bright background (LeClaire et al., 1982), whereas the Brightness Acuity Test (BAT) consists of a 60 mm hemisphere held up to the patient's eye with a 12 mm viewing aperture through which the visual target can be viewed. The white interior surface of the hemisphere is illuminated by an integral light source which can be adjusted to one of three levels: the advantage of this technique is that any type of visual test can be viewed through the aperture (Holladay et al., 1987). There are also a number of factors inherent in glare testing which can cause anomalous results: a point source could produce an after-image, or an extended source cause pupil constriction, each of which could change vision independently of the glare.

Researchers have attempted to correlate the results of these glare tests with the level of subjective complaints or the outdoor acuity, and there is some evidence that there is a higher correlation between the results of glare testing and everyday functional disabilities, than between 'standard' visual acuity (VA) tests and those same disabilities (Elliott et al., 1990). Despite the wide range of tests available, there is no standard protocol for glare measurement (Mainster & Turner, 2012).

Glare testing may be useful for deciding whether cataract extraction was indicated. Surgical intervention would be justified with severe glare disability, even if VA without glare remained good. Such tests may also be useful in evaluating the side-effects of refractive surgery (Aslam et al., 2007).

In terms of providing assistance to the low-vision patient, however, glare testing is not particularly helpful, as the fact that a patient had subjective complaints would be sufficient to warrant a search for a helpful intervention. It should be emphasized that, unfortunately, it is not possible to use 'glare testing' as a way to objectively measure the effect of different management strategies (e.g. the effect of a tinted lens) as overall luminance changes, and pupil size changes, would confound any results which might be obtained.

ADAPTATION GLARE

Adaptation glare is experienced during dark adaptation, the recovery of sensitivity for the detection of a light stimulus which occurs in an individual who has viewed a bright light, and then has been placed in the dark. This is a slow process: full adaptation takes at least 30 minutes in healthy young eyes and far longer in some retinal diseases. The exposure to the bright light has bleached a significant proportion of visual pigment in both rod and cone photoreceptors, and this must regenerate before sensitivity is restored.

Photostress Testing

This recovery of vision after viewing a bright light has been formalized into the 'photostress test', first described by Bailliart (1955) or 'macular dazzling' (Gomez-Ulla et al., 1986). Exact protocols vary, but the optimum method was investigated by Margrain and Thomson (2002). They recommended that the monocular VA is measured, and then the light from the macular stop of a direct ophthalmoscope is shone onto the patient's macula for 30 seconds. Then the time taken for the acuity to recover sufficiently to read the line above the previous threshold is determined. This Photostress Recovery Time (PSRT) is suggested as a marker for the early diagnosis of age-related macular degeneration (AMD) (Severin et al., 1967; Glaser et al., 1977). Margrain and Thomson (2002) determined age-related norms for PSRT by their method: the mean was around 50 seconds, although it is age dependent.

An individual with an extended PSRT may be aware of impaired vision even after relatively more limited changes in illumination (e.g. coming indoors after being outdoors on a bright day). They may also report that after-images from a bright flash are very long-lasting.

During the test, the visual pigments are bleached by the intense light, leading to a scotomatous after-image overlying the letters to be read. Recovery occurs by the resynthesis of visual pigment and this depends on the effective operation of the choroidal circulation, Bruch's membrane and the retinal pigment epithelium. Any disease which affects this relationship slows down recovery (such as AMD or diabetic retinopathy), but a disease which affected the optic nerve, for example, would not be expected to extend the PSRT. Some patients with AMD can have PSRTs from 1 to 8 minutes (using a technique which gives a value of 30 seconds in normal eyes) (Glaser et al., 1977): an asymmetry of measurements between the two eyes would also be highly significant. There is some argument about how well the PSRT correlates with other tests of vision which show deficits in performance in advance of VA changes, which may be explained by the relative involvement of fovea and parafovea in individual patients (Collins & Brown, 1989; Cheng & Vingrys, 1993).

In clinical practice the presence of delayed adaptation in a patient can be determined by careful questioning, without needing to conduct such a test. This has the additional benefit of determining just how disabling the patient finds the problem in 'real life'. A tinted over-spectacle may be helpful outdoors, which can be removed on coming indoors to minimise the change in illumination, and speed adaptation.

On a practical note, if there is an increase in PSRT, this suggests that ophthalmoscopy or other tests involving shining lights into the eye should not be carried out on these patients immediately prior to assessment of their vision. If a patient has reported severe discomfort with bright light during your history taking, you should modify the room lighting and the tests you are going to carry out, where possible, to take account of this.

A CLASSIFICATION OF GLARE

Table 10.1 summarises the different types of glare, and the strategies available to overcome them, (which will be discussed later in more detail). If a patient does report glare, careful questioning is required to determine which type it is, so the appropriate management can be suggested. Some appropriate open questions (without using the word 'glare', to avoid any misunderstanding) would be:

'Do you see better on a bright sunny day, or a dull, cloudy day?'

'Do you ever find lights too bright for you?' or 'Are you ever bothered by bright lights?'

'Does light ever make your eyes uncomfortable?'

POSSIBLE APPROACHES TO GLARE REDUCTION

Increasing or decreasing the illuminance of the task does not influence image contrast so long as the reflection from the task is diffuse: for example, in reading, if the text is printed on matt paper. If the paper were glossy, however, the (specular) reflected light would act as a glare source, thus reducing the contrast as the illuminance increased. In order to remove the effects of disability glare and maximise the contrast of the retinal image, it is necessary to remove any scattered light. There are several ways in which this can be achieved:

Changes in the Environment

Any measures which can move the glare source out of the patient's field-of-view will be beneficial. Difficulties may arise, for example, from a child sitting in a school classroom facing a window, a video display unit (VDU) screen being placed beneath a window, or a bright lamp being positioned on top of a television. Moving the position of the patient's seat will usually be required to avoid this type of glare. Although the need for good lighting and effective use of daylight has been emphasised, it must not be achieved by introduction of a glare source. When drawing curtains back away from the windows, one should be alert to possible difficulties that this may cause

TABLE 10.1   A Classification of Glare in Individuals With Visual Impairment, Summarising the Causes, How the Glare is Quantified or Assessed, and How Adverse Effects of Glare Can Be Ameliorated

	Mechanism	Assessment/Measurement	Strategies
Discomfort glare that causes annoyance, 'squinting', and averting gaze	Retinal signals sent to cortical areas. Illumination is too variable, or too intense, for an individual at that time	Subjective questionnaires (e.g. De Boer index); discomfort threshold with LUMIZ 100	Coloured or grey tints can decrease discomfort, but will impair visual performance in dimmer environments Consider a hat or visor and dipping the head
Disability glare that decreases acuity or contrast sensitivity	Light is scattered within the eye (most commonly due to media opacities) that decreases retinal image contrast	Clinical glare tests to measure light scatter, or to measure vision in the presence of light scatter	Block the light from glare source entering the eyes (e.g. peaked cap, visor)
	Veiling light is shining on an object which reduces the contrast of the retinal image		Reposition object and/or light source; increase object contrast whenever possible
Adaptation glare	Retina has been previously exposed to different illumination level, and adaptation to the new level is delayed	Compare vision before and after exposure to increased lighting	Coloured or grey over-spectacles to be worn during increased light exposure and removed when light exposure ceases
Scotomatic glare that causes after-images (photostress)	Brilliant focal light exposure bleaches photopigment; in the presence of retinal pathology, regeneration of photopigment is delayed	Photostress testing to measure the recovery time to regain a certain proportion of pre-exposure acuity	The situation rarely occurs in everyday life: individuals do not stare into bright lights
Photophobia (this is NOT a type of glare, but is included for comparison)	Anterior segment of the eye has active inflammatory disease, causing acute pain with pupil constriction	Thorough slit-lamp examination of anterior segment of the eye	Dilate pupil pharmacologically

Adapted from Mainster, M. A., & Turner, P. L. (2012). Glare's causes, consequences, and clinical challenges after a century of ophthalmic study. *American Journal of Ophthalmology, 153*(4), 587–593.

for some patients. In the presence of specular glare from glossy white paper, the material can be photocopied onto matt pages which will not produce directional reflections.

Visors and Shields

The aim in this case is to obstruct light from the glare source so that it cannot enter the eye, whilst not obstructing the rays of light which will be forming the required retinal image. Patients may wear a sports eye-shade, a hat with a brim or a pair of clip-on/flip-up sunglasses in the flipped-up position, and may dip their head to block stray light. Shielding at the sides may also be useful, but is more difficult to achieve unless attached permanently to the spectacle frame. Using spectacle frames designed for safety eyewear, with the side-shields tinted, may be one possible option.

Pinholes

The optometrist is familiar with the use of the pinhole in the refractive routine. If the rays of light entering the eye are not focused on the retina, a blur circle is formed, and acuity is less-than-optimal. The use of a pinhole with its limited aperture (approximately 1 mm) reduces the size of the blur circle on the retina, and thus improves acuity. When the corrective lens is optimised, it should be possible to achieve an acuity at least as good as that achieved with the pinhole. In the low-vision patient, however, the situation is rather different. In this case, single or multiple pinholes may improve the acuity by selective occlusion. Taking the case of a patient with a corneal scar, the rays of light which are transmitted by this region of the cornea will be irregularly refracted and scattered. They may therefore contribute to reduced contrast or impaired clarity of the retinal image. If a pinhole is placed in front of the eye such that this region of the optical pathway is covered or occluded, it is likely that the quality of the retinal image will improve, and vision will be increased. Unfortunately, when the pinhole is removed, vision will be impaired again, even if the refractive correction is optimal. In such circumstances, single or multiple pinholes have been proposed as LVAs for constant wear. However, there have been relatively recent studies (Kim et al., 2017) where multiple- (MPH) and single-pinhole (SPH) glasses have been trialed in healthy patients and the authors reported a reduction in contrast sensitivity, stereopsis, visual field and reading speed, as well as severe ocular discomfort particularly with MPH glasses. There are other disadvantages such as the cosmetic appearance, and the loss of field-of-view, although their use may be possible for a sedentary task such as watching TV. The cosmetic problem may be solved by providing the pinhole in contact lens form, using long-term miosis (Schachar et al., 1973), or even tattooing the corneal surface to obstruct light passage (Reed, 1994).

Artificial Iris Contact Lenses

If the iris is absent (as in aniridia, or as a result of trauma), or shields the retina inadequately because of the absence of pigment in its epithelium (e.g. due to albinism), the use of tinted or partially opaque contact lenses may be useful

(Rosenbloom, 1969; Bier, 1981; Phillips, 1989). Soft contact lenses which can be dyed or made completely opaque over the area corresponding to a natural iris (an annulus with outer diameter of about 12 mm, and inner diameter around 3.5 mm) are readily available, and have been found to allow the contrast sensitivity of the wearer to be maintained in the presence of a bright glare source shining onto the surface of the eye (Abadi & Papas, 1987). For optimal maintenance of corneal integrity, a dyed high-water content lens appears to be the best lens design in such cases.

Typoscopes

The typoscope was invented in 1897 by Charles Prentice, and is sometimes known as the 'Prentice typoscope' (Mehr, 1969). It consists very simply of a rectangle of black card with a small central slit. It is designed to be placed over a page of text such that only about two to three lines of print can be seen within the slit area (Fig. 10.9). The aim of the device is two-fold: firstly, it helps the patient to read along lines of text without straying up or down. When reaching the end of the line, the patient can first track back along the line which has just been read and can then move the typoscope down to the next line. The same purpose can be achieved by a simple (coloured) card placed under the text, or the use of the index finger to trace along the words. The second purpose is to increase contrast by preventing scattering from the background and is equivalent to the effect achieved with white-on-black print presented on an EVES. The contrast of the *object* is identical with either the white background or the black background, but scattering of the light from the white surround causes the contrast of the retinal *image* to be reduced. The presence of the black surround therefore increases retinal image contrast.

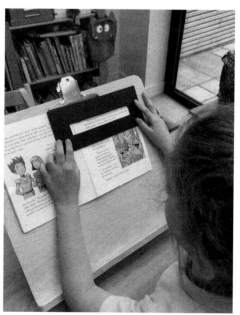

Fig. 10.9 The use of a typoscope to avoid glare from the surrounding page.

Tints

One of the most obvious measures for the patient to take when they find bright light is problematic, is to buy 'sunglasses' and/or to request that a tint be incorporated into their spectacle prescription. In the case of spectacles for constant wear, the patient may have selected, or had recommended, a pale (high transmission-low absorption) tint. Although this is sensible, such a lens with a transmission of 70% to 85% is often totally ineffective. Darker lenses, on the other hand, are useful in bright sunlight, but impair visual performance when used in poorly lit environments, or at night. Photochromic lenses, whose tint darkens in response to high ambient levels of ultraviolet (UV) radiation (present in natural daylight, but not from artificial sources) but fades once the source is withdrawn, appear to offer a solution to this problem. In fact, clinical experience suggests that they are not particularly useful: patients find the tint ineffective in full sunlight, and too slow to react as they move, for example, from a bright street to indoor conditions. By comparison, plano 'fashion' sunglasses can be surprisingly successful. They often have large lenses, and this can create a 'wrap-around' effect, with the lens periphery shielding the eyes from light from overhead and from the sides; when moving indoors, the spectacles can be quickly removed.

Tints for Discomfort Glare

Discomfort from glare can be removed by simply reducing the light level with a tint, and the colour and percentage transmission are often selected on the basis of subjective reports and cosmetic acceptability. Hoeft and Hughes (1981) reported on a study where they allowed patients with a variety of eye conditions to select their preferred lens. Particular diseases did appear to be associated with particular tint characteristics, but it is not clear how significant this is because the choice of tint colour and transmission was limited. It is clear, however, that the patient frequently selects a very dark tint: although this is quite acceptable for comfort, care must be taken not to impair visual performance by the selection of a lens with excessive absorption, especially if the lenses are to be used in a variety of different circumstances.

Selecting Tints for Disability Glare

The question of whether tinted lenses can reduce disability glare and actually improve visual performance is much more controversial. Reduction of the disability glare (and improvement of the image contrast) will require that the tint preferentially absorbs the light which is being scattered by the eye. The use of a nonselective neutral grey filter with equal absorption throughout the visible spectrum will not change the retinal image contrast, as both the light and dark areas within the image will be equally attenuated. This is illustrated quantitatively by using the previous example of high-contrast letters made less visible by glare. Introducing a neutral grey tint with 60% transmission reduced L_{max} to $(1.25 \times 0.6) = 0.75$, and L_{min} to $(0.25 \times 0.6) = 0.15$. Contrast is unchanged by this, being $(0.75 - 0.15)/(0.75 + 0.15) = 0.67$ or 67%.

Scatter occurs when very small particles (a fraction of the wavelength of light) deflect a portion of the incident light beam approximately equally in all directions. Smaller particles (a smaller fraction of the wavelength in size) would have less effect as they form less of a barrier to the wave, and so scatter is wavelength dependent. A given particle size will scatter short wavelengths more effectively than long: Rayleigh's Law states that the intensity of scattered light is inversely proportional to the fourth power of the wavelength $(1/\lambda^4)$.

Applying Rayleigh's law shows that the intensity of scatter for a blue light of wavelength 400 nm is $9.4\times$ greater than the intensity of scattered red light of 700 nm wavelength. This Rayleigh scattering is responsible for the blueish tinge seen when viewing distant mountains in clear weather: as light has travelled a long way through the air, the air molecules have caused scattering, and more blue light has been scattered, giving a hazy blue appearance which increases with viewing distance. In photographing such scenes, a yellow filter can reduce the amount of scatter and increase the contrast and clarity of the image. Whether the situation is quite this simple within the eye is debatable, because it is likely that the protein molecules within the hazy crystalline lens are not all uniformly small. It is known that when light passes along a path interrupted by larger particles, the process is no longer wavelength dependent (Mie scattering) and the scattered light has the same wavelength distribution as the incident light. In such cases, selective filtering will not improve the contrast: the filter will attenuate the image just as much as the scattered light.

From a theoretical standpoint, a tint designed to minimise light scatter would selectively attenuate short-wavelength light. It would usually absorb wavelengths below 500 nm, and would therefore be yellow, amber, brown or even red, in colour. Examples of such tints are the Corning Color Protection Filter (CPF) glass photochromic lenses (clip-on, or prescription spectacles), the Protective Lens Series (PLS) 530, 540, 550 solid-tinted plastic lens (plano or prescription spectacles) and the UV and NoIR shields which are overspectacles with additional overhead and side shielding (Figs. 10.10A and B). These shields can be worn alone, or over prescription spectacles.

Yellow and amber spectacle tints have a long history as 'contrast-enhancing' spectacles: they have often been marketed in the past as 'driving' spectacles, being designed to improve vision under conditions of poor visibility, where atmospheric cloud and rain would tend to scatter the light and reduce image contrast. Despite some early results suggesting that the visual performance of normally sighted subjects does not benefit from the use of such tints (Richards, 1964), they have continued to be popular in some quarters, with some studies measuring improved visual performance (Rieger, 1992). Even if they are not effective for people with good vision, could they improve vision for people with media changes, where the amount of scattering is likely to be considerably greater? Several groups of researchers have tested the potential of such tints to increase retinal image contrast, and hence improve vision. Unfortunately, such experiments have yielded very mixed results. Leat et al. (1990) found the result

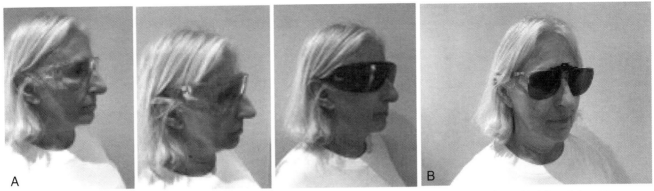

Fig. 10.10 (A) Plano ultraviolet (UV) and short-wavelength–absorbing tinted wraparound spectacles. (B) Patient with 'clip-on' tinted lenses over her spectacle frame.

predicted by the theory: namely, the Corning CPF lenses (which selectively absorb short-wavelength light) improved vision for medium-contrast grating targets in the presence of a glare source. The same improvement was not found using neutral density grey filters which absorbed light of all wavelengths equally, nor were the lenses usually beneficial to those visually impaired patients with retinal disorders. Other studies have not been so encouraging. Steen et al. (1993) could not find any difference in the amount of disability glare with either a red or a blue filter, although the red filter should have reduced the glare by absorbing the short-wavelength blue light which is preferentially scattered. Similarly, Bailey et al. (1978) found that yellow filters actually marginally reduced reading speed, an effect attributed to the reduction in task luminance when viewed through the filter. The same study showed that reading could be improved by the use of a typoscope; this did appear to enhance the contrast of the retinal image by reducing scattered light. Despite this, the suggestion that print contrast can be improved using a yellow overlay still appears: this would only be correct for purple print (such as on a mimeograph) which can be made black by this procedure.

Unfortunately, therefore, it is extremely difficult to show that tints are beneficial at all, and there has certainly been little objective data to suggest which particular tint from amongst those available may be best suited to a particular patient (with a particular pathology, or at a particular stage of the disease). Tints which do not transmit short-wavelength light have also been recommended in a wide range of other pathologies, such as albinism, retinitis pigmentosa and AMD. It is unclear why such lenses are sometimes found to improve acuity in such cases. Silver and Lyness (1985) invited patients with retinitis pigmentosa to compare 'red photochromic glass lenses' (the precise provenance is not given), with a fixed red or brown tinted CR39 lens. Individuals were divided over which correction was 'best', but the preferences were very strongly expressed: these did not correlate with any pathological or visual characteristics of the patients. The lenses are obviously beneficial to some patients, but the prospect of trying all possible tints for all patients is daunting: unfortunately, it appears that the lens ultimately found to be the best is not that selected initially: the patient needs to have a little time to try the lenses in their real environment.

Morrissette et al. (1984) conducted a survey of successful users of the CPF 550 photochromic lenses and compared the results to those of patients who had tried the lenses and rejected them. Bearing out the results of previous studies, the patients reported improved acuity, reduced time to adapt to changing lighting levels and increased comfort: all of these are subjective reports, and there is no objective measurement to support these findings.

In summary, tint prescribing at present is by 'trial-and-error' with the eventual lens choice often based on the patient's subjective judgement, rather than objective measurement of visual performance. If the patient is to try out the lenses under everyday conditions for a period, then this makes a tinted overspectacle or clip-on the most practical form in which it can be dispensed. Examples of the transmission curves are given (Fig. 10.11). The overall luminous transmission factors vary from 49% (bright orange) to 2% (very dark brown) in the models currently available in the UK, although the latter would probably only be used in achromatopsia. If the patient finds the over-spectacles useful, similar tints could be incorporated into a spectacle correction on a long-term basis, although patients may prefer overspectacles due to the glare reduction from over-the-brow and side shielding. It is sometimes possible to have tinted or opaque shields made to fit the patient's own frame by a frame-maker, or to use a frame designed as industrial safety eyewear which already has the required shielding.

Tinted Contact Lenses

An alternative management for disability and discomfort glare is tinted contact lenses. These lenses have been shown to improve cosmetic appearance and to result in a marked reduction of discomfort and disability glare and improved quality of life (QoL) (Terry, 1988; Fernandes, 2005; Rajak et al., 2006; Schornack et al., 2007; Severinsky et al., 2016). There are some advantages to the use of tinted contact lenses including: reduced vertex distance (due to reduced eye-to-telescope distance) leading to an increased field of view (Schornack et al., 2007), for some eye conditions there might be better

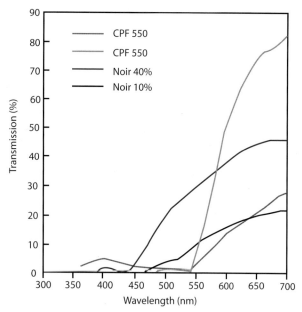

Fig. 10.11 The spectral transmission at visible wavelengths (400–700 nm) of tints which may be recommended for use with visually impaired patients. The NoIR 40% *(grey)* and 10% *(black)* are available as plano overspectacles. The Color Protection Filter *(CPF)* 550 *(amber; brown)* is a glass photocrhomatic which can be glazed to any frame in plano or prescription form.

glare reduction than with tinted spectacle lenses (Terry, 1988), cosmetic appearance might be more important if the patient is a child and they do not want to look different to their peers (Rajak et al., 2006), although improved self-image and interpersonal relationships have also been reported in adults (Severinsky et al., 2016), and in some cases the lenses provide better visual performance than glasses (Vincent, 2017). The disadvantages are related to the potential risks of contact lens wear; custom tinted contact lenses are relatively expensive and patients may avoid replacing them as regularly as necessary—longer replacement intervals are linked with increased risk of papillary conjunctivitis (Donshik & Porazinski, 1999), also oxygen transmissibility (in hydrogel lenses) decreases with the ageing of the lens and this is associated with an increased risk for microbial keratitis (Schornack et al., 2007). In addition to this, as with any tinted spectacle lenses, a darker tint (which is normally preferred by patients) will reduce vision. Another alternative is a plano-tinted contact lens to reduce glare and spectacle correction on top (Vincent, 2017).

REFERENCES

Abadi, R. V., & Papas, E. (1987). Visual performance with artificial iris contact lenses. *Journal of the British Contact Lens Association, 10*(2), 10–15.

Allan, A. C., Garcia-Hansen, V., Isoardi, G., et al. (2019). Subjective assessments of lighting quality: A measurement review. *LEUKOS: The Journal of Illuminating Engineering Society of North America, 15*(2–3), 115–126.

Aslam, T. M., Haider, D., & Murray, I. J. (2007). Principles of disability glare measurement: An ophthalmological perspective. *Acta Ophthalmologica Scandinavica, 85*(4), 354–360.

Bailliart, J. P. (1955). Examen fonctionnel de la macula [Functional examination of the macula]. *Bulletin des societies d'ophtalmologie de France, 85,* 1–81.

Bailey, I. L., Kelty, K., Pittler, G., et al. (1978). Typoscopes and yellow filters for cataract patients. *Low Vision Abstracts, 4,* 2–6.

Bier, N. (1981). *Albinism. International Contact Lens Clinic, 8,* 10–15.

Cheng, A. S., & Vingrys, A. J. (1993). Visual losses in early age-related maculopathy. *Optometry and Vision Science, 70,* 89–96.

Collins, M., & Brown, B. (1989). Glare recovery and its relation to other clinical findings in age-related maculopathy. *Clinical Vision Sciences, 4,* 155–163.

Donshik, P. C., & Porazinski, A. D. (1999). Giant papillary conjunctivitis in frequent-replacement contact lens wearers: A retrospective study. *Transactions of the American Ophthalmological Society, XCVII,* 205–220.

Elliott, D. B., Hurst, M. A., & Weatherill, J. (1990). Comparing clinical tests of visual function in cataract with the patient's perceived visual disability. *Eye, 4,* 712–717.

European Committee for Standardization. (2011). *Light and lighting—Lighting of work places. Part 1: Indoor work places* (pp. 1–57). BSI Standards Publication.

Fernandes, L. C. (2005). Absorptive and tinted contact lens for reduction of glare. *International Congress Series, 1282,* 534–538.

Franssen, L., Coppens, J. E., & Van Den Berg, T. J. T. P. (2006). Compensation comparison method for assessment of retinal straylight. *Investigative Ophthalmology and Visual Science, 47*(2), 768–776.

Glaser, J. S., Savino, P. J., Sumers, K. D., et al. (1977). The photostress recovery test in the clinical assessment of visual function. *American Journal of Ophthalmology, 83,* 255–260.

Gomez-Ulla, F., Louro, O., & Mosquera, M. (1986). Macular dazzling test on normal subjects. *British Journal of Ophthalmology, 70,* 209–213.

Hoeft, W. W., & Hughes, M. K. (1981). A comparative study of low-vision patients: Their ocular disease and preference for one specific series of light transmission filters. *American Journal of Optometry and Physiological Optics, 58,* 841–845.

Holladay, J. D., Prager, T. C., Trujillo, J., et al. (1987). Brightness acuity test and outdoor visual acuity in cataract patients. *Journal of Cataract & Refractive Surgery, 13,* 67–69.

Junker, C. (1976). Contralight testing. *Klinische Monatsblätter für Augenheilkunde, 169,* 21–23.

Jacobs, R. J. (1990). Screen colour and reading performance on closed-circuit television. *Journal of Visual Impairment & Blindness, 84,* 569–572.

Knoblauch, K., & Arditi, A. (1994). Choosing colour contrasts in low vision: Practical recommendations. In A. C. Kooijman, P. L. Looijestijn, J. A. Welling, & G. J. van der Wildt (Eds.), *Low vision: Research and new developments in rehabilitation* (pp. 199–203). IOS Press.

Kim, W. S., Park, I. K., Park, Y. K., et al. (2017). Comparison of objective and subjective changes induced by multiple-pinhole glasses and single-pinhole glasses. *Journal of Korean Medical Science, 32*(5), 850–857.

Kruijt, B., Franssen, L., Prick, L. J. J. M., et al. (2011). Ocular straylight in albinism. *Optometry and Vision Science, 88*(5), 585–592.

Lawton, T. B. (1989). Improved reading performance using individualized compensation filters for observers with losses in central vision. *Ophthalmology, 96,* 115–126.

Leat, S. J., North, R. V., & Bryson, H. (1990). Do long wavelength pass filters improve low vision performance? *Ophthalmic & Physiological Optics, 10,* 219–224.

Lebensohn, J. E. (1934). The nature of photophobia. *Archives of Ophthalmology, 12,* 380–390.

Lebensohn, J. E. (1951). Photophobia: Mechanisms and implications. *American Journal of Ophthalmology, 34,* 1294–1300.

LeClaire, J., Nadler, M. P., Weiss, S., et al. (1982). A new glare tester for clinical testing. Results comparing normal subjects and variously corrected aphakic patients. *Archives of Ophthalmology, 100,* 153–158.

Legge, G. E., & Rubin, G. S. (1986). Psychophysics of reading. IV. Wavelength effects in normal and low vision. *Journal of the Optical Society of America, A, Optics, Image & Science, 3,* 40–50.

Mainster, M. A., & Turner, P. L. (2012). Glare's causes, consequences, and clinical challenges after a century of ophthalmic study. *American Journal of Ophthalmology, 153*(4), 587–593.

Maltzman, B. A., Horan, C., & Rengel, A. (1988). Penlight test for glare disability of cataracts. *Ophthalmic Surgery, Lasers and Imaging Retina, 19,* 356–358.

Margrain, T. H., & Thomson, D. (2002). Sources of variability in the clinical photostress test. *Ophthalmic and Physiological Optics, 22*(1), 61–67.

Mehr, E. B. (1969). The typoscope by Charles F Prentice. *American Journal of Optometry and Archives of American Academy of Optometry, 46,* 885–887.

Montés-Micó, R., Cerviño, A., Martínez-Albert, N., et al. (2020). Performance of a new device for the clinical determination of light discomfort. *Expert Review of Medical Devices, 17*(11), 1221–1230.

Morrissette, D. L., Mehr, E. B., Keswick, C. W., et al. (1984). Users' and nonusers' evaluations of the CPF 550 lenses. *American Journal of Optometry and Physiological Optics, 61,* 704–710.

Neumann, A. C., McCarty, G. R., Steedle, T. O., et al. (1988a). The relationship between indoor and outdoor Snellen visual acuity in cataract patients. *Journal of Cataract & Refractive Surgery, 14,* 35–39.

Neumann, A. C., McCarty, G. R., Locke, J., et al. (1988b). Glare disability devices for cataractous eyes: A consumer's guide. *Journal of Cataract & Refractive Surgery, 14,* 212–216.

Severin, S. L., Tour, R. L., & Kershaw, R. H. (1967). Macular function and the photostress test 2. *Arch Ophthalmol, 77,* 163–167.

Peli, E., Goldstein, R. B., Young, G. M., et al. (1991). Image enhancement for the visually impaired. *Invest Ophthalmol Vis Sci, 32,* 2337–2350.

Peli, E., Fine, E. M., & Pisano, K. (1994). Video enhancement of text and movies for the visually impaired. In A. C. Kooijman, P. L. Looijestijn, J. A. Welling, & G. J. van der Wildt (Eds.), *Low vision: Research and new developments in rehabilitation* (pp. 191–198). IOS Press.

Phillips, A. (1989). A prosthetic contact lens in the treatment of ocular manifestations of albinism. *Clinical and Experimental Optometry, 72*(2), 32–34.

Rajak, S. N., Currie, A. D. M., Dubois, V. J. P., et al. (2006). Tinted contact lenses as an alternative management for photophobia in stationary cone dystrophies in children. *Journal of AAPOS, 10*(4), 336–339.

Reed, J. W. (1994). Corneal tattooing to reduce glare in cases of traumatic iris loss. *Cornea, 13,* 401–405.

Richards, O. W. (1964). Do yellow glasses impair night driving vision? *Optometric Weekly, 55*(7), 17–21.

Rieger, G. (1992). Improvement of contrast sensitivity with yellow filter glasses. *Canadian Journal of Ophthalmology, 27,* 137–138.

Rosenbloom, A. A. (1969). The controlled-pupil contact lens in low vision problems. *Journal of the American Optometric Association, 40,* 836–840.

Schachar, R. A., Pokorny, J., & Krill, A. E. (1973). Use of miotics in patients with cone degenerations. *American Journal of Ophthalmology, 76,* 816–820.

Schornack, M. M., Brown, W. L., & Siemsen, D. W. (2007). The use of tinted contact lenses in the management of achromatopsia. *Optometry, 78*(1), 17–22.

Severinsky, B., Yahalom, C., Sebok, T. F., et al. (2016). Red-tinted contact lenses may improve quality of life in retinal diseases. *Optometry and Vision Science, 93*(4), 445–450.

Sicurella, V. J. (1977). Color contrast as an aid for visually impaired persons. *Journal of Visual Impairment & Blindness, 71,* 252–257.

Silver, J. H., & Lyness, A. L. (1985). Do retinitis pigmentosa patients prefer red photochromic lenses? *Ophthalmic & Physiological Optics, 5,* 87–89.

Silver, J. H., Wolffsohn, J. S. W., & Gill, J. M. (1995). Text display preferences on self-service terminals by visually disabled people. *Optometry Today, 35*(2), 24–27.

Steen, R., Whitaker, D., Elliott, D. B., et al. (1993). Effects of filters on disability glare. *Ophthalmic & Physiological Optics, 13,* 371–376.

Terry, R. L. (1988). The use of tinted contact lenses in a case of congenital rod monochromatism. *Clinical and Experimental Optometry, 71*(6), 188–190.

Vincent, S. J. (2017). The use of contact lenses in low vision rehabilitation: Optical and therapeutic applications. *Clinical and Experimental Optometry, 100*(5), 513–521.

Waiss, B., & Cohen, J. M. (1992). The functional implications of glare and its remediation for persons with low vision. *Journal of Visual Impairment & Blindness, 86,* 28.

Wurm, L. H., Legge, G. E., Isenberg, L. M., et al. (1993). Color improves object recognition in normal and low vision. *Journal of Experimental Psychology: Human Perception and Performance, 19,* 899–911.

Illumination and Lighting

TERMINOLOGY

The amount of light emitted by a light source is called the luminous flx and is measured in **lumens**. The efficacy of a particular light source is the quantity of luminous flx which is created by a given input of electrical energy, and this is expressed in **lumens per watt**. This light now spreads out from the source, and the quantity of light hitting the working surface or task is described as the illuminance, which is defined as the amount of light per unit area. It is measured in lumens per square metre, which are also called **lux (lx)**. Consider a light source emitting a particular amount of light—luminous flx, measured in lumens—and illuminating the working area from a distance d. If the light source is moved further away from the surface, then the area it illuminates (the area over which the amount of light is spread) will increase. As the distance doubles, the area illuminated increases fourfold, and thus the illuminance decreases by a factor of 4. This represents the inverse square law: illuminance of an object is inversely proportional to the square of the distance of the light source from that object. Illuminance of the surface decreases if it is tilted, because this also increases the area to be illuminated (Fig. 11.1). If the surface is tilted by an angle α (or the light source is placed at an angle α with respect to a perpendicular to the surface) the illuminance will be proportional to the cosine of angle α: this is the cosine law.

Combining these two relationships, it is clear that

$$\text{illuminance} = \frac{\text{intensity} \times \cos \alpha}{d^2}$$

Thus, the maximum illuminance is obtained by having the most intense light source, placed as close as possible to the task and perpendicular to the surface rather than obliquely: distance is the most significant factor in determining the illuminance in a given situation. The formula given only applies to the direct illumination from a point source: indirect illumination by reflection can make a significant contribution to the illuminance created by extended sources if the distance from the working plane is greater than 5× the size of the light source.

Luminance describes the intensity of light ('brightness') emitted or reflected in a particular direction by an area which is either self-luminous or is reflecting incident light. It is measured in **candelas per square metre** (cd/m^2). Reflections of a light source from a shiny, smooth surface will all be in the same direction (specular reflection) but from a rough matt surface the reflected rays will be in all directions (diffuse reflection). Diffuse reflection is necessary as that is what allows us to see the object, but it is usually undesirable to have specular reflection from a task because this will obscure the detail near the reflection: it can be impossible, for example, to read text from glossy paper with the light in certain directions.

A 'black body' is a theoretical object which absorbs all radiation which hits its surface. It only emits light when it is heated: when heated to a specific temperature, it emits light of a particular colour, ranging from reddish white (corresponding to a low colour temperature) to blueish white (a high colour temperature). The colour temperatures typically seen in white lights range from around 2800 (red/orange—a 'warm' colour) to 6500 K (blue—a 'cool' colour).

TYPES OF DOMESTIC LIGHTING

Until recently, incandescent filament lamps with their characteristic pear-shaped envelopes of soda–silica–lime glass were the most common form of household lighting. Due to their high energy use, these bulbs are no longer sold in Europe. In these bulbs, a tungsten filament is heated and an inert gas fills the envelope to help slow the evaporation of tungsten from the filament. This increases bulb life and prevents

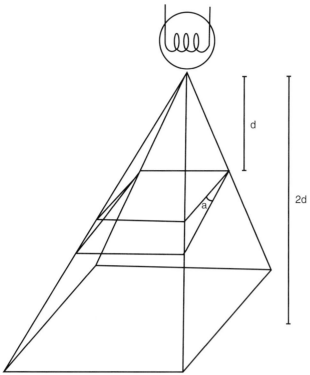

Fig. 11.1 The illumination by a light source onto a working surface. As the distance of the working surface from the light doubles from *d* to 2*d*, the area illuminated increases by a factor of four. The area illuminated also increases (and so illuminance decreases) when it is tilted by an angle *α*.

blackening of the inside of the glass (which would reduce light output). Clear glass envelopes can give harsh shadows and act as a glare source, so it is more usual to have a frosted 'pearl' finish to the glass to diffuse the light without significant loss of brightness. The efficacy of incandescent lamps is approximately 10 lm/W, being higher for higher wattage lamps. This is a very poor rating, with a lot of energy being wasted as heat, but the lamps are very cheap, small and compact, relatively long-lasting and require only simple electronic circuitry. Light output is biased towards longer wavelengths, and this gives a 'warm' light which is favoured for household use.

If a halogen gas is introduced into the bulb to create a tungsten halogen lamp, the filament can be operated at higher temperature to give greater efficacy (up to 25 lm/W). This causes more evaporation of tungsten from the filament, but this combines with the halogen and is redeposited on the filament, rather than on the inside of the glass, leading to increased bulb life. If of high wattage, the envelope is made of fused silica or quartz and can deteriorate if touched with the fingers when oil or moisture can be transferred. Low wattage versions use aluminophosphate glass, but problems of uneven heating and subsequent failure can still occur if the glass envelope is touched.

Tubular fluorescent lamps could also be described as low pressure mercury discharge lamps. An electrical discharge passed through the mercury gas causes its atoms to lose electrons (become ionised) which collide with other atoms. These collisions cause further ionisation, or the absorption of energy with the result that some electrons are raised to a higher energy state. As these fall back, the energy is emitted in the form of

visible and ultraviolet (UV) radiation. The latter is absorbed by the phosphor coating on the inside of the envelope and re-emitted in the form of visible radiation. The radiation emitted from the mercury is at certain discrete wavelengths, but the spectral composition can be broadened by careful choice of these phosphors. Because the output of short-wavelength light is increased over that produced by incandescent lamps, some people consider fluorescent lighting to be too 'cold' for household use. These lamps have an efficacy of at least 40 to 60 lm/W, thus using about one-quarter the power to achieve the same luminous flx compared to incandescent lamps. They also require much less frequent replacement. Some control circuitry is required to limit the electrical current through the lamp, and this can add to the physical size and weight of the installation. Compact fluorescent lamps are available where the long discharge tube is folded or bent into a circular or spiral configuration. The circular tube can be arranged around the large diameter lens in a variable-focus stand magnifier. Limiting the size using the spiral configuration allows it to be used as an energy-saving replacement for an incandescent filament lamp, but this is often not successful because the shade has been designed for an incandescent envelope which gives its maximum intensity straight down, whereas the fluorescent tube emits maximum intensity sideways. It takes up to 3 minutes for the older compact fluorescent lamps to reach maximum brightness from a starting brightness at switch-on of 50% of the maximum: if used for ambient lighting, especially on staircases or corridors where the occupant is passing through, this could create a hazard. The compact fluorescent is extremely successful, however, in purpose-made localised task lighting. The high efficacy means that there is little energy lost as heat, so that the lamp housing does not get as hot as would that surrounding an incandescent bulb. This means that the patient can place their head very close to the lamp without discomfort and can grasp the housing to adjust it without risking burning their hand. However, compact lamps without the covering envelope should not be used closer than 30 cm for more than 1 hour per day, due to a UV hazard.

Light-emitting diode (LED) lamps are becoming consistently more available and for all types of light fittings, rather than those specifically designed for them. They are extremely low power (2 W) so represent an exceptionally efficient lighting system (more so even than fluorescent lamps). The lifetime of these lamps can be up to several years, which is important for a user with visual impairment, due to the practical difficulty for them of changing a failed unit (and the potential safety issue of reaching a wall or ceiling luminaire). LED sources are often in a sealed light fitting, so when the lamp fails, the whole fitting needs to be replaced rather than just changing the LED. These lamps do not get very hot so there is less danger of the patient burning their hands, or there being a fire hazard. The LED lamps can be made to emit various 'white lights' and is now common to also see these used in illuminated hand-held and stand magnifiers. It is possible to have white LED light created by using combinations of red, green and blue LEDs. LEDs offer white light with a variety of colour temperatures by mixing the amount of red, green and blue LEDs that are being used to create each of these different light sources. Schweizer magnifiers, for example, are available with three alternative colour temperatures: 2700 K which is the incandescent equivalent, 4500 K is the fluorescent equivalent and 6000 K which is a bluish light (i.e. overcast sky in the northern hemisphere).

Some LEDs have the facility to tune the colour temperature to individual preference across the range from 2700 to 6500 K. On a table lamp, this may be a manual control, but 'smartbulbs' which can have colour temperature and brightness controlled by a smartphone app, or voice controlled via a digital assistant, are also available. The low power of LEDs means batteries last a long time in these types of magnifiers. Unlike incandescent lamps, where the light gets dimmer as the batteries lose their power, LEDs maintain their brightness over time until the batteries have not got enough power to work them and then the light stops working altogether.

Even table-top LED lamps can be battery operated or connected to a USB socket which means the patient can move them to wherever they are required (or even take them on holiday). LEDs are also available on adhesive strips, which are a cheaper alternative to having lighting installed under kitchen wall cupboards to illuminate the worktop, or inside wardrobes to help in selecting clothes. A miniature LED lamp is also available which can be attached to the side of a spectacle frame to illuminate the reading task (Fig. 7.28).

The design of the luminaire—the housing for the lamp—can be just as important as the light source itself: it controls the amount and direction of the light output as well as offering a simple physical support, the electricity supply and a means of heat dissipation for the lamp. The bare lamp envelope does not necessarily emit light in the required direction, and may also create a glare source if viewed directly, so the lamp housing can be used to control the light. This can be done by obstruction, diffusion, refraction, reflection, or any combination of these. Obstruction is used when the lamp is surrounded by an opaque material which prevents light being emitted in that direction. Light is then only emitted through a limited aperture in the shade—usually at the bottom, and sometimes at the top of a ceiling-mounted lamp in order to create diffuse reflection from the ceiling. Diffusion occurs when a translucent cover is placed over the light, increasing the spread of the light but also usually absorbing a considerable proportion of it. The lamp covering can be made in the form of multiple prismatic elements to refract the light and redirect it into the required position. Reflection of light from the inside of the luminaire is also an extremely efficient way of deflecting all the light into the required direction. At its most extreme, the reflecting surface is specially shaped and highly polished to maximise the effect (such as in car headlamps), but it is frequently used less dramatically by the inside surface of a lampshade having a matt white finish. Dirt and deterioration of the luminaire surfaces can cause light loss over time.

The illuminance on surfaces within a room also depends on the décor. If walls and ceiling are pale, they have high reflectance, then a specific light source creates a greater task illuminance than if the surroundings were dark. If light from a luminaire is directed towards the ceiling, then the ceiling must be light in order to reflect that light into the room.

VISUAL PERFORMANCE AND LIGHTING

Based on the investigations by Boyce (1973), Fig. 11.2 shows schematically how an observer's ability to perform a visual task increases with improvements in the task illuminance: this effect is more dramatic for old compared to young subjects. This general pattern of response can be found with a wide variety of tasks (ranging from laboratory-based studies of searching for a Landolt C of particular orientation among an array of letters of other orientations, to a 'real-life' task of scanning components on a conveyor belt looking for those which are incorrectly manufactured), and with a variety of measures of performance (such as the numbers of errors made, or the time taken to perform a search). If the visual task is very easy—using large objects of high contrast—there will be very little difference between the performance of the different age groups, and the response will appear as in point (c) in Fig. 11.2 even at relatively low luminance. If the detail within the task is small, and contrast is low, the characteristic response is that at point (a) of Fig. 11.2, and the illuminance must be increased to produce an improvement.

Increasing the task illuminance cannot compensate completely for the small size and low contrast of difficult visual tasks, however, and Fig. 11.3 shows that changing the size of the task detail is more effective (Weston, 1945). Thus, the larger size letters always support a better performance, even when illumination is optimised, and the performance with low-contrast targets cannot be improved to match that produced by high contrast letters (although for medium-contrast levels, it can be brought close to it). It is also clear that whilst large increases in performance can be created by improving the contrast, these are not so great as the effects achieved with increases in the letter size (compare the improvement in changing the 1.5 min arc target from a contrast of 0.56 to 0.97, and note that it is less than the improvement of increasing the size to 3 min arc, whilst maintaining 0.56 contrast). Extrapolating these findings to low vision, it can be seen that increasing the illumination is not a replacement for magnification of the image, but only a supplement to it: no matter

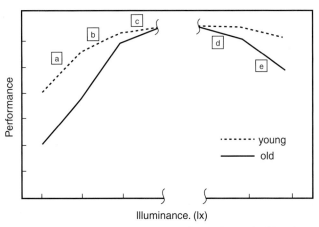

Fig. 11.2 A schematic representation of the change in 'visual performance' as a result of increasing illumination, with more marked effects apparent in older subjects. As illumination increases, performance increases to a peak, but if illumination becomes excessive, glare can cause a decrease in performance.

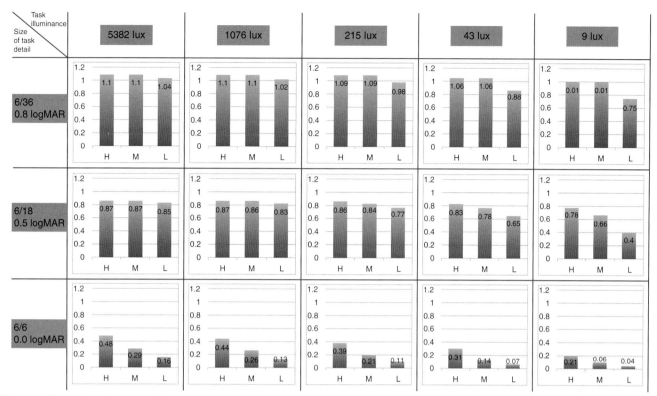

Fig. 11.3 The task performance (% of targets (Landolt C of a specific orientation) correctly detected x detection speed) of individuals with good vision, at a range of illuminances. The targets are presented in a range of sizes and a range of contrasts (H - high contrast 92%; M- medium contrast 68%; L - low contrast 37%). Based on data from Weston HC (1945) The relation between illumination and visual efficiency - the effect of brightness contrast. Medical Research Council Industrial Heath Research Board Report No 87. HMSO, London.

how much the illumination is increased, it does not bring the performance of a visually demanding task (small detail, low contrast) up to the level of a visually easy task. An increase in illuminance will produce a greater improvement in performance on a near-threshold task than on a visually easy task, and the low-vision patient is much more likely to be working near to their visual threshold. Magnifiers can offer a much greater range of improvement in performance compared to lighting alone, but performance will still be limited for large letters if the illumination is suboptimal: no magnifier will produce optimum performance without sufficient light.

Older people are likely to gain more benefit from improved task illumination than the younger age group. The performance of these two groups can be equated if the illuminance is high enough, and it is suggested that the decrease in the amount of light reaching the retina is the cause of the poorer performance in the elderly subjects. There is increased absorption and scattering of light by the ocular media with advancing age, in addition to senile miosis (Werner et al., 1990). Weale (1961) reported a threefold decrease in the amount of light reaching the retina of a 60-year-old compared to that of a 20-year-old: Werner et al. (1990) describe even more dramatically the 22-fold decrease in transmission of light of wavelength 400 nm by the ocular media between the ages of 1 month and 70 years.

Thus, people performing difficult visual tasks (and a given task will always be more difficult for the low vision patient as it will be nearer to the limit of their ability) require the highest level of illumination. A further consideration of

Fig. 11.2 suggests, however, that there are limits to how high this illuminance can be raised. In point (d), the performance has reached an optimum plateau for both age groups, but it may well decrease due to glare if excessive illumination is used. There is also an increase in the amount of light scatter by the 'normal' crystalline lens after the age of 40 years which will contribute to a loss of contrast of the retinal image, even if the object itself is of high contrast. Thus, the decreasing performance with excessive illuminance is represented by point (e), showing that the effect is likely to be more marked in the older subjects. For some low-vision patients, the plateau (c) may not be reached: performance may be affected by glare even at modest levels of illumination.

The effect of slowed adaptation in older eyes is also dramatic: an object has to be 10× brighter to be seen by an 85-year-old compared to a 20-year-old after an equivalent period of dark adaptation (IES, 2020). Light adaptation (going from the dimmer indoor environment to bright outdoor space) is also slowed. So uniformity of illumination, and gradual transitions in illuminance level, are very important to individuals with visual impairment.

NONVISUAL EFFECTS OF LIGHT

As well as the rod and cone photoreceptors, the retina contains intrinsically photosensitive retinal ganglion cells (ipRGC) which contain a photopigment called melanopsin. This has a peak absorption around 470 nm, and the ipRGC are part of the signalling pathway which sets the body clock to its 24-hour cycle (circadian rhythm). The exposure to 'daylight'—intense blue light especially in the morning—increases the production of melatonin towards the evening time, and this causes sleepiness. Some visually impaired individuals with retinal disease may have an abnormality in the circadian system because their ipRGC are also affected, and they experience sleep disturbance, which can have further consequences for physical and mental health. However, some individuals with total vision loss can have a normal sleep-wake cycle because their circadian receptors are preserved (Allen, 2019). To try to reduce sleep disturbance, individuals should have exposure to high light levels (and preferably natural daylight) during the early part of the day. If they need a light to be on continuously at night (in case they need to get out of bed), this should be a red/amber light to avoid stimulating the ipRGC. Melatonin tablets are sometimes prescribed to be taken at night, to regulate the sleep-wake cycle.

LIGHTING LEVELS FOR OLDER AND VISUALLY IMPAIRED PEOPLE

Experimental data obtained by several researchers in a variety of 'performance versus illuminance' studies allowed a determination of the level of lighting required to optimally detect a target of a particular size and contrast. When these studies are applied to subjects with 'normal' vision, the absolute level of illuminance which will allow a task of 'normal' size and contrast to be performed efficiently and safely can

be determined, and these results have influenced the lighting codes developed in various countries. These standards usually relate to the working environment, with regulations for domestic lighting being based on energy efficiency. The Illuminating Engineering Society Aged and Partially Sighted Committee have, however, published detailed recommendations on lighting design for these populations, and selected illuminance values are shown in Table 11.1. Separate values are given for the overall ambient space (A) and the specific task (T). It should be emphasized that these are minimum levels, and may need to be increased in specific cases, especially if visual impairment is more severe.

In contrast to the recommended illuminance levels, it can be seen that surveys which have measured the illuminance in typical unselected households have shown that whether relying on natural light ('Day') or electric light ('Night'), levels are often inadequate, particularly for detailed close-work tasks. The results of these surveys are shown on the right-hand side of Table 11.1. The problem is not just confined to private households, since Lehon (1980) reviews several surveys suggesting that classroom lighting in schools for the visually impaired is usually also below the standard recommended. Levitt (1980) also showed that those surveyed were totally unaware of the inadequacy and felt that the lighting was good. Similarly, almost 80% of the participants surveyed by Eilertsen et al. (2016) reported their home lighting as good, despite the low illuminance levels measured (given in Table 11.1). This is not surprising, as the visual system is

---

TABLE 11.1 **The Left-Hand Side of the Table Shows the Recommended Minimum Illuminance Levels (in lx) From the Illuminating Engineering Society (IES) for Spaces Occupied by Older and Visually Impaired Individuals**

Type of Task	IES Recommendations	SURVEYS Home for Visually Impaired[a]	TYPICAL HOUSEHOLD Day	Night
Living room	A 200	Lounge 500	150[b]	60[b]
	T 750	Dining Table 750	35[c]	
Sewing	T 750	1000	177[d]	100 (range 30–240)[e]
Sustained reading	T 750		225[c]	70[f]
Kitchen work areas	A 300		150[b]	100[b]
	T 500		120[c]	70–80[f]
				90 (range 35–180)[e]
Hall and stairs	A 300 (at ground level)	200	55[b]	40[b]
			30[c]	20–30[f]
				20 (range 5–180)[e]
Bathrooms	A 300		80[b]	100[b]
	T 500		125[c]	
Bedrooms	A 200	300	100[b]	70[b]
	T 750		35[c]	90 (range 5–350)[e]

[a]Boyce (1986a).
[b]Lovie-Kitchin et al. (1983).
[c]Eilertsen et al. (2016).
[d]Silver et al. (1978).
[e]Levitt (1980).
[f]Simpson and Tarrant (1983).
Values are given for the overall ambient space (A—measured at 0.76 m above floor level, unless otherwise stated) and the specific task (T—measured at the task surface). The right-hand side shows the actual mean illuminance recorded in residential locations (in studies by Lovie-Kitchin et al. (1983), Silver et al. (1978) and Simpson and Tarrant (1983), the values are medians, rather than mean).

concerned with the detection of contrast, rather than absolute lighting levels: humans usually do not notice the 10,000-fold decrease in illumination coming from a sunlit city street to a building interior.

It is possible that the advent of LED lighting might have improved these values.

USING LIGHTING FOR VISION ENHANCEMENT

For the optometrist, it is important to recognize that the recommendations in Table 11.1 will apply to many older patients seen in routine clinical practice, who are not identified as visually impaired. Many of those individuals would benefit from improved task lighting for critical visual tasks and improved ambient lighting to reduce the risk of falls. Falkenberg et al. (2019) raised the illuminance level in the living room of a group of healthy 77-year-olds from its habitual mean of 35 lx, to 200 lx, and showed a significant increase in the ability to perform tasks, and in health-related quality of life, in comparison to a control group. This patient group may be the one to benefit most from improved lighting in terms of ability to perform tasks. In a visually impaired group, Brunnström et al. (2004) found improved quality of life from improved lighting in the living room, but less effect on task performance. It may be that this group require additional interventions (e.g. magnification and task modification) in combination with lighting to get a significant effect.

Evans et al. (2010) studied the influence of lighting on performance of activities of daily living in older people with low vision. They selected four different real-life tasks—walking along a corridor with uneven floor, inserting a plug in a socket, sorting pills and reading—and the tasks were performed under three light levels—50 lx (dim), 200 lx (medium), and 800 lx (bright). The patients had cataracts, age-related macular degeneration (AMD) or cataracts and AMD and their best corrected visual acuity (VA) ranged from 6/9 to 6/24. The general trend showed that higher light levels were associated with better performance. Most participants, and nearly all participants with AMD, showed a large (>20%) effect of lighting in at least one task. However, there were some participants in every task who performed best in the dimmest lighting condition. The results indicate the large interindividual variation in the effect of lighting in visual performance. The authors suggest that it is important to test the effect of lighting individually rather than making any assumptions concerning lighting conditions and patient's visual status or disease condition.

Cornelissen et al. (1995) found that the ability of visually impaired patients to detect and recognise everyday objects in a realistic environment was also very dependent on the illuminance. For tasks such as recognising faces, chairs and cups, illuminances over 1000 lx were often required to reach optimal performance (although normally sighted subjects had performed the same task at 1 lx). Boyce (1986a) carried out measurements in a residential home (see Table 11.1) where the lighting was designed with the expectation that the majority of the residents would be visually impaired, and which he concluded was a model of good practice. Despite the fact that the illuminances are higher than those recommended, residents did not find them excessively bright, although (surprisingly) some residents felt that the corridor lighting was too bright. This may simply have reflected the perception that lower illuminance would still have been adequate for navigation, or may have arisen from the uneven nature of the lighting (it varied between 50 and 350 lx at different points within the area when not supplemented by daylight). The corridor lighting will need to be brighter than the minimum required if high illuminance is used in the rooms it serves, in order to avoid problems in adaptation (Boyce, 1986b). Bedhead lights were available for residents which provided up to 4000 lx (presumably for reading in bed), however, and some residents found this too bright. Boyce (1986b) also surveyed a school for the visually impaired and found the daytime illuminance on the classroom desks of approximately 1500 lx (compared to the 300 lx recommended for mainstream schools) to be excessive for some pupils but inadequate for others. The conclusion seems to be that illuminances up to 1000 lx will be generally useful and acceptable, but higher illuminances may be too bright for some visually impaired patients, and when this illuminance is provided it should be by the use of localised, variable and moveable task lighting.

Most studies on low-vision have tested patients with a range of pathologies and found equivalent improvement in acuity with luminance in each case (Lie, 1977; Richterman & Aarons, 1983). However, Sloan et al. (1971) identified a subgroup consisting of some patients with macular disease who benefit disproportionately from greatly increased levels of illumination. This finding was confirmed by Brown and Lovie-Kitchin (1983). Bowers et al. (2001) suggested that the majority of patients with AMD require task illumination of at least 2000 lx to optimize reading performance (the median illuminance for optimum performance was 3500 lx, with two observers requiring 7700 and 9900 lx, respectively.) Eldred (1992) suggests preferred illumination up to 7500 lx (the highest tested in the study) to optimise reading speed in most people with AMD. It may be that such responses to high illumination are not unique to macular disease: LaGrow (1986) investigated the optimal level in patients with various conditions, and found preferred levels ranged from approximately 700 to 15,000 lx, although the median value was about 2000 lx.

Despite the universal agreement that illuminance of task lighting is critical for optimum reading, studies by Haymes and Lee (2006) and Eperjesi et al. (2007) suggested that the colour temperature was not significant. In these studies they used a range of incandescent and fluorescent lamp types, although LEDs were not available, limiting the range of colour temperatures tested. Wolffsohn et al. (2012) were able to overcome this limitation when they studied the effect of illumination colour temperature from LEDs on magnifier reading performance. The study included more than 100 people with a wide range of age (37–96 years), disease type (including AMD, diabetic retinopathy, retinal detachment and other ocular conditions) and VA (from 0.2 to 1.9 logMAR). The magnifiers used were Schweizer (stand-magnifiers) and ranged from +8.00D to +56.00D with colour temperatures of 2700, 4500 and 6000 K. Participants were asked to rank each of the three colour temperature illuminations (best, in between or worst performance) on ease of reading, comfort and overall preference. Reading speed and VA were measured. Performance was no different across all these colour temperatures with each of the different colour temperatures being preferred by about one-third of the group. Patients read smaller print and were faster with their preferred illumination. Although the improvement was statistically significant, patients' VA and reading speed improved only by 0.05 logMAR and 10 wpm, respectively. Colour temperature preference could not be predicted from participant age, cause or severity of visual impairment, which means that it is necessary to demonstrate each colour temperature to every individual patient.

A commercially available instrument LxIQ has been developed which is placed over the text and has controls to vary intensity from 0 to 5000 lx, and colour temperature from 2700 to 6500 K, to allow the optimum light to be identified for that patient whilst reading. This has not been found to be repeatable enough to inform management recommendations (Wittich et al., 2018).

In some rare conditions, such as achromatopsia, acuity is best under low illuminance conditions, perhaps between 5 and 50 lx. In the case of achromatopsia, this is due to the fact that they have only rod photoreceptors in the retina, and these are 'overloaded' by higher levels of illumination. Such patients often appreciate lenses with a transmission around 2% for general wear (see Chapter 10): these are most effective if the transmission is selectively at longer wavelengths to which the rods are relatively insensitive. The absence of cone photoreceptors means that these patients have no colour vision. VA is typically about 1.0 logMAR and nystagmus is common. Achromatopsia is one of the first eye diseases to be treated by gene therapy.

There are many more diseases in which the patient is sensitive to light, and may wear tinted lenses outdoors. Albinism and aniridia are classic examples of such conditions, in which excess light is incident on the retina. Albinism is a group of conditions which are characterised by varying degrees of hypo-pigmentation of the eyes (ocular albinism), or the eyes, skin and hair (oculocutaneous albinism). In the eye, pigment is absent or reduced in the retinal pigment epithelium and the uveal tract, and so light enters the eye through the iris (and sclera) as well as via the pupil. People with aniridia have no iris, again lacking the normal restriction on light entry to the eye. Despite this, for detailed visual tasks, both these groups of patients usually require normal or even increased levels of illumination. They will often appreciate the provision of localised task lighting, although great care must be taken to avoid glare. Likewise, people with cataract may experience more scatter of light as the illuminance increases: nonetheless, they still perform better with higher light levels, so long as measures to avoid glare are adopted (e.g. use of a typoscope).

PRACTICAL ADVICE TO OPTIMISE LIGHTING FOR LOW-VISION PATIENTS

Three aspects of optimising illumination can be considered:
1. Increasing the general ambient level of illuminance
2. Providing adequate enhanced illumination for detailed tasks in a discrete localised area (task lighting)
3. Supplying additional light outdoors, for mobility

Ambient Illumination

Cullinan (1980) found that the median level of ambient lighting in the homes he tested was only 10% of that in the hospital clinic in which the inhabitants were examined, and this will obviously worsen their performance considerably compared to that measured in the hospital clinic. As noted previously, patients are unaware of how poor the lighting is in their home, so do not feel the need to change it. Many patients will have multiple lights available in each room, but may not be switching them on. A great deal can therefore be achieved with relatively simple measures. The following steps could be taken to improve illumination (Anon, 1982):

1. Optimum use can be made of daylight by drawing curtains well back (being careful not to create glare), cleaning windows regularly and avoiding the use of net curtains. Chairs should be positioned sideways on to the window so that light comes onto the task, but not directly into the eyes.
2. Where possible, fluorescent or LED fittings should be fitted. Luminaires with a white reflective interior should be selected. If a pendant fitting is used, this should be open at the top to allow light to be reflected from the ceiling. Lights mounted against a dark background are usually undesirable as the patient would see a marked contrast between the bright light and its surround, and there will also be less diffuse reflection of the light back into the room.
3. From a lamp in the centre of the ceiling, only half the light emitted comes onto the surface directly, with the remainder being reflected by the walls, ceiling and floor. For example, a lamp in a light-coloured room 3 m² and 2.5 m high gives an illuminance of about 70 lx on a table surface immediately below. If the floor covering is dark, this illuminance reduces to 60 lx, if the walls are dark too it decreases to 45 lx, and darkening the ceiling finish as well gives an illuminance of only 34 lx (Jay, 1980). The reflectance of decor finishes can range from 75% to less than 5% depending on the colour, so the importance of choosing pale matt finishes to give diffuse reflection cannot be overemphasised. However, it is important not to make the area featureless, as orientation can only be achieved when corners, intersections and horizons can be detected. Judicious use of dark outlines and borders can create such boundaries, without significantly reducing the total reflected light.
4. Near-uniform light levels should be achieved throughout the area, making sure that corridors and stairs have no less than one-third to one-quarter of the illuminance of the rooms opening onto them: adapting to changing light levels is likely to be slowed in a significant percentage of visually impaired patients. Stairs in particular should be evenly

lit to avoid confusing shadows: entrances and porches, especially with steps, must be adequately lit. This will also allow visitors to be seen from inside the house and aid the householder in finding the keyhole.

Localised Task Lighting

To find out how the individual responds to different levels of task illuminance will require a test to be made in the consulting room. This should begin using dim room lighting (~5–20 lx) then normal room illumination augmented by a task lamp positioned about 1 m from the patient (~100–300 lx) and then the reading lamp should be brought to 20 cm or less to produce high illumination (~2000–5000 lx) (Lovie-Kitchin et al., 1983). Bowers et al. (2001) suggest that a suitable illuminance level for the reading task can be determined subjectively. Whilst the patient is viewing continuous text (and it may be appropriate to choose real-life reading materials rather than high-quality reading charts), they are asked to set a minimum (below which the lighting is too dim) and maximum (above which the lighting is uncomfortable). Then the patient is asked to judge the optimum level within that range, based on 'visual comfort an ease of reading'. If a light meter is not available to measure these illuminances, then an approximate guide to the level of illumination which can be obtained is given in Table 11.2: figures will vary with luminaire designs, and the age of the lamps.

As pointed out earlier, patients are often totally unaware of the inadequacies of the home lighting. Careful questioning may reveal deficiencies, however, such as if the patient reports only being able to read during the day. The effect of the use of localised task lighting should be demonstrated and is normally quite convincing in the consulting room, because the patient will usually acknowledge that the ambient level of illumination is high (and higher than that to which they are accustomed at home) and yet accept that the extra lighting is still beneficial. It can be more difficult, however, to convince a patient that a standard lamp with a heavy dark shade which is positioned several feet behind them will not provide the extra localised lighting which they require.

The following measures will produce optimum localised task lighting:

1. Localised lighting is not just used when reading, but might be necessary in a wardrobe or cupboard, under wall-mounted kitchen cupboards to illuminate work-surfaces, over the dining table, or over a tool shed work-bench. It may be needed during the day to supplement natural daylight.

2. The traditional position for a 'reading lamp' is behind the patient so that light comes over the shoulder onto the task (Fig. 11.4A). This can be very effective for 'normal' reading distances but is difficult to combine with the use of a magnifier and/or a very short working distance, when it is almost inevitable that the patient's body will shadow the task, and the light will create annoying reflections from the magnifier surface (Fig. 11.4B). A better arrangement here is to place the light in front of the face, with the shade arranged so that there is no light shining directly into the eyes (Collins, 1987) (Fig. 11.4C). This inevitably places the lamp housing very close to the face, which can be uncomfortably warm unless a fluorescent or LED lamp is used. Although wishing to avoid direct light, the use of a completely opaque shade can be undesirable: the patient is likely to view it simultaneously with the bright reflective interior of the shade, and this can form too much of a contrast, creating discomfort glare.

3. If the lamp is to be adjusted to different angles, it must have a flexible or jointed arm with sufficient reach and have a heavy base so that it will be stable, even when the arm is fully extended. If this creates problems with portability, a clamp fitting to attach it to the edge of a shelf or table may be considered.

4. A miniature torch or 'penlight', the torch on a mobile phone, or even a head-mounted torch can be carried in the pocket or handbag for seeing detail when the ambient lighting is poor.

Lighting for Outdoor Mobility

Difficulty with vision at night is a common complaint from people with conditions which affect the rod photoreceptors, such as retinitis pigmentosa and other inherited retinal diseases. It is likely, however, to be a problem identified by any patient with severe visual field restriction, regardless of the cause: as the peripheral retina contains a preponderance of rod receptors, they will be preferentially lost as the visual field reduces. There are a number of 'mobility lights' which are commercially available: the Wide-Angle Mobility Light (WAML) which is designed specifically for the visually impaired user is a headlamp attached to a waist-belt, but other aids may be equally effective and more widely available (Morrissette et al., 1985; Wacker et al., 1990). Requirements

TABLE 11.2	The Approximate Illuminance (in lx) Provided on the Task Area at the Specified Distance From Typical Fluorescent, LED and Tungsten Halogen Lamps									
Distance of Light From Task (cm)	15	20	30	40	50	60	70	80	90	100
Illuminance of task (lx)										
11 W compact fluorescent/ LED	8000	4500	2000	1125	720	500	370	280	220	180
20 W tungsten halogen	35,500	20,000	8890	5000	3200	2220	1630	1250	990	800

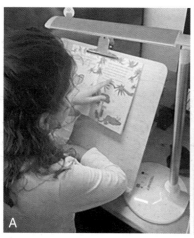
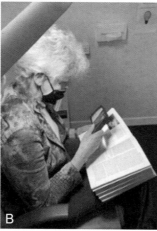
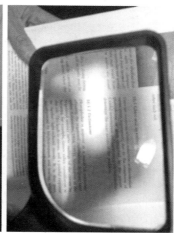
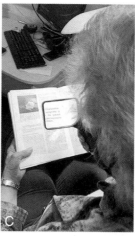

Fig. 11.4 (A) The optimum position for a shadow-free illumination of a near task with a compact light-emitting diode (LED) light. Room lights have been turned off to show this more clearly, but in everyday use would be left on, as discomfort glare may result from wide variations in illumination within the visual field. (B) Reading lamp positioned over the patient's shoulder. Here the patient is trying to use a magnifier but this is creating shadows on the task and the light creates awkward reflections on the magnifier lens' surface. (C) The optimum position for a shadow-free illumination of a near task. The lamp here is positioned in front of the face so that the patient's body or position does not interfere with the lighting and shadows are avoided on the task.

are for a beam with wide even illumination: a wide range of LED headtorches are available which are sold for running and cycling which would be effective. These lamps, which leave the hands free, can also be very useful for a patient when carrying out household tasks, or repairs.

Night-Vision Devices

Light or image intensification using a luminance-enhancing 'night-vision scope' has also been suggested as an aid for patients with difficulties navigating in the dark. Small amounts of light are intensified up to 750× and thus provide a sufficiently bright image to stimulate the cones (Berson et al., 1973). Because of the weight of early devices, these were used handheld in the same way as monocular magnifying telescopes: they are therefore only intermittent spotting aids and would need to be backed up by, for example, a long cane or other such aid.

Technological advances have led to the development of night vision goggles (NVGs), which are widely used by military and security personnel, and for hunting. The only device that is currently commercially available specifically for individuals with vision impairment, is the NiVis-2. This is spectacle-mounted with a camera on the frame, transmitting a monochromatic image to the miniature displays mounted in front of each eye. Infra-red light sources are also incorporated into the frame, and there is a connection to the power supply. It is not possible to wear it comfortably over spectacles, but prescription lenses can be incorporated.

Using night-vision devices has also been proposed (Friedburg et al., 1999; Rohrschneider et al., 2000) to improve nighttime mobility in dark outdoor conditions. NVGs have been shown (Hartong et al., 2004) to only be effective in reducing collisions and increasing walking speed under these conditions. With night-time street-lighting levels (e.g. in shopping streets) between 10^{-1} and 10 lx, this was found to be adequate for mobility without the NVG. Indoor corridors which were very dark were difficult to navigate because of the small field

of view of the device (less noticeable when viewing more distant scenes outdoors), and the lack of depth perception (the same camera is used to provide an image to each eye, making viewing effectively monocular). Although the users were accustomed to a restricted field of view because of their ocular pathology, they were accustomed to making eye movements to compensate. With the NVGs, this was not possible, and head movements were required instead. A further problem with NVGs is the unexpected appearance of a light in the environment, which can be uncomfortably bright when viewed through the device. The pilot study performed by Zebehazy et al. (2005) found that the MultiVision night vision device helped increase the distance at which two adults with retinitis pigmentosa could recognize objects in dark outdoor conditions. New head-mounted electronic vision enhancement system (EVES) have bright screens and can also improve visibility in dark conditions.

REFERENCES

Allen, A.E. (2019). Circadian rhythms in the blind. *Current Opinion in Behavioral Sciences*, 30, 73–79.

Anon (1982). *Lighting for low vision*. The Electricity Council.

Berson, E. L., Mehaffey, L., 3rd, & Rabin, A. R. (1973). A night vision device as an aid for retinitis pigmentosa patients. *Archives of Ophthalmology*, 90, 122–126.

Bowers, A. R., Meek, C., & Stewart, N. (2001). Illumination and reading performance in age-related macular degeneration. *Clinical and Experimental Optometry*, 84(3), 139–147.

Boyce, P. R. (1973). Age, illuminance, visual performance and preference. *Lighting Research & Technology*, 5, 125–144.

Boyce, P. R. (1986a). *Lighting for the partially sighted: Some observations in a residential home (Capenhurst Research Memorandum ECRC/M1980)*. The Electricity Council.

Boyce, P. R. (1986b). *Lighting for the partially sighted: Some observations in a school (Capenhurst Research Memorandum ECRC/M2021)*. The Electricity Council.

Brown, B., & Lovie-Kitchin, J. (1983). Dark adaptation and the acuity/luminance response in senile macular degeneration (SMD). *American Journal of Optometry and Physiological Optics, 60*, 645–650.

Brunnström, G., Sörensen, S., Alsterstad, K., et al. (2004). Quality of light and quality of life—The effect of lighting adaptation among people with low vision. *Ophthalmic and Physiological Optics, 24*(4), 274–280.

Collins, J. (1987). Non-optical low vision aids. *Optician, 32*–33.

Cornelissen, F. W., Bootsma, A., & Kooijman, A. C. (1995). Object perception by visually impaired people at different light levels. *Vision Research, 35*, 161–168.

Cullinan, T. R. (1980). Visual disability and home lighting. *International Journal of Rehabilitation Research, 3*, 406–407.

Eilertsen, G., Horgen, G., Kvikstad, T.M., et al. (2016). Happy living in darkness! Indoor lighting in relation to activities of daily living, visual and general health in 75-year-olds living at home. *Journal of Housing for the Elderly, 30*(2), 199–213.

Eldred, K. B. (1992). Optimal illumination for reading in patients with age-related maculopathy. *Optometry and Vision Science, 69*, 46–50.

Eperjesi, F., Maiz-Fernandez, C., & Bartlett, H. E. (2007). Reading performance with various lamps in age-related macular degeneration. *Ophthalmic and Physiological Optics, 27*(1), 93–99.

Evans, B. J. W., Sawyerr, H., Jessa, Z., et al. (2010). A pilot study of lighting and low vision in older people. *Lighting Research and Technology, 42*(1), 103–119.

Falkenberg, H.K., Kvikstad, T.M., & Eilertsen, G. (2019). Improved indoor lighting improved healthy aging at home— An intervention study in 77-year-old Norwegians. *Journal of Multidisciplinary Healthcare, 12*, 315–324.

Friedburg, C., Serey, L., Sharpe, L. T., et al. (1999). Evaluation of the night vision spectacles on patients with impaired night vision. *Graefe's Archive for Clinical and Experimental Ophthalmology, 237*, 125–136.

Hartong, D. T., Jorritsma, F. F., Neve, J. J., et al. (2004). Improved mobility and independence of night-blind people using night-vision goggles. *Investigative Ophthalmology and Visual Science, 45*(6), 1725–1731.

Haymes, S. A., & Lee, J. (2006). Effects of task lighting on visual function in age-related macular degeneration. *Ophthalmic and Physiological Optics, 26*(2), 169–179. https://doi.org/10.1111/j.1475-1313.2006.00367.

IES (2020). Recommended Practice: Lighting and the visual environment for older adults and the visually impaired. An American National Standard. Illuminating and Engineering Society. ANSI/ES RP-28-20.

Jay, P. (1980). Fundamentals. *Light for low vision: Proceedings of the symposium held at University College* (pp. 13–29). London: The Partially Sighted Society. April 1978.

LaGrow, S. J. (1986). Assessing optimal illumination for the visual response accuracy in visually impaired adults. *Journal of Visual Impairment & Blindness, 83*, 888–895.

Lehon, L. H. (1980). Development of lighting standards for the visually impaired. *Journal of Visual Impairment & Blindness, 75*, 249–253.

Levitt, J. (1980). Lighting for the elderly: An optician's view. *Light for low vision: Proceedings of the symposium held at University College* (pp. 55–61). London: The Partially Sighted Society. April 1978.

Lie, I. (1977). Relation of visual acuity to illumination, contrast, and distance in the partially sighted. *American Journal of Optometry and Physiological Optics, 54*, 528–536.

Lovie-Kitchin, J. E., Bowman, K. J., & Farmer, E. J. (1983). Technical note: Domestic lighting requirements for elderly patients. *Australian Journal of Optometry, 66*, 93–97.

Morrissette, D. L., Goodrich, G. L., & Marmor, M. F. (1985). A study of the effectiveness of the Wide Angle Mobility Light. *Journal of Visual Impairment & Blindness, 79*, 109–111.

Richterman, H., & Aarons, G. (1983). Response of limited residual vision patients to working conditions with varied light and color combinations. *Journal of the American Optometric Association, 54*, 895–899.

Rohrschneider, K., Spandau, U., Wechsler, S., et al. (2000). [Utilization of a new night vision enhancement device (DAVIS)]. *Klinische Monatsblätter für Augenheilkunde, 217*(2), 88–93.

Silver, J. H., Gould, E. S., Irvine, D., et al. (1978). Visual acuity at home and in eye clinics. *Transactions of the Ophthalmological Societies of the United Kingdom, 98*, 262–266.

Simpson, J., & Tarrant, A. W. S. (1983). A study of lighting in the home. *Lighting Research & Technology, 15*, 1–8.

Sloan, L. L., Habel, A., & Feiock, K. (1971). High illumination as an auxiliary reading aid in diseases of the macula. *American Journal of Ophthalmology, 76*, 745–757.

Wacker, R. T., Bullimore, M. A., Dornbusch, H., et al. (1990). Illumination characteristics of mobility lights. *Journal of Visual Impairment & Blindness, 84*, 461–464.

Weale, R. A. (1961). Retinal illumination and age. *Transactions of the Illuminating Engineering Society, 26*, 95–100.

Werner, J. S., Peterzell, D. H., & Scheetz, A. J. (1990). Light, vision and aging. *Optometry and Vision Science, 67*, 214–229.

Weston, H. C. (1945). *Industrial Health Research Board Report 87.* HMSO.

Wittich, W., Amour, L., St., Jarry, J., et al. (2018). Test-retest variability of a standardized low vision lighting assessment. *Optometry and Vision Science, 95*(9), 852–858.

Wolffsohn, J. S., Palmer, E., Rubinstein, M., et al. (2012). Effect of light-emitting diode colour temperature on magnifier reading performance of the visually impaired. *Clinical and Experimental Optometry, 95*(5), 510–514.

Zebehazy, K. T., Zimmerman, G., Bowers, A., et al. (2005). Establishing mobility measures to assess the effectiveness of night vision devices: Results of a pilot study. *Journal of Visual Impairment & Blindness, 99*(10), 663–670.

Aids for Peripheral Field Loss

FUNCTIONAL EFFECTS OF PERIPHERAL FIELD LOSS

Even people with very good visual acuity can be severely visually impaired if their visual field is reduced. When the visual field is constricted to less than 20° in total extent, or there is a hemianopia, the main difficulty for the patient is to gather sufficient information from the environment for effective orientation and mobility: where are they and how do they find a safe path to their destination, avoiding obstacles and hazards? To gain this information a patient must be able to systematically and quickly scan the visual scene in an ordered sequence of eye movements, have sufficient visual acuity to identify what they see, remember it, and coordinate all the information gathered into a coherent picture as quickly as possible: they are correctly and quickly assembling a jigsaw of the scene in their mind. An efficient scanner may only retain a 3° *static* visual field, but have a so-called *dynamic* field of perhaps 20° which can be quickly assessed. A poor scanner is one who uses erratic and inefficient head movements to slowly scan the scene, and whose dynamic field is no larger than their static field. For this patient, it is as if the jigsaw is lying broken up in its box, and a few pieces have been selected at random.

Many patients are very efficient scanners, especially if the field defect is less severe or long-standing, or if they have received training in visual search techniques (see Chapter 13). If the loss is monocular, or binocular but incongruous, intact areas in the fellow eye's visual field will compensate for the missing regions sufficiently to maintain reasonable performance in mobility, navigation and orientation tasks. Formal tests like the Greene Hemianopsia test are used by some people to assess scanning, but it is possible to investigate how well a patient scans by observing their performance on a vision test (e.g. if they always miss letters on one side of the chart, or consistently lose their place on a reading test). Asking the patient to touch a pen held in different positions of the visual field and watching their eye movements can indicate how well they can make scanning movements to non-seeing regions of their visual field.

People are more likely to struggle with orientation and mobility when there is a binocular congruous field defect to within 10° of fixation and when the field loss is of recent onset, so efficient eye scanning technique has not yet developed.

Overall restriction of the visual field is most commonly caused by eye diseases like glaucoma, inherited retinal disease such as retinitis pigmentosa, retinal colobomas or bilateral retinal detachment. These field defects are not usually homonymous.

Homonymous field defects are usually caused by neurological disease or injury. Nearly half of those who survive a stroke and have suspected vision problems show some homonymous field loss, with about a third having a complete homonymous hemianopia (Rowe et al., 2009). As stroke is so common, a large proportion of the adult population have some field loss: 0.8% of those over 49 years old have a homonymous field defect of some kind (Gilhotra et al., 2002).

Clinical experience suggests that those with neurological field loss are usually easier to help with field expansion techniques than people with overall constriction of the visual field. Those with macular sparing and better visual acuity are more likely to succeed with field expansion than those with poor vision, and those without other diseases affecting their mobility also tend to do better. Some people with hemianopia also experience visuospatial neglect, where they are not aware of the existence of the part of the world corresponding to the region of visual field loss (Li & Malhotra, 2015). Signs of visuospatial neglect might include leaving half of a plate of food, or only applying makeup to one-half of the face. It is more difficult to use optical devices to rehabilitate those with neglect, although some successful cases are reported in the literature (Rossi et al., 1990; Houston et al., 2018a). Tests to identify neglect are described in Chapter 3.

Assessing Functional Adaptation

Under British law, people with significant field loss are not usually permitted to drive. However, they may apply to drive as an 'exceptional case' if their field loss is stable and has been present for at least 12 months; if they have no coexisting ocular condition which could cause visual loss; and if they have 'clinical confirmation of full functional adaptation' to their vision loss (Driver & Vehicle Licensing Agency, 2021). Patients with hemianopia are eligible for registration as sight impaired, but this would be incompatible with seeking to obtain a driving licence.

'Functional adaptation' is not defined in the regulations or in published research (Howard & Rowe, 2018) but, in the authors' view, it may be considered if:

- the patient consistently makes scanning eye movements to a target presented in their blind field;
- they are quickly and accurately able to point towards a pentorch or similar target presented in their non-seeing field, when permitted to make eye movements;
- they do not report bumping into obstacles in their non-seeing side;
- they are aware of their hemianopia;
- they are able to scan effectively for other tasks, such as cycling, racket sports or reading; and/or
- they do not experience a positive scotoma, Charles Bonnet hallucinations, distortion, or other visual phenomena in their non-seeing region of field.

Driving regulations are updated frequently and it is essential that the practitioner is fully aware of the current guidance, and seeks professional advice where needed, before advising patients if they are able to drive.

FIELD EXPANDERS

Reverse Telescopes

In order to present more information within the limited remaining visual field of the patient, the objects to be viewed can be minified—that is, they can be viewed with a magnification of less than 1.0. The patient can experience such a system by using a conventional telescope the wrong way round, although this limits the field-of-view because the lens which is now furthest from the eye, and is acting as the objective lens, has such a small diameter. Door viewers, of the kind used in hotel room doors or on some front doors, have long been suggested as field expansion devices, but the high amount of image compression with these systems limits their benefit as field expanders. Designs for purpose-made reverse telescopes have been suggested by several researchers (Drasdo, 1976; Mehr & Quillman, 1979) but there are only limited options

available commercially. The most common approach is to reverse a conventional handheld Galilean telescope or to use a commercially available bioptic minifying telescope.

Visual acuity will be reduced in proportion to the amount of minification: somebody with visual acuity of 0.0 logMAR (6/6) will have an acuity of 0.3 logMAR (6/12) through a reversed 2× telescope; for someone with acuity of 0.7 logMAR (6/30), the same telescope will reduce acuity to 1.0 logMAR (6/60). This poor acuity means that reversed telescopes can rarely be used as full-aperture spectacle-mounted systems, unless the amount of minification is relatively modest. In a case study of one older adult with retinitis pigmentosa, Mehr and Quillman (1979) reported that a low amount of minification (1.3×) was used successfully on a constant basis in a spectacle-mounted telescope, with the wearer demonstrating a threefold increase in visual field diameter on perimetry.

The advantage of using a reversed telescope is that the increased field through the system allows the patient a better appreciation of objects and their relative locations, especially if the scene contains repetitive detail, such as a row of parked cars or a line of shop-fronts. It can also be used to identify obstacles in a corridor, for planning a route across a crowded area such as a railway station concourse, or for sightseeing (Fig. 12.1).

When prescribing a reversed telescope, it is important to match the size of the patient's field to that of the device. A 2×-minification telescope with a 5° field will compress 10° of the visual scene into that 5° image. If the patient's remaining visual field is 5°, they will get the full benefit of this, but if the unaided field is 12°, they will in fact get a larger field without the device. A field-of-view mismatch of this type is particularly likely with a 'normal' telescope used the wrong way round as it was not designed for this purpose.

It is also important to consider the patient's adaptations and their dynamic visual field. For example, if a patient with a 5° field is good at scanning, they might have an effective visual field of 15° by using head and eye movements, outweighing the benefit from a reversed 2× telescope. Sometimes a patient may react favourably in the consulting room, and peripheral field testing might confirm the expected increase in static field, yet the patient rejects the device once it is tried in the real world. The spatial distortion created by the minification will be more obvious under dynamic conditions, which may contribute to dissatisfaction. It is worth noting the very large depth-of-field obtained with any reversed telescope, due to the fact that the accommodative demand is **divided** by the magnification squared, rather than being multiplied by it as in the magnifying telescopes (see Chapter 9).

A reversed telescope could be constructed using a contact lens as the eyepiece lens and a spectacle lens as the objective (Vincent, 2017), although this approach has similar limitations to other contact lens telescopes (see Chapter 9). Reversed telescopes can also be made in bioptic form, so that the wearer drops their head in order to examine the overall scene.

Electronic vision enhancement systems can offer minification, particularly on head-mounted devices (Htike et al., 2020).

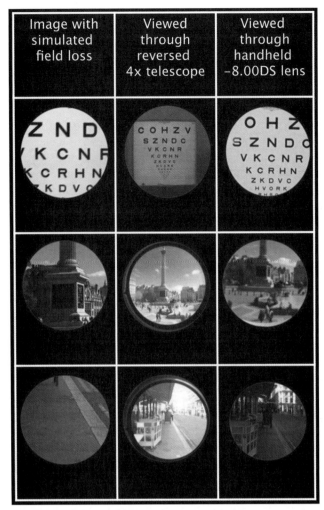

| Image with simulated field loss | Viewed through reversed 4x telescope | Viewed through handheld −8.00DS lens |

Fig. 12.1 Examples of scenes viewed with *(left column)* simulated field loss, *(middle column)* a reversed telescope, and *(right column)* a handheld minus lens. Notice that the obstacles on the pavement in the bottom row are not visible without a minifier, although scanning eye movements or mobility aids would identify them.

Electronic and augmented view techniques which simultaneously slow a minified and a 'real' view can overcome the problem of acuity reduction, as can an amorphic lens which expands the field horizontally without affecting the vertical image size (Hoeft et al., 1985). Although amorphic lenses cause significant image distortion, they have only a small effect on visual acuity and, after training, can improve performance on various detection and mobility tasks (Szlyk et al., 1998).

In practice, reversed telescope systems are most useful for specific tasks, such as a parent watching their child playing football or a commuter trying to navigate a crowded railway station. Very often a similar effect can be obtained by making efficient scanning eye movements or by using mobility aids (see Chapter 15). It is quite rare for patients to continue using a reversed telescope after the initial trial period.

For stationary tasks, such as watching television, or other display screens, increasing the viewing distance (if practicable) will produce minification, and so effectively increase the linear field of view.

Handheld Minus Lenses

A handheld minus lens positioned at about 20 to 30 cm from the eye allows viewing of an image with reduced size but expanded field. This device is in fact also a reverse Galilean telescope, with the handheld minus lens being the objective, and the user's accommodative power providing the positive eyepiece component. The higher the power of the minus lens, and the closer it is held to the eye, then the more accommodation is required. Typically, however, the accommodative demand is modest (<2.50 DS). If the patient's amplitude of accommodation is insufficient, the field expansion is still achieved, but the image is slightly blurred. This positive power can be provided by a small Fresnel stick-on portion in the superior part of the spectacle lens, or the use of the positive segment addition if the patient wears multifocal lenses. Obviously, in either case, the patient will need to tilt their head vertically in order to use the appropriate zone of the lens. This does not normally pose a problem as the device is only intended to be used for short spotting tasks.

Lens powers of up to −50.00 DS have been suggested by some authors (Bailey, 1978a), but relatively low-power lenses are more often used.

Kozlowski and colleagues devised a systematic method of prescribing such minus lenses, which overcomes the rather arbitrary way in which these devices are usually presented (Kozlowski et al., 1984; Kozlowski & Jalkh, 1985). Taking a high-minus lens and holding it at a distance from the eye, it quickly becomes obvious that the greater this distance, the smaller the magnification (or greater the minification) and the larger the field-of-view through the lens becomes. This field expansion occurs at the expense of acuity, so it is important that the field-of-view created by the lens exactly matches that of the patient. This is illustrated in Fig. 12.2, which shows an eye which has considerable constriction of the visual field to a remaining diameter of α degrees. A high-minus lens of diameter d is placed at a distance s from the nodal point (N) of the eye. Position (2) is the optimum position in which to place the lens, because the expanded field exactly fills the patient's own usable field—the edge of the lens subtends an angle at the nodal point of the eye which is equal to the size of the patient's visual field. In Position (1), the lens is held too far away and the view is excessively minified: whilst a very large area of the visual field will be 'sampled' by the high-minus lens, the user will need to move the hand holding the lens around in order to actually use the full extent of his remaining peripheral field. By contrast, in Position (3), the edge of the field-of-view of

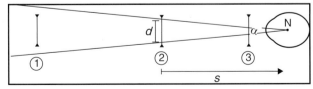

Fig. 12.2 The eye with a constricted visual field of diameter α is to view through a lens of diameter d, held at distance s from the eye's nodal point (N). For a lens of given diameter, there is only one distance *(position 2)* at which it can be held in order to completely fill the remaining visual field.

the high-minus lens is falling onto scotomatous retina, and the user would need to use eye movements in order to scan across the whole of the field-of-view provided by the device.

The optimum distance of the lens from the eye (eye-to-lens distance, s) can be found from simple geometry:

$$\tan(\alpha/2) = (d/2)/s$$

so   (12.1)

$$s = (d/2) / (\tan\alpha/2)$$

where α is the remaining visual field diameter of the patient and d is the diameter of the high-minus lens.

Magnification values of between 0.33 and 0.1 are likely to be most useful. If $M = 0.33$, for example, a field expansion of $3\times$ (from perhaps 5° to 15° in diameter) will be accompanied by a corresponding loss of acuity (e.g. from 0.3 logMAR to 0.9 logMAR). If a device with $M = 0.1\times$ was used by the same patient, the visual field would expand to 50° but the acuity would only be 1.3 logMAR within that field. The smaller the patient's field, and the better the acuity, the lower the value of M which could reasonably be selected.

'Standard' telescope formulae (see section 'The Optical Principles of Telescopes' in Chapter 9) can be used to determine the appropriate objective and eyepiece powers:

$$M = - F_E / F_O$$ (12.2)

and

$$t = f_O' + f_E'$$ (12.3)

where F_O and f_O' are the power and focal length respectively of the objective lens; F_E and f_E' are the power and focal length respectively of the eyepiece lens; and t is the length of the telescope, the separation of F_O and F_E.

These equations are just as applicable to reverse telescopes, although now $0 < M < 1.00$. F_O in this case is the handheld minus lens (F_{HHM}), which is positioned at a remote distance from the eye. The power F_E is provided by the user's accommodation (F_{ACC}) and t is now the eye-to-lens distance s. Therefore:

$$M = (-F_{ACC}) / F_{HHM}$$ (12.4)

and

$$s = f_{HHM}' + f_{ACC}'$$ (12.5)

These formulae can be used in conjunction with Eq. (12.1) to design a customised field expander, appropriate to the patient's individual requirements.

Example:
A 25-year-old patient has a visual acuity of 0.5 logMAR and a visual field with a maximum diameter of 10°. Deciding to use

a 70-mm diameter lens, substituting $d = 70\,mm$ and $\alpha = 10$ into Eq. (12.1) shows that the patient's remaining visual field will be filled by this lens held at a distance from the eye of 40 cm ($s = 400\,mm$): other diameters at other distances would have been equally appropriate. The patient's acuity is 0.5 log-MAR, so moderate minification is selected, $M = 0.33\times$.

Using Eq. (12.4):

$$0.33 = -F_{ACC}/F_{HHM}$$

$$F_{ACC} = -0.33 F_{HHM}$$

$$f_{ACC}' = -3f_{HHM}'$$

Using Eq. (12.5):

$$0.4 = f_{HHM}' - 3f_{HHM}$$

$$f_{HHM}' = -0.2\,m$$

$$F_{HHM} = -5.00\,DS$$

So,

$$F_{ACC} = -0.33 \times -5.00 = +1.67\,DS$$

The required minus lens is therefore, $F_{HHM} = -5.00$, and the accommodation needed is $F_{ACC} = +1.67$, which is easily within the accommodative amplitude of a young person.

Uncut plastic spectacle lens blanks can be used for this task, perhaps with a hole drilled through the lens near the edge and passing a cord through, so that the lens can be conveniently carried around the neck for intermittent use (Kozlowski et al., 1984). The neck-cord can also have its length fixed to match the required eye-to-lens distance: when the patient holds the lens at the maximum extent of the cord it is automatically in the correct position. A later refinement to the prescription of these lenses (Kozlowski & Jalkh, 1985) was to drill a small hole (5–10 mm diameter) in the centre of the lens so that, once objects have been located with the minifying lens, they can be examined through the hole without the loss of detail brought about by minification. This is in fact equivalent to a bioptic system, but in this case, both the minified, expanded periphery and the 'normal' central field are seen simultaneously, rather than requiring a shift of gaze to move between them.

FIELD EXPANSION IN HEMIANOPIA

There are three approaches to expanding visual fields in people with hemianopia: sector prisms, peripheral prisms (also known as Peli prisms) and spectacle reflecting systems. Although they do not technically expand the visual field, full-lens yoked prisms are also sometimes useful in people with restricted fields.

Sector Prisms

The aim of a sector prism, also known as a sectorial prism or partial-aperture prism, is to increase the patient's awareness of objects which fall into the blind field, encouraging them to make a head movement to identify and localise the object using the intact portion of the visual field. The analogy of a car wing mirror is sometimes helpful: people make regular eye movements in to the prism (or wing mirror) to identify objects, although their true position cannot always be determined correctly.

A base out prism is applied to the temporal side of the spectacle lens corresponding to the hemianopia (the right lens in right hemianopia, the left lens in left hemianopia). The prism is placed in such a way that it does not interfere with straight-ahead viewing and the image of the peripheral object initially falls on non-seeing retina. When the patient wishes to scan to see the object (apparently requiring a rotation of the visual axis through an angle α as in Fig. 12.3), however, the amount of eye rotation is reduced (to the smaller angle β). Viewing through the prism allows the subject to detect the peripheral object, but if it were to be examined more closely, the patient would be more likely to use a portion of the lens adjacent to the prism (to avoid aberrations) and so rotate their eye through the larger angle α. It must be appreciated that as the eye moves from viewing without the prism to viewing through the prism, prismatic 'jump' will be experienced: the objects in the peripheral field will appear to move towards the prism apex and the midline. Objects at position B (Fig. 12.3B) will not be seen through the lens with the prism.

The amount of field expansion, E, in degrees, for a prism of power $P\Delta$ is given by the following formula (Apfelbaum et al., 2013):

$$E = tan^{-1}(P\Delta / 100)$$

so approximately 1° of expansion is given for every 1.75Δ of prism power.

The patient will experience diplopia when they make an eye movement to the non-seeing side, hence the need to examine the object through the portion of the lens without the prism. This diplopia does not occur if prisms are fitted binocularly, but binocular fitting leads to a disturbing 'jack in the box' effect as objects suddenly appear, and leads to a prism scotoma. For example, an object at position B in Fig. 12.3 would be seen by the contralateral eye in a monocular prism but would not be seen in a binocular prism.

This effect is illustrated in Fig. 12.4. The street to be navigated is shown in Fig. 12.4A. The patient with a right-sided hemianopia (Fig. 12.4B) would not be aware of the lamp post to the right and would need to be making large scanning movements in that direction in order to notice it. The effect of viewing through the prism (Fig. 12.4C) is that the lamp post appears shifted and the eye movement required is less. However, the clock tower is not seen as it falls into the apical scotoma (Fig. 12.4).

Visual confusion through a unilateral prism can lead to suppression, so the patient's eye dominance and binocular status should be considered when deciding on whether to fit a prism monocularly or binocularly (Apfelbaum et al., 2013). Given the risks of an apical scotoma, the authors prefer monocular fitting.

In people who are monocular, an apical scotoma will always be present. Particular care is needed when dispensing prisms to patients who use only one eye, and the benefit of increased peripheral awareness should be balanced against the risks of a more central apical scotoma. A theoretical method to overcome this scotoma is a multiplexing design, which looks like a conventional Fresnel lens but comprises alternating prismatic and flat segments (Peli & Jung, 2017). At the time of writing these systems are not commercially available.

The poor image quality of Fresnel prisms led Gottlieb et al. (1992) to experiment with a small aperture ground glass prism placed into a hole drilled into a carrier lens (the Gottlieb Visual Field Awareness System). A cemented prism could be employed equally well. A rotated Franklin split lens incorporating 18Δ of prism has been described in one case report (Fig. 12.5, Crossland et al., 2022). The patient had used a Fresnel sector prism but complained of low contrast through the prism. She preferred the Franklin lens, although noticed more chromatic aberration with the solid lens. Very careful spectacle dispensing was required, and discussion with a specialist glazing laboratory.

Positioning the Prisms

Recommendations on the placement of the prisms vary enormously. At the closest, they could be fitted to correspond to an anatomical feature such as the pupil margin or limbus, and the recommendation when fitting upper- or lower-field prisms is to fit to the limbus or lower eyelid margin (as in a bifocal). For lateral prisms, however, most clinicians recommend matching them to the size of the remaining field. At a typical back vertex distance, each 1 mm on the spectacle lens represents approximately 2° of eye rotation and visual field (Bailey, 1978b). Thus, for example, if the patient retains 10° of field on that side, and the prism was not to encroach on straight-ahead gaze, then it

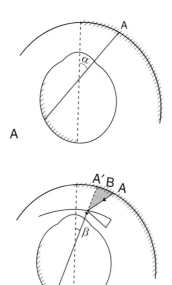

Fig. 12.3 Use of partial-aperture refracting prisms for increased awareness of objects in the non-seeing hemi-field. In the eye shown in (A), the right hemi-field is non-seeing so an object at *A* is not seen unless the eye rotates through an angle ≥ α. In (B), the object at *A* is seen through the prism so that it appears at *A'*, so the eye only needs to rotate through angle β in order to fixate it. An object at *B* falls in the prism scotoma and is not seen.

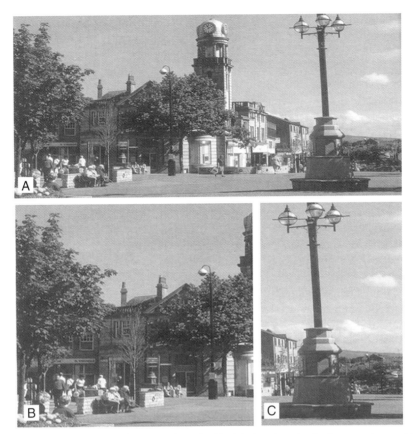

Fig. 12.4 (A) Scene as viewed with no field loss. (B) Scene as viewed with right hemianopia: the lamp post cannot be seen. (C) Lamp post can be seen when an eye movement is made into the prism, but the clock tower falls into the apical scotoma.

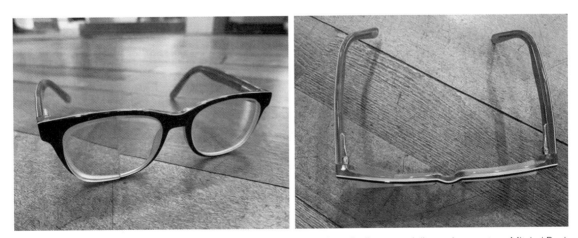

Fig. 12.5 Use of a rotated Franklin split lens with 18Δ sector prism for right hemianopia. (Image and dispensing courtesy Mitchel Reuben, FBDO.)

would need to be positioned 5 mm from the pupil centre in the primary position (Gadbaw et al., 1976; Jose & Smith, 1976). It has been suggested that the prism edge is placed 5° from pupil centre in hemianopia (Hoppe & Perlin, 1993). In quadrantanopia, the prism is placed only over the upper or lower side of the spectacle lens, corresponding to the location of the scotoma.

As the patient's scanning ability improves, the prisms may have to be moved further from the centre of the lens. Hoppe and Perlin adopted the opposite argument, however: they felt that initially the patient will find the prisms annoying, and so positioned the prism such that approximately 20° of ocular

excursion is needed to reach the edge (about 10 mm from pupil centre). With adaptation, they hoped to be able to bring the prism closer (and incidentally also increase its power), in order to use it more quickly, and with a smaller eye movement. Jose and Smith (1976) suggested limiting the prism height to the top of the pupil so that the patient can drop their head slightly and look over the top of it. This may be particularly useful in the higher-powered prisms because of the poor image quality and reflections associated with Fresnel prisms.

Prism position is something which the practitioner should discuss with the patient. As Fresnels can be moved easily, the effect of different prism positions can be demonstrated in the consulting room, or as the patient carefully walks up and down a corridor.

Attaching the Prisms

When applying the Fresnel prisms to the lens, first cut a paper template, checking its positioning against the rear surface of the spectacle lens. Note on the template the base direction of the prism. Place it on the uncut prism with the base in the correct direction and cut smoothly around the template with a razor blade. Apply to the concave surface of the lens under water, pressing the prism surface to expel air bubbles. Alternatively, wipe both contact surfaces with alcohol and place together. Warm the attached prism in frame heater to evaporate any remaining liquid and secure.

Cleaning can be a problem because patients should be advised not to immerse the spectacles in water. A camera blower-brush can be helpful to remove dust. If the lens becomes badly soiled, a cotton bud dipped in detergent solution and rubbed gently up and down the line of the facets is effective.

Success of Sector Prisms

In the authors' experience, sector prisms are most useful for patients with macular sparing, with no other limitations to their mobility and with good motivation and understanding of the purpose of the prism.

They can be helpful for avoiding collisions in crowded environments, and for avoiding being surprised by people suddenly appearing in front of them (the moment of surprise is instead when the person is around 20° to their non-seeing side, which is less alarming than when they are immediately in front of the patient's midline). They are not appropriate for sedentary tasks like watching television or using a computer, where appropriate placing of the screen to the seeing side is more helpful. They are also not useful for near tasks such as reading (see Section 'Help for Near Tasks').

In one small study, Lee and Perez showed improvements on self-reported task activities of daily living for seven of nine patients fitted with sector prisms (Lee & Perez, 1999), although there was no control group. In a further noncontrolled study, Hoppe and Perlin reported that 19 of 22 patients prescribed Fresnel sector prisms were still using them at follow-up (Hoppe & Perlin, 1993).

The unusual appearance of the Fresnel lens can be disguised by ensuring it is attached to the back surface of the spectacle lens and by using a light tint on the spectacles (Nowakowski, 1994).

Peripheral Prisms

To avoid the difficulties of diplopia, Fresnel prisms can be applied to the upper and lower portions of the spectacle lens only. These lenses are often called 'Peli prisms,' after Eli Peli, an optometrist at Schepens Eye Research Institute who popularised their use (Peli, 2000). These lenses are available as pre-cut Fresnel segments, 25 mm wide and 8 mm high, and are placed above and below the pupil on the lens corresponding to the

non-seeing side: like a sector prism, base out on the right lens in a right hemianopia and base out on the left lens in a left hemianopia. A gap of 12 mm is recommended between the prisms, although they can be moved up and down depending on the fit and vertex distance of the patient's spectacles. It is important to ensure that the prism does not fall over the pupil in primary position, so the patient does not experience diplopia when looking straight ahead (Fig. 12.6). It is recommended that the prisms are attached only to single vision distance glasses, with sufficient height that the patient can look under the lower prism. A vertical frame height of 36 mm has been suggested.

Initially 40Δ flexible prisms were used, providing approximately 22° of field expansion (see Eq. 12.6). It is now possible to obtain rigid Fresnel prisms with a power of either 40Δ or 57Δ, with the latter allowing objects from nearly 30 degrees into the blind field to be seen. Prisms are usually fitted horizontally, although oblique prisms have been suggested to collect information from within the area of a windscreen when driving, as the horizontal prisms tend to sit above and below the driver's view of the windscreen. The upper prism is fit with base down and out, and the lower prism with base up and out (Peli et al., 2016). It should be noted that it is not currently legal to drive with peripheral prisms in the UK and many other countries.

Fig. 12.7 shows the view through a 40Δ peripheral prism. In each case, the circle shows the direction of gaze. The person on the right of the corridor would not be visible to someone with a right hemianopia, but they appear through the prism at the top of the lens (top image). The patient makes an eye movement to the right, (lower image), to determine exactly where the obstacle is. They can then walk safely along the corridor without fear of collision.

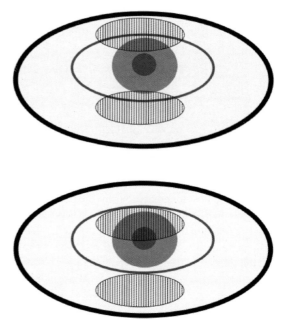

Fig. 12.6 Placement of peripheral prisms. *(Top)* Optimal position, avoiding pupil centre. *(Bottom)* Incorrect positioning, causing diplopia in the primary position.

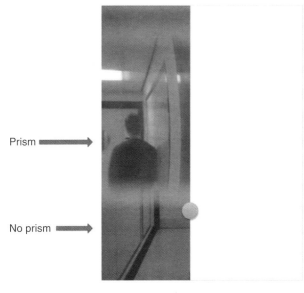

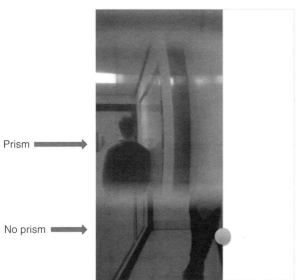

Fig. 12.7 View through a peripheral prism (see text for explanation).

4 weeks, about two-thirds of the participants preferred the 'real' peripheral prism glasses. About 40% of those who completed the trial were still using the prism glasses 6 months later, and these participants reported a significant improvement in mobility, as assessed on a questionnaire (Bowers et al., 2014). Interestingly, about one-third of their participants preferred the sham glasses. Bowers suggests this is due to the increased comfort of wearing very low-power prisms. There was a marked placebo effect: participants reported improved mobility with the sham glasses, as well as with the real prisms.

More recent studies have shown that peripheral prisms can help when detecting pedestrians on a simulated driving task (Houston et al., 2018b) and that they improve obstacle detection when walking, even in people with visuospatial neglect (Houston et al., 2018a).

Spectacle Reflecting Systems

Mirrors can be used to redirect an image into healthy visual field. The basic principle is illustrated in Fig. 12.8 which assumes a right homonymous hemianopia, with the result that images falling on the left (shaded) half of the retina are not perceived.

Unlike prismatic systems, the mirror is placed on the opposite side of the lens to the field defect, and reflects the image into intact retina during straight-ahead gaze. This means that the object will be seen without the need for any scanning eye movement, but unfortunately this is at the expense of the directly viewed field, because the mirror occludes a portion of the nasal field.

The mirror is usually angled at between 34° and 40° to the spectacle lens and can be attached to the bridge of a plastic frame (Nooney, 1986). The mirror occludes a portion of the nasal field, but only in the eye wearing the mirror—the view of the fellow eye is unobstructed and the images are superimposed. The view experienced by the wearer is shown in Fig. 12.8.

The two images are of equal clarity (which is not the case with the prism systems) so tinted mirrors have been suggested to make the reflected image distinguishable by colour. The mirror also causes reversal of movement, which also helps the images of the directly viewed and reflected objects to be distinguished. However, it causes some initial difficulties if the wearer reaches out for an object, as the initial corrective movement they make can be in the wrong direction. Patients can adapt to this reversed motion, in the same way that car drivers do to when using rear view mirrors (Nowakowski, 1994). It has been suggested that a training visit of up to 4 hours is needed for patients to familiarise themselves with the mirror system (Nooney, 1986).

The best cosmetic appearance is achieved when the mirror is mounted behind the lens (often cemented to the back surface), although this limits the physical size of the mirror (which would otherwise touch the patient's eyelashes) and could potentially cause injury in the case of an impact to the spectacles. A safer alternative which has been suggested is to apply a mirror coating to the back temporal side of a spectacle lens (Waiss & Cohen, 1992).

If patients are unhappy with the prism getting dirty or falling off, prisms can be incorporated into the substance of a spectacle lens using a lamination process. At the time of writing, these lenses can only be ordered from one laboratory (Chadwick Optical, Harleysville, PA, USA, chadwickoptical.com), and they are not currently CE-marked for use in the UK or European Union. Alternative methods of mounting the prism include 'hang-ons' which are worn over the patient's current spectacles, or a magnetic mounting system known as SLAM (Single Lens Attached by Magnets).

Success of Peripheral Prisms

In a randomised controlled trial of 73 people with hemianopia across 13 clinics, Bowers and colleagues dispensed patients with a pair of glasses with 'real' 57Δ peripheral prisms, and a pair of glasses with 5Δ 'sham' prisms, in a randomised order. After wearing each pair of glasses for

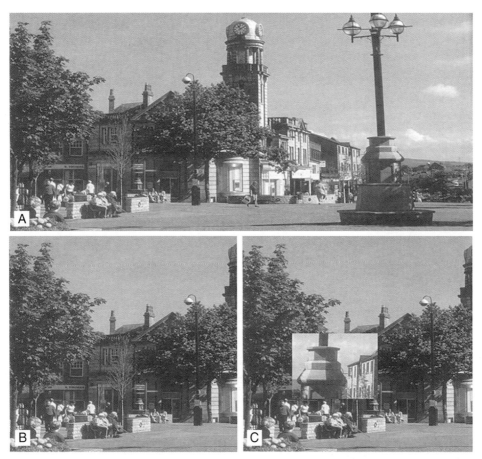

Fig. 12.8 View through a spectacle reflecting system. (A) The unobstructed view. (B) The view as seen with a right hemianopia. (C) The view as seen through a spectacle reflecting system. Note the base of the lamp post is superimposed over the view of the shops.

If the mirror is instead attached to the front surface of the spectacle frame nasal rim, it can be made larger, and there is more scope for its angle to be varied. The smaller the angle, the larger and more peripheral is the reflected field of view, but at the same time this increases the area of the directly viewed field which is obstructed. The use of mirrors which clip onto the front of the spectacle lens and are adjustable is possible. For trial purposes, a dental mirror or cyclist's helmet mirror can be demonstrated.

Although some authors report considerable success with mirror reflecting systems for hemianopia (Nooney, 1986), they are not widely used in the UK, with peripheral prisms being the most commonly prescribed low vision aid for people with hemianopia.

Yoked Prisms

A further technique which can be used in hemianopia is to prescribe Yoked prisms, of equal power in each lens, with the prism base coinciding with the non-seeing hemifield (right hemianopia: base out right, base in left; left hemianopia: base in right, base out left). This system moves the image away from the blind side and is particularly useful for people who experience head or neck pain from using a compensatory head posture to overcome their hemianopia. It should be noted that these prisms are to improve comfort, rather than to increase the visual field or help in the rehabilitation of field loss.

The amount of prism used must be balanced against the increased weight and thickness of the spectacle lenses: about 12Δ is usually the most which can be worn comfortably. Fresnel prisms could be used but will reduce the contrast of the image.

A similar approach can be taken with vertical prisms for people with altitudinal visual field defects. Significant caution is needed if they are to be worn for mobility, but they can be useful for sedentary tasks, such as eating, when the field loss interferes with the tasks or requires an unusual head position.

Recumbent Prisms

Originally designed for reading in bed, recumbent prisms are very high powered base down prisms which move an image upwards by nearly 90° (Keeler et al., 2010). They can be used by people with limited mobility who wish to watch television, read or look at a computer whilst lying on their back. Theoretically, a similar high-power base up prism could be used by someone with an unusual posture caused by arthritis or another disease which causes them to have a stooped gait, so they can see things in front of them despite their head facing the ground. The prescriber should be extremely cautious to ensure that this prism does not affect the patient's balance.

PRISMS FOR EXPANDING CONSTRICTED VISUAL FIELDS

For people with a general constriction of their visual field, a Fresnel prism could theoretically be placed on each edge of a spectacle lens, around a clear central zone, with each lens having a base pointing away from the lens centre. Fig. 12.9 shows two possible placements of the prisms.

Somani and colleagues used this approach for 16 patients with retinitis pigmentosa and visual fields of less than 10°, although they used prisms only on the temporal, nasal, and lower edges of the lens. After a 1-month trial of 20Δ Fresnel lenses, patients demonstrated a significant improvement on their functional field score and a modest improvement in their self-reported peripheral vision (Somani et al., 2006). There was no control group, and they did not report whether any of their 16 participants kept using the prism glasses after the trial period.

A 'trifield' lens is a system where two vertical prisms are glazed, apex-to-apex, in one lens of the spectacles, whilst the other lens has no prism. As long as the patient has binocular vision, they will not experience a prism scotoma (Peli, 2001). The prism is fitted in front of the nondominant eye, and each prism is tinted a different colour to help the patient identify which side the image is being projected from. In a study by Woods and colleagues, 9 of 12 patients using trifield spectacles were still wearing them at a follow-up visit about 6 weeks later, and all 12 had field expansion on perimetry (Woods et al., 2010).

More recently, Peli has described a novel three-dimensional (3D) printed lens design which uses 'multi-periscopic prisms' for field expansion in people with constricted peripheral fields. This system is not yet commercially available, and at the time of writing no clinical trials of these lenses have taken place (Peli et al., 2020).

HELP FOR NEAR TASKS

It is not unusual for patients with limited peripheral fields to also have reduced visual acuity, which means that they may well be candidates for magnifying aids, especially for near vision. If the visual field is smaller than that of the magnifying device, this may limit the benefit of the magnifier: some of the magnified image will fall onto nonfunctional retina so the device may not be as effective as hoped. An electronic vision enhancement system is often more effective than an optical aid of equal magnification. This is probably because the patient can then keep their eyes still and scan the text through the remaining field of vision. Patients can also be taught to utilise this 'steady eye strategy' using optical aids (see Section 'Central Field Loss' in Chapter 13).

Even with good reading acuity, and no requirement for near magnification, following lines of print can be difficult if the field loss extends close to fixation. Minus lens minifiers can theoretically be used to expand the field obtained whilst reading (Weiss, 1991), which may help to navigate the whole page. Relatively modest lens powers (−1.50 DS to −2.50 DS) at 30 to 50 cm from the eye will create a magnification between 0.5 and 1.0.

Nonoptical methods of aiding reading in hemianopia include the use of typoscopes (see Section 'Typoscopes' in Chapter 10), tracing along under the line of text with a finger, or changing the orientation of the text so that the patient reads the lines on the slant, vertically, or even upside-down.

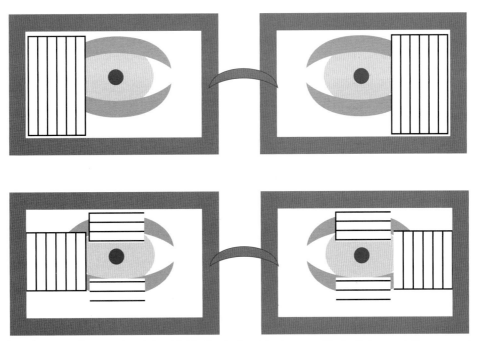

Fig. 12.9 Possible prism placement for constricted visual fields. The horizontal prisms are fitted with base out, the upper prisms with base up and the lower prisms with base down.

Good organisation and placement of objects in the environment should be encouraged: cutlery and tableware, desk accessories and tools should be placed on the side of the still-functional field. The patient can develop strategies such as rotating the plate occasionally whilst eating. Students with visual field loss should be placed on the side of the classroom so that the teacher and whiteboard fall into the best region visual field, removing the need for uncomfortable head movements. Carers should be encouraged to position themselves, and objects of interest such as television, to the most appropriate side of the patient.

Near-Vision Aids for Hemianopia

Binocular full-aperture yoked prisms, with the base towards the field defect, have been suggested to displace the entire field away from the blind side (see Chapter 13). Such a correction is intended to create a linear shift in the field: a portion which was previously missing is gained at one edge of the field, at the expense of an equal segment lost from the opposite edge. If, for example, a patient with a left hemianopia could not see the first three words on the line when fixating on the fourth word, then a prism placed with base to the left would shift the retinal image of these missing words so that they now fell into the functional right field. The patient could, however, achieve this effect without any prismatic correction, simply by shifting their gaze to the left, or moving the book to the right. It must be emphasised that the reading process is dynamic and the eyes are constantly moving: even if a prism was used to shift the retinal image appropriately with the eyes stationary, the eyes will still have to make a saccade from the end of one line to the beginning of the next. If the return saccade is visually aimed, it is then just as likely not to reach the beginning of the line as was the case without the prism. A more useful strategy is often to train the patient to make the return saccade to a point right at the beginning, or even slightly in advance, of the first word on the line, and perhaps encourage them to hold their index finger or a ruler adjacent to the first word, to give them a clear target to aim for. If the return saccade is 'resetting' the eye position to a particular location in space—for example, returning the eye to 'straight-ahead'—then the patient with left hemianopia will miss all the words to the left of this location. The strategy in this case would be to encourage the patient to hold the book to the right of the midline, so that 'straight-ahead' coincides with the start of the line.

Despite reservations concerning the theory behind such devices, they are prescribed and it is claimed that patients benefit because they require less head and eye movement, and read more fluently. It may represent a solution for those who do not succeed with eye movement training or other rehabilitative techniques. Although powers from 6Δ to 20Δ have been recommended by various authors, the maximum prism power generally recommended is around 15Δ, which will produce a shift of approximately 5 cm at a typical reading distance of 0.3 m. More powerful prisms would produce a greater shift but are heavy and thick even when made in high-index material: Fresnel stick-on prisms of this power create unacceptably poor image quality and are not well tolerated for reading, even as a temporary measure.

Near-Vision Aids for Constricted Fields

A difficulty encountered by those with constricted fields in near and intermediate tasks is in seeing the full area simultaneously. A decrease in the size of the retinal image is required in order to fit more information into the available functional visual field. Some of the 'distance' devices can also be used for near and intermediate tasks: for example, a reversed telescope can be used to expand the field to search for a mislaid object on the desk or eat a meal.

Mirrors can be used to increase the viewing distance of an object. In the 1980s, artist Ewert Johns constructed a system where one mirror was placed flat on a table and a second, larger, mirror was suspended above the table, facing the first mirror. In Johns' system, an object is placed on the table, reflected by the suspended mirror, and viewed in the tabletop mirror, at a reduced image size (Johns, 1987). Johns reported that his system would have helped Michelangelo when painting the ceiling of the Sistine Chapel, freeing him from 'regular journeys down the scaffolding'. A simpler approach is to increase the viewing distance, as Michelangelo would have done by climbing away from the ceiling. Today people are more likely to use an electronic vision enhancement system for the same purpose, or a camera.

SUMMARY AND COMPARISON OF AVAILABLE METHODS

Optical field expansion devices are only one component in the rehabilitation of people with visual field loss: scanning eye movements, mobility training, environmental modification and electronic vision enhancement systems are also important.

Prisms reflect or, more commonly, refract light onto non-seeing retina and are attached to the side of the lens nearest the field defect, with base towards the field loss. **Mirrors** reflect light onto seeing retina and are attached to the side of the lens furthest from the field defect.

There has been very little information in the literature regarding a rational prescribing strategy for patients with peripheral field defects: with the exception of Bowers' study of peripheral prisms (Bowers et al., 2014), too many reports have described a limited number of patients, without control groups, and they have rarely compared different techniques.

Success rates have in general been limited, perhaps because patients have too high an expectation when a device is described as a 'field expander'. It is more realistic to consider these devices as 'increasing peripheral field awareness' (Jose & Smith, 1976) or as 'aids to efficient scanning'. However, properly used optical devices can help people with visual field loss maintain independence and navigate more safely.

REFERENCES

Apfelbaum, H. L., Ross, N. C., Bowers, A. R., et al. (2013). Considering apical scotomas, confusion, and diplopia when prescribing prisms for homonymous hemianopia. *Translational Vision Science & Technology, 2*(4), 2.

Bailey, I. L. (1978a). Field expanders. *Optometric Monthly, 69*, 813–816.

Bailey, I. L. (1978b). Prismatic treatment for field defects. *Optometric Monthly, 69*, 1073–1078.

Bowers, A. R., Keeney, K., & Peli, E. (2014). Randomized crossover clinical trial of real and sham peripheral prism glasses for hemianopia. *JAMA Ophthalmology, 132*(2), 214–222.

Crossland, M. D., Reuben, M., & Bedford, S. L. (2022). Novel use of a Franklin split lens for cycling with hemianopia. *Ophthalmic & Physiological Optics, 42*(1), 218–223.

Drasdo, N. (1976). Visual field expanders. *American Journal of Optometry and Physiological Optics, 53*(9 Pt 1), 464–467.

Driver & Vehicle Licensing Agency. (2021). *Assessing fitness to drive: A guide for medical professionals*. DVLA.

Gadbaw, P., Finn, W., Dolan, M., et al. (1976). Parameters of success in the use of Fresnel prisms. *Optical Journal and Review of Optometry, 113*, 41–43.

Gilhotra, J. S., Mitchell, P., Healey, P. R., et al. (2002). Homonymous visual field defects and stroke in an older population. *Stroke, 33*(10), 2417–2420.

Gottlieb, D. D., Freeman, P., & Williams, M. (1992). Clinical research and statistical analysis of a visual field awareness system. *Journal of the American Optometric Association, 63*(8), 581–588.

Hoeft, W. W., Feinbloom, W., Brilliant, R., et al. (1985). Amorphic lenses: A mobility aid for patients with retinitis pigmentosa. *Optometry and Vision Science, 62*(2), 142–148.

Hoppe, E., & Perlin, R. R. (1993). The effectivity of Fresnel prisms for visual field enhancement. *Journal of the American Optometric Association, 64*(1), 46–53.

Houston, K. E., Bowers, A. R., Peli, E., et al. (2018a). Peripheral prisms improve obstacle detection during simulated walking for patients with left hemispatial neglect and hemianopia. *Optometry and Vision Science, 95*(9), 795–804.

Houston, K. E., Peli, E., Goldstein, R. B., et al. (2018b). Driving with hemianopia VI: Peripheral prisms and perceptual-motor training improve detection in a driving simulator. *Translational Vision Science & Technology, 7*(1), 5.

Howard, C., & Rowe, F. J. (2018). Adaptation to poststroke visual field loss: A systematic review. *Brain and Behavior, 8*(8), e01041.

Htike, H. M., Margrain, T. H., Lai, Y. K., et al. (2020). Ability of head-mounted display technology to improve mobility in people with low vision: A systematic review. *Translational Vision Science and Technology, 9*(10), 1–27.

Johns, E. (1987). A tunnel vision aid devised by an artist. *British Journal of Visual Impairment, 5*(1), 35–36.

Jose, R. T., & Smith, A. J. (1976). Increasing peripheral field awareness with Fresnel prisms. *Optical Journal and Review of Optometry, 113*, 33–37.

Keeler, R., Singh, A. D., & Dua, H. S. (2010). Recumbent spectacles: Taking it lying down. *British Journal of Ophthalmology, 94*(5), 535.

Kozlowski, J. M. D., & Jalkh, A. E. (1985). An improved negative-lens field expander for patients with concentric field constriction. *Archives of Ophthalmology, 103*(3), 326.

Kozlowski, J. M. D., Mainster, M. A., & Avila, M. P. (1984). Negative-lens field expander for patients with concentric field constriction. *Archives of Ophthalmology, 102*(8), 1182–1184.

Lee, A. G., & Perez, A. M. (1999). Improving awareness of peripheral visual field using sectorial prism. *Optometry, 70*(10), 624–628.

Li, K., & Malhotra, P. A. (2015). Spatial neglect. *Practical Neurology, 15*(5), 333–339.

Mehr, E. B., & Quillman, R. D. (1979). Field "expansion" by use of binocular full-field reversed 1.3X telescopic spectacles: A case report. *Optometry and Vision Science, 56*(7), 446–450.

Nooney, T. W. (1986). Partial visual rehabilitation of hemianopic patients. *Optometry and Vision Science, 63*(5), 382–386.

Nowakowski, R. W. (1994). *Primary low vision care*. Appleton & Lange.

Peli, E. (2000). Field expansion for homonymous hemianopia by optically induced peripheral exotropia. *Optometry and Vision Science, 77*(9), 453–464.

Peli, E. (2001). Vision multiplexing: An engineering approach to vision rehabilitation device development. *Optometry and Vision Science, 78*(5), 304–315.

Peli, E., Bowers, A. R., Keeney, K., et al. (2016). High-power prismatic devices for oblique peripheral prisms. *Optometry and Vision Science, 93*(5), 521–533.

Peli, E., & Jung, J. H. (2017). Multiplexing prisms for field expansion. *Optometry and Vision Science, 94*(8), 817–829.

Peli, E., Vargas-Martin, F., Kurukuti, N. M., et al. (2020). Multi-periscopic prism device for field expansion. *Biomedical Optics Express, 11*(9), 4872–4889.

Rossi, P. W., Kheyfets, S., & Reding, M. J. (1990). Fresnel prisms improve visual perception in stroke patients with homonymous hemianopia or unilateral visual neglect. *Neurology, 40*(10), 1597–1599.

Rowe, F., Brand, D., Jackson, C. A., et al. (2009). Visual impairment following stroke: Do stroke patients require vision assessment? *Age and Ageing, 38*(2), 188–193.

Somani, S., Brent, M. H., & Markowitz, S. N. (2006). Visual field expansion in patients with retinitis pigmentosa. *Canadian Journal of Ophthalmology, 41*(1), 27–33.

Szlyk, J. P., Seiple, W., Laderman, D. J., et al. (1998). Use of bioptic amorphic lenses to expand the visual field in patients with peripheral loss. *Optometry and Vision Science, 75*(7), 518–524.

Vincent, S. J. (2017). The use of contact lenses in low vision rehabilitation: Optical and therapeutic applications. *Clinical and Experimental Optometry, 100*(5), 513–521.

Waiss, B., & Cohen, J. M. (1992). The utilization of a temporal mirror coating on the back surface of the lens as a field enhancement device. *Journal of the American Optometric Association, 63*(8), 576–580.

Weiss, N. J. (1991). Low vision management of retinitis pigmentosa. *Journal of the American Optometric Association, 62*(1), 42–52.

Woods, R. L., Giorgi, R. G., Berson, E. L., et al. (2010). Extended wearing trial of Trifield lens device for "tunnel vision". *Ophthalmic and Physiological Optics, 30*(3), 240–252.

Special Training Techniques for Visual Field Loss

CENTRAL FIELD LOSS

When someone with bilateral central field loss looks straight at an object, it will fall into the scotoma and not be seen. This effect has been known for centuries: for example, in the late 19th century, friends of the impressionist artist Degas reported that he found it 'torment to draw, when he could only see around the spot at which he was looking, and never the spot itself' (Trevor-Roper, 1997). This method of using peripheral retina to observe something is known as *eccentric viewing (EV)*.

Eccentric Viewing and the Preferred Retinal Locus

Most people with central field loss will use a single region of peripheral retina in place of the damaged fovea to look at a scene (Fletcher & Schuchard, 1997). When this part of the retina is used repeatedly for observation, it is known as the preferred retinal locus (PRL).

The PRL has been shown to develop within 6 months in most people with bilateral macular disease (Crossland et al., 2005), although training may be needed for the patient to use the most effective region for every task. In studies, microperimeters are usually used to identify whether a patient is using a PRL, but careful observation of the patient whilst they fixate a target can also show their fixation behaviour. For example, if the patient is asked to observe a budgie stick in front of the clinician's face, their eye position can often be determined. Asking the patient to switch their gaze between a distance acuity test and the budgie stick can indicate how well established the PRL is: if the patient always quickly adopts the same eye position, they are likely to have a more stable PRL than if they make several scanning movements or use a different position each time.

Another method of determining the PRL location is to use an Amsler grid. The patient is asked to look towards the centre of the chart, and then to report any missing regions. If the top of the chart is missing, for example, it is likely that they are using a PRL beneath the scotoma; if the left hand side is distorted then their PRL is to the right. If the central dot is not visible, or the centre is missing, they are probably not using EV. A similar approach, using a clock, is often used for training EV (see Section 'PRL Training' later).

The best Amsler Grid to use is the recording chart (black-on-white) with an additional diagonal fixation cross drawn on it. The testing must be carried out monocularly, and the nonviewing eye occluded. An appropriate reading addition is used as required, and the patient is allowed to hold the chart at any comfortable distance in order to see it. Even with an acuity of 1.60 logMAR, the chart can usually be seen under these circumstances, but if vision is extremely poor, the chart can be presented on an electronic vision enhancement system, or a hand-drawn enlarged chart can be used. The California Central Visual Field Test (see Chapter 3) can be used if it is necessary to plot the position and depth of the scotoma more precisely.

Systematic errors on a vision test can also indicate the PRL position. For example, if the last letter on a distance acuity chart is always missed, or the patient skips the last word on each line of a reading task, it is likely that the PRL is to the left of the scotoma in visual field space.

Patients are often not aware of using EV, even when they make very obvious head or eye movements to see, or when they move the object they are looking at around. When asked, for example, why they move a reading test around to read it, they often say that it is to get the lighting right or to bring the print into focus.

Someone who does not use EV strategies effectively may report being able to read only a few words before 'all the words run together' or 'it all runs into one'. This person may not perform any better if magnification is used: in fact, they sometimes do worse as fewer magnified letters can be visualised simultaneously. When asked about their reading, they might report that they have just as much difficulty with newspaper headlines as with the small text underneath. A careful history can establish whether a patient has adapted to using a PRL effectively (Table 13.1).

Location of the PRL

Considered in terms of resolution ability, which decreases dramatically with distance from the foveal centre, it makes sense for the patient to 'choose' a PRL on the edge of the scotoma nearest to the fovea. Even with the best area of remaining retina selected, the patient would also be expected to require magnification of the image to compensate for the poorer resolution.

People may use different PRLs for different tasks (Crossland et al., 2011). For example, a smaller, better resolution area of retina may be used for reading single letters on an acuity chart, but a larger PRL with worse acuity may be better for reading with a magnifier, as more letters would be seen at once.

A PRL to the left or right of the scotoma is unlikely to be optimal for reading, as the scotoma would obscure either the start or the end of the line: the patient would be reading 'into' or 'out of' the scotoma (Fig. 13.1). Given the choice between placing the PRL above or below the scotoma, it is slightly better to use a PRL under the scotoma (i.e. to move the eye up to see), as there is a slightly higher photoreceptor density (Curcio & Allen, 1990) and better attentional deployment (He et al., 1996) in that part of the retina, and the upper eyelid is less likely to obstruct the vision. Despite this theoretical advantage, there does not seem to be a systematic difference in reading speed between people who use PRLs in different retinal regions (Sunness et al., 1996; Fletcher, 1999). Other factors such as eye movements and fixation stability may be more important in determining the success of EV.

Fixation Stability

It is less easy to hold the eye steady with peripheral retina than with the fovea. People with central vision loss who are better able to hold the eye still when observing a target—in other words, those with better fixation stability—have better visual acuity (Tarita-Nistor et al., 2009, 2011) and tend to be better at reading (Crossland et al., 2004; Amore et al., 2013) than those who have less precise fixation. Fixation stability tends to decrease as the scotoma increases in size and the PRL becomes more eccentric, although it is often acceptable for scotomas of less than 20 degrees in diameter (Zeevi et al., 1979; Whittaker et al., 1988).

Eye Movements and Steady Eye Strategy

If someone is fully adapted to using EV, they will make an eye movement straight to their PRL rather than to their fovea: that is, they will make the PRL the centre of their oculomotor system. This is relatively rare: in one study, only one-third of patients had made this adaptation (White & Bedell, 1990). In a longitudinal study, one of the authors found that all of their subjects with early-onset inherited macular disease were unaware of using EV, which implies some degree of rereferencing their oculomotor system, but only about half of those with age-related macular degeneration (AMD) had made this adaptation within 1 year of losing central vision (Crossland et al., 2005).

Someone who does not automatically make an eye movement to their PRL will always be aware of using EV. When they read a vision chart and get close to their threshold acuity, they will often start moving their eyes to identify the letters and may spontaneously report 'trying to catch the letter out of the corner of the eye' or 'moving the blind spot out of the way'.

When a patient is unable to make eye movements to their PRL, they may adopt a technique known as steady eye strategy (SES), where the eye is held steady, but the print is moved right to left so that it scrolls through their PRL (Collins, 1987). The patient fixates the first letter on the line of print and is instructed to obtain the clearest possible view of it. This should mean that they are using EV to place the letter on the PRL. As they keep the eye still and move the print, each succeeding letter will be imaged in turn on the PRL and the words are read accurately, letter by letter.

TABLE 13.1 Ways to Identify the Likelihood of an Established Eccentric Viewing Technique

More Likely to Have an Established Preferred Retinal Locus	Less Likely to Have an Established Preferred Retinal Locus
Can see large print, but difficulties increase as print gets smaller	Finds headlines just as difficult to read as smaller print
Accurately ranks magnifiers in terms of power and utility	Has a variety of magnifiers of different strengths but cannot tell any difference between them
Progressive increases in magnification produce predictable improvements in performance	Acuity improvement with magnification is less than expected
Reads single letters, short words, and long words (of appropriate size) equally easily	Can read single letters, or part of a line on a sight chart, but not full words
Can read a whole sentence over multiple lines	Words 'run into one another'
Head and text are held still, and eyes move 'normally' when reading	Moves head, eye and text around in an irregular pattern when attempting to read

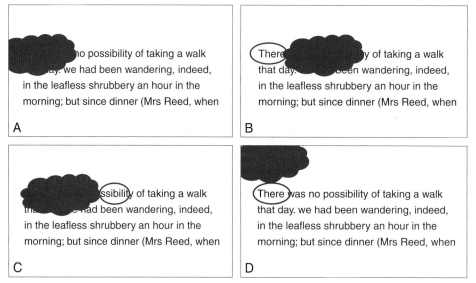

Fig. 13.1 Effect of preferred retinal locus (PRL) position on reading magnified text. (A) Observing the text without eccentric viewing blocks the first word. (B) A PRL to the left of the scotoma affects forward eye movements. (C) A PRL to the right of the scotoma affects movements back to the start of the line. (D) A PRL below the scotoma does not interfere with page navigation for reading.

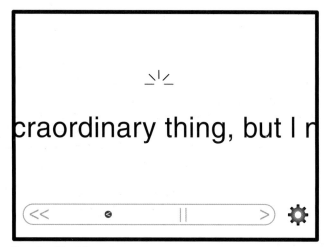

Fig. 13.2 The MD_evReader app. Text is scrolled left to right (or right to left) at a speed selected by the user. Text size, colour and font can be modified. The fixation guide can be turned off and on.

At first, this technique can make reading slow and frustrating: patients often report that it is 'like learning to read again', but when SES is mastered it can support a reading speed which is fast enough for enjoyable leisure reading, of up to about 120 words per minute (Gustafsson & Inde, 2004).

An alternative to asking the patient to move the text themselves is to present scrolled text on a screen. This can be performed using software such as Zoomtext (Gustafsson & Inde, 2004), through an app such as MD_evReader (Walker et al., 2016), Fig. 13.2, or on the EV internet news system managed by Royal Holloway, University of London (http://www.mdevreader.rhul.ac.uk/ev-news/).

It should be noted that even though the patient is being asked to keep their eyes still, and believes this is what they are doing, successful SES does not actually result in eyes which are stationary. The moving text elicits an optokinetic-like or sawtooth eye movement, with alternating fast (saccadic) and slow (pursuit) eye movements. As the text is moved to the left, the eyes fixate (eccentrically) on the letter of interest and match their speed to that of the text, making a smooth pursuit movement. After analysis of that letter is complete, the eyes reset to the correct position relative to the next letter/word (i.e. with the correct EV angle) with a saccade. This appears as the fast phase of the nystagmoid sawtooth movement.

SES can be used without EV, and it has proved to be a fast and efficient method of reading with a magnifier. It has the additional advantage that the task can be aligned so that rays of light from the object of interest always pass through the optical centre of the lens, and image quality is optimised: as the task is moved under the magnifier, the patient is always viewing the object through the optimal portion of the lens. In binocular viewing, an additional advantage is that as the eyes consistently use the same portion of the lens, they experience a constant prismatic effect. This means that there is no need for the patient to alter the degree of convergence, which would be necessary if they were to move the eyes laterally and use different zones on the lens.

Eccentric Viewing Training

As many people with central vision loss do not use EV efficiently, an obvious question is whether better EV techniques can be trained. Many different training programmes have been suggested, including maximising the use of the existing PRL; encouraging people to adopt a new, trained retinal locus (TRL); improving eye movements to the PRL; and improving fixation stability. Some training programmes use sophisticated technology such as microperimeters or scanning laser ophthalmoscopes, whilst others use only basic equipment.

EV training is most commonly provided by rehabilitation officers, but it is sometimes offered by optometrists, orthoptists or by volunteers with macular disease (Dickinson, 2016).

Home-based training has also been offered, using an audio CD or computer programme (Vukicevic & Fitzmaurice, 2009).

There is limited evidence for the benefit of low vision training on improving reading ability (Gaffney et al., 2014; Dickinson, 2016). Despite the absence of high-quality evidence for its benefit, there are many anecdotal reports of success with EV training, and up to half of low-vision clinics in some countries offer this training (Gaffney et al., 2014). It is known that some individual patients do well from training, but this improvement is not universal enough for studies to determine a systematic benefit for everyone with central field loss (Nguyen et al., 2011). In one study, almost three-quarters of participants found EV training helpful, despite not demonstrating faster reading or improvements in visual task performance (Dickinson, 2016). This might indicate that this training confers benefits which are not easily measured in clinical trials.

EV training is usually provided as part of an integrated rehabilitation programme (Fig. 13.3, Palmer et al., 2010). There is considerable variation between professionals on the content of an EV programme, even within the same organisation (Stelmack et al., 2004). The methods described here are based on techniques used by some rehabilitation workers in the United Kingdom and do not require specialist equipment.

PRL Training

To train EV, the patient is made aware of the location of their PRL and encouraged to make eye movements to this location. A clockface is often used to identify the location of their PRL, and the patient is shown how to move their eyes so that the PRL falls on other items of interest (Fig. 13.4). Training is performed monocularly on the better eye, unless both eyes are similar in which case the dominant eye is used (Palmer et al., 2010; Seiple et al., 2011).

For example, if a patient reports that the star in the centre of the clock in Fig. 13.4 is clearest when they direct their eyes towards the number 3, their PRL is likely to be to the left of where they are fixating and it can be explained that they need to move their eyes to the right to see most easily. As they move their eyes further to the right, the number 3 should become clearer. They can then be asked to move their eyes to the left to see the star again, and eventually the number 9. Once horizontal movements can be made effectively, the patient can use the same technique to observe other numbers on the clockface: for example, by making the number 6 as clear as possible by looking to the right of it. Once the patient is aware of

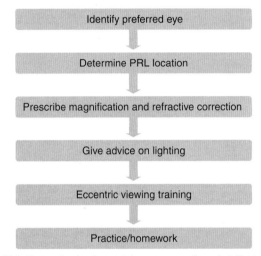

Fig. 13.3 Eccentric viewing training as part of a rehabilitation programme. *PRL*, Preferred retinal locus. (As suggested by Palmer, S., Logan, D., Nabili, S., & Dutton, G. N. (2010). Effective rehabilitation of reading by training in the technique of eccentric viewing: Evaluation of a 4-year programme of service delivery. British Journal of Ophthalmology, 94, 494–497.)

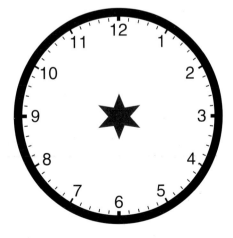

Star clearest when looking towards...	Location of PRL	Move eyes...
12	Below scotoma	Up to use PRL
3	Left of scotoma	Right to use PRL
6	Above scotoma	Down to use PRL
9	Right of scotoma	Left to use PRL

Fig. 13.4 Use of a clockface to determine preferred retinal locus *(PRL)* position.

the principle of 'dragging' their PRL to see more easily, they can practise 'jumping' their eyes to different numbers on the clock, and then to different objects around the room.

Daily practice is usually recommended, and the training is tailored to the patient's interests: if they want to watch television, they are asked to practise EV for the screen; if they are a keen gardener they should try identifying flowers with their PRL. If the training is performed for reading, progressively longer words are introduced (Fig. 13.5).

Multiple training sessions are usually required. The time spent will vary between practitioners, but is often 5 or 6 hours,

split over several sessions (Nilsson et al., 2003; Tarita-Nistor et al., 2009), and in some cases is as much as 5 to 10 hours per week, for 6 weeks (Hassan et al., 2019). The exact content of each session is often based on the patient's response to the previous 'lesson' (Coco-Martín et al., 2013).

To train reading with EV, a sample of print with short words in a large size should be used (see Fig. 13.5A), positioned at a normal reading distance with appropriate presbyopic correction. The patient is asked to look at the first letter on the page and identify it. They are then told either to move their eyes to use the best PRL identified on the clockface or

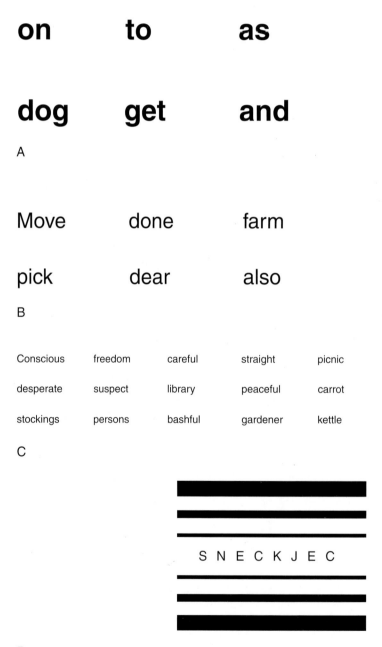

Fig. 13.5 Samples of text used to practice eccentric viewing. (A)–(C) represent reading tasks of progressively increasing difficulty (decreasing letter size and increasing word length). In (D) fixation targets have been added around the letters, to direct the patient's gaze.

(if no EV direction could be identified, or the patient appears to be already viewing eccentrically) to 'make that letter as clear as you can'. The patient is now instructed to keep their eyes still and move the print to the left until the next letter comes into view. They must read along the lines letter by letter, initially without attempting to interpret the letters as part of words. If the patient hesitates or stops, or says that the next letter has disappeared or become blurred, then they are asked to go back to the beginning of the line and start again. Various types of sample text can be used beginning with very large letters in groups of 1 or 2, ultimately progressing to long words of up to 10 letters (see Figs. 13.5B and C). Large spaces between adjacent words make the task easier because there are no surrounding contours to confuse the patient. As proficiency increases, the patient can progress to more closely spaced words which require much better technique to avoid confusion. As the print size decreases the patient will probably need additional magnification in order to read, but as EV ability improves, lower magnification devices can often be substituted. The aim would be to give the patient several practice sheets to use at home, with two 5-minute sessions each day, and return visits to the optometrist every 1 or 2 weeks.

If preferred, early text samples can be produced with fixation asterisks or lines above and below the words to be read. These can be used as fixation targets for the patient: for example, with a text such as Fig. 13.5D: 'Look at the left-hand edge of the first line over the word—how many letters can you see? Do you see more letters, or more clearly if you look at the left-hand side of the middle line?'

With time, the patient can read with verbal reminders rather than fixation lines: (e.g. 'Can you see the first letter? Look slightly above it—do you see it now?'). It is preferable not to be too precise about exactly how far away from the target the patient should view, because although the gaze *angle* remains the same regardless of the task, the precise linear distance will vary with viewing distance. One study (Yap et al., 1986) suggests that when the patient is required to change their eye position by a constant *angular* extent, they will tend instead to use the inappropriate strategy of looking to one side by a constant *lateral* distance regardless of the distance of the target. It can be more appropriate to simply give the patient an instruction such as 'make the first letter as clear as possible' rather than 'look up and to the right' when they begin reading with EV.

If the scotoma progresses, it is possible that the required EV direction may change, and the patient may be concerned that their efforts in mastering the technique will be wasted. The patient can be reassured that the technique remains valid, and again it will be more appropriate here to simply concentrate on teaching the patient to get a clear view of the first letter on the line and then adopt SES, rather than indicating an exact direction of gaze.

EV training is very difficult to perform in people who have ring scotomas and intact central vision. In this case, SES is the most helpful approach.

The PRL 'naturally' selected by the patient may not be optimal: for example, they may have a horizontally shifted PRL and difficulty in reading even with SES. In this case, the patient may be trained to use a different TRL in a better retinal location.

TRL training uses the same techniques as conventional EV training, but rather than selecting their own PRL, the patient is told to move their eyes in a specific direction to use the best possible retinal area for fixation. Usually, this would involve a vertical movement (moving the eyes up to see more clearly) (Nilsson et al., 2003), but in some circumstances, such as a very irregularly shaped scotoma, a different TRL location may be selected, perhaps so that the region of retina with best visual acuity is used for fixation (Déruaz et al., 2006). It is important to note that most people with macular disease select a PRL naturally, and training them to adopt a different strategy for one task, such as reading, may impact their ability to perform a different task, such as to walk around safely.

Techniques to Assist Training Eccentric Viewing

Some people find EV very difficult to understand and achieve. With this in mind, a number of methods have been suggested to try to make the instructions easier to follow.

Asking the patient to centrally fixate an eccentric target is one possibility, and this can be done with a small spot placed adjacent to the aperture of a typoscope (Collins, 1987): the patient looks at the spot whilst attending to the letters which appear in the aperture. If they have an absolute scotoma, the spot should disappear as they fixate it accurately, and this gives them positive feedback that they are carrying out the task correctly.

It has been claimed that EV is easier to establish when looking through a telescope (Woo & Calder, 1987); this may be because the patient sees a physical boundary on the edge of the magnified field, and fixates a point on it, allowing the image from the centre of the field to be seen peripherally. The same effect may be reported on looking through a hand or stand magnifier.

Desktop electronic vision enhancement systems can also help when training EV. In this case, the patient is encouraged to fixate a point on the screen whilst moving the X–Y platform to allow successive words to pass across the optimal retinal region. This is analogous to the use of EV and SES with an optical aid, but it often appears more natural to the patient to read in a 'different' way using an electronic magnifier, because it is a novel device.

Eye Movement Training in Central Field Loss

Even if a patient uses a single PRL, they may not always make eye movements to this location and may have reduced fixation stability when eccentric viewing. Seiple and colleagues devised an eye movement training programme which involved making repeated saccades to a target: initially a dot, then a letter, then short words (Seiple et al., 2005). In a well-designed clinical trial, they found that six 2-hour long eye movement training sessions brought about significant improvement in reading speed, by an average of 27 words per minute. Interestingly they did not find that reading speed improved after PRL awareness training or reading practice (Seiple et al., 2011).

Other Training in Central Field Loss

A randomised controlled trial has shown that reading speed and visual-related quality of life improved in people with dry AMD who performed a structured reading practice programme, but did not improve in a control group who spent the same amount of time doing crossword puzzles (Kaltenegger et al., 2019). The training involved reading words presented on a screen, one word at a time, using the Rapid Serial Visual Presentation technique, which reduces the need for eye movements (Rubin, 1994). Although the study participants did not practise reading on paper, this training improved the ability to read printed text, using a magnifier. The training did not have any effect on PRL location or fixation stability, and it is not clear exactly what mechanism caused the improvement in reading ability. The results of this study, and clinical experience, support the idea that people with central vision loss should be encouraged to practise reading as much as possible. This may well improve their vision-related quality of life.

Prism Relocation in Central Field Loss

A theoretical alternative to EV is for the patient to look directly towards an object with their fovea, and for the image to be relocated onto peripheral retina using a prism. To determine the optimal prism power and position, a four-prism dioptre lens is placed into the trial frame and rotated until the patient reports the best vision. The prism power is then increased, until vision is subjectively most clear (Romayananda et al., 1982).

A further benefit of prisms is to avoid the need to make uncomfortably large eye movements in order to use the PRL (Verezen et al., 1996). In one long-term study trying to reduce eye movements into the PRL, 40% of people prescribed prism relocation glasses kept wearing them, despite reporting negative effects including heavy weight, poor cosmesis, distortion and dizziness (Verezen et al., 2006).

In a careful randomised controlled trial, prism relocation spectacles have been shown to have no effect on visual acuity, reading speed or vision-related quality of life (Smith et al., 2005). Many of the participants in this study reported significant improvements with placebo spectacles, of equivalent weight but without a prism. Reasons for the lack of success may be the fact that people had already developed EV skills, so the prism relocation did not further help their adaptation; or that they just made a compensatory eye movement to overcome the prism, as would happen in somebody with good vision (Leat et al., 2001).

HEMIANOPIA

Training to improve visual function in hemianopia is concentrated within the first year after visual loss, once it is clear that spontaneous recovery will not occur: partial recovery occurs within 2 to 3 months in up to 20% of people with hemianopia (Kerkhoff, 2000). In later stages of the rehabilitation process,

the focus is on optical devices such as those described in Chapter 12, although training can still improve performance.

Hemianopia is very different from other visual deficits, and this must be borne in mind when deciding how to proceed. The vision loss is usually bilateral, sudden, and most frequently the result of stroke or head trauma. It may well be associated with oculomotor defects (e.g. incomitant squint leading to diplopia; or convergence insufficiency causing reading problems) or difficulties with hand-eye coordination or grip, which may affect the manual manipulation of a magnifier. There may be disorders of higher visual functions, such as the inability to name objects even though they can be seen clearly (agnosia), or neglect of one-half of the visual field even though no field defect exists (Li & Malhotra, 2015, see also Chapters 3 and 12). On the other hand, they have often received considerable rehabilitation in hospital and may be more used to training than people with purely ocular causes of visual impairment.

Visual Exploration

Visual exploration is the ability to search for, detect and recognise objects in the nonseeing hemifield (Zihl, 1995). People with hemianopia do not typically make effective voluntary eye movements into the blind area: if any movements are made, they are usually a series of very small stepwise saccades coupled with random head movements. A training programme to encourage large single saccades, preferably overshooting the target of interest, can be devised in which (over several hundred trials, and in response to an acoustic signal) patients with hemianopia learn to eliminate head movement and 'catch' a light target which appears there (Nelles et al., 2001). Patients are often taught a system scanning strategy for the blind area, for example, progressing 'row-by-row' or vertically 'column-by-column' (Kerkhoff et al., 1994; Nelles et al., 2001). Kerkhoff and colleagues emphasise the importance of extending such training (and subsequently measuring success) with 'real-life' search situations, such as improving the search time for an object on a table-top.

More recently, visual exploration training has been performed using computer programmes such as Visiocoach and free web-based applications such as Eye-Search, developed at University College London (eyesearch.ucl.ac.uk; Ong et al., 2015). As well as improving reaction times when making eye movements to the blind hemifield, Eye-Search improves self-reported difficulty on tasks like shopping, avoiding collisions and preparing meals (Szalados et al., 2021).

Reading

Depending on whether the hemianopia is right- or left-sided, the patient might experience difficulty in reading the end or beginning of lines and words. Patients with right homonymous hemianopia must be trained to ensure they have read all of the words on a line before scanning to the start of the next line; those with left hemianopia must make sure they do not miss the first word of a line. A ruler, or the patient's finger, can be placed at the right margin (for right hemianopia) or left margin (for left hemianopia) of the page, and the reader can be told to ensure they can see the ruler or finger before starting to read the next line. A modified typoscope can also be used for this purpose.

An online training system is available which specifically trains eye movements in hemianopia. The Durham Reading and Exploration Training package (DREX) encourages patients to make small precise eye movements to identify words and to read more effectively (Schuett, 2009). After about 7 hours of training, a modest improvement in reading speed is seen (Schuett et al., 2008). Read-Right is another web-based application, which uses scrolled text to train reading for people with right-sided hemianopia (readright.ucl. ac.uk; Ong et al., 2012). Unlike the scrolled text programmes used by people with central field loss, the aim of this system is to train saccadic eye movements into the blind field, rather than just to present text in a more accessible format. Perhaps surprisingly, this programme has also been shown to help people with left-sided hemianopia to read more quickly: after 5 hours of training, reading speed improved by about 15% in those with right- and left-sided hemianopia (Woodhead et al., 2015).

People with hemianopia may be able to read without difficulty for a few lines when they are concentrating for a limited period in the clinic, and this can seem at odds with their reports of severe reading difficulties at home. Having checked that spectacles, low vision aids and lighting are all appropriate, the explanation is probably the considerably greater effort (and therefore fatigue) which they experience when reading for a longer duration. They should be encouraged to practise daily to increase their reading speed and duration.

CONSTRICTED VISUAL FIELDS

Surprisingly little research has examined the effect of training eye movements on people with generalised constriction of their visual field, such as those with glaucoma or retinitis pigmentosa. Anecdotally, it was often expected that the gradual loss of vision in these conditions would mean that the individual could gradually adapt and would spontaneously develop good scanning. Both the Eye-Search and Visiocoach programmes do have specific training for tunnel vision available in them. In one study of 78 people with low vision from various causes, eye movement training was shown to improve visual search times (Kuyk et al., 2010) but only a small number of these people had peripheral field loss. In a pilot study of 25 people with retinitis pigmentosa, Ivanov and colleagues showed that eye movement training improved reaction times and gave small improvements in walking speed and avoiding obstacles (Ivanov et al., 2016).

Despite this relatively small evidence base, scanning and eye movement training is an important part of the rehabilitation of people with peripheral visual field loss. Techniques which are designed for people with other types of vision loss, such as scrolled text and SES, may also be helpful for those with tunnel vision.

REFERENCES

Amore, F. M., Fasciani, R., Silvestri, V., et al. (2013). Relationship between fixation stability measured with MP-1 and reading performance. *Ophthalmic and Physiological Optics, 33*, 611–617.

Coco-Martín, M. B., Cuadrado-Asensio, R., López-Miguel, A., et al. (2013). Design and evaluation of a customized reading rehabilitation program for patients with age-related macular degeneration. *Ophthalmology, 120*, 151–159.

Collins, J. K. (1987). Coping with the rising incidence of partial sight. *Optometry Today, 27*, 772–779.

Crossland, M. D., Crabb, D. P., & Rubin, G. S. (2011). Task-specific fixation behavior in macular disease. *Investigative Ophthalmology and Visual Science, 52*, 411–416.

Crossland, M. D., Culham, L. E., Kabanarou, S. A., et al. (2005). Preferred retinal locus development in patients with macular disease. *Ophthalmology, 112*, 1579–1585.

Crossland, M. D., Culham, L. E., & Rubin, G. S. (2004). Fixation stability and reading speed in patients with newly developed macular disease. *Ophthalmic & Physiological Optics, 24*, 327–333.

Curcio, C. A., & Allen, K. A. (1990). Topography of ganglion cells in human retina. *Journal of Comparative Neurology, 300*, 5–25.

Déruaz, A., Goldschmidt, M., Whatham, A. R., et al. (2006). A technique to train new oculomotor behavior in patients with central macular scotomas during reading related tasks using scanning laser ophthalmoscopy: Immediate functional benefits and gains retention. *BMC Ophthalmology, 6*, 35.

Dickinson, C. (2016). Evaluating the effectiveness of an established community-based eccentric viewing rehabilitation training model-The EValuation Study. *Investigative Ophthalmology & Visual Science, 57*, 3640–3649.

Fletcher, D. C. (1999). Relative locations of macular scotomas near the PRL: Effect on low vision reading. *Journal of Rehabilitation Research and Development, 36*, 356–364.

Fletcher, D. C., & Schuchard, R. A. (1997). Preferred retinal loci relationship to macular scotomas in a low-vision population. *Ophthalmology, 104*, 632–638.

Gaffney, A. J., Margrain, T. H., Bunce, C. V., et al. (2014)., & Binns, A. M. How effective is eccentric viewing training? A systematic literature review. *Ophthalmic and Physiological Optics, 34*(4), 427–437.

Gustafsson, J., & Inde, K. (2004). The MoviText method: Efficient pre-optical reading training in persons with central visual field loss. *Technology and Disability, 16*, 211–221.

Hassan, S. E., Ross, N. C., Massof, R. W., et al. (2019). Changes in the properties of the preferred retinal locus with eccentric viewing training. *Optometry and Vision Science, 96*, 79–86.

He, S., Cavanagh, P., & Intriligator, J. (1996). Attentional resolution and the locus of visual awareness. *Nature, 383*, 334–337.

Ivanov, I. V., Mackeben, M., Vollmer, A., et al. (2016). Eye movement training and suggested gaze strategies in tunnel vision—A randomized and controlled pilot study. *PLoS ONE, 11*(6), e0157825.

Kaltenegger, K., Kuester, S., Altpeter-Ott, E., et al. (2019). Effects of home reading training on reading and quality of life in AMD—A randomized and controlled study. *Graefe's Archive for Clinical and Experimental Ophthalmology, 257*, 1499–1512.

Kerkhoff, G. (2000). Neurovisual rehabilitation: Recent developments and future directions. *Journal of Neurology, Neurosurgery, and Psychiatry, 68*, 691–706.

Kerkhoff, G., Münssinger, U., & Meier, E. K. (1994). Neurovisual rehabilitation in cerebral blindness. *Archives of Neurology, 51,* 474–481.

Kuyk, T., Liu, L., Elliott, J., et al. (2010). Visual search training and obstacle avoidance in adults with visual impairments. *Journal of Visual Impairment and Blindness, 104,* 215–227.

Leat, S. J., Campbell, M. C. W., Woo, G. C., et al. (2001). Changes in fixation in the presence of prism monitored with a confocal scanning laser ophthalmoscope. *Clinical and Experimental Optometry, 84,* 132–138.

Li, K., & Malhotra, P. A. (2015). Spatial neglect. *Practical Neurology, 15*(5), 333–339.

Nelles, G., Esser, J., Eckstein, A., et al. (2001). Compensatory visual field training for patients with hemianopia after stroke. *Neuroscience Letters, 306,* 189–192.

Nguyen, N. X., Stockum, A., Hahn, G. A., et al. (2011). Training to improve reading speed in patients with juvenile macular dystrophy: A randomized study comparing two training methods. *Acta Ophthalmologica, 89,* e82–e88.

Nilsson, U. L., Frennesson, C., & Nilsson, S. E. G. (2003). Patients with AMD and a large absolute central scotoma can be trained successfully to use eccentric viewing, as demonstrated in a scanning laser ophthalmoscope. *Vision Research, 43,* 1777–1787.

Ong, Y. H., Brown, M. M., Robinson, P., et al. (2012). Read-Right: A "web app" that improves reading speeds in patients with hemianopia. *Journal of Neurology, 259,* 2611–2615.

Ong, Y. H., Jacquin-Courtois, S., Gorgoraptis, N., et al. (2015). Eye-Search: A web-based therapy that improves visual search in hemianopia. *Annals of Clinical and Translational Neurology, 2,* 74–78.

Palmer, S., Logan, D., Nabili, S., et al. (2010)., & Dutton, G. N. Effective rehabilitation of reading by training in the technique of eccentric viewing: Evaluation of a 4-year programme of service delivery. *British Journal of Ophthalmology, 94,* 494–497.

Romayananda, N., Wong, S. W., Elzeneiny, I. H., et al. (1982). Prismatic scanning method for improving visual acuity in patients with low vision. *Ophthalmology, 89,* 937–945.

Rubin, G. S. (1994). Low vision reading with sequential word presentation. *Vision Research, 34,* 1723–1733.

Schuett, S. (2009). The rehabilitation of hemianopic dyslexia. *Nature Reviews. Neurology, 5*(8), 427–437.

Schuett, S., Heywood, C. A., Kentridge, R. W., et al. (2008). Rehabilitation of hemianopic dyslexia: Are words necessary for re-learning oculomotor control? *Brain, 131,* 3156–3168.

Seiple, W., Grant, P., & Szlyk, J. P. (2011). Reading rehabilitation of individuals with AMD: Relative effectiveness of training approaches. *Investigative Ophthalmology and Visual Science, 52,* 2938–2944.

Seiple, W., Szlyk, J. P., McMahon, T., et al. (2005). Eye-movement training for reading in patients with age-related macular degeneration. *Investigative Ophthalmology and Visual Science, 46,* 2886–2896.

Smith, H. J., Dickiznson, C. M., Cacho, I., et al. (2005). A randomized controlled trial to determine the effectiveness of prism spectacles for patients with age-related macular degeneration. *Archives of Ophthalmology, 123,* 1042–1050.

Stelmack, J. A., Massof, R. W., & Stelmack, T. R. (2004). Is there a standard of care for eccentric viewing training? *Journal of Rehabilitation Research and Development, 41,* 729–738.

Sunness, J. S., Applegate, C. A., Haselwood, D., et al. (1996). Fixation patterns and reading rates in eyes with central scotomas from advanced atrophic age-related macular degeneration and Stargardt disease. *Ophthalmology, 103,* 1458–1466.

Szalados, R., Leff, A. P., & Doogan, C. E. (2021). The clinical effectiveness of Eye-Search therapy for patients with hemianopia, neglect or hemianopia and neglect. *Neuropsychological Rehabilitation, 31,* 971–982.

Tarita-Nistor, L., Brent, M. H., Steinbach, M. J., et al. (2011). Fixation stability during binocular viewing in patients with age-related macular degeneration. *Investigative Ophthalmology and Visual Science, 52,* 1887–1893.

Tarita-Nistor, L., González, E. G., Mandelcorn, M. S., et al. (2009). Fixation stability, fixation location, and visual acuity after successful macular hole surgery. *Investigative Ophthalmology and Visual Science, 50,* 84–89.

Trevor-Roper, P. (1997). *The world through blunted sight.* Souvenir Press.

Verezen, C. A., Meulendijks, C. F. M., Hoyng, C. B., et al. (2006). Long-term evaluation of eccentric viewing spectacles in patients with bilateral central scotomas. *Optometry and Vision Science, 83,* 88–95.

Verezen, C. A., Volker-Dieben, H. J., & Hoyng, C. B. (1996). Eccentric viewing spectacles in everyday life, for the optimum use of residual functional retinal areas, in patients with age-related macular degeneration. *Optometry and Vision Science, 73,* 413–417.

Vukicevic, M., & Fitzmaurice, K. (2009). Eccentric viewing training in the home environment: Can it improve the performance of activities of daily living? *Journal of Visual Impairment and Blindness, 103,* 277–290.

Walker, R., Bryan, L., Harvey, H., et al. (2016). The value of Tablets as reading aids for individuals with central visual field loss: An evaluation of eccentric reading with static and scrolling text. *Ophthalmic & Physiological Optics, 36,* 459–464.

White, J. M., & Bedell, H. E. (1990). The oculomotor reference in humans with bilateral macular disease. *Investigative Ophthalmology and Visual Science, 31,* 1149–1161.

Whittaker, S. G., Budd, J., & Cummings, R. W. (1988). Eccentric fixation with macular scotoma. *Investigative Ophthalmology and Visual Science, 29,* 268–278.

Woo, G. C., & Calder, L. (1987). Telescopic scanning and age-related maculopathy. *Optometry and Vision Science, 64,* 716–717.

Woodhead, Z. V. J., Ong, Y. H., & Leff, A. P. (2015). Web-based therapy for hemianopic alexia is syndrome-specific. *BMJ Innovations, 1,* 88–95.

Yap, Y. L., Bedell, H. E., & Abplanalp, P. L. (1986). Blind spot "fixation" in normal eyes: Implications for eccentric viewing in bilateral macular disease. *Optometry and Vision Science, 63,* 259–264.

Zeevi, Y. Y., Peli, E., & Stark, L. (1979). Study of eccentric fixation with secondary visual feedback. *Journal of the Optical Society of America, 69,* 669–675.

Zihl, J. (1995). Visual scanning behavior in patients with homonymous hemianopia. *Neuropsychologia, 33,* 287–303.

Rehabilitation Techniques for Nystagmus

Nystagmus is an involuntary ocular oscillation which includes a slow phase eye movement as part of each cycle. Visual impairment can result, either from the oscillation itself, or from an associated visual pathology. Therefore, individuals with nystagmus may benefit from magnifying devices in the same way as other visually impaired individuals. However, nystagmus also has some particular features which can be addressed by unique solutions, and these will be discussed here. Methods of treatment of the nystagmus (e.g. using systemic drugs, or surgery on the extraocular muscles, to reduce the oscillation) are beyond the scope of this book.

Nystagmus can be broadly divided into:

1. Early onset nystagmus (<6 months of age) including infantile nystagmus syndrome (INS) and fusional maldevelopment nystagmus syndrome (FMNS). (Spasmus nutans will not be considered as it disappears within the first 2 years of life and so is unlikely to be seen in a low vision clinic.)
2. Acquired nystagmus, which can occur at any age, but is very rare in young individuals. This is caused by, for example, cerebellar, brainstem or vestibular disorders and needs urgent referral to a neurologist if not previously diagnosed.

The detailed investigation and diagnosis of childhood nystagmus takes place in a few specialist tertiary centres in the UK (Self et al., 2020); and Harris et al. (2019) have proposed a specific local clinical pathway managed by orthoptists. Low vision rehabilitation does, however, form an important part of the care pathway.

A comprehensive set of information on nystagmus for parents and carers has been developed by the University of Sheffield and is available for download (University of Sheffield, 2017). In common with parents of other visually impaired children, the most frequent concerns they raise (and for which they would benefit from advice and signposting) are around education and future employment, and ability to drive. In addition, a video 'The way we see it', presented by individuals with nystagmus, has been produced by the Nystagmus Network (Nystagmus, 2015).

INFANTILE NYSTAGMUS SYNDROME

INS was formerly termed congenital nystagmus, but this was not really an appropriate term, because onset is shortly (typically a few weeks) after birth. Infantile nystagmus (IN) is a binocular involuntary ocular oscillation, almost invariably in the horizontal plane (even on vertical gaze). It is conjugate for frequency in the two eyes (typically 3–4 Hz), but may not be exactly matched in amplitude. Amplitude varies considerably between individuals (<1° to >10°), and in the same individual over time. Some individuals have a variant called periodic alternating nystagmus which undergoes a cyclical change (with a period of several minutes) in amplitude and direction,

In very general terms the rhythmic movement of the eyes has been classified as pendular or jerky. In the pendular waveform, the eye makes a slow movement which causes the retinal image to move away from the fovea and then makes a slow movement back. The waveform could be described as approximately sinusoidal with the position of the fovea corresponding to one peak of the oscillation (Fig. 14.1A).

In a jerk nystagmus, the eyes move slowly away from the target, and then make a rapid saccadic return (fast phase), before the next slow drift away (slow phase) begins. The nystagmus is described as 'left-beating' if the saccadic movements are to the left, and 'right-beating' if they are directed the opposite way. Jerk and pendular waveforms can be distinguished by direct observation of the patient's eyes.

Although the retinal image is constantly in motion, the patient is rarely aware of this and does not report oscillopsia. At most they may notice a horizontal 'smearing' or elongation of bright lights against a dark background. It is surprising that when using a magnifying device (such as a telescope), which presumably magnifies the retinal image motion, the majority of patients are still not aware of the motion. In fact, the success rate of nystagmats using telescopes is almost twice that of non-nystagmats (White et al., 1994): this may be because

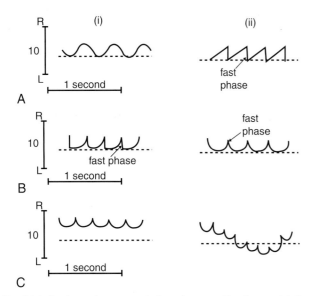

Fig. 14.1 A schematic representation of eye position (upward deflection is movement to the right *(R)*) against time in a patient with horizontal infantile nystagmus (IN). The eye position when the image falls on the fovea is indicated by a dashed line. (A) shows (i) pure pendular and (ii) jerk with fast phase to the left *(L)*, waveforms, illustrating foveation at one peak of the waveform. (B) shows the more common (i) jerk with extended foveation and (ii) pseudocycloid waveforms which have longer foveation times. (C) shows that, even if the eyes are stationary for a prolonged period, this foveation may not place the target on the fovea. In (i) the foveation is consistent, but inaccurate, whereas in (ii) it is variable over time.

nystagmats already have perceptual strategies to cope with a moving retinal image, whereas non-nystagmats are disturbed by the apparent movement of the object as they move the telescope. Exceptionally, an individual with IN *will* find that viewing through the telescope produces oscillopsia and the amount of magnification which can be used may be limited by this: nystagmats should be questioned closely when first using such a device.

Another type of nystagmus which is present from early childhood is latent or manifest latent nystagmus (LN or MLN). This has also been renamed as 'fusional maldevelopment nystagmus syndrome (FMNS)'. In this condition the nystagmus is much more noticeable when viewing is monocular, and it always takes the form of a jerk nystagmus with the fast phase towards the fixing eye. Classically, in 'LN' the nystagmus is not present at all under binocular viewing conditions, but if the patient has a squint, the suppression of one eye even when both are apparently viewing can cause the oscillation to become manifest (MLN). As suggested by the name FMNS, however, the condition is caused by an ocular condition which disrupted binocular vision during early development (e.g. infantile esotropia), so an individual with FMNS who has sufficient 'binocular' vision to experience no oscillation under binocular conditions is rare. It can be diagnosed by the change in beat direction as an occluder is moved from one eye to the other: with the left eye covered and the right fixating, it will be right-beating, but will change instantaneously to left-beating as the cover is moved over the right

eye. IN can also alter its amplitude or frequency on covering, but rarely alters its direction so consistently. The individual with FMNS is more likely to experience oscillopsia than those with IN, and this may be particularly relevant when using low-vision aids, as viewing with devices is more likely to be monocular, leading to a larger oscillation.

IN can be idiopathic or 'isolated' (indicating no known cause or origin, and no association with other conditions) or can be associated with ocular pathology which has been present from birth, such as albinism, aniridia, retinopathy of prematurity or congenital cataract. Less commonly, FMNS is also associated with such conditions. These ocular pathologies have a variety of mechanisms, some inherited, and some idiopathic nystagmus can also be inherited, with X-linked recessive, autosomal recessive and autosomal dominant patterns all being reported. In up to 50% of X-linked idiopathic cases, a defect of the *FRMD7* gene has been identified (Thomas et al., 2018). The associated pathology (if any) does not determine the characteristics of the eye movement, but is likely to affect the visual performance, and some inherited eye disease will have a poor prognosis (e.g. Leber's congenital amaurosis).

In a pure pendular or jerk nystagmus, the image spends very little time on the fovea before the eye movement takes it away, and this is not compatible with good visual acuity. In most infantile nystagmats, the waveform has been spontaneously adapted to one which affords better vision. 'Jerk with extended foveation' or 'pseudocycloid' have a long foveation period before the image drifts off the fovea and would support better acuity than a pure jerk oscillation (Fig. 14.1B). It is not just the length of the foveation period which is important, however, but its consistent placement: if the retinal image is stationary but does not coincide with the fovea (or only does so on a small percentage of the foveation periods), then again the acuity will be more limited (Fig. 14.1C). Thus, the waveform (and the foveation time it allows), foveation accuracy and foveation repeatability are likely to be more important in determining acuity than the intensity (amplitude × frequency) of the oscillation. It is believed that in an individual, the waveform develops from pendular on initial onset, to one with better foveation, during the early years of life (Theodorou et al., 2015)

The eye movement characteristics vary considerably under the influence of a number of factors, and one of the most significant is 'effort-to-see' or 'fixation attempt' (Abadi & Dickinson, 1986). This means that when the patient is relaxed and visual tests are not being conducted, the oscillation is minimal, but as soon as the patient's attention is directed to the letter chart, the oscillation becomes dramatically increased. Stress, anxiety, fatigue and illness have all been reported to increase the intensity of the oscillation.

The patient may adopt a head turn (to left or right, or chin up or down) when attempting a critical visual task. It is believed that this occurs in order to take advantage of an eye position where the ocular oscillation has a less significant influence on vision: if this 'null zone' is in eccentric gaze, and occurs when the eyes are turned to the left, for example, then an equal and opposite head turn to the right will be required to place the eyes in the null zone when viewing a target straight ahead. It may be expected that the head posture would be adopted to take advantage of a minimum intensity of oscillation, but it appears that there are often more subtle factors at work, such as the relative amount of time that the retinal image is maintained on the fovea at each gaze angle (Abadi & Whittle, 1991). Surgical rotation of the eyes can be used to place them in the required position without an accompanying abnormal head posture. Fusional maldevelopment nystagmus (FMN) also has a gaze direction corresponding to minimum nystagmus intensity, and this is usually determined by Alexander's Law. This states that the nystagmus is minimal on looking in the direction of the slow phase—for FMN, this involves adduction of the fixing eye. It may be difficult for the patient to use the optimal head posture whilst using a spectacle-mounted telescope or telemicroscope: the housing of the lenses may obscure viewing when the eyes are at the required eccentric gaze angle.

Visual Performance in Infantile Nystagmus Syndrome

Strategies adopted by the patient (often unconsciously) and methods of treatment proposed are intended to reduce the oscillation, and hence the retinal image motion, and thereby improve acuity. It is important to realise that this is only one of the three factors that can impact the visual performance in IN. These are:

1. The current oscillation
2. The deprivation effect of retinal image motion during early development
3. The associated visual pathology (if any)

With regard to (1), it has been suggested that visual performance does not increase at all when retinal image motion is prevented (Dunn et al., 2014a) but this conclusion is controversial (Dell'Osso, 2014; Dunn et al., 2014b). Even if decreasing the oscillation does not help, then any increase in oscillation should certainly be avoided, and every attempt made to exploit its minimum habitual state. Therefore, the vision should be tested when the patient is as relaxed as possible: as noted previously, 'effort to see' can cause an initial measurement of acuity to be much worse than the habitual level, and it should be measured on several occasions to ensure that an accurate baseline has been reached. If vision is only possible during limited foveation periods, this has led to the concept that nystagmats are 'slow to see' and need to be given much longer to establish fixation and extract visual information. They should be given an extended observation time and allowed to use preferred head positions. When the patient with IN is performing visual tasks, head shaking is often observed. This used to be considered to be compensatory, but is now recognized as a component of the syndrome. If the nystagmus increases in monocular viewing, then complete covering of the eye should be avoided. To test visual performance monocularly, a plus lens sufficient to blur the non-tested eye (but only by one to three lines) is recommended.

Even in idiopathic IN, with no associated ocular disease to impair vision, point (2) above will limit how much improvement is possible. The visual system has never experienced stable retinal images and Abadi and King-Smith (1979) identified an 'orientation amblyopia' which meant that the detection of vertical contours was poorer than for horizontal contours (which would be less 'smeared' by the oscillation). Felius and Muhanna (2013) also identified poorer acuity in those children whose nystagmus waveform took longer, in the first few years of life, to transition from pendular to one with longer foveation times. That is, children who spent more of their critical period of development with uncontrolled retinal image motion had a poorer visual outcome.

With regard to (3), the advent of optical coherence tomography (OCT) has made the diagnosis of idiopathic IN less common, as subtle ocular abnormalities (such as foveal hypoplasia) are often identified that would previously have gone undetected. However, many of the conditions associated with IN are stable throughout life (e.g. aniridia, albinism).

Optical Strategies Specific to Infantile Nystagmus Syndrome

Although surgery can be used to remove the need for a head posture in INS, if the gaze angle is not extreme, then bilateral prisms can be used instead to produce the required gaze deviation (Fig. 14.2A). The beneficial effect of prisms (or surgery) is often greater than would have been predicted by simply measuring the nystagmat's acuity whilst adopting their abnormal head position: it appears that the more relaxed head posture with treatment decreases the 'effort-to-see' (Dell'Osso, 1973). The amount of prism required means that Fresnel prisms may have to be used to avoid excessive weight and thickness: unfortunately, these create chromatic aberrations, a loss of image contrast and linear reflections from the prism bases.

The nystagmus in INS is often also attenuated with convergence in near vision, and if the effect is clinically significant, the patient's eyes can almost become stationary when converging to ~20 to 30 cm. This same reduction in the oscillation whilst the patient fixates a distant acuity target can be stimulated with the use of base-out prisms to produce a converged eye position even for distance viewing (Fig. 14.2B). A standard amount of 7Δ base out for each eye is suggested as a starting point, along with modifying the distance refractive correction by adding -0.75 or -1.00 DS to allow for the slight amount of accommodation which may have been stimulated by the convergence (Hertle, 2000). If this amount of prism is sufficient, the use of a small eyesize, and high index lenses, may allow the use of lenses with surfaced prisms (rather than Fresnel prisms). If a larger prism is required, the prism can be used binocularly or monocularly because symmetrical or asymmetrical convergence is equally effective (Dickinson, 1986) and this may mean that only one eye has to suffer the poor image quality inherent in the Fresnel prisms.

Even without optical or surgical intervention, the use of a null zone in INS should be encouraged as required: reading

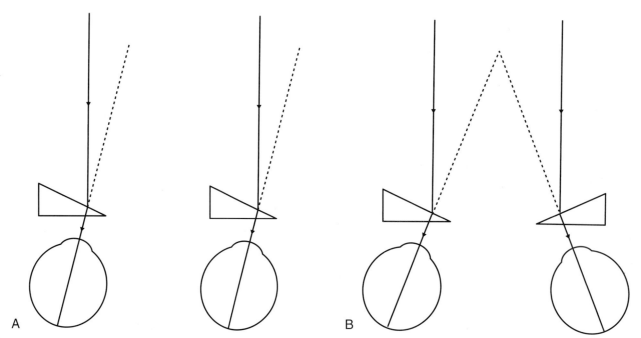

Fig. 14.2 The use of prisms to change eye position in infantile nystagmus (IN). (A) illustrates prisms base-left inducing a gaze deviation to the right to maintain fixation of an object straight ahead. (B) shows bilateral base-out prisms inducing convergence to maintain fixation of a distant object.

may be more comfortable with the book held laterally rather than straight ahead, or a child with a null zone to the left may see much better when viewing the board from a seat on the right of the classroom, compared to one on the left. If the nystagmat has strabismus, then using prism to correct the deviation may be worth trying. If this is able to support any degree of binocular vision, this can sometimes reduce the oscillation.

Individuals with IN invariably have a high refractive error with a marked (usually >3.00 DC) corneal astigmatism with-the-rule (Dickinson & Abadi, 1984). Correction of these significant refractive errors often makes little difference to the recorded visual acuity (for the reasons discussed previously), but full refractive correction should be strongly recommended (Hertle, 2000). A number of writers have suggested that the patient may benefit from contact lenses rather than spectacles (Ludlam, 1960; Abadi, 1979). Bier (1978) suggested the use of rigid scleral lenses because their bulk would physically damp the oscillation. Rigid corneal lenses may be the best choice because of their suitability for correcting the corneal astigmatism and the possibility of increased proprioceptive feedback from the eyelids leading to modification of the oscillation as the nystagmat becomes more aware of it (Taibbi et al., 2008). Other benefits of contact lenses are reduced aberrations as the lens moves with the eye, which remains looking through the optical centre, and a slightly increased amount of convergence required if the patient is a myope as they will no longer experience base-in prismatic effect from the lenses during near viewing. In fact, a randomized trial of rigid versus soft contact lenses in comparison to spectacles found there was no difference in the nystagmus characteristics between the different conditions. However, visual acuity at distance and near was significantly worse in soft contact lenses compared with

rigid lenses or spectacles (Jayaramachandran et al., 2014): it was suggested that the eye movement caused the soft lens to rotate on the eye. Glare control using contact lenses for those with albinism is discussed in Chapter 10.

ACQUIRED NYSTAGMUS

A nystagmus acquired later in life (usually due to some neurological defect) can be distinguished from IN by several characteristics: it will invariably have a pure jerk waveform (without the adaptations found in IN), may be vertical rather than horizontal (and change direction on vertical gaze), will be associated with severe oscillopsia, and have associated systemic neurological symptoms. The eye movement produces an equal and opposite movement of the image across the retina, of which the patient is constantly aware. This oscillopsia often creates feelings of nausea and disorientation and impairs vision because the image of contours perpendicular to the movement is 'smeared'. As in IN, a gaze direction can usually be found in acquired nystagmus which corresponds to minimum nystagmus intensity, and this is governed by Alexander's Law: the nystagmus intensity is minimal on looking in the direction of the slow phase. The patient can be encouraged to adopt an appropriate head position to minimise oscillopsia, or prism can be used to shift this null, as discussed earlier for IN. As the nystagmus increases away from the null zone, the sufferer may find it particularly distressing to look towards the fast phase. Whereas it can be helpful to encourage viewing into the null zone, viewing in the opposite direction should be avoided. If symptoms are extreme, it may be beneficial to suggest partial occlusion of the spectacle lenses so that viewing in this direction has to be avoided (Berrondo, 1975).

An Image Stabilisation System

A more complete solution would be to use an optical system capable of 'stabilising' the retinal image: as the eye moves, the retinal image should move by an equivalent amount so that it falls on the same point on the retina (Rushton & Rushton, 1984; Rushton & Cox, 1987; Rushton, 1989). If the object is initially imaged on the fovea, and the eye rotates, the target should appear to move to the same side so that the observer feels that they are still looking straight at the target. To specify the performance of such a system it is necessary to consider the angular rotation of the eye (θ) and the resultant amount of retinal image movement (θ'). In 'normal' vision, if the eye rotates about its centre of rotation, and the object stays still, the retinal image would be expected to move across the retina by an equivalent amount and $\theta'/\theta = 1$. Partial stabilisation is represented by $1 > \theta'/\theta > 0$, and perfect stabilisation by $\theta'/\theta = 0$. Retinal Image Stabilisation (RIS) is often expressed as a factor or percentage, and by definition this is $(1 - \theta'/\theta)$, or $(1 - \theta'/\theta)100\%$. Perfect stabilisation also means that if the eye was stationary, and an object moved in the visual field, the retinal image of this object should **not** move across the retina: although the object subtends a different angle at the centre of rotation of the eye, it should subtend the same angle at the nodal point of the eye so that it does not appear to have changed its position relative to the fovea. In Fig. 14.3 the target moves in the visual field from A to B, and looking at the angle subtended by these two positions at the centre of rotation of the eye, this is an angular movement of θ.

Considering the change in the angle subtended at the nodal point of the eye, this is θ': the eye would need to rotate by an angle θ' in order to put the retinal image back onto the fovea. In 'normal' viewing the two angles are the same—if the target moves x degrees, then the eye must rotate x degrees in order to fixate it again. In optical stabilisation, however, θ' should be zero: no matter where the object is moved to in the visual field, the image should not move and the angle it subtends at the nodal point should stay the same. This occurs when the image is formed at the centre of rotation of the eye because the image position does not change as the eye moves. As this point is approximately 13.5 mm behind the cornea, it requires a very powerful positive spectacle lens in order to focus the image at this point. This obviously then makes the image on the retina

very blurred, and a method of diverging the rays onto the retina without changing their direction is needed. This is accomplished by using a high-minus contact lens. The negative power produces the correct focus, and the fact that it moves with the eye means that objects are viewed through its optical centre and so the angle of those rays is not altered. The high plus spectacle lens and the high-minus contact lens are in fact a Galilean telescope, and for this to be afocal, the focal points of the two lenses must be coincident. Thus, the focal point of the contact lens must also be at the centre of rotation of the eye, approximately 13.5 mm behind the cornea (Drasdo, 1965) (Fig. 14.4).

$$F_{CL} = \frac{1}{f'_{CL}} = \frac{1}{-f_{CL}} = -\frac{1}{0.0135} = -74.07 DS$$

If the vertex distance $v = 0.015$ m

$$F_{SPEC} = \frac{1}{f'_{SPEC}} = \frac{1}{r + v} = \frac{1}{0.0135 + 0.015}$$
$$= \frac{1}{0.0285} = +35.09 DS$$

This Galilean telescope system is also producing angular magnification, as would be expected, and this will also aid the patient's vision.

$$M = \frac{-F_E}{F_O} = \frac{-F_{CL}}{F_{SPEC}} = \frac{-(-74.07)}{+35.09} = 2.11x$$

These powers are quite extreme, and could be difficult to achieve practically, but total stabilisation may not, in fact, be required (Leigh et al., 1988). There is commonly partial physiological compensation for the eye movement and the patient often perceives an apparent target movement which is less than the extent of the eye movement. For this patient, adequate stabilisation is achieved if the degree of retinal image movement produced by the oscillation is equal to the amount that is spontaneously compensated. In order to determine the amount of oscillation which the patient can compensate,

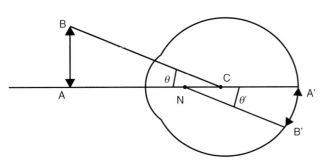

Fig. 14.3 The comparative change in the position of the object and its retinal image in normal viewing. The object shifts from **A** to **B**, showing an angular shift of θ at the centre of rotation **C**. The corresponding retinal image moves from **A'** to **B'**, through an angle of θ' subtended at the nodal point **N**.

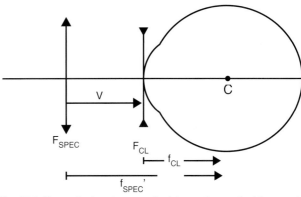

Fig. 14.4 The optical system required to produce retinal image stabilization. The Galilean telescope system consists of a contact lens F_{CL}, and a spectacle lens F_{SPEC} at a vertex distance **v**, whose focal points both lie at the centre of rotation **C** of the eye, which is 13.5 mm behind the corneal vertex.

Rushton (1986) suggests that the patient's fundus is observed with an ophthalmoscope, and the amplitude of the movement estimated relative to the horizontal disc diameter, which is approximately 5°. The patient should then observe the oscillation of a target in the visual field. An Amsler chart can be used which has squares which subtend 1° at a viewing distance of 28.5 cm, so the amplitude of the perceived movement can be estimated by judging across how many squares the fixation spot moves. Then the stabilisation required can be determined as:

$$RIS = \frac{\text{amplitude of oscillation perceived by patient}}{\text{amplitude of nystagmus observed during ophthalmoscopy}}$$

The contact lens power should then be determined as:

$$F_{CL} = -74.00 \times RIS$$

or the maximum obtainable, if this is lower.
Then

$$F_{SPEC} = \frac{1}{-f'_{CL} + v}$$

where v is the vertex distance of the spectacle lens (in metres).
Example:
A patient has a 5-degree amplitude of oscillation and perceives a 3-degree target movement. To stabilise the image sufficiently to remove the oscillopsia will require

$$RIS = \frac{3}{5} = 0.6$$

$$F_{CL} = -74.00 \times 0.6 = -44.50 DS \; (to \, nearest \, 0.25 DS)$$

The vertex distance of the spectacles is measured as 15 mm, so

$$F_{SPEC} = \frac{1}{-(-0.022) + 0.015} = \frac{1}{0.037} = +27.00 DS$$

This correction should be mounted at the correct vertex distance and verified subjectively to provide optimum acuity.
Yaniglos and Leigh (1992) perfected a −58.00 rigid gas permeable (RGP) contact lens of diameter 9.5 mm which was found to give good stabilisation of the retinal image. The front surface of the contact lens will probably be nearly plano, or even concave, over the optic zone to give the required power, and it is difficult to ensure acceptable comfort and adequate blinking. A soft contact lens could be even better, but its dimensional stability may be insufficient in the required power.

It must be realised that even if the stabilisation is successful in reducing oscillopsia and increasing vision, the optical system produces other less desirable effects. The stabilisation only exists within the field of view of the spectacle lens: beyond that will be an annular ring scotoma created by the high-powered positive lens, and then a region in which image movement can still be seen. When a normal subject makes

an eye movement, such as a saccade, the retinal image moves but the subject is not aware of it because of central compensation mechanisms. The image stabilisation device interferes with this process, as there is internal cancellation of a retinal image motion which has not occurred, so natural head and eye movements will create the perception of movement in the visual field. It is thus a system which is designed for a long-duration sedentary task, such as watching TV or reading. As with all telescopic magnifying systems, the depth-of-field is poor, and a different spectacle correction will be required to focus for near vision. It is usually necessary to restrict the system to monocular use, as the image stabilisation also disables the convergence mechanism.

REFERENCES

Abadi, R. V. (1979). Visual performance with contact lenses and congenital idiopathic nystagmus. *British Journal of Physiological Optics, 33*(3), 32–37.

Abadi, R. V., & Dickinson, C. M. (1986). Waveform characteristics in congenital nystagmus. *Documenta Ophthalmologica, 64,* 153–167.

Abadi, R. V., & King-Smith, P. E. (1979). Congenital nystagmus modifies orientational detection. *Vision Research, 19*(12), 1409–1411. https://doi.org/10.1016/0042-6989(79)90215-3.

Abadi, R. V., & Whittle, J. (1991). The nature of head postures in congenital nystagmus. *Archives of Ophthalmology, 109,* 216–220.

Berrondo, M. P. (1975). Occlusions en secteurs par parésies, vertiges, nystagmus, cyphoses, torticolis, latéralisations [Sector occlusion for paresis, vertigo, nystagmus, kyphosis, torticollis, and laterality]. *Bulletin des Societes d'Ophtalmologie de France, 75,* 149–160.

Bier, N. (1978). Contact lenses in children with nystagmus. *Metabolic Ophthalmology, 2,* 165.

Dell'Osso, L. F. (1973). Improving visual acuity in congenital nystagmus. In J. L. Smith & J. S. Glaser (Eds.), *Neuro-ophthalmology* (Vol. VII, pp. 98–106). CV Mosby.

Dell'Osso, L. F. (2014). Grating visual acuity in infantile nystagmus in the absence of image motion. *Investigative Ophthalmology & Visual Science, 55*(8), 4952–4954. https://doi.org/10.1167/iovs.14-14756.

Dickinson, C. M. (1986). The elucidation and use of the effect of near fixation in congenital nystagmus. *Ophthalmic & Physiological Optics, 6,* 303–311.

Dickinson, C. M., & Abadi, R. V. (1984). Corneal topography of humans with congenital nystagmus. *Ophthalmic & Physiological Optics, 4,* 3–13.

Drasdo, N. (1965). An experimental and clinical system for producing retinal image constraint under quasi-normal viewing conditions. *American Journal of Optometry and Archives of American Academy of Optometry, 42,* 748–756.

Dunn, M. J., Margrain, T. H., Woodhouse, J. M., et al. (2014a). Grating visual acuity in infantile nystagmus in the absence of image motion. *Investigative Ophthalmology & Visual Science, 55*(4), 2682–2686. https://doi.org/10.1167/iovs.13-13455.

Dunn, M. J., Margrain, T. H., Woodhouse, J. M., et al. (2014b). Author response: Grating visual acuity in infantile nystagmus in the absence of image motion. *Investigative Ophthalmology & Visual Science, 55*(8), 4955–4957.

Felius, J., & Muhanna, Z. A. (2013). Visual deprivation and foveation characteristics both underlie visual acuity deficits in idiopathic infantile nystagmus. *Investigative Ophthalmology & Visual Science, 54*(5), 3520–3525. https://doi.org/10.1167/iovs.13-11992.

Harris, C. M., Owen, J., & Sanders, J. (2019). Arguments for the adoption of a nystagmus care pathway. *British and Irish Orthoptic Journal, 15*(1), 82–88. https://doi.org/10.22599/bioj.126.

Hertle, R. W. (2000). Examination and refractive management of patients with nystagmus. *Survey of Ophthalmology, 45*(3), 215–222. https://doi.org/10.1016/S0039-6257(00)00153-3.

Jayaramachandran, P., Proudlock, F., Odedra, N., et al. (2014). A randomized controlled trial comparing soft contact lens and rigid gas-permeable lens wearing in infantile nystagmus. *Ophthalmology, 121*(9), 1827–1836.

Leigh, R. J., Rushton, D. N., Thurston, S. E., et al. (1988). Effects of retinal image stabilisation in acquired nystagmus due to neurologic disease. *Neurology, 38*, 122–127.

Ludlam, W. M. (1960). Clinical experience with the contact lens telescope. *American Journal of Optometry and Archives of American Academy of Optometry, 37*, 363–372.

Nystagmus Network. (2015, November 4). *Nystagmus The way we see it* [Video]. YouTube. https://www.youtube.com/watch?v=Ey-UD5Vzu_Q.

Rushton, D. N., & Rushton, R. H. (1984). An optical method for approximate stabilisation of vision of the real world. *The Journal of Physiology, 357*, 3P.

Rushton, D. N. (1986). Oscillopsia and retinal image stabilisation in patients with nystagmus. *Journal of Neurology, Neurosurgery and Psychiatry, 49*, 729.

Rushton, D., & Cox, N. (1987). A new optical treatment for oscillopsia. *Journal of Neurology, Neurosurgery and Psychiatry, 50*, 411–415.

Rushton, D. N. (1989). Geometrical optics of the retinal image stabilisation device. *Journal of Neurology, Neurosurgery and Psychiatry, 52*, 137–138.

Self, J. E., Dunn, M. J., Erichsen, J. T., et al. (2020). Management of nystagmus in children: A review of the literature and current practice in UK specialist services. *Eye (London, England), 34*(9), 1515–1534. https://doi.org/10.1038/s41433-019-0741-3.

Taibbi, G., Wang, Z. I., & Dell'Osso, L. F. (2008). Infantile nystagmus syndrome: Broadening the high-foveation-quality field with contact lenses. *Clinical Ophthalmology, 2*(3), 585. https://doi.org/10.2147/opth.s2744.

Theodorou, M., Clement, R., Taylor, D., et al. (2015). The development of infantile nystagmus. *British Journal of Ophthalmology, 99*(5), 691–695. https://doi.org/10.1136/bjophthalmol-2014-305283.

Thomas, M. G., Maconachie, G., Hisaund, M., et al. (2018). *FRMD7*-related infantile nystagmus. In M. P. Adam, G. M. Mirzaa, & R. A. Pagon (Eds.), *GeneReviews [Internet]* (pp. 1–17). University of Washington.

University of Sheffield. (2017). *Nystagmus Information pack.* Retrieved January 2, 2022, from https://www.sheffield.ac.uk/health-sciences/our-research/themes/eye-movement/nystagmus-information.

White, J. M., Porter, F. I., & Goldberg, J. (1994). Rehabilitation with telescopic spectacles in low vision patients with nystagmus. *Investigative Ophthalmology & Visual Science, 35*, 1554.

Yaniglos, S. S., & Leigh, R. J. (1992). Refinement of an optical device that stabilizes vision in patients with nystagmus. *Optometry and Vision Science, 69*, 447–450.

Sensory Substitution

NONVISUAL STRATEGIES: AUDITORY AND TACTILE INFORMATION

The most effective intervention for someone with vision impairment (VI) is usually the optimum use of residual vision, and several ways of achieving this have already been described, including magnifiers, increased contrast and improved illumination ('bigger, bolder, brighter'). An alternative, though usually more limited, approach is 'sensory substitution'; the use of a nonvisual alternative (hearing or touch) as a means of obtaining information from the environment. Of course, for an individual patient, it is not an all-or-nothing choice: use may be made of both visual and nonvisual strategies, depending on the circumstances. For example, the patient may use a magnifier for reading their mail, but for leisure 'reading' prefer to listen to audio books. The systematic use of taste or smell as useful alternative senses has not been explored, although the patient may get a useful clue about their location in the high street by the smell of fresh bread from the bakery!

THE ROLE OF SMARTPHONES, DIGITAL ASSISTANTS AND APPS

Historically, devices designed to use sensory substitution were very much identified as 'equipment for the blind'. They were only useful to a small population, often designed by enthusiasts who identified a perceived need and addressed it with great ingenuity. However, spreading the use of their device to a wider population was difficult. Often the technology was costly, needed extensive training to use, and was difficult to maintain and service: therefore, commercial companies in this field found it difficult to survive. There was also the unfamiliar appearance of the device, and the public perception of it as 'for the disabled'.

A major development in mainstream technology, the smartphone, which could be used without vision, overcame many of these difficulties, and it has the potential to be life changing for people with VI. It should be noted that the device also has many 'vision enhancement' features. Smartphones are suitable for VI users for several different reasons; they have a whole range of accessibility options in terms of changing text to speech (e.g. VoiceOver, Speak Selection) and speech control (Siri, Dictation). They have a camera so the user will be able to take a picture and magnify the view to be able to see the image more clearly or just to record information that the person cannot write down. There are also a whole range of different applications (apps): general apps that are useful for people with VI or specific apps written for people with VI. Some of these apps will allow the person to recognise an object, colours or barcodes; there are apps that work as electronic magnifiers; and those for orientation and location. Appendix 1 includes an up-to-date list of apps.

A smartphone also has a torch that can in itself be a very useful tool. But perhaps one of its greatest assets is its acceptability, as the vast majority of the population uses smartphones and the individual with VI is not going to feel singled out by using it as well. Not everybody has a smartphone available to them, however, and this also depends on age. Table 15.1 shows the difference in media use by age. Currently 86% of UK adults use a smartphone (Ofcom, 2021): this was almost zero prior to 2010.

However, if we have a look at users who are blind or VI, they are not as technology confident as the general population. Table 15.2 shows that the VI and blind population is a

TABLE 15.1 Use of Smartphones, and Media Literacy and Use by Age

16–24 Years Old	66+ Years Old
96% use a smartphone	55% use a smartphone
12% only use a smartphone to go online	2% only use a smartphone to go online
45% watch on-demand or streamed content	22% watch on-demand or streamed content
88% have a social media profile	59% have a social media profile
54% correctly identify advertising on Google (amongst search engine users)	58% correctly identify advertising on Google (amongst search engine users)
28% are aware of all four surveyed ways in which companies can collect personal data online (amongst internet users)	39% are aware of all four surveyed ways in which companies can collect personal data online (amongst internet users)
1% do not use internet	51% do not use internet

Data from Ofcom. (2021, April 28). Adult's media use and attitudes report. https://www.ofcom.org.uk/research-and-data/media-literacy-research/adults/adults-media-use-and-attitudes.

TABLE 15.2 Personal Use of Communication Devices and Services—Comparison of Blind and Vision-Impaired Population Versus Nondisabled Population

	Vision Impaired/Blind	Nondisabled
Landline	57%	56%
Internet	63%	92%
Games console	12%	24%
Computer (including PC, laptop and tablet)	53%	77%
Smartphone	46%	75%
Other phone	25%	18%

From Ofcom. (2019). Disabled users access to and use of communication devices and services—Key points. Research summary: vision-impaired people. https://www.ofcom.org.uk/__data/assets/pdf_file/0023/132962/Research-summary-all-disabilities.pdf.

TABLE 15.3 Prevention and Limitation of Use of Communications Services and Devices Amongst People With Vision Impairment (VI) or Blindness

	Personally Use	Limited by Disability	Prevented by Disability
Television	76%	20%	13%
Landline	57%	6%	4%
Internet	63%	9%	3%
Computer (including PC, laptop and tablet)	53%	10%	8%
Smartphone	46%	8%	5%
Other phone	25%	6%	7%
Games console	12%	3%	3%

From Ofcom. (2019). Disabled users access to and use of communication devices and services—Key points. Research summary: vision-impaired people. https://www.ofcom.org.uk/__data/assets/pdf_file/0023/132962/Research-summary-all-disabilities.pdf.

little behind in terms of personal use of different devices: they are more likely to have a simple mobile phone and less likely to use smartphone, computer or the internet (Ofcom, 2019).

However, those people with visual impairment or blindness who use these different technologies or services, appear to do so without limitations (Table 15.3) (Ofcom, 2019).

Individuals with visual impairment are just as likely to benefit from 'mainstream' apps as any other user, and as mentioned earlier, there are also specific apps that have been written for people with VI. Although smartphones have immense potential for users with VI, it can be very difficult to break through the barrier to reach new users: they may not be used to using technology or have (incorrect) preconceived ideas about it. It is important to bear in mind that although these apps are free, smartphones are not and some individuals may be resistant to investing in a smartphone, particularly if they are unsure if it will be suitable for them. In addition, some of the apps are not available for all phone types (or

older models). It is important not to assume that traditional sensory substitution technology is no longer useful or that 'stand-alone' devices are not as good as a phone. However, it may be that, increasingly, very specialised devices 'for the blind' are discontinued in favour of apps.

It is not a good idea to have a friend or relative who is very familiar and proficient with the device showing someone how to use the device: it really needs specialist training to be able to introduce the accessibility features of the device in the right sort of way and give helpful instructions. Local societies and Social Services departments may have specialist staff (e.g. a Digital Inclusion Officer) to offer this service. Some devices may just be too sophisticated and have too many functions, in which case a good option is the Synapptic phone (www.synapptic.com). Synapptic phones and tablets have been specifically designed for people with visual impairment and they are very intuitive and simple to use.

In addition to using voice commands to control smartphones, there are also stand-alone digital assistants which are voice controlled. The Amazon Echo, and Google Home, are examples. These devices have the advantage that they do not have controls to manipulate and all the information delivered is in auditory form. To interact with the device, the user starts their request with a key word—in the case of the Amazon Echo, this is 'Alexa, …'. It does require an initial set-up, however, and this is likely to need sighted assistance.

A digital assistant uses natural language processing to recognise what is said, and then natural language understanding to separate it into identifiable questions it can answer, or tasks it can perform. It can access multiple sources via the internet to answer questions, but (as with any internet search) it can also pick up misinformation and advertising at the top of its list of hits. Digital assistants can have specific extra programmes written for them to perform certain tasks: in the case of the Amazon Echo, these are called 'skills'. There are several thousand skills available, and the Royal

National Institute of Blind People (RNIB) have produced several of these to give verified information (e.g., '**Alexa**, how do I register as sight impaired?') or to connect to services (e.g. '**Alexa**, open RNIB Talking Books'; '**Alexa**, call RNIB Helpline'). Digital assistants can also control 'smart' household appliances such as heating or lighting, give reminders for taking medication, keep an appointment diary, check transport timetables, order food, make shopping lists, play music and many other activities.

The three major fields in which sensory substitution is used are personal communication (reading and writing), other activities of daily living (home, work, leisure and sport) and mobility and orientation.

PERSONAL COMMUNICATION

Tactile Methods

Braille and Moon Languages

The best known sensory substitution method is the tactile *Braille* alphabet. This is a written language which was invented by the Frenchman Louis Braille in 1824, but it was not universally accepted until after his death many years later. There are 63 symbols in the English version which can substitute for letters of the alphabet (with an additional symbol used to indicate a capital letter), punctuation marks and numbers. Each symbol is produced by particular combinations of up to six raised dots arranged as with the number six on a dice. Grade 1 Braille is the basic code with a substitution of the print letter for a Braille symbol, but contracted Braille (previously known as Grade 2 Braille) uses symbols for frequently recurring groups of letters or words (Fig. 15.1A). Braille is approximately 150× the bulk of inkprint, but the use of contracted Braille can reduce this by one-quarter. Space can also be saved by printing Braille in 'interpoint' style—character dots on one side of the paper between the dots on the reverse—as opposed to 'interline', where the symbols on opposite sides of the paper are on separate lines. The latter will be easier to read because the separation between successive lines of symbols will be greater. There are obviously many different foreign languages in Braille, and also some specialist international languages such as those for mathematics or music.

There are relatively few active Braille users in the UK: less than 10% of the blind population can write Braille, with double that number reading books or magazines. Most users have learnt Braille at school and are congenitally blind, but it can be learnt by people of any age or by parents of children with VI.

Learning Braille from an early age assists with literacy, as Braille is a much better method to understand punctuation, grammar and spelling than audio (RNIB, 2021e).

There are distance-learning courses, self-teaching audio-recordings, books and computer programmes available from the RNIB, there are free online training courses (Unified English Braille [UEB] Online), and it can be taught by Braille teachers and some rehabilitation officers, or in adult education classes. A difficult stage in learning Braille is the development of sufficient sensitivity in the fingertips, and 'jumbo' Braille can be used in the early stages. Decreased tactile sensitivity is often a complication of diabetes, and such patients may find the development of sufficiently sensitive touch difficult.

A machine is needed to write Braille, but this can be quite cheap and simple. A Braille Writing Frame holds the paper in position whilst a pointed metal 'dotter' or stylus is used to punch indentations through from the back. These form the raised Braille dots on the opposite side, so writing is backwards, from right to left across the page, with the symbols reversed: although the technique is very slow, the reversal does not seem to cause undue difficulties. A Braille Writing Machine (the most common of which is the Perkins Brailler) is the equivalent of a typewriter, and electronic versions are available. Such machines have six keys, each of which corresponds to one of the dots of the Braille symbol. They do not require writing in reverse, but in some the sheet produced cannot be checked until it is taken out of the machine: they are often too noisy to be used by a pupil in class, for example.

For labelling there are Braille Dymo embossing machines, and the adhesive tape which is used can also be embossed in a writing frame.

Between 500 and 800 Braille books are published each year in the UK. The RNIB Library is the major source of books, magazines and journals for adults and children. The ClearVision project based at Linden Lodge School, London, has developed a series of children's inkprint books with the standard printed pages interleaved with clear plastic sheets embossed with Braille: these allow sighted and blind siblings to share the same story, or blind parents to read to sighted children. There are a number of transcription services which can convert inkprint letters, documents, or books into Braille, but there is a time delay in getting access to material in this way. Bank statements and utility bills can be provided in Braille on request, and medicine labels (and some food packets) are now labelled in Braille.

Compared to a 'normal' visual reading speed of 200 to 300 words per minute (wpm), a good braillist is likely to achieve about 100 wpm. Even if Braille reading is too slow or requires too much effort to read for pleasure, it can still be useful in, for example, labelling, writing lists and messages, and marking dials on household appliances. There are Braille playing cards, dice and dominoes, knitting patterns and puzzles. Braille clocks and watches are also available. These usually have a hinged cover glass over the watch face. To tell the time the cover is opened, and the position of the strengthened hands is felt: the numbers are indicated by one dot on each hour, two dots at the quarter-hours, and three dots at the '12' position.

Moon is another embossed, tactile reading system, invented by Dr William Moon in 1845 (Fig. 15.1B). It has a Grade 1 form which does not abbreviate any of the words, but Grade 2 (which is usually used for books) has 45 common-sense contractions. Although it is simpler to learn than Braille (because the symbol shapes resemble those of simplified letters) and easier to feel, it has never been widely adopted. There are currently around 240 active readers borrowing Moon titles from the RNIB's National Library Service. Moon can be written on a handframe using a stylus rather like a pen or with the Moonwriter (similar to

Word	Grade 1	Grade 2
the		
understanding		
education		

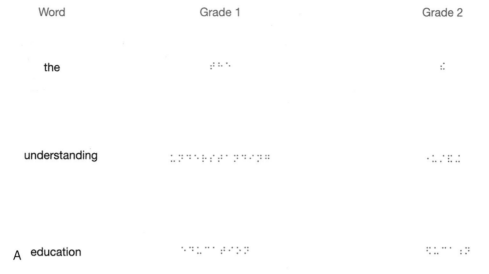

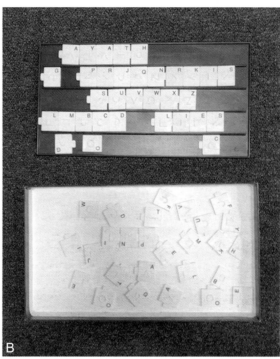

Fig. 15.1 (A) Some example words written in Grade 1 and contracted Grade 2 Braille. (B) Tiles showing Moon symbols to be used for teaching the alphabet. (A) Adapted with permission from Royal National Institute of Blind People (RNIB). (1993). Access technology: a guide to educational technology resources for visually impaired users (1993/1994 ed.).

a typewriter): in both, the symbols are embossed onto plastic sheets rather than paper. Moon is not easy to use for labelling: it is difficult to make the labels at home, and some indication needs to be present to show which way is up (a Moon comma at the end of the word is suggested). The RNIB do not currently produce Moon; however, some Moon materials are still produced in the UK for children by schools and the ClearVision project. The RNIB have decided to focus on teaching and promoting Braille but are not planning to return to active production and promotion of Moon, in line with other organisations world-wide (RNIB, 2021b). However, the RNIB remains committed to supplying existing users with books and other publications free of charge. Currently there are 1750 titles in Moon,

including leisure reading and reference books. Around 20 of these are children's titles (Cryer et al., 2009).

Auditory Methods
Audio Reading

This time, the auditory sense is the substitute for vision, with the information being delivered in verbal form. Patients can be encouraged to record letters to their family, for example, if having difficulty writing, and many public information leaflets (such as guidance on eligibility for benefits, crime prevention, or health information) are available in this format upon request. Commercial audio-transcription services can produce recordings from written documents if required. Popular messaging services have made audio delivery of information far easier.

Smartphones have free apps that can be downloaded to the phone in order to record conversations or, in this case, to record your voice—a podcast, thoughts, a shopping list, or a letter to family or friends. Communication apps, such as WhatsApp or Instagram, allow people to leave audio messages (and even video messages) to each other (rather than text messages) and this is currently a very common way of communication between sighted people.

The *RNIB Talking Book Service* was made free to access for anyone who was registered as severely sight impaired (SSI) and sight impaired (SI) in the UK in 2015. Today, there are over 30,000 SSI and SI adults and children using Talking Books. The RNIB library is the largest of its kind in Europe and contains 60,000 accessible items including their 23,000 Talking Books. Readers can access the audio books on Daisy CD, USB or as a digital download, so that they can listen to them how they choose, nowadays increasingly 'on-the-go'. Daisy CDs have the advantage of being able to search for, and bookmark, specific sections in the text: they do require a special player, or specific computer software. Anyone who is registered as SSI or SI can now borrow up to six Talking Books at any time, completely free of charge.

Calibre is a free postal lending library which is open to anyone with reading difficulties (such as dyslexia) and not just people with vision impairment. There is no fee for membership if the inability to read print is certified by a GP or ophthalmologist, or if the patient is registered. This library also lends books internationally to countries that have ratified the Marrakesh Treaty (the 2013 international copyright exceptions for people with visual impairment or those who are print disabled). Again, these books can be borrowed by members in different formats; memory stick for a period of 3 months, with a maximum of five memory sticks borrowed at one time. The books can be listened on streaming or downloaded to a smart phone device, laptop or tablet and they can be listened to on a Google Home speaker or Alexa.

The RNIB Newsagent service offers the full text of the major national daily and weekend papers. The full text is available electronically and can be read using a screen reader. Alternatively audio selections from newspapers and magazines (both general interest and specialist publications) are available in various formats such as CD, Daisy CD, USB stick, or digital download. There are currently about 200 titles, available on subscription.

The *Talking News Federation* (TNF) supports over 300 local Talking Newspapers to deliver local news and information in audio to people who are registered as SI, SSI or are print disabled. The newspapers can be listened to on CDs, memory sticks or they are available on streaming through a website or smartphone, computer or tablet. If the person has not got their own player, their local Talking Newspaper might be able to lend them one. There is also a Talking Newspaper app.

Audiobooks are available for sale in bookshops or online (via CD, USB or as a digital download), and many libraries are now lending audiobooks and e-books using an app such as Overdrive. Audiobooks are spoken by a professional actor, or even the authors themselves, whereas e-books are usually electronic speech.

Reading Machines and Desktop Scanners

Talking books offer a very useful service in leisure reading, but they are less useful in accessing technical literature or textbooks and do not allow the patient to read their own letters, for example. This would require the use of a reading machine. Such a machine can convert an image of inkprint text into synthesised speech. The input stage is via a photograph or scan of the text which is obtained by the camera on the device and this is done at a very high resolution (about 300 pixels per inch) so that print as small as N5 can be recognised.

It is, however, in the *processing stage* that the success of such devices rests, as the reading machine must perform effective optical character recognition (OCR) (Mori et al., 1992). This is typically a five-stage process:

1. Preprocessing—designed to optimise the image to compensate for poor quality, or features in the original image which will make recognition more difficult. In the latter category, any small imperfections which do not appear to be part of the letters are removed, as is any underlining of the text which might cause letters to appear joined. The image is digitised into black and white areas, but the threshold for this may be set individually for each small area of the image if there are variations in image contrast, such as in a newspaper.

2. Layout analysis—to distinguish the areas which cannot be read (such as diagrams and photographs) from those which can (text), and to arrange the text sections into a logical sequence. Photographs, for example, are often identified by the high percentage of consecutive black pixels, with very few white pixels between them.

3. The sections of text are now segmented. If this operates perfectly, then each segment should contain one whole letter, although if letters are poorly printed and touching, then two may be joined. Alternatively, a letter may be erroneously split in two.

4. Character recognition is now carried out, and there are several alternative strategies for this. Template matching is one common method, in which the unknown character is compared to all possible alternative characters, pixel by pixel. Each time a pixel matches (e.g. it is black in the unknown and black in the test), the similarity rating increases, and each time it does not match the similarity diminishes. After all possible templates have been tried, the unknown is identified as the character to which it is most similar. Alternatively, feature or structural analysis can be used. Each character is described in terms of the number and orientation of strokes, holes, arcs (concavities), cross points and end points and this analysis is unique to that particular character.

5. Ambiguity resolution allows the character recognition to be tested for feasibility and allows possible uncertainties to be resolved. This involves checking words for their appearance

in the dictionary, and spelling. For example, if there was uncertainty in segmentation about whether the character was a single 'm' or the two characters 'rn' which had become joined, then looking up the words 'harnstring' and 'hamstring' would resolve the issue. Context can also assist: if there was confusion about whether a character was '5' or 'S', then considering the characters around it and comparing '£S00' and '£500' would show that the latter was more likely. OCR systems for print reading are designed to be omni-font devices, able to handle any printed text, but they are not as successful with handwritten samples. This is partly due to the difficulty in segmenting letters which are joined together. OCR systems which recognise handwriting do exist in other fields (e.g. postcode recognition in mail-sorting operations) but the methods used are different and not transferable.

Having performed these operations, the signal is passed to the *output stage*, which uses synthesised speech to process the identified letters into word sounds. Suffixes and prefixes are identified so that, for example, the word 're-sort' would be distinguishable from 'resort'. The word is then compared to a dictionary to identify those words whose overall sound is not simply a combination of the individual letter sounds: if a special pronunciation guide is not found, the word will be pronounced phonetically. If the user has difficulty interpreting the speech, the words can be repeated, or spelt out letter-by-letter.

The earliest and most famous of these devices, introduced in 1974, was the Kurzweil Reading Machine (Kurzweil, 1976). Early versions had a high error rate in OCR but that was soon rectified, although successful handling of newsprint, the availability of a portable version with a handheld camera, and foreign language capability all took a little longer to develop. Original costs were very high with the Mark IV version of the 1980s costing over £30,000 and these machines were physically very large in size and almost exclusively based in public libraries. Current systems are dramatically more portable and available for a fraction of this price. It is also possible to add a desktop scanner accessory to a personal computer. The advantage of the reading machine is the instant access it permits to any kind of literature, including technical documents, and private letters. It is usual for the document to be scanned first and then read back at a speed (up to several hundred wpm) and with a voice (several female and male versions) which can be chosen by the user. Although some users dislike listening to synthesised speech, or find it difficult to interpret, this is normally overcome with increasing exposure. Output can be to a speech synthesiser, recorded for storage as an audio file, or to a Braille printer. It is now increasingly common for high-end desktop electronic vision enhancement systems (EVES) to have an additional text-to-speech alternative so that those who have enough remaining vision to read visually can switch to synthesised speech if they get tired.

The OrCam is a wearable (cordless) device with a smart camera, and in some versions, an LED light (that can light the text as the patient reads) that responds to a point of the patient's finger or the tap or the press of a button to read books, documents, letters, newspapers, magazines, etc. This device is also capable of recognising objects, people, colours, reading numbers, telling the date and the time, or barcode scanning, amongst other features. The device is very light and attaches to the patient's spectacles and the cost is between £2500 and £3500.

Similar functions are available using a variety of smartphone apps such as SeeingAI (available for Apple devices), Speak! (for Android devices) and EnvisionAI (for Apple and Android). SeeingAI is a free app which includes a suite of applications, all of which use the camera on a smartphone or tablet. These functions include reading printed text and handwriting, describing scenes, recognising people, identifying banknotes and colours, and identifying products using barcode recognition.

Writing is another communication problem for the visually impaired, and typing is the most effective way to produce printed documents. Vision is not needed to touch-type: once the location of four 'home keys' has been identified, the location of the other keys is known. The sighted typist would find these four keys using vision, but the blind person normally uses the keys F and J which contain some tactile marking that allows them to reset their fingers at the home row. When in a classroom or workplace, typing notes on a tablet or laptop is very practical: output from this could be inkprint, synthesised speech or Braille, if required. Smartphones and computers now allow users to dictate documents (speech-to-text) and full voice control of computers can be performed easily.

Computer Access via Speech and Braille

An excellent guide to current equipment is published by the RNIB (2021d) which produces regular reports comparing the features of similar products.

It is possible to obtain an electronic Braille display that connects to the user's phone, tablet or computer and which converts typing from either a Braille or QWERTY keyboard into Braille symbols. Also known as soft, paperless or refreshable Braille, these displays are light, compact and quiet. If built into a stand-alone computer, the tactile display is placed next to the computer keyboard to enable the user to read the contents of the screen (if present) by touch (Leventhal et al., 1990). Each 'cell' on the display line corresponds to a character on the screen and contains small plastic pins corresponding to the dots of the Braille symbol. These are moved up or down to correspond to whether a dot is present or absent in that position. To have access to the full screen simultaneously would require approximately 2000 characters and this is impractical, so the usual choice is a 40- or 20-character linear display. The half-line 40-character display requires approximately the same extent of movement as when reading a Braille book. These displays allow users to read books or textbooks, communicate with anyone, do the grocery shopping online or take notes when they are in class. The user is able to text, send emails, transcribe music or do anything their sighted peers would normally do. For this reason, some people talk of a renaissance in Braille use.

Alternatively (or sometimes additionally), the characters typed on the screen can be read using a screenreader feeding into a speech synthesiser. The screenreader is used to select which part of the screen will be spoken: keys are usually spoken as they are pressed, and words can be spelt letter-by-letter, and individual words, lines or pages read, depending on the requirements. The equipment required for speech synthesis is usually cheaper than the Braille display, and the 'reading' is quicker which may be very important for long documents. The presence of noncharacter information (such as screen colour, highlights and underlining) can be vocalised, and the device can be set to read the status bar whenever it changes. This is much more difficult in the Braille display: the status bar may only appear for a few seconds, or the user may be unaware that it has altered. The user can carry on with another task whilst listening to the speech output, and could even be away from the computer. Whilst auditory access can be extremely useful, it is not inevitably the best option. Braille is particularly helpful for checking mathematical symbols which are difficult to convert into speech and is silent in operation: the user could be talking on the telephone whilst referring to items on the screen. As noted previously, it also has the advantage that the user can immediately check the spelling, punctuation, grammar and layout of the screen information in addition to just the words: it is only through this use of a written language that the blind person can develop literacy. An inkprint or Braille printer/embosser can be attached to the computer for appropriate output.

Speech synthesis is part of all modern operating systems and additional software is not always needed. It could be argued that with effective speech synthesis, Braille has been made redundant by modern technology. This is, however, equivalent to a sighted person saying that they will never need to use a pen and paper again: even though, it seems unsophisticated, the hand writing frame and stylus are still used by many blind people to make labels or jot down lists (Johnson, 1989; Schroeder, 1989; Stephens, 1989). It is also possible using a Braille printer to get access to Braille very much more easily and quickly than was previously the case, thus enhancing the use and popularity of the medium. In 2011, the chair of the Braille Authority of North America (BANA) highlighted some of the reasons why she thought the use of Braille was declining, such as: decisions about Braille and Braille instruction for schools often being made by administrators and others who have misconceptions about Braille being expensive, bulky and slow in coming; the general belief that Braille is complicated, outdated and only read by a few blind people; and misleading statistics on Braille readers, which have the effect of discouraging manufacturers (Dixon, 2011). The use of new technology has also been underlined as another reason for the decline in the use of Braille, as well as the increase in age and late onset of the visual impairment (Goudiras et al., 2009), the overuse of audio books, and the growing number of children with multiple disabilities and the need for them to use their remaining vision (Spungin, 1990; Castellano, 2010). Braille is no doubt the way to go for children who are blind or with very poor remaining vision; it is a crucial tool that enables children to grow in literacy, self-esteem and personal independence (Koenig & Holbrook, 2000). Learning Braille from a young age will have a great impact on their future academic success and employment opportunities (Zabelski, 2009; Bell & Mino, 2013; Bell & Silverman, 2018). The earlier that a child is introduced to Braille, the more likely that they will become a fluent reader (Willoughby & Duffy, 1989; Ryles, 1996).

Graphical user interfaces (GUI) in computer applications presents considerable challenges in adaptation for people with visual impairment. When the interface between the computer and the user is based on text input, display and output, those text characters can be converted when necessary to synthesised speech or Braille. In GUI, however, the information is often presented in the form of pictures, and the user issues commands by clicking on menu items, or dragging objects around the screen with a mouse. This is not feasible for the blind user, and the Commission of the European Union funded a project to consider possible solutions. A report was issued in 1995 (GUIB Consortium, 1995) detailing the situation, but this will be an area of considerable change in the next few years. The GUIB uses a new input/output device, called GUIDE, which integrates vertical and horizontal Braille displays, two loudspeakers and a touch-sensitive tablet. This device allows blind users to experiment with direct manipulation and two-dimensional (2D) spatial sound presentation. There is another interdisciplinary research project focused on solving the GUI issues and this is The Mercator for X Windows. The Mercator replaces the spatial graphical display with a hierarchical auditory interface, adding speech synthesis system to the standard desktop configuration. Both approaches provide a way of translating a graphical interface into a nonvisual medium that will satisfy different type of users (Mynatt & Weber, 1994).

Desktop accessibility describes the hardware and software solution technologies that help people with visual impairment to use a computer: some are based on vision enhancement and some on sensory substitution. Microsoft Windows and Apple macOS have built-in accessibility available on desktop and laptop computers. The content from the computer can be accessed by a screen reader which will provide speech output (Windows Narrator and VoiceOver), magnification (Windows Magnifier and Zoom) or by changing the colour of how things appear on screen (i.e. high contrast, inverted colours). Other elements of the display can also be changed to suit personal preferences such as size, shape and texture of the cursor and reduction of animations. Virtual assistants (e.g. Cortana, Siri) allow the user to use their voice to perform tasks like sending emails, conducting web searches and opening applications and files. Voice recognition or dictation can also be used to compose emails and documents (RNIB, 2021c). All these features make day-to-day activities such as shopping, emailing, web browsing, accessing documents, banking or navigating the device accessible to people with severe sight impairment or sight impairment. There are other speech-recognition software available that can be installed on the user's computer. One example is Dragon NaturallySpeaking (https://www.nuance.com/en-gb/dragon.html), which was not developed or marketed for people with VI, and although, these systems can be helpful, they need training before acquiring optimum effectiveness and the set-up might require useful vision.

TABLE 15.4 Comparison of the Advantages and Disadvantages of Audio Versus Braille Access

	Audio	Braille
Advantages	High speed	Silent operation
	Reading letter by letter, by word, sentence or page	Useful for symbols with no spoken equivalent
	Simultaneous access to status bar and display information	Grammar, spelling, punctuation, layout can be all checked
Disadvantages	Disturbing to others in office or classroom (limited with bone conduction headphones)	Expensive Braille display
		Limited size of display (40 characters maximum)

Table 15.4 shows a comparison of the advantages and disadvantages of audio versus Braille access.

OTHER ACTIVITIES OF DAILY LIVING

There is a wide variety of personal and household items available which have the option of an auditory read-out of the usual digital or analogue visual display. A popular example used by many people with VI is the talking watch: other examples include an alarm clock, timer, calculator, scales, thermometer and compass. For those users with hearing difficulties, it is also possible to have a vibrating alarm clock or watch: the time is indicated by periods of vibration of the device which uses short pulses for hours, long for tens of minutes, and short for minutes.

For television, *audio description (AD)* provides narration on the details on screen. This system is becoming far more widespread, and many cinemas and theatres across the UK, as well as museums and galleries are equipped with a system that delivers AD through a headset, which is provided when the person collects their ticket. Some theatres offer audio descriptive tours and the opportunity to experience the highlights of an exhibition as part of a group and may include the option to touch or handle artefacts. Museums may offer live audio-descriptive tours on request. At the cinema, the AD normally runs every time the film is shown and is undetectable to anyone not wearing a headset (RNIB, 2021a). The majority of video on demand (VOD) platforms also offer AD on their films and programmes (e.g. BBC iPlayer, ITV Hub, All 4, My5, Netflix, Amazon Prime Video, Apple+, Disney+, iTunes, AMI Player) and more information on how to access these or how accessible they are can be found on the RNIB website (www.rnib.org.uk) (RNIB, 2021a) or the Henshaws website (www.henshaws.org.uk) (Henshaws, 2019). AD in Europe is not as well established as in the UK, although there are plans to coordinate an effective mechanism to monitor the implementation of AD to audiovisual media, at the moment the, legislation is weak (European

Broadcasting Union [EBU], 2020) and the European AD landscape is still fragmented and countries are at different stages of development (Reviers, 2016).

Research shows that 60% of adults in the UK were spontaneously aware of AD in 2013 (Ofcom, 2013). Awareness was higher amongst younger respondents (73% amongst 25- to 34-year-olds, compared to 55% amongst those aged 55 to 64, 51% amongst those aged 65 to 74 and 42% amongst those aged 75+). Spontaneous awareness of AD increased significantly from 37% in 2008 and 45% in 2009 when similar surveys were conducted.

There are many board games which have a tactile adaptation for the visually impaired. In chess, for example, the dark squares on the board are slightly raised, each square has a hole in the centre, and all pieces are the same height. Each has a peg in the bottom to be fitted into the holes in the board, and the white pieces each have a point on the top. There are many toys available for sighted children which are equally suitable for children with vision impairment: a variety of tactile stimuli, which when manipulated are rewarded with interesting sounds, makes the perfect combination.

Around the house, there are various tactile methods available to organise, label and identify items. Dials on domestic appliances can be adapted using 'Bump-ons' (which are self-adhesive plastic raised dots, also available in bright orange for an added visual stimulus) to indicate frequently used settings. Various home-made markings include matchsticks, metal nuts, or buttons, or (if a new appliance is being selected) audible click settings may be obtainable. For comestibles, there are many methods of organising and labelling which can be used. Examples might include taking the labels off dog food tins so that they can be distinguished from others; putting one elastic band round the jar of marmalade and two round the jar of jam; buying plain flour in small bags and self-raising flour in large bags, and many other possibilities. A common difficulty experienced by the visually impaired is judging when a cup has been filled. The liquid level indicator (Fig. 15.2) has prongs which hook over the edge of the cup. When the cup is almost full the circuit is completed and there is an intermittent tone and vibration (in case hearing is impaired). Then the milk is added until the cup is filled, when a continuous tone and vibration occur. Working on a similar principle is a 'rain alert' whose sensor plate is placed outdoors to give an audible warning to bring in washing.

Patients can often distinguish clothing by the feel of the material, and small items such as socks are best bought always in the same colour. For larger items whose colour must be identified, colour indicating buttons can be used. These are produced in 16 distinctive shapes, each representing a particular colour. One would be sewn inside the garment in an inconspicuous place, and the blind person could then identify colour by touch. Smartphone apps including SeeingAI can recognise colours, although at present, only bright and clear colours can be reliably identified.

Other nonvisual strategies for performing household tasks can also be found in the Knowledge Village by Henshaws

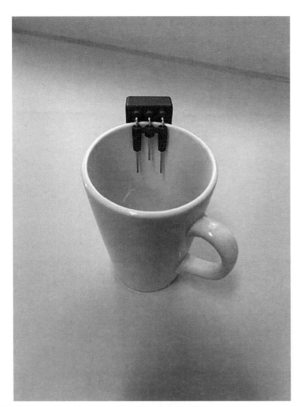

Fig. 15.2 A liquid level indicator in position for use.

(www.henshaws.org.uk/knowledge-village) and on the SightAdviceFAQ website (https://www.sightadvicefaq. org.uk/).

MOBILITY

Mobility can be defined as the physical process of independently navigating from the present position to a desired location in another part of the environment in a systematic, safe and comfortable manner. The adjective 'independently' describes a situation which, whilst desirable, is often not achievable: the person with VI will often need help crossing a busy road because they cannot distinguish individual cars approaching.

Mobility aids can be divided into two distinct categories: obstacle detectors (clear path indicators) and environmental sensors (Kay, 1974).

Obstacle Detectors

The first possibility is that the obstacle detection is carried out using the vision of another person (a *sighted guide*) or a *guide dog*: it is their direct physical contact with the person with vision impairment which then signals the presence of the obstacle, and the direction they need to travel to move around it.

Sighted Guide Technique

The purpose of this technique is for the person with vision impairment to follow half a step behind the sighted guide, with their hand holding the guide's arm slightly above the elbow. In this way, if the guide stops, or steps up or down,

this will be clearly transmitted to the follower. Usually the guide holds their contact arm bent with the hand at waist level, but if the space is narrow, the guide extends their arm backwards, and the person with visual impairment slides their hand down to grip the wrist and moves a full pace behind. This position with the arm extended should be used all the time when guiding a child, who should grip the guide's wrist, or finger. In passing through a door, the person with vision impairment should be on the same side as the hinge so that as the sighted guide pulls the door open towards them, the person with the VI can then hold it until they have both passed through. When arriving at a seat, it should be approached from behind and the sighted guide should grip the centre of the backrest: the person with vision impairment slides their hand down to the back of the chair and then moves around the chair keeping their leg in contact with it until standing with the back of the knees against the edge of the seat when they can sit down. If the person with the VI is required to wait or stand, they should always be positioned in contact with a wall whenever possible. It may help to maintain their orientation if they can 'trail'—that is, keep the back of their hand in contact with a wall as they move along.

Guide Dogs

Many people consider guide dogs synonymous with blindness, but only a small percentage of people with VI have them: about 4800 at the present time. The individual must be fit, healthy and active enough to work and care for the dog properly. Training with a guide dog is called 'new partnership training'; it takes a minimum of 5 weeks to complete and is delivered in two stages: *core skills training*—which lasts 10 days at a residential centre, where applicants will learn the skills needed to care for and work the dog; this training occurs in both group and individual settings, and *development training*—which lasts 3 weeks (minimum) and consists of 'establishing the new partnership' on known working routes and is carried out in the applicant's home and work area. The guide dog owner does not need to pay anything towards the dog or its care (i.e. food and vet bills) but there are people who decide to contribute to some or all of their dog's on-going care, although this is not expected.

White Sticks

An equally familiar 'obstacle detector' is a *white stick or cane* of which there are in fact four distinct types (any of these may be striped red and white to indicate that the user is deaf as well as blind):

1. The symbol cane is a lightweight folding cane, made from sections of hollow metal tubing joined by elastic cord (Fig. 15.3). It can be used in a limited fashion as a probe to find obstacles, but it is designed primarily to indicate that the user has a visual impairment and, for example, may step out unexpectedly to cross the road, or may require help to know which bus is coming. When not in use the cane folds up to be carried in a pocket or handbag. As a similar indication of impairment, it has been suggested that patients who have a VI should wear a lapel badge

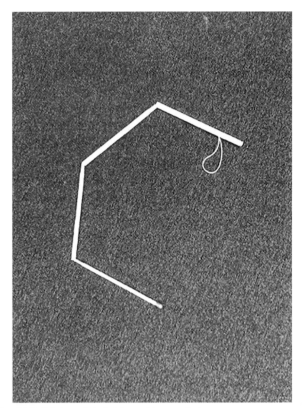

Fig. 15.3 A lightweight folding white symbol cane.

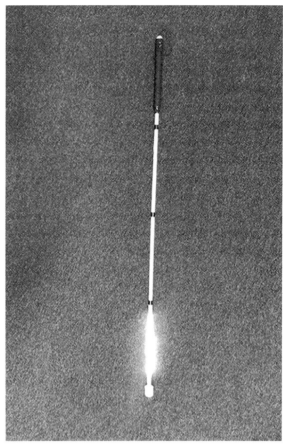

Fig. 15.5 Folding graphite long cane with LED light to make it more visible.

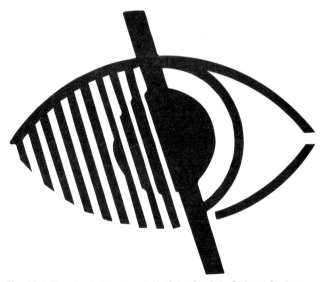

Fig. 15.4 The shaded eye symbol of the Partially Sighted Society.

bearing the shaded eye symbol (Fig. 15.4). A patient who openly uses either of these is one who has come to terms with their visual disability and will be quite willing to use low vision aids (LVAs) in public as well. The white cane in particular, however, is a powerful symbol of blindness, and many patients will completely reject its use.

2. A white walking stick is used by the patient who needs the support of a walking stick regardless of their visual impairment. These are usually available with length adjustment, and this should be set by a physiotherapist or other professional who will make sure that it offers maximum help.

3. The long cane (Fig. 15.5) and its use were developed by a group of enthusiasts at the Veterans Administration Hospital at Valley Forge in the United States in the years following World War II. By 1960, the work had progressed to the stage where a university master's course had been initiated to train 'orientation and mobility specialists' who could teach people with VI this travel technique on a one-to-one basis. Although the device itself is inexpensive, there are considerable indirect costs in the training: it may take 150 hours of tuition over several months, working from the patient's home with a mobility/rehabilitation officer of the local Social Services Department. The cane itself is a lightweight aluminium tube with a crook handle on the top, covered by a rubber grip. It reaches mid-chest height when held upright, but in use in unfamiliar surroundings, the cane is held in front of the body at an angle of about 30° to the ground and moved from side to side in an arc slightly greater than the width of the body. The cane is swung to left as user's right foot moves forward, and it touches the ground at each extreme of its travel. Some canes are fitted with roller tips, and these stay constantly in contact with the ground which helps mobility over uneven ground.

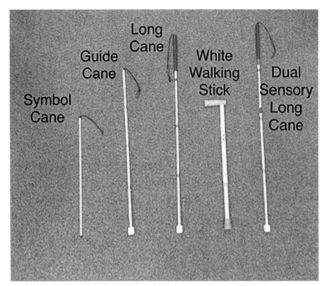

Fig. 15.6 Mobility canes. Image from Wilberforce Trust (http://www.wilberforcetrust.org.uk/) with permission from Tom Watson IT & Digital Communication Coordinator.

4. The guide cane is shorter than the long cane but longer and sturdier than a symbol cane. It is used by those patients who have some useful guiding vision, and it backs up their visual appreciation of the environment by, for example, checking the depth of steps.

Fig. 15.6 shows the different types of mobility canes.

Trailing

In a familiar or more restricted environment, the patient may not need so much advance warning and may be able to gain adequate information by following a parallel path close to the wall. In trailing, the hand nearest to the wall is held with fingers curled into the palm and with the knuckles against the wall. As the patient travels forward, the hand is moved smoothly along the wall to maintain a straight line of travel, and to detect doorways and handrails, for example. If the patient is worried about contact with an object straight ahead, the other arm can be held in front of the body with the hand placed palm towards the body, fingers pointing down, at waist height. Precautions can be taken against an obstacle at head height by raising the forearm in front of the face: this position can also be used when bending down to protect the head from the edge of a table or cupboard.

Ultrasonic and Laser Aids

Many inventors have developed 'echo-location' obstacle-detecting devices to be used by blind people, but few have been marketed commercially and none have achieved great popularity. It was initially hoped to offer a universal panacea for all the mobility problems of the blind, as these devices were likened to providing users with a navigation system similar to that of the bat. All the systems involve directing a light (laser) or ultrasound wave from an emitter on the device, which will then be reflected from nearby objects in the environment. The radiation arrives back at a detector on the device, and the distance of the reflecting object is measured by the time taken for return of

the signal. This distance is coded in an auditory or tactile form (vibration). The latter is best because the user is being bombarded by 'natural' sound cues from, for example, footsteps, echoes and traffic. In either case, the distance is usually coded by frequency (higher frequency indicating shorter distance and changing in proportion to it). The distances at which obstacles are detected are very short—a maximum range of about 5 m, but it is the closest object which generates the reflections—and it is important that the information should be as accurate as possible over such short distances. For this reason, laser sources are less useful than ultrasound because the time delays are very short (nanoseconds) and difficult to measure accurately. Sound waves are slower and therefore more accurate for distance, but they cannot detect such small objects.

Various devices have been used in the past, including the Mowat Sensor, the Sonic Pathfinder, the Sonic Guide, and the Laser Cane, but none of these systems proved as effective as a long cane or guide dog, especially in detecting objects at ground level. Both the long cane and guide dog have the disadvantage that they are unable to detect obstacles above waist height and beyond arm's length, however, and the ultrasonic aids are used to give additional information concerning these (Blasch et al., 1989). It is important that this secondary aid delivers very simple and easily understood information, as the user is already concentrating on information from the primary aid and on interpreting natural sounds from the environment.

The UltraCane (www.ultracane.com) invented by Prof Brian Hoyle's research group at the University of Leeds in 2004, for example, is an electronic long cane, which emits ultrasonic waves from two sensors to detect objects ahead (at 2 or 4 m) at chest and head height. Then, it gives tactile feedback to the user in the form of vibration from two buttons located on the cane handle, over which the user places their thumb. If the obstacle is at waist height, the bottom sensor will vibrate and if the object detected is above the waist, the top sensor will vibrate. The strength of the vibration will indicate the proximity of the object.

Another interesting gadget is the Sunu Band (www.sunu.com), a smart band that uses ultrasound to interact with the environment and feedbacks the user by vibrating. This band allows the user to navigate, together with a long cane or a guide dog, and locate objects, warning through vibration when these are too close and protecting the user's head and upper body, where the long cane and guide dog miss overhead objects. The Sunu band is worn like a watch, allowing the user to rotate their wrist to direct the ultrasound as required. It allows the user to walk around more confidently, knowing that they are not going to bump into people, walls or other objects like tree branches and also allows them to keep at a safe distance from the next person in a queue, for example. The Sunu Band app is available for iOS or Android but the Sunu Band can be used with the app or without it. Although the app is free, the Sunu Band is around £217. When used with the app, the Sunu Band is not just an object detector but also a smart watch. Some of the features that it offers are time/date telling, connection to navigation apps like Compass app to be able to navigate around the city or go to a specific address, information about places around the user's location (e.g. restaurants, museums) by connecting to Google Maps, phone finder or activity tracker amongst others.

Some high-specification smartphones now include LIDAR (light-detection and range) lasers which can provide obstacle detection with an app such as 'Super Lidar'.

Sensory Substitution Devices

Many devices considered for mobility so far have simply indicated whether there was an obstruction in the path, with perhaps some limited information about what it was, and it is necessary in most cases to get additional assistance with another aid if more detailed information is required. Sensory substitution devices (SSDs) are an attempt to provide more comprehensive information about the environment in a single device, in either tactile or auditory form, to allow the user to recognise objects and navigate independently. Equivalent devices are suggested for individuals who are profoundly deaf in order to 'hear' using other senses (Paterson, 2021).

Such SSDs for vision comprise three separate components (Kaczmarek et al., 1985):

1. Input Stage—an optical sensor or camera with the additional facility to produce a digital image. The image is focused onto an array of photodetectors, each of which converts incident light into an electrical signal. This allows the picture to be broken down into individual picture elements (pixels) and each of these gives rise to a signal proportional to its brightness.

2. Processing Stage—image processor using appropriate software to modify the image to give better representation. In the simplest case, if the signal corresponding to a given pixel brightness is above a certain threshold value, this is called 'white' and assigned a maximum value; if below threshold, the value is reduced to zero and this is 'black'. The image data are stored sequentially from a row-by-row scan down the image (top row, second row … bottom row). Some devices can process greyscale information, and vary the stimulus intensity relative to the brightness of the element of the image.

3. Output Stage—delivery of image in tactile or auditory form. Auditory devices have not been produced, but a tactile stimulator array which can deliver electrical or mechanical stimulation through a matrix of points on the skin is feasible. In the simplest system, there is a 1:1 mapping of the image onto the skin, with each stimulated point corresponding directly to a pixel in the image. In an electrical system, a matrix of electrodes is used, and the current to each is proportional to the brightness of the pixel it represents. Alternatively, mechanical stimulation uses a matrix of vibrating pins, with the amplitude of the vibration being proportional to the brightness of the corresponding pixel.

A 2D tactile stimulator array would be necessary to create point-by-point transfer of the 'image' onto a suitable area of skin, and the back of the observer was first used for this in experimental studies (Bach-y-Rita et al., 1969). Unfortunately, the skin has very poor spatial discrimination, and two adjacent stimuli must be well separated (12 mm in the Bach-y-Rita et al. [1969] experiment) before they can be individually appreciated. This means that the image can only be created from a limited number of 'points' (~400 in total). This is obviously very different from the millions of individual photoreceptors which could respond visually to an image in the retina. This difficulty of reducing a complex image to a pattern of relatively few on-off signals is also shared by the developers of bionic implants (Eiber et al., 2013).

Much of the research interest in SSDs has been in the area of brain plasticity (can the visual cortex gain access to nonvisual information?), and users need considerable training to learn how to interpret the information, so commercial rehabilitation devices have been limited.

The Optacon (**OP**tical-to-**TA**ctile **CON**verter: Cole, 1978) was an SSD designed specifically for reading, which was used around the world, but is not currently produced. This digitised an image into a display felt by the fingers, on an array of 144 miniature metal rods over an area of approximately 2 × 1 cm, to form the shape of the letter.

Several parts of the body have been used for the output device (Auvray et al., 2007) but the tongue has been found to be very sensitive: electrode separation is only 1.32 mm in the commercial Brainport Vision Pro (Grant et al., 2018). The electrode array placed in the mouth delivers stimulation to the tongue with a sensation described as gentle vibrations, tingling, or like bubbles from a fizzy drink (Stronks et al., 2016).

Object identification with audio notification can be performed with image recognition algorithms built in to apps like SeeingAI or by using human assistance, as in BeMyEyes.

ORIENTATION

This could be defined as 'the process of integrating sensory information about the environment with existing knowledge to allow one's position to be known and optimal routes of travel to be planned'. To gain such information, a sighted person would use street signs or familiar landmarks to assess the immediate area, and maps to give a longer-range picture. In the residential environment, the use of a *sound beacon* can allow the user to return to a chosen location from where the device is emitting a constant whistling or bleeping sound. This can also be used to mark the position of an object laid aside which must be collected later; an example might be a box of tools in the garden. Patients can learn to use 'natural' sound sources in this way as well: the ticking of the clock or hum of the refrigerator can give useful clues.

A basic problem can be 'am I still heading in the right direction'? A simplified version of the SSD using tactile stimulators arranged around the waist can be used. The one at the navel can indicate the required direction, and if the individual veers off course, the sensors to either right or left are triggered (Durá-Gil et al., 2017; Brandebusemeyer et al., 2021).

Even combining a navigation aid and an obstacle detector cannot always help with unpredictable obstacles such as temporary road-crossing lights, broken kerbs, or puddles. These challenges are yet to be fully solved with technology.

To gain an appreciation of the spatial relationship of locations requires the use of a 2D tactile map, presented in the usual plan view (Luxton et al., 1994), although there are limitations to these maps for some people who have never had vision: the plan view is not the intuitively obvious way in which to present information, and it is a view never seen by the traveller! Users of such maps report that they should be as simple as possible. Attempts to give extra information (such as the features of stations on a railway map) must be resisted because this information is better understood when presented on a separate sheet. Although a 2D tactile map has advantages for route planning, the 'linear' sequence offered by AD can be much easier when physically travelling the route. One-dimension linear tactile 'strip' maps are sometimes useful and are the tactile equivalent of the spoken message. Information is presented sequentially on sections of a lengthy route. Each section represents a straight section of the route, and for each new section, the user has to establish which way to orient at the start of the section (Golledge, 1991).

Global positioning system systems can locate people to within a few metres—many smart assistant devices on smartphones can answer the question 'where am I?' with accuracy. A phone app such as BlindSquare (www.blindsquare.com) determines the user's location and obtains information about the surrounding environment from FourSquare and Open Street Maps. The algorithm determines the most relevant information (current address and details about the nearest intersection and venues around) and then voices it out using high-quality speech synthesis, for example, 'found five restaurants within radius of 70 m' and will describe each of them and direct the person to the one they choose to go to. If the user is riding a bus, it will report their location (e.g. the next bus stop or the next street crossing). This app works also in indoor places, for example, shopping centres, and will guide the user around these, giving them auditory cues in advance. The app is very detailed; it alerts about intersections, location of doors, how many sets there are and where they are located in relation to the user, or the location of the lift and escalators in relation to the user's position. The user will know their options in advance and the app allows them to navigate independently and confidently without having to ask for help. This app can also access the user's Instagram, Facebook or Twitter accounts, for instance, so they can check into their favourite venues, sharing their check-ins on Facebook, Twitter and Instagram or keep them private if they wish.

Soundscape is a further app which can set audio beacons at a location such as a bus stop or corner shop. When wearing stereo headphones, the user hears the location of the beacon in the correct place in space. This system does not provide directions for how to approach the beacon but will give an indication of its relative position. Soundscape also provides a commentary of what places of interest are in the near area and can narrate what the person is passing as they walk along a street. The developers recommend using bone-conduction headphones to avoid the dangers of not being able to hear the surroundings when the ears are blocked with earphones.

SPORT FOR INDIVIDUALS WITH VISUAL IMPAIRMENT

Sensory substitution is important in adapting many sporting activities so that individuals with visual impairment can participate successfully. Several sports (e.g. skiing or triathlon) use a sighted guide, and cycling takes place on a tandem bike with a sighted pilot. In swimming, competitors may learn to count strokes or can be touched on the back by their 'tapper' as they near the edge of the pool, to give them the signal to turn. There are many different sizes and types of ball which have mechanical (ball bearings) or electronic devices to produce a sound. These ball games may also have amended rules (e.g. cricket, where the ball has to bounce twice before reaching a blind batter, rather than (usually) once as in the sighted game. In some competitive sports, to ensure parity, participants are blindfolded (e.g. all players in goalball, except the goalkeeper). Some sports use additional equipment: archers with a VI will position themselves using foot-locators to help them stand in a consistent place. They will also use a tactile sight (a rest against which to place the back of their hand which holds the bow), mounted on a tripod.

British Blind Sport (www.britishblindsport.org.uk) has details of local clubs across the UK offering a wide range of activities. Sport is generally acknowledged to be important for both physical and mental health, and it is important to make individuals with VI aware of the possibilities. There are only very rare occasions when someone with VI may be discouraged from participating: for example, if there was a high risk of retinal detachment in someone wishing to play a contact sport. Many children are introduced to sport when at school, but the opportunities may be less for the child who may be the only one with VI within a mainstream school. At the elite level, disabled sport has a high profile, and the development pathways are equivalent to those for nondisabled sport. However, overall participation in sport is relatively low. Sport at the grassroots level is not well publicised, and travelling to take part can be a major barrier for an individual with VI. If a sighted partner needs to be found this can be a further impediment, but England Athletics and British Blind Sport have developed a training and licence scheme for sighted runners wishing to become guides, and there is a national database of guide runners known as 'Find a Guide' to help individuals with VI find someone who can support them to run (https://runtogether.co.uk/get-involved/find-a-guide/).

'Parkruns' are free 5k runs which take place weekly on Saturday mornings in many local parks and open spaces. They are open to individuals with or without any experience, either walking, jogging or running, and there is no competitive element or time limit. Many local events are recruiting existing parkrunners who are willing to act as guide runners for participants with a visual impairment.

Classification in Disability Sport

If the individual with visual impairment wants to go beyond sport as a leisure activity, and enter competition, then they need to be classified with regard to the degree of their visual

TABLE 15.5 **The Visual Acuity and Visual Field Criteria for Classification of Visual Impairment Used for Competitive Disability Sport**

Classification	Status	Visual Acuity	Visual Field Diameter
B1	International	No LP, LP, perception of movement logMAR >2.60	
B2	International	≤2/60 logMAR 1.5–2.60	<10°
B3	International	>2/60–6/60 logMAR <1.5–1.0	<40°–10°
B4	British national/local	>6/60–6/24 logMAR <1.00–0.6	
B5	British national/local	>6/24–6/18 logMAR 0.59–0.48	

The standard is reached if either the visual field or visual acuity criteria are met. In Snellen visual acuity, < is used to indicate 'worse than' and > indicates 'better than'.
LP, Light perception.

impairment. This classification system is familiar across all disability sports and is the method used to place athletes in a competition against individuals with similar impairments. This is intended to ensure that the best athlete wins rather than the one with the least impairment. This sort of classification is also common in nondisabled sport, such as sex-specific races, and different weight divisions in boxing.

The classification criteria for visual impairment are shown in Table 15.5. Performance is based on the eye with better acuity, wearing optimum corrective lenses. Individuals can be classified into a particular category based on either visual acuity (VA) or field (the latter tested with an automated instrument such as the Humphrey Visual Field Analyser): if these results fall into two different categories, then the more impaired category is taken. Individuals requiring classification for recreational sport may approach their optometrist or ophthalmologist with a request to complete the relevant documentation.

It will be obvious that not all sports have the same visual requirements, and so this uniform classification system across all sports is considered to be unfair. The International Paralympic Committee is committed to sport-specific classifications, and evidence-based methods of classification (Tweedy & Vanlandewijck, 2011). This will obviously require a great deal of experimental research to determine how a particular degree of reduction in vision (impairment) affects performance in different sports (activity limitation). It is important that the tests used are likely to be repeatable (so long as the underlying eye condition does not change) and cannot be affected by training: they should be tests of the visual system and not tests of the ability to use vision. Other factors to be investigated are whether testing should be binocular (if this is usually the way in which the sport is performed) rather than based on the better eye and whether lighting needs to be taken into account. For example, an individual with albinism would have very different VA when tested outdoors in bright sunshine rather than in the consulting room.

The research into visual impairment classification is coordinated by Dr David Mann at the Faculty of Human Movement Sciences, Free University Amsterdam, Netherlands. Mann and Ravensbergen (2018) have described the process for determining sport-specific visual requirements. The first stage is to determine 'minimum impairment criteria (MIC)', which is the level of vision at which the performance of an athlete in the nondisabled (nonadapted) sport would be affected. This can be done by taking elite-level sighted athletes and having them compete with simulation spectacles to create different levels of VA, contrast sensitivity and visual field loss and find out at what level their performance deteriorates (Allen et al., 2016; Allen et al., 2018). All potential participants whose visual performance is worse than the MIC are then entitled to compete in the disabled sport, which may well be adapted, and use special equipment. Then it has to be determined whether those individuals need to be subdivided into different categories: for example, do those individuals with some vision have an advantage over those who are totally blind? This was investigated by Myint et al. (2016) for the sport of rifle shooting. They looked at elite VI competitors and correlated their performance with their visual status. As all the competitors were reliant on auditory stimuli to guide their shots, it was found that vision did not give any advantage, and all competitors within the adapted form of the sport could be within a single classification.

REFERENCES

Allen, P. M., Latham, K., Mann, D. L., et al. (2016). The level of vision necessary for competitive performance in rifle shooting: setting the standards for paralympic shooting with vision impairment. *Frontiers in Psychology, 7*, 1–8. https://doi.org/10.3389/fpsyg.2016.01731.

Allen, P. M., Ravensbergen, R. H. J. C., Latham, K., et al. (2018). Contrast sensitivity is a significant predictor of performance in rifle shooting for athletes with vision impairment. *Frontiers in Psychology, 9*, 1–10. https://doi.org/10.3389/fpsyg.2018.00950.

Auvray, M., Hanneton, S., & O'Regan, J. K. (2007). Learning to perceive with a visuo–auditory substitution system: localisation and object recognition with 'The Voice'. *Perception, 36*(3), 416–430. https://doi.org/10.1068/p5631.

Bach-y-Rita, Collins, C.C., Saunders, F. A., et al. (1969). Vision substitution by tactile image projection. *Nature, 221*, 963–964.

Bell, E. C., & Mino, N. M. (2013). Blind and visually impaired adult rehabilitation and employment survey: final results. *Journal of Blindness Innovation and Research, 3*(1).

Bell, E. C., & Silverman, A. M. (2018). Rehabilitation and employment outcomes for adults who are blind or visually impaired: an updated report. *Journal of Blindness Innovation and Research, 8*(1).

Blasch, B. B., Long, R. G., & Griffin-Shirley, N. (1989). Results of a national survey of electronic travel aid use. *Journal of Visual Impairment and Blindness, 83*, 449–453.

Brandebusemeyer, C., Luther, A. R., König, S. U., et al. (2021). Impact of a vibrotactile belt on emotionally challenging everyday situations of the blind. *Sensors, 21*(21), 7384. https://doi.org/10.3390/s21217384.

Castellano, C. (2010). *Getting ready for college begins in third grade: working toward an independent future for your blind/VI child.* Information Age.

Cole, J. (1978). Optical tactile converter. *The Optician, 27*, 7–8.

Cryer, H., Gunn, D., Home, S., et al. (2009). *International survey of tactile reading codes (Research report #6).* RNIB Centre for Accessible Information. https://www.google.com/url?sa=t&rct=j&q=&esrc=s&source=web&cd=&ved=2ahUKEwi5iNq_iIj5AhUZQkEAHT3WCCcQFnoECAUQAQ&url=https%3A%2F%2Fwww.rnib.org.uk%2Fsites%2Fdefault%2Ffiles%2F2009_08_International_survey_tactile_reading.doc&usg=AOvVaw1AU2GBNrzcFzEDgdugPgm.

Dixon, J. M. (2011). Braille: the challenge for the future. *Journal of Visual Impairment & Blindness, 105*(11), 742–744. https://doi.org/10.1177/0145482X1110501103.

Durá-Gil, J. V., Bazuelo-Ruiz, B., Moro-Pérez, D., et al. (2017). Analysis of different vibration patterns to guide blind people. *PeerJ, 2017*(3), 1–10. https://doi.org/10.7717/peerj.3082.

EBU. (2020). Describing audio description. https://www.euroblind.org/newsletter/2016/july-august/en/describing-audiodescription.

Eiber, C. D., Lovell, N. H., & Suaning, G. J. (2013). Attaining higher resolution visual prosthetics: a review of the factors and limitations. *Journal of Neural Engineering, 10*(1), 011002. https://doi.org/10.1088/1741-2560/10/1/011002.

Golledge, R. G. (1991). Tactual strip maps as navigational aids. *Journal of Visual Impairment & Blindness, 85*, 296–301.

Goudiras, D., Papadopoulos, K., & Koutsoklenis, A. (2009). Factors affecting the reading media used by visually impaired adults. *British Journal of Visual Impairment, 27*(2), 11–127. https://doi.org/10.1177/0264619609102214.

Grant, P., Maeng, M., Arango, T., et al. (2018). Performance of real-world functional tasks using an updated oral electronic vision device in persons blinded by trauma. *Optometry and Vision Science, 95*(9), 766–773. https://doi.org/10.1097/OPX.0000000000001273.

GUIB Consortium. (1995). *Textual and graphical user interfaces for blind people.* Royal National Institute for the Blind.

Henshaws. (2019). Video-on-demand services: How accessible are they? https://www.henshaws.org.uk/video-on-demand-services-how-accessible-are-they/.

Johnson, L. (1989). The importance of braille for adults. *Journal of Visual Impairment & Blindness, 83*, 285–286.

Kaczmarek, K., Bach-y-Rita, P., Tompkins, W. J., et al. (1985). A tactile vision substitution system for the blind: computer controlled partial image sequencing. *IEEE Transactions on Biomedical Engineering, 32*(8), 602–608.

Kay, L. (1974). Orientation for blind persons: clear path indicator or environmental sensor. *Journal of Visual Impairment & Blindness, 68*(7), 289–296.

Koenig, A. J., & Holbrook, M. C. (2000). *Foundations of education: Instructional strategies for teaching children and youths with visual impairments*: Vol. 2 . (2nd ed.). American Foundation for the Blind.

Kurzweil, R. (1976) A technical overview of the Kurzweil Reading Machine. *Proc National Comp Conf USA.*

Leventhal, J. D., Schreier, E. M., & Uslan, M. M. (1990). Electronic braille displays for personal computers. *Journal of Visual Impairment & Blindness, 84*, 423–427.

Luxton, K., Banai, M., & Kuperman, R. (1994). The usefulness of tactual maps of the New York City Subway system. *Journal of Visual Impairment & Blindness, 88*, 75–84.

Mann, D. L., & Ravensbergen, H. J. C. (2018). International Paralympic Committee (IPC) and International Blind Sports Federation (IBSA) joint position stand on the sport-specific classification of athletes with vision impairment. *Sports Medicine, 48*(9), 2011–2023. https://doi.org/10.1007/s40279-018-0949-6.

Mori, S., Suen, C. Y., & Yamamoto, K. (1992). Historical review of OCR research and development. *Proceedings of the IEEE, 80*, 1029–1058.

Myint, J., Latham, K., Mann, D., et al. (2016). The relationship between visual function and performance in rifle shooting for athletes with vision impairment. *BMJ Open Sport and Exercise Medicine, 2*(1), 1–7. https://doi.org/10.1136/bmjsem-2015-000080.

Mynatt, E. D., & Weber, G. (1994). Nonvisual presentation of graphical user interfaces: contrasting two approaches. *CHI '94: Proceedings of the SIGCHI Conference on Human Factors in Computing Systems, April 1994*, 166–172. https://doi.org/10.1145/191666.191732 Association for Computing Machinery.

Ofcom. (2013). *Research into the awareness of audio description.* Marketing Sciences Limited. https://www.ofcom.org.uk/research-and-data/tv-radio-and-on-demand/tv-research/audio-description-2013.

Ofcom. (2019). Disabled users access to and use of communication devices and services—Key points. Research summary: vision-impaired people. https://www.ofcom.org.uk/_data/assets/pdf_file/0023/132962/Research-summary-all-disabilities.pdf.

Ofcom. (2021). *Adult's media use and attitudes report.* https://www.ofcom.org.uk/research-and-data/media-literacy-research/adults/adults-media-use-and-attitudes.

Paterson, M. (2021). Hearing gloves and seeing tongues? Disability, sensory substitution and the origins of the neuroplastic subject. *Body and Society, 28*(1–2), 180–208. https://doi.org/10.1177/1357034X211008235.

Reviers, N. (2016). Audio description services in Europe: an update. *Journal of Specialised Translation, 26*, 232–247.

Royal National Institute of Blind People (RNIB). (1993). Access technology: a guide to educational technology resources for visually impaired users (1993/1994 ed.)

RNIB. (2021a). *Audio description (AD).* https://www.rnib.org.uk/information-everyday-living-home-and-leisure-television-radio-and-film/audio-description.

RNIB. (2021b). *Braille and Moon tactile codes.* https://www.rnib.org.uk/practical-help/reading/braille-and-moon-tactile-codes?gclid=Cj0KCQjwz96WBhC8ARIsAATR250x3g8EJnWjjohPg8odki70cON0L0HFN90OCeC8C1aCA7w-7XLpjgwaAjOaEALw_wcB.

RNIB. (2021c). *Desktop accessibility.* https://www.rnib.org.uk/sight-loss-advice/technology-and-useful-products/technology-resource-hub-latest-facts-tips-and-guides/desktop-accessibility.

RNIB. (2021d). *Technology resource hub: the latest facts, tips and guides.* https://www.rnib.org.uk/practical-help/technology/resource-hub.

RNIB. (2021e). Why is Braille important? https://www.rnib.org.uk/living-with-sight-loss/education-and-learning/braille-and-moon-tactile-codes/why-is-braille-important/.

Ryles, R. (1996). The impact of braille reading skills on employment, income, education, and reading habits. *Journal of Visual Impairment & Blindness, 90*(3), 219–226.

Schroeder, F. (1989). Literacy: the key to opportunity. *Journal of Visual Impairment & Blindness, 83,* 290–293.

Spungin, S. J. (1990). *Braille literacy: Issues for blind persons, families, professionals, and producers of braille.* American Foundation for the Blind.

Stephens, O. (1989). Braille—Implications for living. *Journal of Visual Impairment & Blindness, 83,* 288–289.

Stronks, H. C., Mitchell, E. B., Nau, A. C., et al. (2016). Visual task performance in the blind with the BrainPort V100 Vision Aid. *Expert Review of Medical Devices, 13*(10), 919–931. https://doi.org/10.1080/17434440.2016.1237287.

Tweedy, S. M., & Vanlandewijck, Y. C. (2011). International Paralympic Committee position stand-background and scientific principles of classification in Paralympic sport. *British Journal of Sports Medicine, 45*(4), 259–269. https://doi.org/10.1136/bjsm.2009.065060.

Willoughby, D. M., & Duffy, S. L. M. (1989). *Handbook for itinerant and resource teachers of blind and visually impaired students.* National Federation of the Blind.

Zabelski, M. (2009). A parent's perspective on the importance of braille for success in life. *Journal of Visual Impairment and Blindness, 103*(5), 261–263.

Inclusive and Universal Design

Definitions

Universal design has been described as a design method to achieve the inclusion of as many people as possible throughout their life. The British Standard Institute (BSI, 2005) defines inclusive design as 'The design of mainstream products and/or services that are accessible to, and usable by, as many people as reasonably possible without the need for special adaptation or specialized design'. 'Design for all' and 'Universal design' both have the same meaning. These approaches aim to build environments and websites or products that are accessible to all regardless of age, sex, capacities or cultural background. On the other hand, inclusive design acknowledges the commercial restrictions linked to fulfilling the requirements of an intended audience (Engineering Design Centre [EDC], 2017). Inclusive design suggests that it is not always possible to design a single product that addresses the needs of the entire population. However, it is recognized that what makes a product essential for some particular users will often make it more accessible and easier to use for everyone else (Persson et al., 2015). As a simple example, consider a ramp which leads to a shopping centre. It might be designed for wheelchair users, but will also help people pushing prams, those with shopping trolleys, and cyclists wheeling their bike.

Inclusive design involves developing a family of products which between them cover the majority of the population, with each product targeted to specific users. This design process should involve much more than just adding a Braille label.

The University of Cambridge have developed guidelines to assist product designers (http://www.inclusivedesigntoolkit.com/). The Royal National Institute of Blind People (RNIB) have a 'Tried and Tested' certification for some products whose accessibility and usability has been checked by a panel of visually impaired users.

There are a few principles that comprise universal design (World Blind Union [WBU], 2015):

Equitable use—The design is usable and saleable to individuals with different characteristics and income.

Flexibility in use—The design is aimed to accommodate a wide range of people with diverse abilities and preferences.

Simple and intuitive use—The use of the design is easy to understand, independently of the individual's experience, knowledge or language skills.

Perception information—The information provided by the design is sufficient so the individual can use it effectively, independently of their environment and their sensory abilities. In the case of vision, the advice given to designers is based on the size, colour and contrast of visual stimuli.

Tolerance for error—The design reduces adverse consequences from accidental or unintended actions.

Low physical effort—The design is used with minimal fatigue and in a competent and comfortable manner.

Size and space for approach and use—The size and space to use the design need to adapt to the individual's characteristics and circumstances (e.g. body size, posture, mobility).

A good example of the need for universal design is in health testing. For example, current pregnancy tests are not usable by blind women, which means that very private results have to be shared with others. The RNIB has therefore developed a prototype for a more suitable design, in the hope that it will be taken up by a commercial supplier. Another example is COVID-19 self-testing (i.e. lateral flow tests), which is not possible without sighted assistance.

Equality legislation (the *Equality Act 2010*) already requires websites to be accessible, but this is often not the case for users of screen readers or screen magnification software. The Web Content Accessibility Guidelines (WCAG) (https://www.w3.org/TR/WCAG21/) provide guidance to web designers to ensure that their content is universally accessible. Good design ensures that webpages can be accessed by all users, including those using screen readers, magnification or Braille displays.

Basic requirements for visually impaired users are to optimise text size and contrast, preferably in a way which can be selected by users. Good contrast is important, particularly for forms, tick boxes and edit fields.

More specific requirements must be met for users who access the website using screen-reader software. A logical heading structure is vital so that the user can establish a clear understanding of the overall page layout. Speech users also need to be given (audio) feedback on any actions they have executed, for example, when selecting an option or placing an item in a basket. Images and icons should come with their own short accurate spoken description ('alt text'). Decorative rather than informative images can have alt text set so that it will be ignored by the screen reader. Any video content should have audio-description, and transcripts should be available for video and audio content, with clear information added about nonverbal content.

'The Public Sector Bodies (Websites and Mobile Applications) (No.2) Accessibility Regulations 2018' came into force in 2019, with the aim of ensuring that public sector websites and mobile apps are accessible to all users, especially those with disabilities.

New public sector websites must meet these accessibility standards and publish a statement to that effect.

Recommendations for Good Practice in the Built Environment

The possibilities for improving visibility of objects or for modifying their indoor environment can be suggested and demonstrated to the patient, to be adopted as the opportunity arises: they will obviously not have their whole house reequipped and redecorated immediately, but the next time they choose wallpaper may think of choosing a pale colour to reflect light and to contrast with the carpet, for example. Occasionally, however, it is possible to make major recommendations for a complete environment, taking into account all possible factors which could make the environment more appropriate. Many care homes for older people will have a substantial proportion of their residents experiencing visual problems, and many mainstream schools will have a small number of visually impaired pupils: in either case, a low vision practitioner may be asked for advice or recommendations. These factors should also be considered when designing healthcare facilities, including optometric practices.

General Layout

Rooms should be regular rectangular shapes of moderate size, with all surfaces matt so there is no specular reflection to create a glare source. In general, the decor should be light to give ample diffuse reflection of light, with contrasting (darker) floors and doors/doorframes. The difference in reflectance between pale and dark walls is considerable, and it is desirable

to use pale decor because much of the light falling on surfaces in the environment is reflected. It is not good, however, to create large featureless white spaces: we align ourselves in our environment with reference to corners, horizons and edges, and a large area without such features is difficult to orientate in. Such orienting features can be added by using a contrasting frieze at the top of the wall, with a contrasting dado rail and dado (Fig. 16.1). The floor covering may be coloured differently to 'divide' the floor space into sections, or a route across it may be defined by contrasting surface colour or texture. It is essential that this path is free of obstructions such as chairs or tables (especially those which are low and have sharp corners).

The location of reception desks, stairs and lifts should be obvious. They should not be hidden around corners, and if the visitor is required to approach an enquiry window, the floor in front of that should be a different colour to mark its location. If there is a clear glass screen at the reception

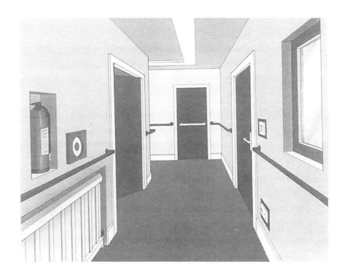

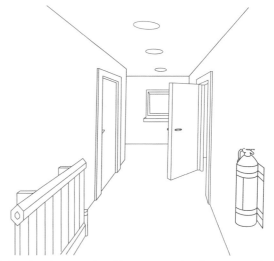

Fig. 16.1 An example of how contrasting features can be used to aid orientation within the indoor environment. In the top photo, the decor is mostly pale to increase reflectance of the natural light and the protruding objects have been enclosed to avoid a person bumping into them, contrasting with the bottom image.

window, this should not be located so that the visitor could bump their head into it. There should be a direction-finding guide in a public building—this may be a tactile or auditory map, or a telephone line to an information service, or to summon a sighted guide.

All corridors should be the same constant width, and travel in straight lines. All changes in the direction of corridors should be right-angled to maintain orientation. It is not desirable to have a zig-zag in the middle of the corridor: if it cannot travel in a straight line then a gentle curve is more acceptable. A contrasting band painted on the wall can provide orientation, and it will have breaks in it to indicate the location of doorways. The same contour could be provided by a contrasting-coloured handrail if one was required. Tactile markings on the handrail can be used to give information: at the break for a doorway, one raised dot could indicate a classroom door, two raised dots a lift door, for example. Different colours can be used for doors or walls on different floors: for example, every door on the ground floor might be red and every door on the first floor blue.

The choice of floor covering can allow use to be made of the sounds produced by footsteps or a tapping cane, to aid in orientation. The usefulness of this will be lessened if there is a lot of background noise to mask it (e.g. the sound of an escalator or machinery), and too much echo (such as in a swimming pool) makes it impossible to tell where sounds are originating. The change in texture of flooring or paving (which might, for example, be grooved or studded near a doorway) can be used to give information about an approaching hazard, or indicate a route through the area. If a building is carpeted throughout, there is no possibility of using sound clues to location, and there is no possibility of using a change in texture as a signal. It is essential to have a matt (to avoid specular reflection), nonslip floor surface with no loose coverings (such as rugs or mats).

There should be no change in floor level within a room or corridor. If one is unavoidable, warning should be given of its presence by a change in the colour or texture of the floor covering, and on a corridor the handrail or contrasting wall band should begin to slope before the step is reached. Conversely, it can be undesirable to have a change in colour or texture just for aesthetic reasons if there is NOT a difference between adjacent areas: the visually impaired person will usually think that there is a step at this point. It is better that all changes in level should be at a doorway.

Obstacles and Obstructions

Very narrow corridors and passages should be avoided because collision with wall-furniture or other people is more likely. All circulation routes should be free of obstacles: if these cannot be avoided, they should be of contrasting colour, or with rounded edges so they do not constitute a hazard. If possible, they should be extended down to ground level so that there is a greater chance of the lower part being touched with the cane or foot before the patient's body contacts them. The long-cane user cannot detect an obstacle above 0.7 m from the floor with their cane, so it will only be located when they bump into it.

It should be possible to walk down a passage close to the wall without encountering free-standing columns or pillars. This is important if the patient uses the technique of 'trailing' their hand along the wall to locate landmarks—for example, to count down the number of doorways when given an instruction such as 'it's the fourth door on the right'. Protruding display cupboards or stands should be avoided, or at least extend to ground level so that the user of a long-cane would detect them. Coat-hooks, litter bins and fire-extinguishers may be unavoidable but could be recessed into the wall: a protrusion greater than 10 cm is not acceptable (Fig. 16.2). An upper height clearance of 2.2 m from ground level should apply to awnings, signs, ladders and light fittings. Light fittings are often best recessed into the wall or ceiling, as this should also avoid a potential glare source. Shelves or cupboards should be continuous from wall to wall, so that it is not possible to

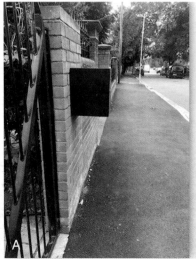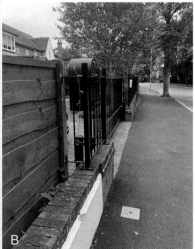

Fig. 16.2 Protruding objects can be a problem particularly if the patient uses trailing but also if they use long-cane because they will not be able to detect them. (A) Protruding mail box. (B) Recessed mail box.

walk into the edge. Windowsills, balustrades and guard-rails should not be lower than waist high. All heating appliances which constitute a fire risk should be guarded.

Lighting

Lighting should be as uniform as possible throughout the building. If daylight is to be used in some areas but not others, then the artificial light in the latter must be strong, otherwise the patient will be further impaired by the time taken to adapt when moving between these rooms. Light switches must clearly contrast with the wall or have a dark surround. Light fittings should be chosen to shield the eyes from direct light. If an area is lit by daylight, it must be possible to sit facing away from it, such as in a resident's lounge or a classroom. There must be sufficient plugs and the seating must be close enough to the walls to allow provision of localised portable task lighting as required.

The way in which the lighting changes from natural to artificial at the entrance to a building should be carefully considered, for both daytime and night-time use. There should be a 'transition zone' where possible so the change is not too sudden, and time for adaptation is provided. For example, a lobby or waiting area with tinted windows or blinds can provide a transition between a sunny street and an artificially lit doctor's surgery.

Staircases, Lifts and Escalators

Staircases should be enclosed so that it is not possible to walk into the underside (Fig. 16.3) (although access could be prevented by a trough of plants if necessary) or to step off the edge. It should not be possible to accidentally step out onto a staircase without some warning of the approach. All the steps should be equal in height and width, and preferably be in a single flight, rather than in two with a landing between. If a landing is provided at a turn in the stairs then it should be in a contrasting colour. The 'nose' of the stair treads can be highlighted in contrasting white or yellow (on both its horizontal and vertical edges) but arrangements must be made for

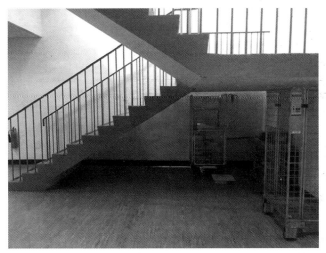

Fig. 16.3 Staircases should be enclosed to avoid the person accidentally walking underneath.

regular maintenance or cleaning if this is to be effective. Open treads, or treads which overhang the risers, should be avoided for safety reasons.

Handrails should be provided, preferably on both sides, continuing about 30 cm beyond the bottom and top steps then curving inwards to the wall to avoid injury. Raised and braille numbers placed on the handrail at the top and bottom of each flight can be used to indicate the floor number (especially when it is possible to travel many flights in a multistorey building). Glazed stairwells are common but are not desirable because at some times of day this will involve walking towards direct sunlight which can create severe discomfort glare and disorientation. The patient will also be dazzled and unable to adapt to the lower illumination level when moving into the building's interior rooms.

A change in the texture and/or colour of the flooring can be used at a sufficient distance from the top and bottom of a flight of stairs, to warn of its presence. The warning of a hazard needs to be far enough in advance for the patient to sense it, react to it, and then come to a complete stop (if required) before the hazard. Steinfield and Aiello (1980) determined that the optimum tactile signal was an area 0.5 to 1.0 m wide with ribbed contours perpendicular to the direction of travel, and on a staircase they recommended that the signal ends about 0.3 m before the staircase begins (Fig. 16.4). They emphasised that such tactile signals must be consistent, and quite unlike any floor texture being used in areas without a hazard. Such signals must be used selectively in the areas described: used indiscriminately they will lose their impact and be aesthetically unacceptable.

In the case of an escalator, it is very difficult to indicate whether travel is up or down without approaching closely enough to touch the adjacent handrail. Clear visual signs should certainly be provided, and if the risers are painted in white or yellow the direction of movement may be visible to a person standing at the bottom. When waiting for a lift car, there should be an auditory signal as it arrives, with some indication of direction such as a spoken voice announcing 'lift going up'. Lifts should have tactile large floor numbers adjacent to the buttons, and that corresponding to the main entry floor level should be in contrasting colour and shape. Emergency buttons should be of contrasting shape and colour, and separate from the floor buttons although still situated on the same panel. Ideally, the control panel should be near to eye level, but this conflicts with the need for access to be possible for a wheelchair user. There should be auditory confirmation of the floor selected, and of each floor as the lift arrives. If this is not available, then the lift door casing can be marked with braille and tactile floor numbers—as the lift arrives and the door opens the traveller can reach out to check the door frame marking and confirm their destination (Fig. 16.5).

Doors and Doorways

Glass doors and a wall glazed from floor to ceiling should have a contrasting coloured band which can be clearly seen against the background, about 1.5 m from the ground (lower if the occupants are much younger and shorter, as in a children's

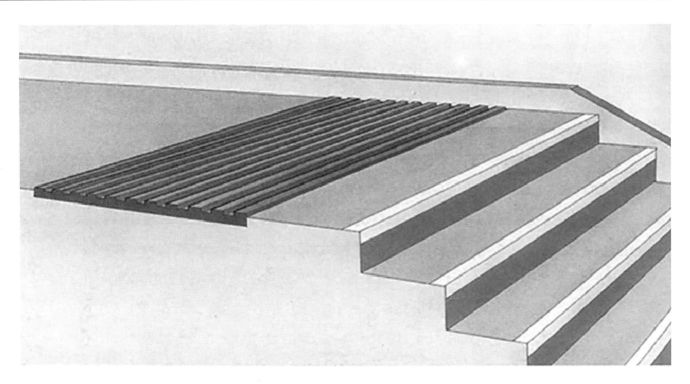

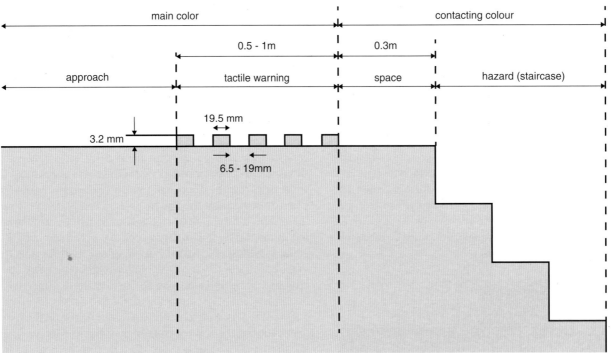

Fig. 16.4 The location and characteristics of the horizontal tactile floor ribbing recommended as a hazard indicator.

hospital). Very large windows may let in too much light and create glare: it may be better to have more smaller windows to create more even illumination. It is particularly difficult (especially for a patient with media opacities) to navigate along a corridor towards a glazed wall or large window at the far end. Doorways should be flush against the wall, because if recessed, they can appear to be the start of a corridor. Doors should open from the busier area into the less busy one (such as from a corridor into an office). A busy door which has people travelling

both ways can be disturbing, and a double-width door may well have the two halves designated for 'in' and 'out'. It is better if the door cannot be left half-open—a swing door which closes in a slow controlled manner is best, but if it can be left open it should open against a wall. This, and marking the edge of the door in a contrasting colour can avoid the patient bumping into it. Sliding doors are preferable on cupboards, especially those above waist height. Revolving doors (particularly automatic ones which stop if the pedestrian gets too close or

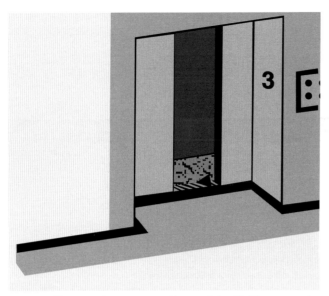

Fig. 16.5 The use of contrast to aid use of the lift. The contrasting floor colour helps to locate the interior and the door edge is marked. All symbols and indicators are contrasting and raised.

touches them) are extremely difficult, and horizontally opening automatic doors are better so long as sufficient time is allowed to navigate them. Doorways need to be wide enough for the patient to pass through with a guide dog or at the side of their sighted guide. Doors should be painted in a contrasting colour to the wall or should have a dark surround. Door handles should be large, easily gripped and clearly visible: they may be in a contrasting colour, or fixed against a coloured panel. Colour coding can be used to distinguish, for example, internal and external doors, lift doors or male and female toilet doors. If colour is being used for coding as well as contrast, then these will need to be saturated bright colours—pastels and dark shades will not be discriminated. Fine discrimination of similar colours should not be required, but would dictate the use of lighting with good colour rendering properties. Doors which open into hazardous areas may have tactile warnings on the handle, such as a roughened or ribbed surface.

Information Signs

Signs and information should be placed so that the person with low vision can walk right up to them, and touch them if possible: they should not be behind railings or high overhead. A suitably large letter size with good contrast should be chosen, and displayed in relief to provide tactile back-up: the further away the sign is, the larger the letters will need to be.

Ideally letters would be at least 16 mm high, with a narrow stroke width (<2 mm) so that the letter is not too 'crowded', and it should be raised by more than 0.8 mm. Shiny or mirrored signs are not appropriate as reflection may obscure the wording. If a floor plan or map is provided (such as at the entrance to a public building), this should be in clearly contrasting colours, and in relief. Door entry systems (such as alarms or intercoms) should have large clear keypads, and preferably audible signals to indicate that, for example, the door has opened, or the alarm has been disabled.

Outside the Building

If lighting is provided outdoors it should be even and not form isolated 'pools' under the lamps. Playgrounds must be enclosed so the patient cannot accidentally walk in: there is not only a hazard from the more obvious swings and roundabouts, but also from blundering unaware into the innocuous sand-pit. Litter bins and statues should be set to the side rather than in the centre of a concourse. For crossing roads, a safe island should be provided in the middle, which is designated by colour and texture or height change so that it is an obvious refuge. It is essential here that there is no doubt when the user has reached or left this safe location, so kerbs and steps are often required. A sloping kerb is easier to walk up and down but does not provide this safety clue: if this must be used, then grooved or studded paving should be used to indicate its location (Fig. 16.6). The slope of a kerb must be in the direction of travel, and not at an angle which would take the pedestrian in a different direction.

Under the principles of universal design, adapting the environment to make it more suitable for people with visual impairment also makes it easier for everyone else, so all these recommendations are generally applicable. It is important to consider the aesthetic appearance though, and if the suggestions are to be acceptable to an architect, the changes must be those whose benefit is clearly demonstrable. There need not necessarily be extra expense—if, for example, a staircase is planned well, it may not need a safety rail added to it. Additional costs may well be involved if the scheme includes the use of special technical aids (e.g. talking signs or sound beacons) but these have not been considered here. If technical aids are used, the costs of ongoing maintenance, and the consequences of any breakdown, must be considered in addition to the initial installation.

Roads, Footpaths and Public Spaces

There are key characteristics that are common and crucial to be able to create an inclusive and obstacle-free environment for people who are blind and partially sighted. These common features refer to colour contrast, acoustics, signage, protruding objects, detectable warning surfaces, audible pedestrian signals (APS), quiet vehicles, automatic teller machines, transport ticketing and similar machines and kiosk equipment, and transport hubs.

For the majority of the visually impaired population, driving is not permitted and cycling might be unsafe, so they rely on public transport and on walking. These are important activities for independent living, and for physical and mental health, so should be encouraged whenever possible. The design and usability of pavements, roads and crossings are therefore important, but do not always match the requirements of these users. Many individuals with visual impairment use sound to provide awareness of other road users. Therefore, cycles, e-scooters and electric cars can all be missed by pedestrians. Shared pavements where cycles and pedestrians are freely mixed (by accident or design) are particularly problematic. From mid-2019, all new electric cars registered in the UK and in the European Union had to be fitted with an

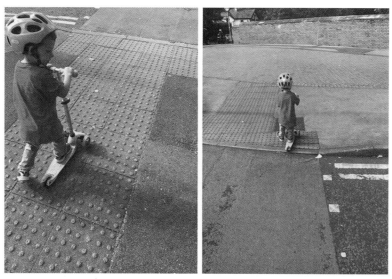

Fig. 16.6 Tactile studded paving to indicate the slope down to the road. The line of the studded paving keeps the walker in a straight line, despite the curve on the edge of the paving.

Acoustic Vehicle Alert System (AVAS) to produce sound at a certain level. Unfortunately, there is no requirement that it actually sounds like a car, which may create some confusion.

Tactile information is also very important, and this is most commonly provided by kerbs, which must be at least 60 mm high in order to be detected (Childs et al., 2009). The kerb forms a clear barrier between the pavement and the road, which is detectable by cane users, and guide dogs are also taught to stop at kerbs. A 'dropped kerb' is used to indicate a place where pedestrians are expected to cross the road. However, the safety of this location is not guaranteed: it may simply be a location where there is a pedestrian refuge halfway across the carriageway, or it may be a courtesy crossing (at neither of which are drivers legally required to stop), or a zebra crossing, or a crossing controlled by traffic lights (and drivers are legally required to stop at both of these).

Zebra crossings also have flashing orange Belisha beacons at each end, which will assist some pedestrians who cannot see the road markings. Parallel crossings (or tiger crossings) combine a zebra crossing with an adjacent lane for cyclists to ride across the road. Pelican crossings are those most adapted for the visually impaired user: the visual indicators are visible from both sides of the road (so are close to the viewer); there is often an auditory signal as well; and there may be a rotating cone under the control panel which spins when it is safe to cross.

In the effort to make urban spaces more appealing, design concepts have been introduced which have been strongly resisted by RNIB on behalf of the visually impaired population. 'Shared spaces' level out all the surfaces, removing the distinction between pavement and road, and remove all traffic signals. Pedestrians are required to establish eye contact with drivers to understand their intention, which is clearly not possible for someone who is visually impaired. In response to campaigning, the UK Government in 2018 introduced a moratorium on any new shared space schemes in England, pending further research on their consequences.

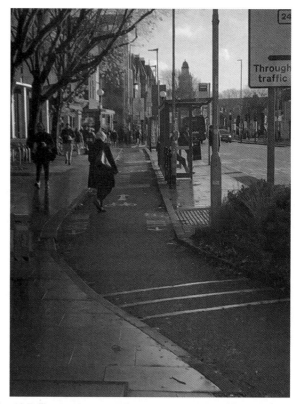

Fig. 16.7 Floating bus stop. The cycle lane veers away from the road and passes between the pavement and the bus stop. Observe how the pedestrian has to cross the cycle lane to get from the pavement to the bus stop.

The introduction of cycle lanes has led to more 'bus stop bypasses' (also known as 'floating bus stops'). Here the cycle lane veers away from the road at the bus stop, and passes between the pavement and the bus stop (Fig. 16.7). A pedestrian therefore has to cross the cycle lane to get from the pavement to the bus stop, and at best there will only be a mini-zebra crossing to assist. Another feature which can cause confusion to a pedestrian with visual impairment is the so-called 'Copenhagen crossing'. This happens at a T-junction when the pavement of the main road carries on across the side road which is joining. Although drivers are required to give way to pedestrians who have begun to cross the road, this could be alarming for the user who does not even realise that they are crossing a road.

Even with traditional pavements, there are many obstacles which can impede safe passage: parked cars, temporary road-works, café outdoor seating, advertising boards and wheelie bins are all common examples. Overhanging bushes and branches are particularly challenging because they are not detectable by the long cane or guide dog user.

Tactile Paving

The use of different textures on the ground surface, particularly outdoors, can allow the visually impaired user to identify certain features to keep them safe. For example, 'blister' paving with raised round dots is used to distinguish footpath from road in areas where the kerb has been removed (e.g. the dropped kerb at a pedestrian crossing) (Fig. 16.8). The paving is often coloured red to provide an additional clue (although there is usually little luminance contrast in the colour change). Adding different colours to other tactile paving to increase its visibility is recommended, but the red colour should be reserved for blister paving. Not all individuals are able to detect the change in texture: the shapes do need to be sufficiently raised (about 5–6 mm), but not enough to cause a trip hazard. Users of a long cane with a roller tip may find textured paving easier to interpret. People should be aware that different parts of the country use tactile markings in different ways.

The 'corduroy' surface consists of raised rounded bars, oriented perpendicular to the direction of travel, and is used to indicate a hazard (Fig. 16.9). This is used at the edge of ramps, or approaching steps, or at the junction of a footpath and shared route. A pattern of raised flat-topped circular domes is used for the edge of rail platforms, with lozenge shapes at the edge of on-street platforms (Fig. 16.10). For platforms, the tactile indicators are set back 0.5 m from the edge to allow the walker to react and stop in time. If a shared cycle track and footpath is used, it is recommended that there is a central raised strip (about 20 mm high) to help the visually impaired user to keep on the correct side. Each side of the line are raised flat-top bars: those on the footpath side in a 'ladder' formation, perpendicular to the direction of travel and those on the cycle side in a 'tramline' design, oriented the opposite way. The tactile profile is used at the start and end of the shared way, and where it joins other routes. A final tactile profile indicates a guidance path, and consists of elongated flat-topped bars running in the direction of travel. This is used to identify a pedestrian route when there are no conventional pavements: for example, through a pedestrian precinct or across a transport hub.

An 'information surface' (in a contrasting colour) can be used near to any amenity (e.g. an ATM, or post box) so that the pedestrian knows when they have reached the correct point as they walk down the footpath. This is made of

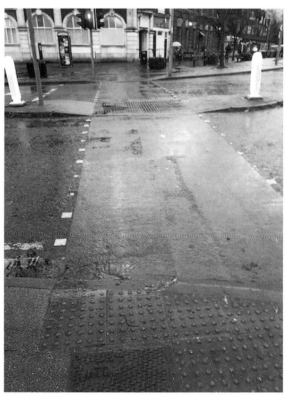

Fig. 16.8 'Blister' paving with raised round dots, used to distinguish footpath from road in areas where the kerb has been removed.

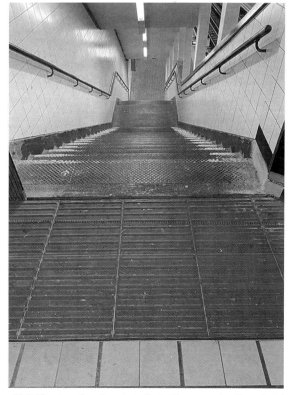

Fig. 16.9 'Corduroy' surface to indicate the approximation of stairs.

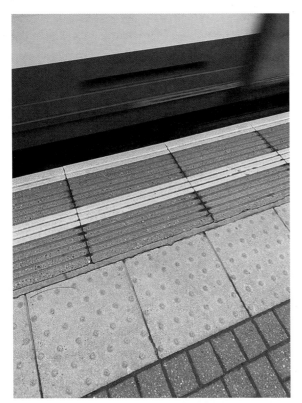

Fig. 16.10 Raised flat-topped circular domes *(yellow)* to indicate the edge of the platform and the corduroy surface (closer to the edge) to indicate imminent hazard (also observe the *bright yellow* and *grey pattern* to increase the contrast).

a rubber material which feels softer underfoot, and is flush with the normal paving surface. As with all of these modifications, it is important the user knows what the tactile marking indicates.

REFERENCES

British Standard Institute (BSI). (2005). *Design management systems—Managing inclusive design. Guide.* BSI Standards. https://knowledge.bsigroup.com/products/design-management-systems-managing-inclusive-design-guide/standard.

Childs, C., Boampong, D., Rostron, H., et al. & Accessibility Research Group. Civil, Environmental, and Geomatic Engineering University College London. (2009). Effective Kerb Heights for Blind and Partially Sighted People. UCL ARG for Guide Dogs, (October).

Engineering Design Centre (EDC). (2017). *What is inclusive design?* University of Cambridge. http://www.inclusivedesigntoolkit.com/whatis/whatis.html#p30.

Persson, H., Åhman, H., Yngling, A. A., et al. (2015). Universal design, inclusive design, accessible design, design for all: Different concepts—One goal? On the concept of accessibility—Historical, methodological and philosophical aspects. *Universal Access in the Information Society, 14*(4), 505–526. https://doi.org/10.1007/s10209-014-0358-z.

Steinfield, E., & Aiello, J. (1980). *Accessible buildings for people with severe visual impairments.* US Department of Housing and Urban Development, Office of Policy Development and Research.

World Blind Union (WBU). (2015). Universal design. *Engineers Australia, 73*(7), 13. https://doi.org/10.5100/jje.38.79.

The Low Vision Assessment

SCHEDULING THE APPOINTMENT

Depending on the clinic setting, the content and format of a low vision assessment will vary. For example, in a hospital eye service (HES) clinic, fundus examination will often have been performed in a separate clinic, so the low vision assessment comprises only history, visual assessment, refraction, prescription of magnifiers and advice. In some third-sector clinics there may be a rehabilitation worker or eye clinic liaison officer (ECLO) present, so the low vision practitioner can pass some discussions onto this other professional. For the purposes of this chapter, it will be assumed that the patient has already received appropriate ophthalmological care, is aware of their diagnosis, and that their ocular health has been assessed recently.

In community optometry practice where the practitioner is responsible for the entire eye examination, it often makes sense for the low vision assessment to be performed on a different day to the eye examination. There are three reasons for this: first, it allows the patient to plan for the low vision assessment and to bring samples of tasks they would like to perform, and any magnifiers or spectacles they have at home. Second, the additional time a low vision assessment takes can prove arduous for the patient. Finally, the bright lights used in indirect ophthalmoscopy, for example, can cause long-lasting dazzle and after-images in people with visual impairment, and it would be unreasonable to then expect reliable measurements of vision to be taken.

Funding of the assessment will also vary depending on the setting. In most hospital low vision clinics, the examination, and loan of optical magnifiers, are provided at no cost to the patient. A similar system exists in Wales: under the Wales Low Vision Scheme, accredited optometrists and dispensing opticians provide low vision assessments and loan optical (and in some cases electronic) magnifiers in community practice without charge to the patient. In other settings, the entire cost of the examination and magnifiers will be provided on a private basis. In this case, it is important that the patient is aware of the examination fee, and likely cost of any devices, before attending the appointment.

It is good practice for the patient to be aware of the purpose of the low vision assessment. Some may not see themselves as visually impaired and, if the purpose of the low vision assessment is not made clear, may choose not to attend the appointment. Others may have unrealistic expectations that medical or surgical treatment will be offered or, more commonly, that a new pair of spectacles will restore their sight. Examples of letters explaining the purpose of a low vision assessment can be found in Appendix 3.

PREPARING FOR THE ASSESSMENT

Detailed records must be kept, and a scheme devised for this. Samples of possible record forms to be used with adult and child patients can be found in Appendix 2, but each practitioner will have their own preferred format. It is unlikely that the usual practice record cards will be suitable: a great deal of information, which is quite different to that usually gathered during an eye examination, must be recorded.

People with low vision are often older adults, and in this age group the frequency of hearing loss is high: more than half of those over 80 years old have significant hearing loss. The examination should be performed in a quiet room, and a hearing loop should be considered. To facilitate lip reading, the practitioner should be well lit and not sit with a light source behind them (such as an illuminated logMAR chart), and all of the information should be explained before the patient removes their spectacles. Even slight visual impairment reduces speech-reading (i.e. the ability to interpret speech using facial expressions and body-language cues).

The room used for an assessment should be uncluttered without trip hazards or obstacles, and where possible it should be on the ground floor. The clinic should be well signposted from the main entrance of the building, it should be easily accessible by public transport, and there should be car parking (Low Vision Services Model Evaluation Collaboration, 2009).

The room lighting should be adjusted so it is comfortable for the patient: people with conditions like congenital stationary night blindness see very little in the dark so a light should be left on whenever possible. Conversely, people with achromatopsia might be extremely light sensitive, so the room light should be dimmed before they enter the room. Patients sometimes ask for the vision chart to be switched off for their acuity test; it is best to politely explain that it is important vision is measured under standardised and repeatable conditions so the chart must be switched on for this test. In this case, make sure it is turned off again after the acuity measurement is completed.

When assessing children, it is usual that a parent or carer is present during the assessment. For adults, it can be helpful for a friend, partner or carer to be present, with the patient's permission. Family members can be both a considerable hindrance to the patient's rehabilitation (perhaps trying to take tasks away from them) but are also the greatest help, and a potential partner in the rehabilitation process (e.g. by reminding the patient how to use the magnifier, buying a new reading lamp or repositioning an armchair to be nearer the television). You need to get to know the social circumstances of the patient and meeting the family in this way is very useful. They, in turn, are often confused about the patient's condition—why can he not read, and yet can see small objects dropped on the floor?—and it is often useful for them to appreciate exactly what the patient's visual standard really is—why is he registered 'blind' when he can still see? You should try and answer their questions, as well as those of the patient, whilst not letting the family become the subject of the assessment: it is the patient's needs which are paramount. All questions should be addressed to the patient themselves and not to a carer, family member or interpreter.

Make sure that everyone in the room introduces themselves to the patient, including any students or observers.

Of course, some information gathered during your assessment may be very personal medical information, and the person accompanying the patient may only be a casual acquaintance. In this case, the patient may not want that person to come into the consulting room, and this would always be respected. This can be achieved by the optometrist going to the waiting area to collect the patient and asking if they wish to be accompanied: if the patient suggests to their companion that they get some refreshments, or sit and read their newspaper, then the optometrist must be sensitive to this hint and see the patient alone.

Collecting the patient from the waiting area is a useful strategy to adopt, because it allows the first stage of the assessment to begin: the general observation of the patient.

GENERAL OBSERVATION OF THE PATIENT

This begins when first seeing the patient in the waiting room and continues throughout the assessment. It should include the following points:

- What are they doing in the waiting room? If they are reading a book or looking at their phone, note what distance they are holding it at, whether they seem to be relying on one eye, and what spectacles or magnifiers they are using.
- Are they able to hear your voice when you call their name, and do they make eye contact when you introduce yourself? Do they appear bothered by bright light, perhaps holding their head or eyes down, screwing up or shading the eyes, wearing a hat with the brim pulled down, or tinted spectacles? This suggests that the use of tints or visors, or a typoscope when reading, may need to be considered.
- Can they travel from waiting room to consulting room chair alone? Do they navigate easily across the room (suggesting moderately spared peripheral vision) alone, or do they hold their companion's arm? Can they find and position themselves in the chair easily? You need to be prepared to help the patient here and should know how to guide the patient using a 'sighted guide technique' (see Chapter 15). You would ask the patient to grasp your arm just above the elbow, and they would then follow you. If you pass through a door, the patient should be on the side on which the door is hinged so that they can hold it as you both pass through. You should also be offering a 'running commentary' in describing the route to them ('We are just approaching two steps up'; 'We are going to turn into the next door on the left'). When you arrive at the consulting room, tell them where the chair is and what colour it is. If they have been walking unguided, note their ability to locate it. If you are guiding them, take them to the chair and stand facing it, and place their hands on the arms of the chair. From this they will be able to determine the position of the seat. If the patient or their carer does not seem familiar with correct 'sighted guide' procedures, then the opportunity may be taken later to suggest how it may help them.
- Do they have an obvious tremor, or limited movement? This may limit the range of tasks which they are able to

perform, or the type of low vision aids they will be able to manipulate.

- Do they look directly at you when talking, or do they appear to view eccentrically? If they appear to be eccentrically viewing, does it seem to be by adopting one consistent direction?

CASE HISTORY

This has been described as the most important part of a low-vision assessment. It is essential to find out exactly what the patient needs and wants, and what they are expecting you to do for them: you must also use this opportunity to build a rapport with them. At the end of this appointment you will be asking them to trust your advice and recommendations, and these may not be exactly what they wanted to hear. Ask the person what they would like to be called, for example, Dr Smith or Mary? Allow the person to lead the conversation a little, so that you can get a sense of what they are most interested in and what is important to them. Try and avoid the 'interrogation' technique of repeated closed questions.

Each practitioner will adopt their own opening question (the authors' are: 'Tell me about your eyesight at the moment', 'What brought you here today?' and 'How long has your vision been affecting what you can do?').

Helpful guidelines to conducting a successful assessment are:

1. Begin the examination with easy and familiar questions, such as name, date of birth, telephone number. This allows a gross assessment of the patient's mental faculties and memory and gives the patient the opportunity to gain confidence in recognising your speech. Speak slowly and in short sentences, seeking frequent responses to be sure the patient has understood.
2. Do not randomly and repeatedly change the subject of your questioning, and when you change topics try to signal and emphasise to the patient that you are now going to talk about a different subject. This is particularly important when you are asking something personal, when a bridging phrase like 'I'm now going to ask about your family situation' can help.
3. Encourage the patient by words or sounds, rather than gestures such as nodding your head.
4. If you wish to make it clear that you are addressing the patient rather than someone else in the room, address them by name.

This history is inevitably going to take a little time: the patient must not feel rushed, or afraid to raise any matter which concerns them. It is important to explain the rather personal nature of the questions that will be asked about their everyday life, and the reason why these are necessary. It is usually better to go through the full range of questions before beginning the examination, but if answers seem contradictory or the patient becomes restless, you may wish to move on and return to some of the questions later. The topics to be covered should include:

1. Duration of condition and onset. The question 'how long have you had problems with your vision' can produce a long account of every pair of spectacles prescribed, so 'when did you start having difficulties managing with your spectacles' can often be more productive. If the condition is very recent the patient may be too upset to accept any assistance, whereas if the condition has been present for many years, they may have developed nonvisual methods and again be unmotivated to use their vision. The patient might associate their vision loss with some traumatic event such as a bereavement, illness, burglary or fall, even though this will rarely be the direct cause of their vision impairment.
2. Stability of condition and difference between the eyes. If the vision is constantly changing then you might need to consider a variety of different approaches for different days. Ask whether the day of the assessment is a 'good day' or a 'bad day' for them. If the patient feels one eye is significantly better, you need to confirm that this is the case, and then concentrate on maximising the vision of that eye.
3. Patient's knowledge of condition and prognosis. It is unlikely that the ophthalmologist has deliberately withheld information from the patient, but the patient might have forgotten or misunderstood what they were told. As well as finding out what pathology is present, this also gives you a guide to the patient's capacity to remember details accurately: you may well be giving them instructions related to magnifiers later which you will require them to remember when they arrive home, or be asking them to make contact with a local service.
4. Ongoing hospital monitoring and/or treatment. It is essential that any patient who has not had medical assessment of their visual impairment should be referred, as should the patient who appears to have deteriorated significantly since their last visit to the ophthalmologist. In your enthusiasm for prescribing magnifiers, do not forget that medical or surgical treatment may be appropriate, although you may consider prescribing something temporarily.
5. Registration status. As discussed previously, eligible patients are often not registered. This should be encouraged whenever possible as the best way to make them aware of the range of services available to them, and to help the societal impact of visual impairment to be measured.
6. Education and/or employment, in the past, at present and in the future. This will be a major factor in defining the patient's requirements. If an adult patient was visually impaired during childhood, find out whether they learned touchtyping and Braille. If not in employment at present, find out what job the patient left, and why, and if they wish to return to it. Include voluntary and unpaid roles and remember that a 'retired' patient may still be involved in their previous profession: a retired accountant may, for example, want to work for friends and relatives occasionally. Experienced practitioners would never

assume that a patient in their 90s has stopped work! Do they have caring responsibilities?

7. What hobbies and other activities do they enjoy? Have they had to stop doing these because of their vision loss?

8. What is their home situation? Do they live alone, or with family? Are they a carer themselves? Find out whether people the patient live with have good vision, and whether they can drive or help with correspondence. Do they own their flat or house, or is it rented from the council or a housing association? This will affect the provision of altered lighting or other adaptations. If they live in a flat, find out whether it is on the ground floor—if not, is there a lift?

9. Present aids and spectacles. It is important to find out what the patient has already, if it is successful, what it is used for and how it is used. It may be that spectacles which are not worn at present may be useful in conjunction with an aid, or that a magnifier which is 'no use' is being used incorrectly. Spectacle prescriptions should be determined and recorded, and magnifiers described as accurately as possible. If there is no label on the magnifier, its equivalent power could be accurately measured if required (see Chapter 7), but within the constraints of the assessment it is sufficient to obtain a general indication. This can be judged from the size of the lens: in general, the larger the diameter of the lens, the lower will be the power. A better indication can be obtained by imaging a distant light target through the lens onto a surface below: this could be done by moving the lens into a position where it creates an image of the ceiling light-fitting on the desk (Fig. 17.1). The image distance from the lens to the desk is now approximately equal to the focal length (if the object is assumed to be at infinity), and this distance can be estimated. The reciprocal of the distance in metres is the power of the magnifier in dioptres.

10. Current methods of performing tasks. Questions such as 'what happens when you get a bill in the post?' or 'what is your strategy for finding the right platform at the station?' indicate the level of support which someone has, and whether they are the sort of person who is willing to ask a stranger for help.

11. What technology do they use, and have they modified it? If they use a smartphone, do they ever use the camera to magnify things, or the LED light as a torch? Do they use large print or speech on their computer? Do they use an e-reader like a Kindle, or a home assistant like Alexa?

12. General health and medication. This may influence the patient's ability to perform everyday tasks or to use a magnifier in the required way. As well as noting the presence of the condition, find out how much it affects the patient: for example, if they have arthritis, does it affect their grip or ability to travel independently? When discussing medication, the opportunity arises to ask the patient if they can distinguish their tablets visually, by shape and/or colour. Are people with diabetes able to see their monitoring equipment?

13. Are there any safety concerns? For example, have they fallen, or burned themselves due to their visual impairment? Do they still drive, or cycle?

14. What does the patient hope or expect to obtain from the appointment? Gently advise them whether their expectations are realistic. Often the patient will have attended only because it was suggested by family or friends, it may be that they are seeking improvement for the patient, rather than the patient wishing it themselves. If the appointment was suggested by another professional (e.g. an ophthalmologist, GP or teacher), then ask the patient for permission to write back to the referrer to keep them informed of progress.

VERBAL AND NONVERBAL COMMUNICATION

Seeing faces is a task of great practical significance to the patient: this applies both for recognising friends in the street, but also for its role in face-to-face communication where head nods, eye contact and mouth shapes corresponding to letters are all useful cues, especially to an older person whose hearing may also be impaired. Erber and Osborn (1994) found that with a 1 m viewing distance and acuity better than 6/24, even subtle facial cues such as eye contact were seen by all subjects. For acuity less than 6/180, however, even the most robust facial cues (head nodding and shaking) could not be seen. For acuities between these two extremes, there was not a good correlation to the ability to perceive facial cues, and the authors recommend a 'real-life' test of function for any patients who are suspected to have communication difficulties. Into this acuity range will fall the majority of low-vision patients who must interpret the nonverbal communication

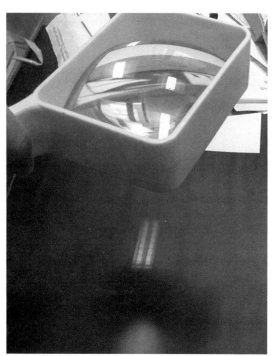

Fig. 17.1 Method of assessing the approximate power of an unknown magnifier.

of those around them. To make this as easy as possible in the consulting room, auditory and tactile back-up to visual gestures must be used: whereas the patient's attention would usually be engaged by eye-contact, this might be backed up by a gentle touch on the arm; encouragement during history-taking might be given by both head nodding and verbal signals.

REACTION TO THE LOSS OF SIGHT

Most of those seen for low vision assessment have acquired visual loss (rather than having the condition from birth), and all the time you are talking to the patient you should try to assess their feelings (and those of their family and friends) about this traumatic event in their life. When assessing children who have had their visual impairment from early in life, consider the emotional response of their parents, who may feel guilty, particularly if the visual impairment is linked to an inherited condition (Lairy, 1969). The attitudes of all carers should be noted because they are crucial to patient success: as already pointed out, the carer may want to do everything for the patient, removing the need for them to manage independently, or may be a staunch ally who will arrange the lighting at home and encourage the patient to persevere.

Depression is extremely common in people with visual impairment (Nollett et al., 2016) and their partners (Strawbridge et al., 2007). The Whooley Questions are recommended for primary care practitioners to screen for depression in adults (Bosanquet et al., 2015). These questions are:

1: In the past month have you felt down or depressed or hopeless?

2: In the past month have you been bothered by little interest or pleasure in doing things?

If the answer to both questions is 'no' it is unlikely that the individual is depressed: a 'yes' response to either questions suggests referral for a further investigation.

A third question ('is this something you feel you need or want help with?') has been suggested, which does not appear to add anything to the screening effectiveness, but may be a practical way for the optometrist to introduce the possibility of referral.

The mental health of the patient and their family should be considered throughout the examination, and referral for counselling services or for professional psychological support should be offered when needed. In very rare cases, urgent medical or psychiatric help is needed, and a plan should be in place for this eventuality (often initiated by telephoning the patient's general medical practitioner).

Vision loss has been likened to bereavement in the effect it has on a patient, and the way in which they cope with it is said to follow the Kubler-Ross model of bereavement, which was initially developed for people with life-limiting conditions. This model describes a series of emotional stages which the patient must go through as they come to terms with their loss (Crossland & Culham, 2000):

1. Shock

Shock is the most common response to being told that vision loss is permanent and untreatable. In this initial stage, it can be difficult to engage the patient in the assessment process: they often do not answer the question they are asked and can only talk about one thing. Denial, guilt and anger are common emotions during this phase. For example, the individual may deny reading problems, saying they have given up buying newspapers because 'they only print rubbish'; they may blame themselves for their sight loss ('if only I hadn't read so much under the covers as a child'); or may attribute their sight loss to professionals ('the cataract operation must have caused this'; 'if my optician had referred me sooner I wouldn't be in this position'). It is important not to criticise the other professional, but defending them may risk losing the patient's trust. A detached view is needed, emphasising that regardless of how the vision loss occurred, this is the situation which now exists, and the aim of the examination will be to try and help the patient find ways to use that vision to its best advantage. Referral for a second opinion may be needed: for example, in the case of a patient who ceases taking prescribed medication due to their disillusion with the treatment received. People may not be willing to accept help, and are unlikely to use magnifiers, in this stage of the adaptation process.

2. Depression

Shock is classically followed by a period of reactive depression: the patient may feel that the situation is hopeless and is bound to get worse; there is nothing which can be done to help, either by them, or by any of the professionals; and a low vision assessment is just a waste of time. If their family and friends are trying to be kind by doing everything for them, this will reinforce their helplessness. Although a certain degree of distress is to be expected, it must be recognised that some patients do suffer from a degree of depression for which counselling or psychotherapy would be beneficial.

During this phase, people may express disbelief. They may rationalise their problem as a failure to find a competent professional; they have often seen several ophthalmologists and optometrists in a short space of time. They typically have many pairs of spectacles and magnifiers, and inevitably none of these are found to be useful because none can restore the vision to its previous 'normality'. Eric Berne describes the 'Yes, but ...' game: the patient accepts that they are able to be helped (perhaps with a low vision aid), but refuses to accept it, saying 'yes, but I could never wear anything that looks like that' or 'yes, but I couldn't hold the book so close' (Berne, 1964). You can insist that they rationalise this by asking 'why not?', and you may be able to make them realise that their reasoning sounds rather feeble, even to themselves. If this is not successful, one approach is demonstrating to them a wide possible range of solutions, with a full explanation of the advantages and disadvantages of each. If they find each unacceptable, then prescribing is unlikely to work at that stage. The patient should be asked to contact you again in the future if they wish to try the aids, and such contact may be made within hours but can take several years!

3. Realistic acceptance

This is seen as the final stage of the process of coming to terms with the visual disorder. The patient understands and accepts the eye condition and its prognosis, trying not to worry unduly about what may happen in the future. They make the most effective use they can of their remaining vision, using whatever aids and strategies are necessary. They are not embarrassed to acknowledge their visual status and do not mind being seen using an aid in public. This is the earliest stage when someone might use a white cane, which often requires a tremendous effort of adjustment by the patient as it is such a strong symbol of blindness (as are Braille and guide dogs).

This 'loss' model of adjustment to visual impairment leads to useful descriptions of patient behaviour, and is most convincingly applied in cases of sudden loss of vision through trauma (Dale, 1992). In the tradition of the 'loss model', the patient will pass through each of these stages, and if they do not they are considered to be suppressing that particular emotion. It is only on reaching the stage of 'realistic acceptance' that the patient will unreservedly accept help and be fully motivated to use all available aids. It has been suggested that in the earlier stages there is little that can be done until the patient works through that stage and progresses onward. On the contrary, the patient can in fact still be helped in the earlier stages of adjustment, providing that you are aware of the problem and adjust your routine accordingly.

Of course not every person with sight loss follows this pattern, and it is important to deal with each patient as an individual, adjusting your approach to that person's needs, rather than following the theoretical guidelines too slavishly. It is difficult to predict how an individual will respond to sight loss: research has shown that personality type is more important than visual acuity in determining the level of acceptance to visual impairment (Tabrett & Latham, 2012).

GIVING INFORMATION AND ADVICE

The aim of the consultation has been to establish what practical help the patient might require in the form of aids, visual strategies, training and onward referral. In a survey of low-vision clients two years after being registered as blind, however, the main need which they identified was for psychological support: someone to talk to, and an explanation of the pathological condition rather than purely practical assistance (Conyers, 1992). The increased time usually available in a low vision assessment represents an ideal opportunity to give the patient information about their eye condition: many patients do know the name of their eye disease but have very little extra information. You can offer a valuable service here: the patient may well have been too agitated and upset when they saw the ophthalmologist to remember what they were told and cannot read or interpret what is written on letters

or documents which they have received. It is also important to correct information which they have read on inaccurate websites.

Explaining the disease process to them and their family can be extremely helpful. Many low vision practitioners use a poster or model of the eye for this purpose. An interesting although dated guide to such explanations is given by Fine (1993). People often ask questions about new advances in technology and disease treatment. It is important to give accurate advice about possible future treatments without giving false hope that surgery, drugs, gene therapy or stem cell treatment will provide an immediate cure for any vision loss.

Some practitioners use simulation spectacles to demonstrate the effect of various eye conditions to relatives and carers who may be present. Although there are many limitations with these glasses, they can help to explain why, for example, the patient can see a small piece of dust on the carpet but not a face right in front of them. Simulation apps use a smartphone camera to simulate different types of vision loss, with similar limitations.

It is important to provide honest advice about the limitations of help which is being provided: it is unlikely (although not impossible) that someone will read James Joyce's *Ulysses* from cover to cover with a 15× illuminated stand magnifier, for example. A child with albinism and visual acuity of 1.0 logMAR (6/60) is unlikely to ever be allowed to drive a car, and even with counselling, people can still be angry or depressed about their vision loss. Giving false hope that all the patient's problems can be solved by a low vision assessment is unfair and unhelpful.

Formed Visual Hallucinations

An example of when the low vision practitioner can provide valuable advice is when discussing Charles Bonnet syndrome (CBS): a very common cause of visual hallucination in people with sight loss. It is wise to discuss CBS with every person with sight loss, regardless of whether they report hallucinations or not. Some practitioners ask about hallucinations in the history taking process, but others wait until the end of the examination when more of a rapport exists.

The images experienced can range from colours and regular patterns (like tiles, checks or brickwork) to fully formed objects such as animals, faces or flowers. Although the images are not usually frightening (although faces are often distorted or grotesque), people can find it upsetting to experience hallucinations, at least initially. The origin of this condition is uncertain, but one hypothesis is that it is caused by the lack of the normal signals along the retino-cortical pathway ('deafferentation') leading to a reduction in inhibition of spontaneous activity in the striate and extrastriate cortex. This is supported by functional magnetic resonance imaging (fMRI) studies which show activity in the areas of the brain responsible for processing images with these features at the same time that the hallucinations are occurring (Ffytche et al., 1998), even though no real visual stimuli are present at that time.

It can be difficult to broach the subject of hallucinations. One approach is to describe CBS and then ask 'do you ever see coloured or flashing lights or shapes?' An alternative strategy is to ask 'do you think your eyes ever play tricks on you?' and follow up with 'I am asking this because it is something that people with visual impairment quite often report'. This will sometimes produce a full description of these symptoms, although patients may still be reticent to 'admit' to seeing things which are not there. Even if people deny having hallucinations, it is important to relay the information that CBS is common (some studies suggest almost two-thirds of people with visual impairment will experience this) and that these visions are not associated with psychosis or dementia (Ffytche, 2009).

Of course, people with sight loss can experience hallucinations for other reasons: psychosis, substance abuse, prescribed medications, sleep disorders and dementia could all be possible causes. The key ways to differentiate Charles Bonnet type hallucinations are that they never involve other senses and the patient is aware the image is not present: that is, they have 'insight' and do not try to interact with the illusion (e.g. reach out and touch it). In a small prospective study, 2/12 individuals with CBS, but no controls, developed dementia after 1 year (Russell et al., 2018). At the initial diagnosis, these individuals had only partial insight and had atypical hallucinations which involved familiar or recognised individuals.

Flashing lights or floaters (which might be interpreted as cobwebs or spiders) should also make the practitioner consider the presence of retinal detachment. Therefore, the practitioner needs to question the patient carefully, before classifying the condition as entirely benign. Sometimes reassurance is all the treatment which is needed for CBS: it is suggested that patients can be encouraged to conceptualise it like a 'phantom limb' (Carpenter et al., 2019). In some cases improving vision as much as possible, and then making eye movements or changing the room lighting when the hallucinations appear, can reduce or remove hallucinations. Individuals who are very affected may require counselling: cognitive behavioural therapy (CBT) or relaxation therapy have also been suggested (Carpenter et al., 2019). There is no current evidence to support other proposed treatments (O'Brien et al., 2020). Esme's umbrella is a UK charity which provides information and support for people with CBS and maintains an excellent website (charlesbonnetsyndrome.uk).

ADAPTING THE ASSESSMENT FOR A CHILD WITH VISUAL IMPAIRMENT

It is important to discuss the impact of visual impairment on the child's education, and to work as part of an integrated team with the teacher for visual impairment, the class teacher, habilitation workers and the child's ophthalmologist.

Ask the child how they are managing at school and what support they receive to access to curriculum: for example, do they have a one-to-one learning support assistant, a relay screen for the whiteboard or enlarged worksheets? When did

they last see their teacher for visual impairment, and do they have mobility, Braille or touch typing lessons?

Ask them about their school day: how they get to and from school, and whether they enjoy school. What is their favourite lesson and which do they not enjoy? Is this because they struggle to see it, or because they do not like it for other reasons? Can they manage in sports lessons, in music and in the lunch hall? Who is their best friend, and can they find them in the playground? It is good practice to ask the child each question first, perhaps turning to the parent or guardian for clarification if needed.

Ask to see examples of their work, and always praise them on it. Measure the print size of any enlarged text they show you. Ask teenagers whether they have any special provision for exams, such as enlarged print, additional time, a reader or a scribe.

It can be helpful to ask the child to write something in a pencil and then a black felt-tip pen. Notice how close they are to the page and how neat the writing is. If the writing is much clearer in pen, this may indicate that they struggle to see the thinner, lower contrast pencil writing. A letter to the class teacher requesting that the child is allowed to write in pen can help.

Ask the child about their hobbies and any clubs they are part of. Some young people are far happier to talk about their climbing lessons, or their cricket club, than about school.

Try and make the appointment fun: younger children would rather look at 'toys' than 'magnifiers'. Having posters in the consulting room makes it brighter and can help when showing a child how to use binoculars. Make sure that you have a selection of books and magazines for different ages.

If the child needs to have a cycloplegic refraction, remember that they will not be able to read afterwards, so low vision aids should be demonstrated before this. Consider performing the refraction on a different day, and perhaps ask another professional to put the eyedrops in: you do not want the child to be scared of you.

Make sure that the child's teacher for visual impairment receives a copy of the report from the low vision assessment, with the family's consent.

ADAPTING THE ASSESSMENT FOR SOMEONE WITH LEARNING DISABILITY

It is important to understand the level of understanding of the person with learning disability, and how the consultation can be made easier for them. Some clinics will send the patient a questionnaire before the visit, and ask the person and their carer to fill it in (Fig. 17.2) with questions like:

- What do you like to be called?
- What do you particularly enjoy doing?
- What do you particularly dislike (such as being touched, or the room lights being turned off)?

Have a selection of vision tests, perhaps Cardiff cards, Kay pictures, and a single line Snellen chart, and be quick to change the test if the patient finds it too hard or too easy.

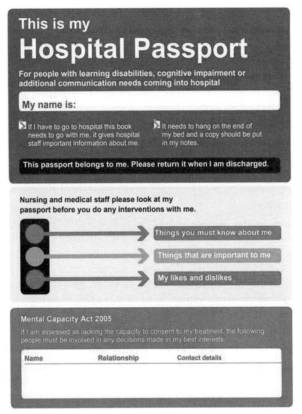

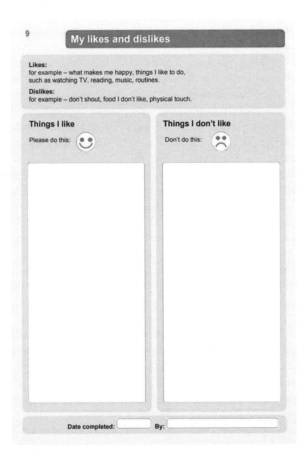

Fig. 17.2 The cover and an example page from a learning disability passport.

Always congratulate the person with learning disability on how well they are performing.

You can often learn a lot about someone's vision by showing them a tablet computer playing a favourite television programme. Looking at where they hold the screen, which eye they use to see it and whether they look through or over their glasses can show an approximate visual acuity, binocular vision status and the accuracy of their spectacle correction.

Be prepared to split the assessment over multiple visits: at the first appointment it may only be possible to measure vision and perform a cover test. A second consultation may be required for refraction and ophthalmoscopy, and low vision aids may be demonstrated at a third visit. Try and ensure that the same practitioner assesses the person at each visit, and that the consultation is performed in the same room.

FOLLOW-UP

It is important not to overwhelm the patient with information at their first visit. It may be that some tasks are addressed at the initial assessment, perhaps reading, and assistance with distance vision is offered at a subsequent appointment. It can be tempting for practitioners who are new to low vision to try

and 'show off' all of their knowledge of visual impairment to every person they see with low vision.

At the follow-up visit it is good practice to check whether the patient or their carers have implemented any suggestions you have made: for example, making modifications to lighting or the arrangement of furniture at home, using different colour plates when eating to increase the contrast, or downloading new apps. Check whether they have heard back from any referrals which you have made—perhaps to the hospital, local sensory team or a sight loss charity.

The ability to offer follow-up appointments will vary depending on the setting and funding of the low vision clinic, but it is particularly important to offer follow-up to people with progressive conditions, to children with low vision and to those of working age. Some clinics use telephone appointments to check how patients are getting on and use this consultation to decide whether a further face-to-face appointment is needed.

The Need for Follow-Up

Short-term follow-up (within a few weeks) is useful for people who have been prescribed low vision aids, so that any problems can be rectified before disillusionment occurs. If the low vision aid is successful and all of the patient's needs have been met, they could be discharged from the clinic until there was either an alteration in the visual or personal circumstances such that the aid was no longer appropriate, or the patient's requirements had changed. However, Jackson et al. found that of a group of patients supplied with aids, 28% needed replacement or repair of the aid, or identified the need for an additional aid when seen 6 months later. Of the group continuing to use aids for a further year, 24% required different aids when seen again (Jackson et al., 1987).

If a rigorous system of review appointments is used, with all patients being booked at fixed intervals, then the service rapidly becomes overwhelmed by numbers, and many patients who are coping well may feel that the appointment is unnecessary and fail to attend. Patients can be given (perhaps written) information on how an appointment can be made for them on demand at any time if they feel that there is a need. Despite this facility, many patients will not make such an appointment, even though they may be experiencing problems and not be finding the aid as useful as it was initially. This is illustrated by the results of Robbins (1994): when patients were sent a reminder letter, about 30% of those seen 1 to 2 years before returned for review, but without prompting this percentage fell to 12%.

WRITING REPORTS

If the patient has been referred to you by another professional, then it is good practice to write a report to the original referrer, with the consent of the patient. This will give you the opportunity to notify the ophthalmologist, GP, optometrist or social worker of what aids you provided, what advice you gave and what you consider the prognosis for success to be. This report should also be copied to the patient for their own records.

Even if the patient has self-referred, a letter is helpful to remind them of what happened in the assessment and for them to explain what happened at their low vision appointment to other people. The report provides a good opportunity to reiterate advice which might otherwise be forgotten: for example, 'Dr Anderson will use this magnifier with her reading glasses', or 'I have suggested that Mr Root moves his armchair closer to the television'.

Remember that other professionals may not be familiar with optometric terminology. Provide information in simple terms, for example:

With both eyes open and her glasses on, Miss Guha can see letters of 0.8 logMAR (6/48). This means things in the distance need to be 8 times larger, or she needs to be 8 times closer, for her to see them as well as someone with perfect sight.

In some areas, a 'Low Vision Passport' containing information about the aids dispensed and the acuities achieved is given to the patient for them to show to any of the professionals involved in their care.

Example reports and letters are given in Appendix 4.

REFERENCES

Berne, E. (1964). *Games people play*. Penguin.

Bosanquet, K., Bailey, D., Gilbody, S., et al. (2015). Diagnostic accuracy of the Whooley questions for the identification of depression: A diagnostic meta-analysis. *BMJ Open, 5*(12), e008913.

Carpenter, K., Jolly, J. K., & Bridge, H. (2019). The elephant in the room: Understanding the pathogenesis of Charles Bonnet syndrome. *Ophthalmic and Physiological Optics, 39*(6), 414–421.

Conyers, M. C. (1992). *Vision for the future: Meeting the challenge of sight loss*. Jessica Kingsley Publishers.

Crossland, M. D., & Culham, L. E. (2000). Psychological aspects of visual impairment. *Optometry in Practice, 1*(1), 21–26.

Dale, B. (1992). Issues in traumatic blindness. *Journal of Visual Impairment and Blindness, 86*(3), 140–143.

Erber, N. P., & Osborn, R. R. (1994). Perception of facial cues by adults with low vision. *Journal of Visual Impairment and Blindness, 88*(2), 171–175.

Ffytche, D. H., Howard, R. J., Brammer, M. J., et al. (1998). The anatomy of conscious vision: An fMRI study of visual hallucinations. *Nature Neuroscience, 1*(8), 738–742.

Ffytche, D. H. (2009). Visual hallucinations in eye disease. *Current Opinion in Neurology, 22*(1), 28–35.

Fine, S. L. (1993). Advising patients about age-related macular degeneration. *Archives of Ophthalmology, 111*(9), 1186–1188.

Jackson, A., Silver, J., & Archer, D. (1987). An evaluation of follow-up systems in two low vision clinics in the United Kingdom. In G. Woo (Ed.), *Low vision principles and application* (pp. 396–417). Springer-Verlag.

Lairy, G. -C. (1969). Problems in the adjustment of the visually impaired child. *Journal of Visual Impairment & Blindness, 63*(2), 33–41.

Low Vision Services Model Evaluation Collaboration. (2009). *Low vision services assessment framework: A tool for service providers*. Royal National Institute for Blind People.

Nollett, C. L., Bray, N., Bunce, C., et al. (2016). Depression in visual impairment trial (DEPVIT): A randomized clinical trial of depression treatments in people with low vision. *Investigative Ophthalmology and Visual Science, 57*(10), 4247–4254.

O'Brien, J., Taylor, J. P., Ballard, C., et al. (2020). Visual hallucinations in neurological and ophthalmological disease: Pathophysiology and management. *Journal of Neurology, Neurosurgery and Psychiatry, 91*(5), 512–519.

Robbins, H. (1994). Low vision care: Is ongoing assessment really necessary?. In A. C. Kooijman, P. L. Looijestijn, J. A. Welling, & G. J. Van der Wildt (Eds.), *Low vision: Research and new developments in rehabilitation* (pp. 485–493). IOS Press.

Russell, G., Harper, R., Allen, H., et al. (2018). Cognitive impairment and Charles Bonnet syndrome: A prospective study. *International Journal of Geriatric Psychiatry, 33*(1), 39–46.

Strawbridge, W. J., Wallhagen, M. I., & Shema, S. J. (2007). Impact of spouse vision impairment on partner health and well-being: A longitudinal analysis of couples. *Journals of Gerontology. Series B. Psychological Sciences and Social Sciences, 62*(5), S315–S322.

Tabrett, D. R., & Latham, K. (2012). Adjustment to vision loss in a mixed sample of adults with established visual impairment. *Investigative Ophthalmology and Visual Science, 53*(11), 7227–7234.

The Eye Examination

There are a number of tests which could be carried out at this stage to confirm what the patient has told you about their ocular condition, or what you have discovered from your questions to the patient. Direct or indirect ophthalmoscopy, external examination, slit-lamp biomicroscopy, tonometry, motility, colour vision and others could be usefully employed to fully assess the health of the eyes and visual system. This can, however, take considerable time (and a major toll on the patient's stamina), and it has no direct bearing on the patient's functional performance, or on the types of assistance which you might offer the patient. Such examination also often involves bright light being directed into the patient's eye, and the recovery time from such dazzling is often extended. It is therefore better to delay any other tests which are required until the end of your examination. Such tests must not be neglected, as the diagnosis of one disease does not make the patient immune to a second unconnected disorder, although the primary disease may render other tests uninformative. The patient with macular degeneration, for example, should still have their intraocular pressure and optic disc appearance checked to rule out the presence of glaucoma, but their visual field assessment is likely to be unreliable.

VISUAL ASSESSMENT

Visual acuity (VA), contrast sensitivity and visual field tests should be performed with both eyes open and using the patient's habitual correction, so that their current performance is measured. The effect of lighting, altered contrast and tints can be demonstrated at this stage.

Refraction should be performed, including the demonstration of high power adds.

DETERMINING REFRACTIVE CORRECTION

At this stage, it is not usually productive to measure vision without spectacles as it will almost invariably be less than the optimal acuity, and thus gives the patient a negative impression. Instead, if a small prescription is found, the difference with and without glasses can be demonstrated at the end of the refraction when deciding whether to prescribe spectacles.

The subjective routine should begin with an approximately correct prescription in place whenever possible: a reliable retinoscopy result or (if this cannot be achieved) the result from neutralising previous spectacles. There can be risks in taking a prescription from old spectacles: one of the lenses may, for example, be a balance lens: a spherical lens of the same average power as its partner prescribed to the eye with poorer acuity. Alternatively, the patient may have become confused about their old spectacles and, as lenses appear to have little effect on vision, now be wearing reading glasses for distance tasks. It is therefore particularly important to assess the refractive error objectively if possible, as subjective responses may be less reliable. If the reflex is dim, so-called radical retinoscopy can be performed by getting very close to the patient to brighten the reflex. This requires a change to the correction made for the retinoscopy working distance. Keratometry or keratoscopy may give an indication of the cylindrical correction, particularly in corneal disease. Optometrists know it is important to refract along the visual axis, because errors in refraction can be induced if not. This is because the astigmatic error changes in an unpredictable way when measured in the periphery (Gustafsson & Unsbo, 2003). It has been suggested that this could contribute to the optimum prescription not being correctly determined in patients with eccentric viewing. For example, when carrying out retinoscopy on the right eye of a patient, the gaze would be controlled by the left eye. On subjective refraction, the right eye would be fixating. The practitioner should be aware that this phenomenon may cause unexpected changes in prescription, or differences between retinoscopy and subjective measurements. Clinical judgement should be used to decide which prescription is more appropriate, but it has been suggested that optimising the prescription for the eccentric gaze direction does improve acuity (perhaps by about 0.2 logMAR) (Lundström et al., 2007) so care should be taken to ensure that eccentric viewing is adopted consistently during refraction.

For subjective confirmation, the patient will need to view a letter chart. Due to the Snellen chart's limitations (see Chapter 3), a logMAR chart is generally preferred. Computerised test charts can be useful as long as the screen and viewing distance are sufficient to allow large letters—of at least 1.3 logMAR—to be displayed, preferably with crowding bars. It is also important that the screen has high contrast and luminance, which may not be the case with older systems. Methods which allow lines of letters also allow the patient's localisation of visual targets to be judged: can they find the third line down, or the second letter?

If the acuity is not known, starting vision testing at 1 m is a good idea. It is then easy to retreat to 3 m if the letters viewed from 1 m are obviously well within the patient's capabilities, or to move to 50 cm (or even 25 cm) if needed. The aim should be to encourage the patient, always giving them the impression that they are doing better than expected. The patient should be given longer to make judgements and encouraged to view eccentrically if this helps: reassure the patient that this is not 'cheating'. You need to objectively measure the acuity of each eye as accurately as possible. If no optotypes can be read from 25 cm, then hand movements and light perception should be measured. Finger counting should not be used as it is not repeatable, has variable size and contrast (depending on the examiner's hand size and skin colour, and the colour of their shirt), and is often disliked by the patient. Someone who can count low-contrast fingers at 50 cm would also be able to see letters at the same distance. A number of 'ultra low vision' tests are available, such as the Berkeley Rudimentary Vision Test, which can measure acuity down to 2.9 logMAR (6/4800) (Bailey et al., 2012; see Chapter 3).

The acuity of the poorer eye should also be measured precisely, and not simply categorised as, for example, '<6/60': any future change in vision which might be a sign of active pathology must be detected, and this eye may end up with better vision in some circumstances. Neither should you simply accept the patient's assurance that they 'can't see anything' with one eye. There are considerable differences between patients in what they mean by such a statement, and a long-standing 'lazy' eye can be surprisingly successful when vision deteriorates in the previously dominant eye. A phrase like 'can you see movement with this eye?' or 'could you tell if a light is off or on?' may gently encourage the patient to allow acuity measurement in their poorer eye.

Trial lenses placed in a trial frame should be used in preference to a phoropter or refractor head, because it is important that you can see the patient's head posture and eye position, and that the patient should be able to change these at will. Full-aperture trial lenses can allow a better view of the patient's eyes. If the current spectacle prescription is $>\pm10.00$ DS it may be more appropriate to conduct an over-refraction, placing any additional trial lenses in a Halberg Clip. This ensures that prescription changes are genuine and not simply the result of a difference in the vertex distance between the

trial frame and the spectacle frame. With the final prescription present, the resultant combined power of trial lenses and spectacles can be measured using a focimeter.

Subjective testing should begin with steps of at least ±2.00 DS (but sometimes up to ±6.00 DS) in order to produce a response from the patient. The lens power used is usually determined by experience but can be approximated by dividing the denominator of the Snellen fraction at 6 m by 60: thus, 6/60 acuity would suggest $60/60 = \pm1.00$ DS steps; 2/60 when converted to 6 m would be 6/180, giving $180/60 = \pm3.00$ DS steps (Rosenthal & Cole, 1996). An alternative method using logMAR acuity is 'MAR/10': find the MAR by calculating 10^{logMAR} and then divide by 10. For example, for logMAR 0.7, $10^{0.7} \approx 5$, so the step change required would be ±0.50 DS. Theoretically, when using a cross-cylinder, the one selected could have a power equal to half of this calculated value, as the power change from 'position 1' to 'position 2' is doubled. However, clinical experience suggests using a cross-cylinder with powers equal to the sphere steps calculated (if available) is most effective.

The test chart should be placed at a reduced distance so that the patient can read at least three to four lines of letters as this will give a better basis for comparison. All lens choices offered should be successive comparisons for a defined visual target within a short space of time ('is the second line of letters clearer with lens 1 or lens 2?', 'Is the letter T more distinct with this lens or without it?') because alterations in the patient's gaze angle may produce spontaneous changes in acuity which do not relate to the lenses used. All results should be checked several times, and the size of the changes in lens power can be reduced if the patient is giving confident and repeatable responses. Nonetheless, it may only be possible to 'bracket' the final prescription: to determine, for example, that with a +4.00 lens in place the patient reports that an extra −1.00 improves vision, but with +3.00 in place they prefer an extra +1.00, leading to a final prescription of +3.50. Any attempt to use smaller steps of power change to confirm this (e.g. ±0.50) can cause the patient to become unsure.

To check the cylindrical component, an appropriate cross-cylinder can be used to optimise the clarity of a circular letter of a size two lines above the lowest read. Alternatively, if the objectively determined cylinder is ≥1.00 DC, simply increase the axis by 20 degrees from its current position, and ask the patient to compare the shape and clarity of the target in the two positions; that is, at the original axis, or 20 degrees from that. Repeat by rotating the cylinder between its original position and one with an axis decreased by 20°. If the patient is confident in their responses, the rotation can be reduced to 10 degrees. When the axis has been fixed by bracketing, power increases and decreases at that axis can be tried.

The patient should be given more opportunities to make each subjective judgement, allowing them to compare two alternatives repeatedly. Reassurance should be given that they are 'making sense' and not contradicting themselves.

Other refractive techniques for checking cylindrical correction are less successful. The difficulty in obtaining a handheld version of the fan and block target usually makes this technique impractical. It is also possible to obtain unreliable results when irregular refraction in the media causes randomly oriented target lines to appear clear. A stenopaeic slit may produce much better acuity than can be obtained with lenses alone: it may occlude sections of the ocular media which are distorted or hazy and prevent them causing deterioration of the retinal image. The refractive result obtained may not then offer such good acuity, as the distorted media is now scattering light. For the same reason, the use of a pinhole aperture to determine the effect of correcting any refractive error may not be reliable. This test relies on cutting down the size of the blur circle from the out-of-focus image on the retina (indicating what level of vision could be achieved by focusing the retinal image) but there may be an additional effect in which rays of light passing through irregular or partially opaque media are occluded. The improvement achieved in this case would not be replicated with lenses alone. Nonetheless, the pinhole may have diagnostic use, in determining whether symptoms which the patient complains of are due to scattering by the media. If, for example, the patient complains of seeing multiple images (polyopia) with an eye which suffers from cataract, and only one image when seen through the pinhole, this suggests that the multiple images are produced by light scatter from the opacity: cataract extraction, reversed contrast text, tinted spectacles, or a clear pupil painted contact lens may help. Confirmatory refractive tests such as the duochrome test or the +1.00 DS blur test are also not usually helpful, as the vision is not usually good enough to see the required targets.

It is important that both eyes are carefully refracted. In a patient with a progressive disease, the better eye may change: in some cases, an amblyopic eye, previously prescribed a balance lens, may become the better eye and require full spectacle correction. When the optimum refractive correction has been determined, the monocular acuity of each eye can be recorded, along with any comments on performance (e.g. 'using eccentric viewing to the right,' 'slowly,' or 'better at the start of the line').

If the refraction has been carried out with the test chart closer than 6 m, the final spherical component of the refractive error will be over-plussed. Testing at 2 m gives a refractive result +0.50 DS stronger than for distance, and at 1 m the refraction will be +1.00 more than at optical infinity. This may need to be modified for distance spectacles, although the over-plussed 'intermediate' prescription may be more appropriate for some tasks such as watching TV.

For near vision, the acuity should be determined for the patient's preferred working distance, using any reading addition which is required for the patient to focus at that distance. The closer the patient can be persuaded hold the reading material, the larger the retinal image, but increasing the reading add to +4.00 DS (at 25 cm) is considered to be the maximum 'normal' reading addition for presbyopes. The acuity with this addition, in conjunction with appropriate lighting, is determined. The reading chart should contain words of various sizes, and these may be in the form of paragraphs or isolated words (see Chapter 3). A word chart should be used

rather than letters, because the spacing of the letters within a word is closer, and thus can be more difficult. If words in meaningful sentences are used, this gives the additional clue of context to the reader, which is absent in isolated word texts.

This procedure should also be followed for young, prepresbyopic patients. Children and teenagers may use relative distance magnification successfully to read small print, but the close working distance required may not be sustainable for long durations. With the patient holding the print at their required distance, extra plus lenses are introduced binocularly to relax the accommodation, until the point where the patient finds the print has now blurred, and or they need to bring the print closer to focus it again.

If the near word acuity achieved does not comfortably reach the required print size, then magnification will be required (see Chapter 5). This magnification may be in the form of a spectacle-mounted high addition (see Chapter 7), if the patient is willing to hold the reading material closer.

Contrast sensitivity will give an indication of task performance, in particular for reading (see Chapter 3). Interpreting the results in terms of the contrast reserve can give an indication of whether the patient will be able to achieve spot reading or survival reading, or whether sensory substitution might be necessary. It also allows some of the patient's difficulties to be explained (e.g. reading coloured text on coloured backgrounds; seeing steps and kerbs); and for lighting recommendations (e.g. task lighting; illuminated magnifiers) to be targeted. When VA is equal in each eye, monocular contrast sensitivity testing can reveal which is the better eye, to guide which eye to use with monocular low vision aids.

BINOCULAR VISION

Having determined the best acuity in each eye, it is now possible to consider whether an assessment of binocular vision is required. A possible incomitant deviation, suggested by a report of diplopia which varies with gaze direction, should be investigated using motility and cover tests. Gross binocular vision can be demonstrated in people with vision impairment, and sometimes difficulties in reading can be caused by binocular vision problems rather than the visual impairment itself (Rundström & Eperjesi, 1995). More subtle binocular vision problems such as convergence insufficiency or decompensated phorias should be considered if the acuity in the two eyes differs by a factor of two or less, and binocular correction is being considered.

Binocular VA should be measured, as this will reflect visual performance under real-world conditions. People with low vision can still show binocular summation of VA (so the binocular VA is better than the VA of the better eye), even when each eye has a different level of vision (Tarita-Nistor et al., 2006). However, contrast sensitivity is often better monocularly than with both eyes open (Faubert & Overbury, 2000; Valberg & Fosse, 2002).

In practice it is best to demonstrate vision on real-world tasks with both eyes open and with the poorer eye covered. An Amsler chart can also be used to determine whether the vision is clearer with both eyes open or with one closed. If tasks are significantly easier with one eye covered then a frosted or occluded lens may be useful. When looking at a reading test at a close distance, some patients will use their dominant eye, or the eye corresponding to their dominant hand, rather than using the eye with better vision. On questioning, patients may sometimes be aware that they have to close or cover one eye in order to see more clearly and should be encouraged to try reading with the better eye.

Binocular vision tests which rely on good VA—such as many stereopsis tests—will not be appropriate for people with low vision. More gross tests of binocularity, such as a bar reading test are more likely to produce relevant results. To carry out this test, a bar (e.g. a pen) is placed midway between the patient (viewing binocularly) and the reading task. If lines of text can be read without any interruption, then both eyes are contributing: if only one eye is being used, then the pen will cover part of the text and a full line cannot be read. The Bagolini test can also be used successfully in people with low vision.

Visual Assessment of People With Nystagmus

People with nystagmus often have far better VA with both eyes open and measuring only monocular VA will underestimate their visual ability. To test visual performance monocularly, a plus lens sufficient to blur the nontested eye (but only by one to three lines) is recommended.

In some people with nystagmus, the oscillation can appear minimal, but as soon as their attention is directed to the letter chart the oscillation becomes dramatically increased. Therefore, an initial measurement of acuity can be much worse than the habitual level, and it should be measured when the oscillation has settled down, to ensure that an accurate baseline has been reached. Alternatively, as the examination progresses and the patient gets more tired, their nystagmus may increase and their vision may get poorer. This can be confusing or demoralising for the practitioner: the vision with an updated refraction may be less clear than the presenting acuity measured earlier in the examination. They may also be 'slow to see' and need to be given much longer to establish fixation and extract visual information.

It is important that any family members accompanying a person with nystagmus are aware that the vision will fluctuate, otherwise they may leave the examination with an unrealistic expectations of the persons' visual ability.

Look carefully for a compensatory head posture and encourage them to use this during the vision testing, or move the letter charts into a suitable position. If the person moves their head to the right to read the distance acuity chart, for example, then it would be better if the chart was moved to the left (and for them to sit so their television [or whiteboard at school] is to their left). Similarly, if they turn their head to the left when reading, you could position the chart to their right (and suggest that they hold a book, or position their laptop, in the same way). This may reduce the chance of neck or back pain and should improve the vision (as the person is using their null point).

ADDITIONAL TESTS

The use of additional tests of vision at this stage is for functional rather than diagnostic purposes, and their use will be dictated by the particular circumstances of the patient. The different strategies for testing different visual functions in a patient with visual impairment are discussed in Chapter 3.

The most common would be tests of the absolute dimensions of the peripheral visual field using a manual confrontation technique, a large white target on a perimeter, or a binocular Esterman test. Testing for a central scotoma using an Amsler chart or California Central Visual Field Test may be indicated in other cases.

Testing colour vision may be informative, particularly in people with retinal disease. Standard colour vision tests may be less accurate when acuity drops to lower than about 0.8 logMAR (Thyagarajan et al., 2007). Larger versions of some colour vision tests are available.

There are some patients who appear to present with visual problems, who in fact have disturbed visual *perception* yet may have relatively normal acuity or visual fields to conventional testing. Additional tests to confirm the nature of the defect should be used if the patient has a history of neurological disease or cortical lesion and has symptoms which do not correlate with the visual performance measured (see Chapter 3).

SPECTACLE DISPENSING

Under the *Opticians Act 1989*, spectacle dispensing for people who are registered as sight impaired or severely sight impaired can only be performed by a General Optical Council registered optometrist or dispensing optician. It is important for the person dispensing spectacles to have an understanding of the special lens and frame requirements for someone with vision impairment.

Although it is important that the patient is happy with the appearance of any glasses, larger spectacles are often better for people with nystagmus, especially if they use a compensatory head posture, and for those who need to use eccentric viewing to see.

When dispensing high power reading spectacles, the patient should be reminded about the close and specific working distance at each stage: prescribing, dispensing and collection. It is common for patients to complain that these glasses 'don't work' when they are merely holding the page too far away. If binocular correction at near is dispensed for any patient, the correct near centration must be provided: extra decentration/inset or base in prism may be required (see Chapter 7). A single vision near correction will also be preferred if the patient may use it with a magnifier: it is very difficult to combine positioning the magnifier close to the eye to get the required field of view, and looking down to use the reading area of the lens.

Bifocal spectacles with high reading adds can be very useful under other circumstances: it is possible to obtain bifocals with adds of up to +25 DS (see Chapter 7). These glasses can be suitable for someone who wants to, for example, watch television and read a book at the same time. However, the bifocal is also very useful for a patient who only requires a reading correction: it avoids the extreme blur experienced when looking up, and is a much thinner and lighter lens. It is wise to ensure that the patient also has another pair of spectacles—either single vision distance glasses, or some with a lower powered add—for everyday use. Progressive addition lenses (PALs or 'varifocals') are not ideal for patients with visual impairment, although they are very commonly used. Reasons for this include the variation in power across the pupil compromising image focus; difficulty in using the correct part of the lens when using unusual head or eye positions/movements; limitation in add power available (or excessive aberrations when such adds are possible through freeform surfacing). Despite this, some people (particularly teenagers and young adults) prefer the cosmetic appearance of a multifocal lens and sometimes refuse bifocal lenses.

Thirty percent of people aged 65 and over will fall at least once a year, as will half of those over 80 years of age. A fall can lead to pain, distress, loss of confidence, lost independence and even death: in around 5% of cases a fall leads to fracture and hospitalisation (Falls Consensus Statement). People with visual impairment are more likely to fall than those with good vision. Large changes in spectacle prescription (>0.75 DS) and wearing multifocal glasses (either bifocals or PALs) are associated with an increased fall risk (Elliott, 2014). Practitioners need to weigh up the risks of making large changes in the spectacle correction with the benefits of visual improvement. Patients need to be counselled that a sudden gain (or loss) of vision in one eye makes them vulnerable to misjudging distances and falling: Meuleners et al. (2014) found a twofold increase in falls after first-eye cataract surgery. Elliott (2014) suggests that active individuals spending time outdoors should have a separate distance correction: those who go out rarely can stay with multifocals if well adapted to them. Multifocal wearers with a minimal distance prescription should be recommended not to use them outdoors. Monovision corrections should also not be recommended to visually impaired patients because of an increased fall risk.

Tinted prescription lenses should be ordered using the colour and light transmission factor (LTF) (e.g. '20% LTF grey,' or '50% LTF, 500 nm orange'). It is sensible to demonstrate tints outdoors before prescribing them, and to ensure that patients are aware of what colour the glasses will look ('you realise that people will see that you are wearing yellow glasses?'). Wrap around frames or side shields will reduce glare from around the lenses. However, the patient does need to have colourless lenses available when lighting is low, or when reading, so may find an overspectacle more versatile (see Chapter 10).

Multilayer antireflection (MAR) coatings improve the cosmetic appearance of lenses, but do not have any effect on glare: in fact, as more light passes through, discomfort glare could be worse. They should under no circumstances be described as 'antiglare' coatings to the patient, who may be misled into thinking they have visual benefits.

Make sure that the patient is aware if you are using a balance lens in one eye, and the reasons for this being prescribed. If you choose to frost one lens, it is sometimes better to use a removable filter in case the patient dislikes this, or the vision changes. Blenderm or a Bangerter foil can be used: the foils have the advantage of being available with different degrees of fogging.

REFERRAL AND SIGNPOSTING

During the assessment, it is likely you will have identified concerns which cannot be addressed solely by the low vision clinic: for example, problems with lighting, social isolation, or depression. Consider referral to other services where they are needed, such as local sensory teams, counsellors, the general medical practitioner, or sight loss charities. It is important to have information on other services available in a variety of formats including audio, large print and electronic versions.

If the vision has changed or there are any concerns with disease progression, or if the patient requires registration as sight impaired or severely sight impaired, then referral to a hospital ophthalmology clinic may be needed.

THE NEXT STAGE

A significant minority of patients (10%–20%) need only a good refraction, coupled perhaps with advice about lighting, in order to meet their requirements (e.g. see Sunness & El Annan, 2010). Although it could be argued that any improvement which can be offered will be worthwhile, experience suggests that an increase of around two lines of acuity will be needed in order for the patient to subjectively appreciate the improvement in everyday viewing.

The initial assessment allowed the patient to identify their visual difficulties and to list the tasks for which their VA was inadequate. By considering this list, you can now determine if these are dealt with by the refractive correction just determined.

If the refractive correction does not improve visual performance sufficiently, then additional aids can be considered to prevent the impairment from becoming an activity limitation. Patient requirements can then be divided into three categories, and you must be quite honest with the patient about how you intend to approach each task:

1. No aid is suitable for the task. This may be because the amount of magnification required will be beyond a practical range, or because their VA does not meet a legal requirement for a task: for example, if the patient is registered as severely sight impaired and they want to drive a car. Some tasks are not amenable to low vision aids, such as face recognition or reading very low contrast subtitles on a television. In these cases, other strategies can be suggested such as letting their friends know that they may not recognise them and using television audio description.
2. The task may be tackled most effectively by nonvisual aids such as sensory substitution devices. For example, it may be easier to read a newspaper on a tablet computer with

speech activated, or a talking thermostat may be the best solution.

3. The task can be approached by trying to overcome visual impairment using an optical or electronic low vision aid (LVA). The LVA may work in isolation, or the task may require a combination of strategies (e.g. an optical magnifier plus increased lighting, or with an eccentric viewing technique) and the patient must be fully trained in their use.

REFERENCES

Bailey, I. L., Jackson, A. J., Minto, H., et al. (2012). The Berkeley rudimentary vision test. *Optometry and Vision Science, 89*(9), 1257–1264.

Elliott, D. B. (2014). The Glenn A. Fry award lecture 2013: Blurred vision, spectacle correction, and falls in older adults. *Optometry and Vision Science, 91*(6), 593–601.

Faubert, J., & Overbury, O. (2000). Binocular vision in older people with adventitious visual impairment: Sometimes one eye is better than two. *Journal of the American Geriatrics Society, 48*(4), 375–380.

Gustafsson, J., & Unsbo, P. (2003). Eccentric correction for off-axis vision in central visual field loss. *Optometry and Vision Science, 80*(7), 535–541.

Lundström, L., Gustafsson, J., & Unsbo, P. (2007). Vision evaluation of eccentric refractive correction. *Optometry and Vision Science, 84*(11), 1046–1052.

Meuleners, L. B., Fraser, M. L., Ng, J., et al. (2014). The impact of first-and second-eye cataract surgery on injurious falls that require hospitalisation: A whole-population study. *Age and Ageing, 43*(3), 341–346.

Rosenthal, B. P., & Cole, R.G. (1996). *Functional assessment of low vision.* Mosby Year Book.

Rundström, M., & Eperjesi, F. (1995). Is there a need for binocular vision evaluation in low vision? *Ophthalmic & Physiological Optics, 15*(5), 525–528.

Sunness, J., & El Annan, J. (2010). Improvement of visual acuity by refraction in a low-vision population. *Ophthalmology, 117*(7), 1442–1446.

Tarita-Nistor, L., González, E. G., Markowitz, S. N., et al. (2006). Binocular function in patients with age-related macular degeneration: A review. *Canadian Journal of Ophthalmology, 41*(3), 327–332.

Thyagarajan, S., Moradi, P., Membrey, L., et al. (2007). Technical note: The effect of refractive blur on colour vision evaluated using the Cambridge Colour Test, the Ishihara Pseudoisochromatic Plates and the Farnsworth Munsell 100 Hue Test. *Ophthalmic & Physiological Optics, 27*(3), 315–319.

Valberg, A., & Fosse, P. (2002). Binocular contrast inhibition in subjects with age-related macular degeneration. *Journal of the Optical Society of America A, 19*(1), 223.

19

Prescribing Magnification

Once it has been concluded that refractive correction alone will not be sufficient to improve vision to the required level, magnification will be needed. This may be combined with other strategies, such as training in eccentric viewing, nonoptical aids or tints, in order to optimise performance. Multiple aids and strategies are likely to be required: it is unlikely that one approach would be appropriate for all tasks.

Each task will require consideration, so it is important to prioritise the most significant concerns at the first assessment. For example, if someone is struggling to stay at work or is unable to manage their medication then this should be addressed at the first visit, with less important tasks left for a future assessment.

For each task, the following routine should be followed:
1. Determine the strategy most likely to help (e.g. an optical low vision aid, electronic magnification, sensory substitution, or another approach).
2. In the case of magnification, predict the likely magnification required.
3. Determine whether binocular or monocular correction would be preferable.
4. Select an appropriate low vision aid, if required.
5. Demonstrate the device on the required task, and modify it if necessary.
6. Determine the required spectacle correction.
7. Provide instruction for the low vision aid, and consider if training is required.
8. Issue the aid for trial in the 'real world'.
9. Make any referrals needed to other services.
10. Plan a suitable review visit.

It may be that some tasks, such as driving, cannot be safely performed with any aid for legal or practical reasons. This should be sensitively but clearly discussed with the patient. If a task cannot be performed with magnification, then it is far better to explain this in the consultation room rather than to prescribe an aid which is unlikely to help: 'false hope is a cruel deception'. It can also be helpful to manage patient expectations with an explanation of the nature of magnifiers: for example, that these change the way the task is performed, or make the task slower, and that some practice is needed to get the best performance.

DETERMINE THE STRATEGY MOST LIKELY TO HELP

Consider the task that the patient would like to perform, their level of vision, and their ability to use different approaches. For example, if someone would like to read printed bank statements, would they find it easiest to use online banking and a screen reader? If an academic is struggling to see slides at scientific conferences, would it be more plausible for her to use a distance telescope or to take and enlarge pictures using her iPad? Would a retired person wanting to read paperback books be more likely to succeed with a text-to-speech system like Orcam, or with a high-powered hand magnifier?

Discussing the possible options with the patient will help identify the best strategies: the approach would be very different for someone who enjoys trying new things on their computer, for someone who falls asleep when listening to audiobooks, and for someone who does not own a mobile phone.

PREDICT THE MAGNIFICATION REQUIRED

Predicting what magnification will be required for a task means that you can more quickly select a magnifier from the many possibilities you have. Showing a magnifier which is too weak and cannot perform the task can cause the patient to become disillusioned; showing a device which is too strong might be difficult for the patient to align and give the false impression that low vision aids are hard to use.

Predicting the likely magnification required also helps to check how the patient responds to magnification. If the acuity achieved with a device is less than expected, it may be that other strategies such as eccentric viewing training are required; if the acuity is better than predicted, the presenting acuity may have been measured incorrectly and it should be assessed again, perhaps with more encouragement. For example, if acuity is much better than predicted using a telescope, it may suggest glare problems which are aided by the restricted aperture; if much worse than expected for reading, it often suggests a central scotoma.

Although predictions are useful to assess the magnification level, they should only be taken as a first approximation and will not determine the success with using a magnifier. Vision is complex and success with a magnifier is multifactorial: contrast sensitivity, scotoma size and position, eye movements, fixation stability, binocular interactions, magnifier handling and cognitive factors will all affect the final performance of everyday tasks with a device.

Distance Magnification

For distance tasks, the Snellen equivalent of the visual acuity (VA) can be used to predict magnification. If someone wants to read television subtitles of size 6/9 and their acuity is 6/18, then they will need 2× magnification, or to halve their viewing distance, to be able to resolve the target. They might be able to see the subtitles with a 10× telescope, but this would have an unnecessarily small field of view and higher aberrations than a 2× or 4× system, which may be perfectly adequate for the task.

The calculation performed is simple:

$$\text{Magnification required} = (\text{required VA})/(\text{present VA})$$

For example, in Snellen notation to improve from 6/60 to 6/6:

$$\text{Magnification required} = (6 \times 60)/(6 \times 6) = 10\times$$

Or to improve from 2/36 to 6/18:

$$\text{Magnification required} = (6 \times 108)/(6 \times 18) = 6\times$$

(note that the Snellen value was converted to 6 m, by multiplying 36 by (6/2)).

The same method can also be used to assess the improvement which might be achieved with a particular device:

$$\text{Magnification used} = (\text{achieved VA})/(\text{present VA})$$

so

$$\text{Achieved VA} = (\text{magnification used}) \times (\text{present VA})$$

For example, a patient with VA of 6/36, using a 4× telescope, should achieve VA of:

$$\text{Achieved VA} = 4 \times (6/36) = 6/9$$

Note that performing this calculation on a calculator gives a decimal acuity (in this case 0.67). The lower value of the Snellen fraction can then be found using the sum (6/0.67). Someone with a VA of 6/18, using a 2× telescope to view a letter chart at 3 m, should have an acuity of:

$$\text{Achieved VA} = 2 \times (6/18) = 6/9 = 3/4.5$$

so the final acuity would be 3/4.5 (or 3/5 as that is the next largest letter size on a standard chart).

These calculations are easy to make when using Snellen notation. When using a logMAR chart, it can be remembered that the angular size of letters halves after three lines: for example, 0.7 logMAR is half the size of 1.0 logMAR, and 0.1 logMAR is half the size of 0.4 logMAR.

Each line on the logMAR chart is 1.25 times smaller than the line above, so an alternative way to calculate this is to use the formula:

$$\text{Magnification} = (1.25)^n$$

where n is the 'number of steps'.

As noted earlier, the change of three lines in logMAR VA is a magnification = $1.25^3 = 1.95 \approx 2\times$

For example, if the current acuity is 0.5 logMAR, and 0.1 logMAR is required, then:

$$\text{Magnification required} = (1.25)^4 = 2.44\times$$

Alternatively, these acuities could be converted to Snellen equivalents:

$$\text{Magnification required} = (6 \times 19)/(6 \times 7.5) = 2.5\times$$

Note that these values do not agree exactly, as Snellen equivalents are only approximate, and the actual letter size progression between each line is 1.2589×. Nevertheless, there is no clinically important difference in these results.

To assess the improvement which might be expected with a particular device, the formula is

$$x0.1 = \log M$$

Where x is the number of lines change in VA, and M is the magnification of the device. For example, using a 5× telescope,

$$x = \frac{\log M}{0.1} = \frac{\log 5}{0.1} = \frac{0.7}{0.1} = 7$$

So the individual with VA of logMAR 1.0 would be expected to improve to logMAR 0.3.

Near Magnification

If one considers only the angular subtense of the individual letters, distance acuity can be used to predict the near acuity. Despite the equality of the letter sizes, however, the two tasks are not equivalent because reading involves the discrimination of groups of letters, rather than single isolated characters. Thus, word reading may be significantly worse than letter acuity because of the contour interaction effect of adjacent letters or may be better because word shape and the context effect of meaningful sentences allow the patient to guess some words.

Eye disease can also influence near vision. Acuity at near may be worse than at distance due to the presence of central crystalline lens opacities which impair vision more as the pupil constricts, or central scotomas may make it more difficult to read words because the full sequence of letters cannot be imaged simultaneously in a functional area of the visual field.

Nonetheless, distance acuity can be converted to an approximate reading acuity using the 'denominator divided by 3' rule. This rule states that if distance acuity is expressed as a Snellen fraction based on a viewing distance of 6 m, the denominator divided by 3 is equal to the N-point print size which can be read at 25 cm with any appropriate add.

For example:

Distance acuity = 3/18 = 6/36

Predicted near acuity = (36/3) = N12

This person should be able to read N12 print at 25 cm with a +4.00 DS add if presbyopic, or without any add for a young person with normal accommodation.

The equivalent calculation of near acuity at 25 cm, from distance logMAR VA is 'MAR multiplied by 2'.

For example:

Distance acuity = 0.8

Predicted near acuity = $10^{0.8} \times 2 = 12.62 \approx$ N12

It is interesting to consider that these formulae create an expected print size of N2 for someone with 6/6 (logMAR 0.0) vision. Although clinicians tend to think of N5 print as very small, and at the size limit for comfortable long-duration reading, it should be noted that it is considerably above the threshold of someone with perfect sight. Most people would find reading N2 size print slow and uncomfortable, which illustrates the need for an acuity reserve so people are not asked to function at their acuity limit.

It is best to use a comfortable word reading size as the 'present acuity' for these calculations, so that the acuity reserve is accounted for. Alternatively, if a detailed reading speed function has been measured, then the critical print size (see Chapter 3) should be used. Alternatively, the threshold acuity can be used, but the target acuity can be reduced by a factor of 1.3× for spot/survival reading (one line on a Bailey-Lovie word reading chart) or by a factor of 2× for leisure/high fluent reading (three lines on the reading chart).

Near VA will vary depending on where the text is held and what reading addition is used. The magnification formula $M = F_{eq}/4$, assumes that a standard '1×' magnification is achieved by using a viewing distance of 25 cm, which is the focal length of the 'standard' +4.00 add. This means that you must test the vision at 25 cm, with whatever reading correction is appropriate (from no add in a young adult with good accommodation to +4.00 DS in someone who has had cataract surgery). The value of the addition does not affect the calculation.

Some reading tasks involve print sizes which are very familiar, such as newspapers or large print books. It is useful to ask the patient to bring samples of visual tasks which they find difficult, so the size can be measured. If the height of a lower case letter x (the x-height) is determined, then this value can be looked up and its notation determined in whichever system is desired (see Chapter 3).

Being precise about the required 'target' acuity can be difficult even for a reading task: it will depend on contrast, the shininess of the paper, the colour contrast and whether the print is handwritten or printed. N5 is often used as a target acuity to overcome these difficulties and to provide an acuity reserve for most text.

The assignment of an acuity level to a nonreading task such as knitting or wiring a plug is even more difficult. It can be estimated, and achievement of the acuity confirmed with the reading chart, but the magnification required should then be 'fine-tuned' with the actual materials. A wide selection of such items should be available in the clinic, perhaps including newspapers, maps, medicine prescriptions, playing cards, DIY tasks, restaurant menus, theatre tickets, books, crossword and sudoku puzzles, labels from food packaging, a bus timetable, and a needle and thread. People are often more enthusiastic about a magnifier when they see that it can be used on a task which is important to them.

There are multiple ways of determining font size and care should be taken when converting between different formats: font 14 Arial does not have the same print size as font 14 Times New Roman, and neither are exactly equivalent to N14 on a reading card. This size discrepancy is one reason why some fonts have a reputation as being easier to read than others (Rubin et al., 2006).

N-Point Notation

N-point notation is the most common system in use in the UK and is used on most reading charts employed in optometric practice. The point system uses printing terminology for the size of letters with 1 point being equivalent to approximately 1/72 inch. Digital typography systems on computers (like PostScript or OpenType) define font size using exactly 72 points to the inch. Despite this, it is not possible to create one rule to convert computer font size to x-height directly, as each font design has a different relationship between x-height and point size (Legge, 2007).

Within the same font, there is an approximately linear relationship between height and font size, so a letter labelled '10-point' (or N10) is approximately twice the size of a '5-point' (N5) letter.

Word reading cannot always be predicted from letter acuity size, particularly in people with scotomas. Field loss can make word reading poorer than letter reading ability, but clues from the context and word shape can encourage an 'educated guess' about the correct word, sometimes giving a surprisingly good word reading acuity. The Bailey-Lovie Word Reading Chart attempts to solve this problem by presenting unrelated words of varying lengths, in sizes ranging from N80 to N2 (see Chapter 3).

For any N-point notation chart:

$$\text{Magnification required} = (\text{present VA})/(\text{required VA})$$

For example, if someone can read N48 at a standard distance of 25 cm (equivalent to magnification = 1) but wants to read N12 print in a book with a 2:1 acuity reserve (so target acuity is N6), they will require at least 8× magnification (48/6).

Near LogMAR Charts

The same method is used to calculate magnification as for the distance logMAR charts. The main difficulty is in determining the size of the print in the required task, as these are not as familiar as the N-point sizes.

As was seen previously with calculations using distance VA:

$$\text{Magnification} = (1.25)^n$$

where n is the number of steps of improvement required.

If someone can see logMAR 1.4 print, for example, and requires improvement to logMAR 0.7, the number of steps of improvement needed is 7, and they will require at least 4.75× magnification (1.25^7).

Sloan M System

In M notation, the letter size is expressed in terms of the distance, in metres, at which the overall height of the lower case letter subtends 5 min arc. 1 M print size is approximately equivalent to newsprint. These charts were originally designed to be used at a standard distance of 40 cm, but the relationships between the letter sizes are the same no matter what viewing distance is used. The required magnification is simply calculated from:

$$\text{Magnification required} = (\text{present VA})/(\text{required VA})$$

Jaeger Notation Charts

Jaeger charts were calibrated so that a 'J5' letter subtended 5 min arc at 1.02 m, which is approximately newsprint size. Jaeger reading charts are no longer widely used nowadays because there is no consistent relationship between the numerical notation and the letter size.

An Alternative Method for Determining Near Magnification

The equivalent power method is an alternative way to determine near magnification using the table shown (Table 19.1,

Bailey, 1981). An advantage of the method is that the initial baseline acuity (referred to as 'present acuity' in the previous formulae) can be taken at any working distance and with any reading addition, rather than using a potentially unrealistic 'standard' working distance of 25 cm and an addition of +4.00 DS. The method then uses a logarithmic scale to plot changes in reading acuity, working distance and equivalent power.

The number of steps on this scale between the presenting acuity and the target acuity (in point size) is used to calculate the amount of magnification needed. The working distance of the patient (in centimetres) will then need to *decrease* by that same number of steps.

For example: A young adult sees N32 print at 25 cm but would like to read newsprint (N8). From '32' to '8' is six steps on the scale, you can see that there are six steps between them (32 to 25, 25 to 20, 20 to 16, 16 to 12, 12 to 10, 10 to 8). The reading distance will therefore have to decrease by six steps as well. As it is presently at 25 cm, this will need to become 6 cm (25 to 20, 20 to 16, 16 to 12, 12 to 10, 10 to 8, 8 to 6).

If accommodation is insufficient, the patient may need a reading addition to maintain clear vision at this distance. The reading addition will *increase* by the same number of step sizes. This can be illustrated in the following example:

Someone with pseudophakia reads N40 at 40 cm with a +2.50 reading addition. What reading addition will be needed to read N12 print?

Locating '40' and '12' on the scale, you can see that there are five steps between them. The reading addition will therefore have to increase by the same five steps. As it is presently at +2.50, this will need to change to +8.00 (2.5 to 3.2, 3.2 to 4, 4 to 5, 5 to 6, 6 to 8). This gives a working distance which has decreased by five steps (from 40 to 12 cm), which is of course the focal length of the +8.00 reading addition.

Assessing magnification for intermediate tasks requires that these be considered in the same way as either near or distance tasks. If it is a task where the working space cannot be reduced, it should be considered as a distance task, but if the working space could be varied, it may be approached as a near task.

Testing the Prediction of Near Magnification

An additional, very simple, step at this stage is to confirm that the predicted magnification does actually improve the reading acuity as expected. This can be done by using a trial lens with the required plus power and positioning the reading chart at the focal length of that lens (with appropriate illumination). For example, if the predicted magnification was 5×, then a +20.00 DS lens, with the object held at 5 cm, can create this condition. An individual with some accommodation may not require the full reading add for the distance or may bring the object slightly closer than expected (and get even better VA!).

TABLE 19.1	The Bailey-Lovie Logarithmic Scale									
	1	1.2	1.6	2	2.5	3.2	4	5	6	8
10	12	16	20	25	32	40	48	64	80	100

Although the prediction was only a starting point, and can be changed, any major shortfall in the acuity actually achieved needs to be investigated before proceeding further with magnifying devices. In the case of a central scotoma, for example, the individual may be able to read the first letter on each line down to the predicted size but may not read full words. In this case, eccentric viewing training may be required in order to benefit from magnification (see Chapter 13).

A second point which can be explored in this test is the reaction of the patient to a close working distance (as would be required if a spectacle magnifier is suggested). The patient can be asked directly whether they would consider a magnifier of this type (and many initially say 'yes' if asked 'would you like a magnifier which was built into your spectacles?'), and the advantages and disadvantages discussed.

BINOCULAR OR MONOCULAR?

It is usually visually beneficial to use binocular viewing. Even if the acuities are unequal, and no visual advantage will accrue, it is generally more comfortable to keep both eyes open and there is often a psychological benefit from binocular viewing.

When there is distortion in one eye, it may be better for the patient to close that eye. This will often depend on whether the distortion is in the dominant or nondominant eye. An Amsler grid is helpful to determine how much the poorer eye will interfere: the patient is asked to view the chart with each eye individually and with both eyes open and is asked when the chart is clearest and easiest to see. Comparing the better eye's VA to the VA with both eyes open is also helpful.

In some cases, the design of the magnifying device or its viewing distance mean that it must be used monocularly. It is important to explain the reasons for this to the patient, who must be reassured that ignoring one eye will not cause it to deteriorate, nor will using the fellow eye exclusively cause it to be put under excessive strain.

SELECTING A MAGNIFIER

Once the amount of magnification and design of magnifier has been predicted, an appropriate device can be demonstrated, to see if it brings about the expected improvement in performance. The four possible ways in which this can be achieved (relative size magnification, relative distance magnification, transverse, angular) must be considered to determine which is most appropriate for the particular task involved. Table 19.2 summarises the effect of these approaches on field of view, working space and on task.

As Table 19.2 shows, for distance visual tasks angular or transverse techniques are most useful. In contrast, for near viewing, bringing the object closer (perhaps using plus lenses) can be very effective as the working distance is usually more flexible. Magnification for some tasks can be achieved in several different ways: improvements for watching TV could be accomplished by using a telescope, buying a larger television, or by moving closer to the screen. Magnification methods can be used in combination; if, for example, an enlarged object is viewed from a closer working distance, the two individual magnification values would be multiplied together to find the total magnification. An example of this might be the patient who doubles the magnification of their electronic vision enhancement system by halving the viewing distance.

Distance Tasks

Relative distance magnification can be demonstrated in the consulting room: the patient can be asked to move closer to a picture on the wall, or the practitioner can move closer: 'Imagine if I were on the TV, could you see my face? How about if I move here, so I am just a metre in front of you?'. A magnification of 2× or 3× could easily be achieved without restriction in the field-of-view, and without wearing a heavy and uncomfortable spectacle-mounted aid.

If it is not possible to get close to the task (e.g. going to the theatre or airport destination boards), then electronic or telescopic devices must be used. Distance magnification is only possible for a sedentary task (such as going to the theatre or watching a football match) or for a moving task where the patient pauses momentarily to use the telescope (looking at bus numbers, station arrival/departure boards). These systems can only be worn on spectacles if they are fitted using a bioptic approach, so the patient dips their head to look through the magnifier. Table 19.3 shows the types of telescopes used as low vision aids and can be used to select a telescope based on the required magnification and task.

Although the device is being considered purely for a distance task, each telescope has the potential to be used at other viewing distances. Consider if this is an essential feature and will allow you to prescribe a single aid that can be used for two different tasks. Alternatively, it may be a hindrance if the

TABLE 19.2	A Summary of the Characteristics of the Four Available Forms of Magnification		
Type of Magnification	**Field of View**	**Working Space**	**Distance (D), Intermediate (I), Near (N)**
Relative size	No change	No change	Usually N only
Relative distance (reduce working distance)	No change	Decreased	D, I or N
Relative distance (plus lenses)	Decreased	Decreased	N only
Transverse	Decreased	No change	D, I or N
Angular	Decreased	No change	D, I or N

TABLE 19.3 A Summary of the Characteristics of the Different Types of Distance Telescope Available

| | ASTRONOMICAL | | GALILEAN |
	Monocular	Binocular	
Typical magnification	2x–10x	3x–20x	1.5x–3x
Format	Handheld, finger ring, spectacle (to 4x)	Handheld, binocular, spectacle mounted	Monocular or binocular, spectacle mounted, fixed or clip-on
Focus range	Infinity to about 20 cm	Limited	Infinity to about 1 m
Examples	Specwell 8 × 20 monocular, Eschenbach 4 × 13 Microlux	RSPB 6 × 17 binoculars, Eschenbach spectacle mounted telescope	Eschenbach Max TV

patient does not have the dexterity to adjust focus quickly and accurately, or mixes up the reading caps.

The clinician should view through the telescope to check that it is adjusted and focused for the distance to be viewed and then present it to the patient to try out. This allows the patient's reaction to the limited field and unusual cosmesis to be noted, and the ease of manipulation and ability to hold it in the correct position can also be monitored.

Near Tasks

For near tasks, the same four methods of magnification can be considered. Text can be made larger by selecting large print books or a larger font size on a Kindle, for example.

Electronic vision enhancement systems offer the most versatile method of magnification for near images, with a very wide magnification range possible. Near vision telescopes can be useful if the patient wishes to perform some manipulative tasks and requires a long working distance and free hands. It is wise to consider simpler devices at the first assessment, moving on to more complicated approaches only if these do not work. For example, using a pair of high addition spectacles and reducing the viewing distance is far simpler than using a spectacle-mounted Galilean telescope with a near vision cap.

The most common magnifier for near tasks is the plus lens in its various forms, producing its effect by allowing the object to be brought close to the lens without creating accommodative demand. It is this close lens-to-object distance which is the major drawback of these magnifiers, as often they do not allow enough working space for a manipulative task or to get sufficient light onto the task. The plus lens is found in spectacle-mounted, hand and stand forms, and each has relative advantages and disadvantages, depending on the task to be performed. These are listed in Table 19.4, as are other systems for near vision magnification.

DEMONSTRATE THE DEVICE ON THE REQUIRED TASK, AND MODIFY IT IF NECESSARY

The most appropriate magnifier will be determined by careful trial on the task it has been prescribed for. The major factor in

the final decision is the patient's own evaluation of the aid, so it is important they feel free to make comments and choices without pressure from the clinician.

The patient should be briefly shown how to hold the device, and should be advised what spectacles to wear with the aid. The device is then handed to the patient and they are asked to comment on how well they see with it, as well as the working distance, field-of-view, weight, and effort required to maintain the magnifier position. The patient's reactions to the magnifier are as important as their performance, because any reservations about the magnifier will reduce their motivation.

Testing performance with the aid may begin with the patient being assisted with positioning the magnifier and holding the task in the correct position, but at the earliest opportunity leaving them to do this alone. When the patient picks the magnifier up after taking a break, it can be seen whether they could remember how to position it correctly without guidance (which they will need to do at home), or whether they need to have the correct use demonstrated to them again.

The device should be demonstrated on an acuity test first, so that the performance can be measured objectively. Performance should be recorded not just in terms of acuity but also the manner of reading. Examples of some of the comments one might record would be: 'fast', 'easily', 'missing some lines', 'difficulty aligning', 'inaccurately' or 'slow but sure'. If the acuity needed is not achieved, consider whether this is because the magnification is too low, or the device is too difficult to use.

After this, the aid should be shown on the task for which it will be used. While the patient uses the device, additional lighting can be demonstrated if appropriate, to encourage the use of additional task lighting at home. The best way to position the task can be demonstrated: for example, placing a letter against a clipboard or on a table rather than holding it in the hand. Demonstrate nonoptical aids at this time: if the task is writing, demonstrate the effect of thicker felt-tip pens instead of ordinary ballpoints; if carrying out a manipulative task, try improving the contrast (using a sheet of coloured card as a background).

If the task cannot be performed easily with any device, consider whether additional techniques are required (such as

TABLE 19.4   A Summary of the Advantages and Disadvantages of Various Forms of Near Vision Magnifier

Type of Magnifier	Advantages	Disadvantages
High addition spectacles	Hands free Wide field-of-view Intuitive Similar appearance to 'ordinary' spectacles	Close working distance Working distance may block light Blurred distance vision Difficult to use binocularly above about 2×
Hand magnifier	Wide range of magnification and illumination available Intuitive Portable Relatively cheap	Difficult to maintain correct position Less useful if held at wrong distance or with incorrect (reading) spectacles
Stand magnifier	Wide range of magnification and illumination available Easy to hold steady, even with mild hand tremor Easy to use correct working distance	Can only be used on flat surfaces Less portable than hand magnifiers Cannot always be used in books with tight spines Special reading correction may be needed
Near vision telescope	Some can be used for intermediate or distance tasks too Long working distance	Limited field of view Limited depth of focus Requires practice to use May be cosmetically unacceptable
Electronic vision enhancement system	Wide range of magnification Contrast enhancement possible May be more cosmetically acceptable	Expensive Require regular charging or power supply Some may find difficult to use

eccentric viewing training), or if a different approach will be more successful (perhaps using relative size magnification on an iPad rather than a supplementary magnifier).

The last question should be whether the patient is happy with the cosmetic appearance of the device: would they be happy using it in public?

DETERMINING THE REQUIRED SPECTACLE CORRECTION

Distance telescopes which are handheld or clip-on can be held over the distance spectacles. The patient may find it difficult to position, especially if the vertex distance is large, and may appreciate the larger field-of-view when the telescope is held right up to the eye (see Chapter 9). If the telescope is a focusing design, then the separation of the lenses can be altered to compensate for moderate degrees of spherical ametropia.

If the telescope is of variable focus and is used without spectacles, then some of the eyepiece lens power is 'borrowed' to correct the refractive error (see Chapter 9).

With high degrees of ametropia, there may, therefore, be either increased or decreased magnification in using the telescope over the spectacles. Any significant cylindrical correction must be worn as a spectacle behind the telescope or be incorporated into the eyepiece. In practice, astigmatism of less than about 1.50 DS has minimal effect on the vision achieved with a telescope for low vision. Fixed-focus telescopes must be used over the spectacles in order to produce focussed images at the expected distances.

For near vision devices, a general rule is that handheld magnifiers should be used with distance spectacles, whereas stand magnifiers should be used with reading spectacles. A full discussion of the rationale for this is given in Chapter 7. A near telescope is designed to be worn over the *distance* correction because the correction for the close working distance is built into the telescope.

In the case of a spectacle-mounted plus lens, the lens is worn instead of the refractive correction, so this will need to be taken into account. For example, if the distance prescription is −4.00 DS and a +12.00 DS add is needed, this will be provided by a +8.00 DS lens (−4.00 + 12.00); for someone with +4.00 DS of hypermetropia, a +16.00 DS lens would be needed. Cylinders can be incorporated into such lenses: their effect can be demonstrated subjectively with the patient. If both eyes have similar acuity, then base-in prism may make the spectacles easier to wear; if they rely on one eye, then they may prefer the poorer eye's lens to be frosted or opaque. The effect of occlusion or prism should be measured as the patient performs the task which the aid is prescribed for.

PROVIDE INSTRUCTION AND TRAINING FOR THE LOW VISION AID

The patient should be given full instruction in the optimum use of the device (see Chapter 20) and the need for training should be considered. Before the aid is dispensed, ensure that the patient remembers how to use it: which spectacles should be used, which eye it should be used with, and how to hold it. Demonstrate how to replace or charge any batteries and ensure that the patient can operate any switches comfortably. It is important that the patient is aware of the limitations of the device: for example, that they should not walk around using spectacle mounted telescopes, and that they should not use a hand magnifier for chopping vegetables.

Consider giving written instructions, showing a relative or carer how to use the device, or providing a telephone number for patients to contact for help.

ISSUE THE AID FOR TRIAL IN THE 'REAL WORLD'

At this stage the patient should be given the device to take home. There are many differences between using a device under supervision in a well-lit clinic room and using the same device alone at home. Lighting is often significantly poorer at home: sometimes by a factor of 10 when compared with the hospital (Cullinan et al., 1979). The patient may find it harder to use a device in the more cluttered home environment and might have not reported the distances and sizes of their tasks accurately in the assessment. Some clinics offer domiciliary appointments which overcome these problems, while others work with rehabilitation officers for visual impairment who can give advice on lighting and device use in the home setting.

In many clinics, low vision aids are issued on a loan system so patients are able to return or exchange any device which is not helpful. In settings where patients are required to buy devices, it may be prudent to offer a trial period before full payment is made, to ensure that the low vision aid prescribed is useful.

There are several reasons why low vision aids may not be helpful after a real-world trial. First, the vision may have deteriorated since the device was prescribed. If the acuity has fallen, then different magnifiers should be demonstrated, and referral made to investigate the cause of the change in vision.

Second, the aid may not be used properly: perhaps being positioned too far from the eye, at the wrong distance from the task, with inadequate lighting, used with the wrong eye, or used with the wrong spectacles. In this case, the patient should be reminded of the correct way to use the low vision aid, or a simpler device should be issued. If the initial device still seems to be the best option, then a training programme may be necessary to ensure it is effective.

A third reason for failure with a device is that the aid is being used for a different task than that for which it was intended: the patient may be trying to read the newspaper whereas large-print books had been the designated goal, or trying to read with a telescope designed for knitting. Explain again what the magnifier is to be used for, checking with the patient that the task for which the magnifier is intended is still a priority. If it is not, the prescribing routine should be carried out for the newly identified priority task.

PRESCRIBING IN SPECIAL CASES

As each individual low-vision patient presents a unique mix of visual impairments, requirements and solutions, an individually tailored solution must be found in every case. Nonetheless, there are two special patient groups where a few general guidelines may be possible: children, and those with other disabilities.

Prescribing for Children

Children with vision impairment often use a very close working distance to magnify images: it is not uncommon for them to hold something at 5 cm, creating 5× magnification when compared with holding something at a more conventional distance of 25 cm. Consider whether magnification is any better than this: if the child is now given a 3× (+12.00 DS) stand magnifier, for example, the focal length will be 8 cm, so she will get less magnification than before!

Spectacle adds should be demonstrated to see whether this makes holding print close any more comfortable: children with vision impairment may have reduced accommodation, and even those with good accommodation may not be able to read comfortably at a close distance for a long period of time. As a rule of thumb, two-thirds of the total amplitude of accommodation can be exerted for an extended period. If the amplitude of accommodation can be measured, the addition can be determined in the usual way. If this is not possible, calculate the full reading addition required to focus at the viewing distance used, then present the child with an addition +2.00 DS less than this. If blurring of the print occurs, or if the child brings the reading material closer still, then its value can be reduced until the print is clear at the original working distance.

Dome and bright field magnifiers are often very successful for children with vision impairment as they allow a longer viewing distance to be maintained, reducing the chance of neck or back pain.

Children often find binoculars easier to handle than a monocular telescope, and even quite young children can use small binoculars on days out and school trips.

Ensure that the child is allowed to use any low vision aids whenever they are needed: reassure them (in front of the parent or carer) that the devices belong to the child, and that they can be replaced if they are broken, damaged or lost. It is far better for a device to be used every day (but lost once a year) than to be kept in a special drawer and only brought out on special occasions! It is good to provide advice and devices before they are needed: the summer before a child starts school is a good time to provide advice, some devices to become familiar with, and to ensure that referral has been made to the Specialist Teacher for Visual Impairment.

Teenagers and young adults are likely to use technology instead of optical devices: they will often be far happier using a smartphone to photograph and zoom in on a fast food restaurant menu than to use a monocular telescope for the same task. Despite this, it is important that they have access to optical magnifiers as well, for times when their technology is not available or cannot be used (perhaps in an exam), or when their phone's battery has run out.

Do not forget to copy your report to the Specialist Teacher for Visual Impairment, the school or college's Special

Educational Needs Coordinator (SENCo), and the class teacher or Head of Year.

Prescribing for People With Other Disabilities

Consider the presence of any relevant physical or learning disability when prescribing magnifiers. If someone has hand weakness, for example, they may respond better to spectacle-mounted telescopes than a stand magnifier; if they have limited head movement then perhaps an electronic magnifier with scrolled text will help. People with hand tremor may prefer stand magnifiers to hand or spectacle mounted devices.

When someone has dual sensory loss with poor hearing, ensure that the correct interpreter is available: do they require someone to provide British Sign Language, a different language, or a tactile (hands-on) sign language? Ask the patient where they would like you to sit, and where the interpreter should sit. Remember that you will probably need to explain tests such as retinoscopy before you switch the lights off. Sign language interpreters usually appreciate a quiet, uncluttered room to work in, and plenty of time should be made available for the assessment. As with any interpreter, always ask the patient questions directly: 'can you see this letter?', never 'can she see this letter?' Providing written advice is particularly important.

It is very worthwhile to learn some simple signs in British Sign Language and Makaton. It is also useful to know the finger spelling alphabet so you can quickly check which letters the patient is reading on an acuity chart.

When someone lives in residential care then remember the person accompanying them to the appointment may not be the primary carer. It will be important to give written advice for any low vision aid dispensed, for example, 'Mr Warne should use these special glasses for the television but not for walking around' or 'Viv's larger magnifying glass is for her to look at photos but will not help for reading'.

In some cases, it is better to conduct the low vision assessment in the care home, day centre or school where the patient spends most of their time, so their needs and activities can be assessed in detail. It is likely that the patient will also be more relaxed and cooperative in their own environment, and the primary staff will be on hand to discuss clinical findings and possible solutions.

Do not underestimate how helpful simple advice can be: asking for someone to be allowed to sit closer to the television or by a window can make a big difference, as can reassuring a carer that it is OK for a child with myopia and learning disability to take their distance glasses off when they watch films on their iPad.

REFERENCES

Bailey, I. L. (1981). Prescribing low vision reading aids—A new approach. *Optometric Monthly, 72*, 6–8.

Cullinan, T. R., Gould, E. S., Silver, J. H., et al. (1979). Visual disability and home lighting. *Lancet, 313*(8117), 642–644.

Legge, G. E. (2007). *Psychophysics of reading in normal and low vision*. Lawrence Erlbaum Associates.

Rubin, G. S., Feely, M., Perera, S., et al. (2006). The effect of font and line width on reading speed in people with mild to moderate vision loss. *Ophthalmic & Physiological Optics, 26*(6), 545–554.

20

Instruction and Training in the Use of Magnifiers

INSTRUCTION IN THE USE OF LOW VISION AIDS

A task-oriented approach has been adopted throughout the low vision assessment, with the patient identifying what they want to do and a specific aid being prescribed for that purpose. It is important that the final stage of the process—instruction in using the low vision aids—also uses this task-oriented approach and that the assessment ends with ensuring that the patient knows how to use the low vision aids supplied for the specific task they wished to carry out. As Collins writes, the examination should not merely involve: 'the clinical assessment of the optics required and then the patients (being) left to their own devices to learn to use the appliance' (Collins, 1988).

To use a parallel from another area of optometry, someone would not be prescribed contact lenses then sent home without knowing how to insert and remove their lenses, assuming they will discover how to do this by trial and error.

It should be remembered that although the practitioner may think using a low vision aid is simple, in many cases, the patient will find them complicated. It is not uncommon to see someone trying to view a distance chart with a hand magnifier, holding a monocular device to a blind eye, or being unsure which end of a telescope to look through.

The patient should not go home with any aid until they are comfortable and competent in its use. If they use the aid incorrectly and fail to achieve their required goal, this may cause them to reject all low vision aids completely. Written instruction sheets to reinforce verbal instruction can sometimes be useful (see Appendix 3).

At each follow-up appointment, the patient should be asked to demonstrate how they use each of their low vision aids, so the practitioner can check the handling of the device.

As well as technical challenges like knowing how to switch the magnifier on and how to change the batteries, device users must learn to coordinate their eye, head, hand and body movements (Mehr & Freid, 1975).

Instruction in Near Low Vision Aid Use

The patient should be advised:
1. how to position the magnifier and the task material: for example, showing the patient to see that the shorter the eye-to-magnifier distance the greater the field-of-view (Fig. 20.1) and how the lighting should be arranged. Demonstrate how to locate the optimum focal distance with a hand magnifier (Fig. 20.2): with the magnifier touching the page there is no magnification, but it increases as the magnifier moves away, to reach a maximum when the object is at the focal point: move the magnifier further away and the image distorts;
2. which spectacles (if any) should be worn with the magnifier;
3. the location of the on/off switch and other controls, if present; and
4. how to change the batteries, if relevant.

Instruction in Distance Low Vision Aid Use

Distance low vision aids can be less intuitive to use than near magnifiers, so more detailed instruction is likely to be needed (and perhaps training, see Section 'Training for Distance Vision Aids' later).

The patient should be advised:
1. How the aid is mounted (spectacle-mounted; permanently or clip-on), or how carried (wrist or neck strap).
2. Which end goes towards the eye. Often the device will have a rubber cup around the eyepiece, so the patient should learn that the 'squishy end' goes towards the eye.

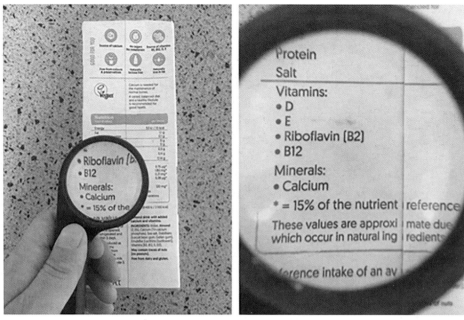

Fig. 20.1 Demonstrating that field of view increases as the magnifier is brought closer to the eye.

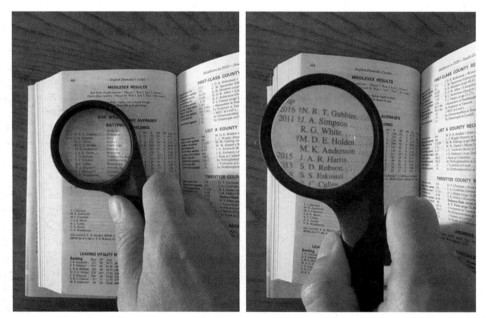

Fig. 20.2 Demonstrating the effect of task distance on magnification: no magnification is given with the magnifier flat on the page; it must be slowly raised to where the object is at the focal point and magnification is optimal.

3. Whether to use the aid with the distance spectacles. If it is to be used as an outdoor spotting aid, this must be with the spectacles if worn: for such an intermittent task, the patient cannot keep taking their spectacles off. For longer tasks, such as watching theatre performances or cricket matches, it will depend on whether the patient has significant astigmatism.

4. In the case of a monocular device, what to do with the nonviewing eye? Can it be ignored and suppressed, or must it be covered? It is often easier to hold the aid with the hand on the same side of the body as the eye being used. If the hand on the opposite side is used, however, this can sometimes be placed up to the eyes in such a way that it acts as an occluder for the unused eye.

5. How to position the aid to minimise device movement. The supporting arm can be braced against the upper body, or the elbow cupped in the opposite palm. If sitting, the elbow can be supported on a table or chair arm. Explain that any tremor of the aid will lead to magnified image motion, which must be avoided if optimum performance is to be obtained.

6. How the aid should be positioned as close to the eye (or spectacles) as possible to increase field-of-view. To achieve this, the thumb and first finger can be placed in a ring

around the eyepiece, and these are then held against the bones of the orbit to steady it. With practice the patient may be dextrous enough to focus the telescope with the middle, ring or little fingers of the same hand. This should not be practised at too early a stage, because the focusing mechanism of new telescopes is often rather stiff and it may need two hands to carry out fine manipulation until the mechanism becomes smoother. It can be helpful to have the telescope looped around the neck on a cord, just in case it is dropped. Show the focusing range of the telescope, showing how a minimum separation of the component lenses produces optimal focus for long distance, whilst the longest telescope length corresponds with the closest viewing distance.

TRAINING IN THE USE OF LOW VISION AIDS

Although many people can use simple low vision aids after instruction (Cheong et al., 2005), some may need extra training. One study showed that 25% of people who were unhappy with their low vision clinic appointment would have liked more device training (McIlwaine et al., 1991) and highlighted that even a small clinic spends thousands of pounds on low vision devices which are issued but not used.

In their scoping review of low vision aid use, Lorenzini and Wittich (2020) associated higher amounts of device training with more success: they pointed out that in a clinic for US military veterans, at least 20 hours of device training and practice was provided, contributing to a very high success rate (Watson et al., 1997).

Training may be carried out by the prescriber, or by other personnel within the clinic such as dispensing opticians, optometric assistants or ophthalmic technicians. A limit of training in the clinic or practice is that practitioners rarely have time to travel outside with their patients or to visit them in their homes. Rehabilitation officers may be able to offer training in the home or workplace, and mobility instructors will usually work with their clients outdoors.

Simple devices such as dome magnifiers may not require any training, whereas electronic magnifiers and telescopes may need more in-depth training. The limited amount of training time available in NHS hospital clinics may be one reason that few spectacle-mounted telescopes are prescribed in these services (Crossland & Silver, 2005).

Training for Near Optical Low Vision Aids

Training is best performed when the patient is comfortable and in a home-like environment. The ideal set up would include an office desk and chair, a table and dining chair, a kitchen surface and an armchair. Various light sources should be available including task lights, desk lights, and a reading lamp. Nonoptical aids such as rulers and typoscopes should be kept in the same area, along with needle-threaders, felt or fibre-tip pens, writing frames and samples of large print.

A variety of reading tests and real-world reading material should be available, including menus, magazines, books, letters, food packets and medicine labels, as well as intermediate tasks such as music, sewing, jigsaws, DIY equipment, playing cards and a computer screen.

The exact format of the training programme will vary for each individual patient and trainer and may be very informal in some cases. A comprehensive device training routine would follow the following stages (adapted from Freeman & Jose, 1997):

1. Observe the patient to determine any physical difficulties and limitations in the use of the low vision aid.
2. Review the objectives to be achieved by use of the aid and remind the patient of related tasks which the aid is definitely not suitable for. Point out the advantages and disadvantages of the aid (e.g. 'it allows you to see your knitting, but you need to hold it closer than you did before').
3. Review other strategies which will be used with the device, such as eccentric viewing and steady eye strategy.
4. Discuss the successes and problems revealed when the patient first used the aid during the initial assessment (e.g. 'You were able to read very small print but found it difficult to find the beginning of each new line').
5. Assess performance with the aid. Measure the patient's present performance: for reading, a timed test will be useful to act as a baseline standard.
6. Review the positioning of the aid.
7. Determine the best physical setting. Discuss lighting, posture and appropriate seating (with or without a table or work surface on which to lean), and the best way to hold and support the magnifier and the task (perhaps considering a reading stand, clipboard, or double-ended clamp for the magnifier). Decide if nonoptical aids might help, such as fibre-tip pens and a writing frame, or a typoscope for reading.
8. Assess the individual skill elements which go to make up the task. Ask the patient to perform the task, breaking it down into its component sections and assessing whether each of these individually is optimally performed. For example, for reading individual skill elements would be to spot and localise the area of interest (the beginning of the first line on the page, the headline of an article) within the task area, to track along the full line of text right to the end (but to realise where the blank spaces are between columns), to return to the start of the next line without repeating or missing a line, and to appreciate when the end of the article/page has been reached.
9. Practise based on revealed weaknesses. Particular practice tasks can be devised which can be performed repetitively to allow the patient to improve that skill. For example, if the patient struggles to find the start of each line, they can be asked to follow a zig-zag pattern by tracing each line back and then going to the next line down. The patient should also be given the opportunity to demonstrate and reinforce their strengths so as not to become anxious by concentrating only on what they cannot do.
10. Repeat assessment of performance. This would be a repeat of the assessment which was carried out in step 5 above, to measure any improvement. This can be very motivating to the patient and demonstrates the importance of practice.

11. Review the patient's understanding of how the aid(s) are to be used.

12. Evaluate the patient's feelings about how successful the aid is in relation to the required aims. Demonstrate how much their performance has improved during the training session. Remind them how difficult these tasks were previously and reassure them they can expect further improvement with continued practice. Daily practice with aids is known to be associated with optimal performance but the patient may decide that this effort is not worth the potential gain: they may, for example, have set the goal of reading novels, but decide that it is always going to be challenging to read with a magnifier no matter how much practice they do, and choose to use talking books instead.

13. Encourage the patient to practice at home, give them written instructions if appropriate. Reassure them that it is normal to become tired or frustrated when first using a magnifier, and that it may feel like they are 'learning to read again'. Frequent short practice sessions are generally preferred.

14. Plan the next training session, perhaps in one or two weeks. Give an indication of how many more visits are likely to be needed, how long each visit will last, and what the final goal is at the end of this series of visits.

Training for Distance Vision Aids

Training is more likely to be required for distance vision aids such as monocular telescopes. The devices themselves are more complex, and the concept of focusing can be challenging for people with longstanding visual impairment. Devices are likely to be used in settings which are more crowded: for example, finding a platform indicator board in a large railway station is a visually demanding task. They are more likely to be used outside, with variations in lighting and contrast, and whilst the user is standing. They are also more dangerous to use: if someone tries to walk when using spectacle-mounted distance telescopes they are likely to fall; if they look at the sun with a telescope they may develop severe retinal disease.

It is useful to demonstrate the device indoors (first sitting, and then standing) before moving to an outside training session.

Equipment which can help the patient use a telescopic device includes a brightly coloured ball (for tracking moving targets), hollow cardboard tubes (for practising lining up the telescope with the object of interest) and even a slide projector to demonstrate the concept of 'focusing' an image.

A complete training package will mirror that offered for near low vision aids earlier. Specific additional skills for telescope use are localisation, focusing, spotting, tracing, tracking and scanning. Unlike the skills involved in reading, none of these are familiar skills to the patient, as they are skills related to the aid rather than to the task to be performed. It is likely that all patients will need at least some instruction to make the best use of the device.

Localisation involves lifting the telescope into position as quickly and accurately as possible, so that the object can be seen. This can be most readily achieved with a single bright object against an uncluttered background, such as a torch light in a darkened room. This can then progress to aligning the telescope to view the instructor, where auditory cues can also be used to assist. Patients often find the task difficult because as they move the telescope to their eye they drop their gaze to it. On the contrary, the patient should keep fixating all the time on the distant object of interest, and interpose the telescope along their line of sight. A lower-powered telescope with wider field-of-view could be substituted temporarily for training purposes, or the patient could practice whilst viewing through hollow cardboard tubes.

Initially the patient may find it easier with the nonviewing eye covered, but should progress to having both eyes open, and ignoring the unmagnified view from the nonviewing eye. It can sometimes be arranged that the view of this eye is obscured by placing the hand holding the telescope across in front of it.

As the patient becomes more skilful, several objects can be placed together, and the patient is instructed to align the telescope to view just one of them: to accomplish this they must lift the telescope to their eye, and then move in precise fashion between the various objects to find the one required.

Focusing involves the subject exploring the whole range of image distances for which a clear image can be arranged. The instructor positions the target at a variety of distances and encourages the patient to refocus the telescope each time. A guide to whether this is being done correctly can be obtained from the visual acuity (because letters of half the size could be read at half the distance) and from the clinician viewing through the telescope to check the clarity of vision. If in doubt, the concept of focus may need to be explained by blurring and clearing a target on a slide projector.

Spotting combines localisation and focusing skills: the distant object is seen without the telescope, then the telescope is raised so it is aligned between the eye and the object and focuses the telescope to view the target. Brightly coloured shapes stuck onto a plain white wall can be used, and if numbers are written on the shapes, these will monitor the accuracy of focusing. As the patient's skill increases, the shapes and numbers can be made smaller. Photographs from magazines, cut out and placed against the plain background, can be used to test the patient's ability to interpret the magnified image.

Tracing involves following a stationary line in the environment, such as the edge of a shelf or a line drawn on a wall. A similar task which also involves refocusing of the telescope can be set by laying coloured tape or rope across the floor or table-top in a random way. Along its length (at progressively increasing distances from the patient) cards containing written words are placed: the subject must trace along the rope, constantly altering the focus of the aid in order to read the cards.

Tracking is the same principle using a moving object. For example, the instructor walks around the room carrying a picture which can be moved side-to-side or vertically or rolls a coloured ball across the floor. The patient will need to learn to move their head smoothly at the same speed as the object they are watching (and may need to practice this without a telescope first of all). If the object moves towards the patient, they will need to constantly refocus as well as track the object.

Scanning is the most difficult skill to learn. This involves searching the environment for an object which **cannot** be seen without the telescope: in previous spotting tasks, the object could be seen without the telescope, although its fine detail was indistinguishable. An orderly sequence of overlapping horizontal sweeps of the telescope must be used to systematically search the designated area. In early training the area should be defined by a clearly seen border (black lines on a wall), with a small picture placed within the boundary. The time taken to locate and identify the picture can be recorded. Alternatively, an object could be placed on a large table-top, and the patient scans to locate and identify it.

Application to everyday tasks is the ultimate aim and will involve elements of all the skills practised. They are usually outdoor rather than indoor requirements, and it can be useful to train outdoors because it gives the realism of the 'uncontrolled' environment of different colours and luminance with randomly moving targets. Each task should be discussed with the patient to decide how it might best be performed. For example, in looking for the number of an approaching bus, it is difficult to both align and focus the telescope within the limited time available. A more effective technique is to focus the telescope in advance, using a lamp-post, street sign or shop frontage which the bus will pass. When the bus is seen approaching, a sweep of the telescope across the visual field should allow the destination board to be seen. The motion of the telescope must then be matched to the movement of the bus for long enough to allow reading of the sign. Alternatively, if the patient wished, for example, to locate a street sign at the junction of two roads, a knowledge of its likely location could guide the scanning routine. It may well be near to ground level, below the ground floor window, or higher on the wall below the first-floor window. Beginning at ground level, focusing on the building wall, and then using systematic overlapping side-to-side sweeps will allow the clear image of the sign to be found. Mobility instructors will be familiar with the layout of street signs in the relevant borough.

Training for Aids for Increasing Peripheral Field Awareness

A reversed telescope or handheld minifier is used as a spotting aid. To become familiar with this, the patient is first asked to look around the clinic room with the minifier without moving their eyes and to report on what they can see. The instructor can move around the room and ask the patient where they are standing and what they are doing (e.g. waving or standing on one leg). The patient can then move to the end of a corridor and be asked to use their device to find obstacles such as fire extinguishers and litter bins, and to plan their route along the corridor. Training can progress to route planning

in complex environments such as railway station concourses, initially when they are quiet, then finally at busy times.

To use sector or peripheral prisms, patients should practise making head movements so they can see the target through the unobstructed (prism-free) portion of the spectacle lens (see Chapter 12). Patients adapt quickly to the prism, after only a few minutes (Giorgi et al., 2009). Although hand-eye coordination can be improved further with additional computer-based training (Houston et al., 2016), many patients benefit from peripheral prisms with minimal extra training.

Training for Electronic Vision Enhancement Systems

It was previously thought that extensive training was needed to use electronic magnifiers, but a recent randomised controlled trial has shown that there is no benefit from additional training, beyond that provided by the device supplier (Burggraaff et al., 2012a, b). This is probably due to improvements in the design of these devices and patients' increasing familiarity with technology.

Training for Accessibility Settings on Consumer Electronic Devices

Training and support for consumer devices, such as smartphones and tablets, may be offered by rehabilitation workers for visual impairment and by many local sight loss charities: such individuals may be called 'Digital Inclusion' specialists. Patients might have tech-savvy relatives who are happy to work through the accessibility settings with them, perhaps using online videos for the specific operating system used. Some device manufacturers have staff trained in supporting people with vision impairment in their shops, and larger shops (such as Apple Stores) run sessions for people with low vision to explore their device settings. However, do not forget that patients may not have even basic technology skills, they may be anxious about using these devices, and they might find environments like an Apple Store quite alien.

REFERENCES

Burggraaff, M. C., van Nispen, R. M. A., Hoeben, F. P., et al. (2012a). Randomized controlled trial on the effects of training in the use of closed-circuit television on reading performance. *Investigative Ophthalmology & Visual Science, 53*(4), 2142–2150.

Burggraaff, M. C., van Nispen, R. M. A., Knol, D. L., et al. (2012b). Randomized controlled trial on the effects of CCTV training on quality of life, depression, and adaptation to vision loss. *Investigative Ophthalmology & Visual Science, 53*(7), 3645–3652.

Cheong, A. M. Y., Lovie-Kitchin, J. E., Bowers, A. R., et al. (2005). Short-term in-office practice improves reading performance with stand magnifiers for people with AMD. *Optometry and Vision Science, 82*(2), 114–127.

Collins, J. (1988). Low vision services. *British Journal of Visual Impairment, 6*(3), 111.

Crossland, M. D., & Silver, J. H. (2005). Thirty years in an urban low vision clinic: Changes in prescribing habits of low vision practitioners. *Optometry and Vision Science, 82*(7), 617–622.

Freeman, P. B., & Jose, R. T. (1997). *The art and practice of low vision* (2nd ed.). Butterworth-Heinemann.

Giorgi, R. G., Woods, R. L., & Peli, E. (2009). Clinical and laboratory evaluation of peripheral prism glasses for hemianopia. *Optometry and Vision Science, 86*(5), 492–502.

Houston, K. E., Bowers, A. R., Fu, X., et al. (2016). A pilot study of perceptual-motor training for peripheral prisms. *Translational Vision Science and Technology, 5*(1), 9.

Lorenzini, M. -C., & Wittich, W. (2020). Factors related to the use of magnifying low vision aids: A scoping review. *Disability and Rehabilitation, 42*(24), 3525–3537.

McIlwaine, G. G., Bell, J. A., & Dutton, G. N. (1991). Low vision aids—Is our service cost effective? *Eye, 5*(5), 607–611.

Mehr, E. B., & Freid, A. N. (1975). *Low vision care*. Professional Press.

Watson, G. R., L'Aune, D., Stelmack, W., et al. (1997). National survey of the impact of low vision device use among veterans. *Optometry and Vision Science, 74*(5), 249–259.

Evaluating Low Vision Services

Optometrists may find it unusual to consider the concept of 'success' in relation to one of their prescribing strategies, because the supply of spectacles for the correction of refractive error is almost invariably successful. It has always been clear, however, from a large number of surveys carried out in several countries over many years, that one cannot expect to achieve 100% success in the prescription of low vision aids (LVAs). Whilst surveys of whole populations are very useful to determine the effectiveness of low vision care, it is helpful for the practitioner to consider how this relates to an individual patient they are assessing. Why are some patients unsuccessful, and could this have been predicted (and even prevented) if the assessment or prescribing routines had been modified?

PROGNOSTIC FACTORS FOR THE SUCCESSFUL USE OF LOW VISION AIDS

It is very difficult to generalise which patients will do particularly well with low vision rehabilitation and which will struggle. Although each patient should be treated as an individual, clinical experience suggests that some groups of people are more likely to respond well to LVAs (Table 21.1).

Those patients with a moderate visual acuity (VA) loss are most likely to benefit from magnification. In severe vision loss, the choice of LVAs is more limited and they are more difficult to use (they usually have high magnification, associated with short working distance and small field-of-view). Those with vision better than about 0.4 logMAR are also often difficult to help as they are more likely to assume that spectacles can completely 'cure' their vision loss. When asked what tasks they have difficulty with, they often identify an extensive list: it is not that their vision is insufficient to perform any of these tasks, but that it is not as good as the patient believes it could (or should) be.

Low contrast sensitivity (CS) has a severe effect on functional performance, and optical aids do not enhance contrast. Poor CS (such that contrast reserve is less than 3:1) makes using any optical device for reading difficult. A contrast reserve greater than 10:1 means that magnification and lighting are often very effective. People with CS of better than 1.05 log units read more fluently with magnifiers (Latham & Tabrett, 2012).

It is much more difficult to prescribe LVAs to aid peripheral field loss than it is to prescribe magnifying devices: and if a magnifying aid is required by a patient with extensive field loss, there must be sufficient field remaining to appreciate the magnified image. With an annular or ring scotoma, there may be good acuity for single letters but a very small visual field, which makes reading words almost impossible: it is very difficult for these patients to use eccentric viewing. The patient is more likely to quickly adapt to viewing eccentrically if an absolute central scotoma is present.

Rapidly changing vision makes rehabilitation challenging, whether in a progressive condition, like retinitis pigmentosa, or a condition where the vision fluctuates, like diabetic retinopathy. If the condition is stable, the LVA will not require frequent changing and the patient will have the opportunity to become proficient in its use. If there are rapid changes in vision, major changes in the type of aid may need to be made at every visit in order to provide the increasing magnification required. One of the advantages of electronic vision enhancement systems (EVES) in such cases is the ability to deliver increasing magnification without the need for a change in the device or the way it is used. If the condition is active, the patient may be seeking or receiving medical or surgical treatment, which may cause their vision to fluctuate and make the patient uninterested in LVAs whilst there is the prospect of a 'cure'.

As a general rule, people with lifelong, stable levels of low vision are better candidates for help, as they have not previously

TABLE 21.1 **Factors Which Have Been Found to Influence the Likelihood of Individuals Being Successful With the Use of LVAs**

Factor	Likely to Respond Better to LVAs	Likely to Respond Less Well to LVAs
Visual acuity	0.5–1.3 logMAR	Better than 0.5 logMAR Poorer than 1.3 logMAR
Contrast sensitivity	Better than 1.05 log units	Poorer than 1.00 log units
Visual field	Well defined, small scotoma	Ring scotoma Extensive peripheral loss 'Patchy' fields
Stability	Stable condition	Progressive or fluctuating condition
Current treatment	No ophthalmological treatment	Undergoing medical or surgical treatment
Employment situation	Computer based Based in one workplace Students	Skilled manual work Extensive work-related travel Dynamic tasks
Comorbidity	No comorbidity	Poor memory Poor dexterity Poor mobility Other sensory loss
Acceptance	Accepting of sight loss	Not accepting of sight loss In denial/disbelief

LVAs, Low vision aids.

relied on good vision to perform a task. On the other hand, they might have little visual experience and have become experienced with tactile and auditory methods. A patient with an acquired loss of long duration must be questioned carefully to find out why they have never sought help before: they could also have well-developed nonvisual strategies which they will not abandon, or simply have become accustomed to not performing particular tasks. There may be a very good reason for their action, however, such as the recent death of a spouse who had previously performed many visual tasks for them.

Having specific and realistic aims is important. Fortunately, the most common requirement identified by people attending a low vision clinic is difficulty with reading and writing (Shuttleworth et al., 1995). Brown et al. (2014) asked patients who were attending a low vision service for the first time, 'What are your chief complaints about your vision?' Two-thirds of the patients responded that reading was their major concern. However, more than a quarter responded 'driving'—something which low vision clinics are not generally able to help with (apart from those areas where driving with bioptic telescopes is permitted). It is interesting that 11% of patients in this study identified no complaints: it is not uncommon to find that a patient cannot name any specific task when asked 'what would you like to be able to improve'. This patient, who is perhaps looking for a general improvement in their vision, is much more difficult to manage than the patient who brings in a written list of specific requests.

The patient must be willing to accept the restrictions on the performance of the task imposed by the use of an LVA, which may be physical (such as the close working distance) or optical (such as aberrations when viewing through the lens periphery). The choice of which aid will be most appropriate for them often depends on which they perceive to create the least restriction.

The level of psychological adjustment to, and acceptance of, vision loss is probably the single most important factor in successfully using LVAs. Someone who accepts their vision loss is likely to present to the low vision clinic, to engage with suggestions which are made, and to be comfortable using LVAs in public. Interestingly, the best predictor of adjustment is personality type and not visual ability, severity of visual impairment or duration of sight loss (Tabrett & Latham, 2012). This study showed that people with high levels of conscientiousness (the desire to carry out tasks carefully and diligently) and lower levels of neuroticism (less likely to experience anxiety, or to be overwhelmed by minor frustrations) were most likely to be successful.

Even if the prognosis does not seem to be encouraging, much can be achieved if the patient is sufficiently motivated and the practitioner adjusts their own and the patient's expectations. If the patient is only motivated to do something which cannot be assisted with aids, however, then no further action can be taken. For these patients, then, aids are simply not appropriate and it is perhaps misleading to call them 'unsuccessful'. Even if a magnifier is not prescribed, it is unlikely that the assessment was a waste of time. It is difficult to tell someone that they will not be able to perform some tasks, such as driving, but this awareness can help the patient adjust to their eye condition. They may be willing to accept further low vision help in the future and an open invitation to reattend the clinic should be offered.

DEFINING SUCCESS

One of the major difficulties in conducting evaluations to determine 'success' is in deciding exactly what this is. If considering the success of a treatment, or intervention, it is important to have a clear idea exactly what it was intended to achieve, such that it is clear whether that aim has been achieved. Often, in a medical field, a treatment is evaluated initially under very closely controlled conditions, with carefully selected participants who have no other health conditions (comorbidities) which might influence how well the treatment works. This gives a measure of efficacy: if and how it works under ideal conditions. In more normal clinical circumstances, these ideal conditions may not be met. The individuals being treated may present with mitigating factors that make the treatment less likely to succeed, or they may not comply with the instructions for optimum use of the device, or they may prefer alternative means to carry out the activity. Measuring what happens as a result of the treatment under these conditions tells us about its effectiveness. To put this in the context of low vision, efficacy may be measured by asking the patient to use a magnifier to read standard texts with optimum lighting in a clinic, but effectiveness is how well the patient can use the device in their everyday life.

A major complication when considering low vision rehabilitation is that it is a so-called 'complex intervention'. This means that it consists of many overlapping and complementary aspects, each of which may have both direct and indirect influences in many areas of daily life. This means that the true effect may not be captured by a single 'outcome measure': for example, if providing a magnifier allows the patient to remain in employment, it is unlikely that a measure of reading speed is enough to represent the full effect on that patient's life. If an attempt is made to single out one element of the intervention to study in isolation, the effect may be very small, and be judged to be insignificant.

In fact, Binns et al. (2012) identified 47 different outcome measures in their systematic review of the effectiveness of low vision rehabilitation. Unfortunately, if each intervention is evaluated using a different outcome measure, it is not possible to compare the effectiveness of competing methods of rehabilitation (Ehrlich et al., 2017).

As the use of magnifying devices is at the forefront of much provision, improvement in acuity is one possible outcome measure. This is not as helpful as it seems, however, because this is much more a function of the device than of the user: it is relatively straightforward to improve single letter acuity by altering the magnification selected. Even extending this to word reading acuity is not sufficient: just because a patient can 'see to read' (i.e. they can recognise words of newsprint size) this does not necessarily mean that they will regularly read the newspaper for pleasure (Rumney, 1995). This was demonstrated by Leat et al. (1994), who found that whilst 75% of the patients surveyed could read 1 M (approximately newsprint size) print in the clinic, only 35% admitted to reading normal print at home.

It may be that this difference is related to the reading speed achieved. It is suggested that to read for education, work or leisure over an extended period requires a fluent speed of at least 80 words per minute (wpm), whereas a much slower speed (40 wpm) could support survival reading (see Chapter 3 for further details). This important distinction has led to reading speed being considered an important outcome measure for rehabilitation using magnifiers. A much broader definition of success could be used, such as that of Hall et al. (1987) who suggested that low-vision care is successful when more independence is gained, when more understanding of the eye condition and the way it affects daily life is gained, and when the patient feels that all possible avenues have been explored, whether or not increased independence is possible. Considering the use of magnifiers specifically, Nilsson (1990a) used a more functional definition of success, asking the patient if they could read newspaper text and see TV pictures and subtitles. Various studies (Leat et al., 1994; Bischoff, 1995) have emphasised the fact that relatively modest gains in ability may be useful for some individuals. Leat et al. found that 79% of patients used an aid for 'reading-related tasks' but 23% could only read for 1 minute or less. Nonetheless, 81% used their aid at least 1× daily, and 86% kept it with them constantly, or within easy reach. They conclude that

> 'short frequent bursts of activity can be useful, and patient expectations modified accordingly … Extended reading should be considered a bonus'

presumably suggesting that for many patients, 'survival' reading is a useful endpoint. The Manchester Low Vision Questionnaire (MLVQ) is an attempt to quantify the usefulness of devices for that particular individual in a structured way, in terms of how much they are used (if ever), for how many tasks, and with what degree of difficulty (Harper et al., 1999).

To try to capture potential improvements in everyday functioning as a result of vision rehabilitation, in a quantitative method, various patient-reported outcome measures (PROMs) have been suggested for use. These include both vision-related (VR) and health-related (HR) quality of life (QoL) instruments (see Chapter 4), which describe the individual's ability to perform everyday tasks: the so-called Activities of Daily Living (ADLs) or Instrumental Activities of Daily Living (IADLs). ADLs are fundamental abilities, regardless of the person's circumstances, and include the ability to eat and maintain personal hygiene. IADLs are not so necessary for life, but they are important for living independently and functioning well within society. They include, for example, preparing meals, managing finances and using transport. VRQoL often concentrates heavily on these IADLs, so many of which rely on the ability to read. They are therefore likely to be more sensitive to the intervention as they relate specifically to vision. The HRQoL questionnaires are more general and often relate to ADLs and so are less relevant to vision impairment (VI). However, they do allow vision rehabilitation to be compared to interventions and treatments in other healthcare specialties. The most common method used to make these comparisons at the present time is the EQ-5D instrument (Euroqol Research Foundation, n.d.). The currency for such comparisons is Quality Adjusted Life Years (QALYs), which is a product of the length of time an individual lives with the condition, and their QoL during that time (Kirkdale et al., 2010). To establish whether a treatment offers 'value for money' the QALYs gained can be judged against the cost. This will include the direct cost of equipment, staff time and healthcare resources (e.g. clinic visits). The time contributed by informal carers (family members and friends), which might be reduced if the patient becomes more independent, is also accounted for. This will allow an incremental cost-effectiveness ratio (ICER) to be calculated: this is a measure of the extra cost for the extra QALY. Such health economic evaluations are rare in vision rehabilitation studies (Binns et al., 2012) but Bray et al. (2017) evaluated the ICER for portable EVES magnifiers being provided in addition to optical aids in a hospital clinic. If a new intervention is both better and cheaper, it will obviously be adopted, but if it is more expensive, then such economic evaluations can be used by healthcare providers in deciding whether to allocate limited resources to it.

Improvements in functioning and independence are likely to increase feelings of well-being and decrease depression in patients, and these characteristics have also been the subject of questionnaires used to evaluate the success of rehabilitation.

A further consideration is the timing of any measurement taken to judge success. It should be far enough removed from the initial consultation that the patient has had the opportunity to obtain full benefit from it but is also over the initial positive effect from the contact itself. It would be hoped that any effect measured would be sustained over a prolonged period, but for many patients, their condition is advancing in addition to their age, which could mitigate this to some extent.

A further problem with studying the effectiveness of low vision rehabilitation is an ethical one: having a control group with no access to low vision services is unfair to those randomised to this group. This means that many published studies are case series, which are confounded by many other effects (such as increased contact time, natural adaptation to vision loss and practice in living with low vision). Some of these concerns can be overcome with waiting list control studies, but these can only take place in centres where there is a long delay before appointments can be offered.

Evidence for the Success of Low Vision Rehabilitation

As noted previously, the methods of evaluation are varied but can be summarised as performance-based (e.g. reading speed) or patient-reported (using validated PROMs) (Ehrlich et al., 2017). If the rehabilitation involves provision of devices (e.g. magnifiers), then an additional measure would be usage of the devices.

A very traditional approach is that reported by Nguyen et al. (2009), who found significant improvement in reading speed after provision of magnifiers (from a mean of 20 to 72 wpm for the whole group). A total of 94% of patients were able to read newsprint-sized text with aids, compared to only 16% without. However, this observational study design is considered as low-quality evidence, because there is no comparison of alternative types of magnifiers, or even

of no intervention. A systematic review of optical and electronic aids (Virgili et al., 2018) found that there was modest evidence that reading with stand-mounted EVES was faster than with optical devices. Electronic aids also support longer duration reading but are less versatile (tend to be used for fewer tasks) than optical aids, as evidenced by use of the MLVQ (Taylor et al., 2017).

In a telephone survey of 88 patients from different clinics who had been prescribed with various types of magnifiers approximately 1 year previously, 71% of the aids had been used during the previous week, but 19% had not been used in the past 3 months (Dougherty et al., 2011). The most common reasons for abandonment included worsening vision, the aid no longer being effective, and use of an alternative device for the task: there was no association with patient age, acuity level or type of magnifier. Watson et al. (1997) reported 85.4% of devices still in use between 1 and 2 years after supply, in their telephone survey of users. They found that continued use was associated with the presence of a supportive helper at home: in fact, in their rehabilitation setting, many spouses had received education on the importance of family support. All the patients had also received extensive training (median >20 hours) in the use of devices.

Although low vision rehabilitation differs substantially in its scope (the range of services incorporated) and its organisation ('one-stop-shop' multidisciplinary vs multiagency), the primary aim is to improve overall functioning and independence for patients. It is therefore necessary to measure this directly in order to assess effectiveness of an intervention. LOVIT (The Veterans Affairs Low Vision Intervention Trial) was an evaluation of a comprehensive outpatient rehabilitation programme for individuals with macular disease causing moderate to severe loss of vision (worse than 6/30; 0.7 logMAR) (Stelmack et al., 2008). The comprehensive intervention included optical and electronic magnifiers, training and homework using aids (five 2-hour in-practice sessions, each followed by 5 hours homework exercises) and advice on environmental modification. Outcomes were measured with the Visual Functioning Questionnaire-48 (VFQ-48), which asked participants to describe their activity limitations in reading, mobility, visual information processing and visually guided movement. Importantly the study had a control group who received no care: individuals were randomly assigned to a 'waiting list' or to immediate intervention. This study provided the first robust evidence of a significant benefit of rehabilitation in all the activity domains, but particularly on reading ability. In contrast, the waiting list group showed small losses in functioning, suggesting that it is beneficial to begin rehabilitation as soon as possible. Despite the strengths of this research, it should not be assumed that its results will be replicated by every low vision clinic: it is an evaluation of a particular protocol, in a specific group of patients. An evaluation of the Welsh Low Vision Service, which is a much less intensive intervention, and delivered on a multi-agency basis, also found very significant improvements in functioning and high usage of aids reported by patients immediately (Ryan et al., 2010) and 18 months later (Ryan et al., 2013). There have been a number of recent studies which have suggested that the finding of a significant improvement in vision-related functioning (VRQoL) as a result of vision rehabilitation can be replicated in several settings (Goldstein et al., 2015; Liu et al., 2021). There is not, however, any consistent evidence of an improvement in HRQoL (Binns et al., 2012; van Nispen et al., 2020; Liu et al., 2021). To tackle the issue of improving psychological well-being, the use of self-management programmes has been advocated. Such a programme is intended to provide the patient with the skills to manage their condition more effectively, by teaching problem-solving skills and goal setting. It is often delivered over a 6- to 8-week period involving weekly meetings and targets (Rees et al., 2015). However, these programs have not been found to offer any additional benefit when combined with a standard rehabilitation intervention (Liu & Chang, 2020).

A specific component of UK low vision rehabilitation is an assessment of need by a rehabilitation officer from the local council's sensory team or a charity, followed up by a number of visits to deliver targeted training and support. This might involve, for example, lighting advice, household tasks, emotional support and long cane training. In a study by Acton et al. (2016), participants who were also accessing optometric low vision assessments were randomised to receive this home visit intervention or to a waiting list control. There was a significantly greater increase in visual function (based on the VFQ-48) in those who received home visits compared with those who did not. The participants also reported their satisfaction with the help received, with only 2/34 participants reporting it as unhelpful. There was, however, no effect on depression, well-being or loneliness, which have been suggested to be improved by the enhancement in visual functioning (Horowitz et al., 2005)

DOES TRAINING WORK?

In the UK, low vision care was initially concentrated on the supply of optical aids from hospital-based clinics, and these did not always achieve success. A survey at Glasgow Eye Infirmary (McIlwaine et al., 1991) found that 33% of patients never used their LVA. Humphry and Thompson (1986) found that of 72% of patients who were provided with a spectacle-mounted LVA, only 23% found it useful at home. These findings were contrasted with surveys from outside the UK (Nilsson 1986, 1989; Virtanen & Laatikainen, 1991; Neve et al., 1992) which showed much higher success rates. As these non-UK clinics routinely provided a training programme in the use of the aids, it could be suggested that this training is generating the enhanced success. In fact, Shuttleworth et al. (1995) repeated the McIlwaine et al. (1991) 'patient satisfaction' questionnaire in a low vision clinic where training was an integral part of the service. On this occasion, 92% of patients stated that the service was sufficient to meet their needs, which compares favourably to the 55% of patients in the original survey who had expressed satisfaction when asked the same question. Training obviously requires a major commitment of the service in time and personnel, but with

a lower wastage rate of LVAs the overall cost of the service is not excessive: the increased benefit to the patient is more difficult to quantify.

There are few studies which have isolated the effects of training from other aspects of their service. Goodrich et al. (1977) monitored the reading speed and duration of 12 patients over a period of 10 consecutive days as they underwent training in using the aids. Improvement occurred throughout the period, and it appeared that it had not reached a final plateau at the conclusion of the study; it was suggested that 15 to 20 days would be needed to achieve that. There is the possibility, however, that the same improvement would have occurred with practice alone and that the training was not a significant factor. This obviously needs to be evaluated with a randomised controlled trial, such as that reported by Burggraaff et al. (2012) and Burggraaff, van Nispen, Knol, et al. (2012). In this study, patients received a new EVES and were randomised to either receive only the instructions provided by the manufacturer, or to receive weekly training in their home with a series of exercises involving realistic tasks performed with the EVES. Although the use of the EVES increased reading performance and decreased patient-reported difficulty on a VRQoL measure, in both groups, there was no evidence for an additional benefit of training.

A positive benefit for the effect of training in the use of optical aids was reported by Nilsson (1990b). A population of 40 consecutive elderly patients, all with age-related maculopathy and acuity less than 6/60, were randomly assigned to two experimental groups—'trained' and 'untrained'. The results are given in Table 21.2.

In the 'trained' group, no subject could read newspaper text before the aid was prescribed, although 65% could read headlines. After a full series of training visits had been made, all the patients could read headlines and text. For the 'untrained' group, it again had 65% of patients reading headlines before the study started, but none reading text. After being given instruction on how to use the magnifier (but not 'training'), the patient went away for a month, before returning for reassessment. At that stage, 25% of the patients could read newspaper text, but they then started on the full training routine, and all patients were able to read newspaper text after completing the training. These dramatic results lead Nilsson (1990a) to say

> 'improvements in visual and near acuity obtained with aids cannot be translated directly into improvements in visual performance in daily life, such as reading longer sections of newspaper text. For successful results in these respects, educational training … is necessary, at least for elderly patients with poor acuity'.

However, it is important to note that these patients were using high-powered, spectacle-mounted plus-lens magnifiers, which require a very short working distance. It is possible that equivalent results would not have been found if hand and stand magnifiers had been used. This suggestion is supported by the results of Pearce et al. (2011) who compared usual low vision care in a UK hospital clinic (providing an aid within a single clinic appointment) with the effect of adding

TABLE 21.2 **A Comparison of the Effect of Training on the Percentage of Patients Who Could Read Newspaper Headlines and Newspaper Text With LVAs**		
Trained Group—Aid prescribed by optometrist, then full training routine with specialist trainer	**Read Newspaper Headlines**	**Read Newspaper Text**
Prior to assessment and prescribing	65%	0%
After training—average of ~5 weekly 1-hour visits (50% had eccentric viewing training)	100%	100%
Untrained Group—Aid prescribed by optometrist		
Prior to assessment and prescribing	65%	0%
After full instruction from prescribing optometrist, and 1 month using aid	70%	25%
Then started on full training routine (55% had eccentric viewing training), result on completion	100%	100%

LVAs, Low vision aids.
From Nilsson, U. L. (1990b).

a follow-up appointment to offer the patient advice on device handling. They found that whilst provision of simple hand and stand magnifiers produced a highly significant improvement in the self-reported ability to perform everyday tasks, there was no additional benefit from the additional training session. There are other possible reasons for the result: this may be insufficient training to have an effect, or the control group may have made particular efforts to use their aids because they were aware their performance was going to be checked later. The study did find that low vision clinic visits improved task performance by the same amount as a VA improvement of more than 0.5 logMAR, showing that a single low vision appointment has dramatic effects on VRQoL (Pearce et al., 2011).

The LOVIT II study (Stelmack et al., 2017) compared the effect of a comprehensive rehabilitation programme (similar content to that in LOVIT (Stelmack et al., 2008) which involves some 35 hours of training and structured practice) to 'Basic LV', which is provision of devices only. It was found that for patients with corrected logMAR VA better than 0.5, there was no difference in results of the two groups, but training was beneficial for those with VA from logMAR 0.5 to 1.0.

Should Training Be Provided?

As can be seen, the evidence on a population basis appears contradictory, so each patient should be evaluated individually. If the patient has been provided with a limited number of simple low-powered aids, can remember instructions, and appears to readily perform realistic tasks unaided after instruction in the clinic, then training is probably not required.

If these conditions are not met, and the practitioner decides that training is required, then it should not be perfunctory: both practitioner and patient have to commit to follow through on the planned protocol of clinic visits and homework. If the patient is struggling to use the aid at the initial dispensing, it should not be assumed that they will suddenly become successful when using this on their own at home without guidance. A full training protocol can be found in Chapter 20.

WHAT ARE SERVICE EVALUATION AND AUDIT?

Clinical audit and service evaluation are restricted to local investigations, use existing data and do not involve new knowledge. This is in contrast to 'research' which involves deriving new knowledge which is generalisable across communities and often involves generating and testing hypotheses. Service evaluation asks, 'What are we doing now?': this might consist, for example, of identifying how many LVAs of different types were dispensed during the past year. It might involve simple questionnaires: for example, gathering patient opinions about the different forms of communication used in the service (website, newsletters, leaflets). Lindsay et al. (2004) describe such an evaluation (although they do describe it as an audit). Service evaluation can also include measuring the effectiveness of the service (e.g. 'can patients read the print size they require, with the LVAs provided by the service?'). This latter study does get close to being defined as research, but in a research project, there should be strong evidence that the performance showed a definite improvement from a baseline measurement without the aid and that the result did not occur spontaneously, or as a result of a placebo effect (i.e. there should be a comparison or control group of patients who do not receive the intervention).

Audit shares some characteristics with service evaluation but measures what is happening in the service against a predetermined standard. This standard would be expected to represent 'best practice', and so the audit process may start with a literature review to determine what that best practice should involve. Alternatively, there may be published guidelines as to what a service should include (Vision 2020 UK, 2003; Dickinson et al., 2011). The audit would then involve a retrospective review of patient records to find out if this optimum protocol was always followed. Unlike the situation with service evaluation, audit then proceeds to try to identify the reasons underlying the results. That is, why is best practice not being achieved, and then the cycle would proceed to make some changes (to procedures) to try to improve matters. To give one example, best practice would suggest that patients with VI are offered certification/registration as sight impaired (SI)/severely sight impaired (SSI) when they are eligible (in this case, best practice is derived from expert consensus (Vision 2020 UK, 2003; RNIB, 2016) rather than published scientific data). Savage et al. (2018) carried out such an audit, and compared the number of registrations in their NHS trust to national and regional averages. They identified lower numbers of registrations due to age-related macular degeneration (AMD) than the national average and attributed this to clinicians not considering certification for patients undergoing active (anti-vascular endothelial growth factor [anti-VEGF]) treatment. They introduced a reminder to the clinician (in the form of a stakeholder meeting at which audit results were discussed), but this did not have any impact on the number of registrations when they conducted a reaudit. The next improvement proposed was the introduction of an Eye Clinic Liaison Officer (ECLO) to lead the certification effort, although the effect of that change is not reported.

If the reaudit shows that new practices have improved the performance of the service, then it is necessary to have a plan to ensure that this standard continues to be maintained in the long term. The next target for improvement is then identified: in this way, the audit process can be very beneficial for the continuous improvement of patient care (Yorston & Wormald, 2010). In a large organisation, the audit policy, priorities and methods will be determined centrally, by a planning group that involves all the stakeholders (e.g. representatives of different staff groups, patients and those commissioning and funding services) (Healthcare Quality Improvement Partnership, 2020). However, for any organisation, it can form an important tool in the range of quality improvement methods available.

In reality, the difference between audit and research can be nuanced. Different levels of ethical approval are required for research studies and audits. Advice should be sought from relevant regulatory authorities before embarking on a research project, or an audit which might be construed as research.

How to Carry Out an Audit

There are many helpful guides to carrying out clinical audits, including those produced by the College of Optometrists (2019). The audit process can be thought of in four stages:

1. Preparation and planning
2. Measuring performance
3. Implementing change
4. Sustaining improvement

1. Preparation and planning

This is the most critical part of the process, and itself consists of a number of stages. It is important to choose a suitable topic, and this should be something which is important for patient care. It might be suggested because it involves some new development in the field, or it has been raised as a concern: this might have been informally by a patient or staff member, or from a more formal meeting of a 'service advisory group' which has representation from all stakeholders. It should be a topic which is important (it forms a significant percentage of the work of the service or affects a large number of the patients) or high cost (in terms of staff numbers, time or equipment). It is important to be specific and not try to cover too much in the single audit. It must also be an area where performance can be measured (without increasing workload unduly), and where changes could potentially be made, and where those changes would have the potential to positively affect patient outcomes. The next stage is to find evidence to support the protocol that is to be used in the service in this topic area. It may be that there already is a clear protocol/expectation in place, but it would be beneficial to very clearly write this down at this stage, to make sure that it is understood by all staff and that there are no misunderstandings. A target of 100% compliance with the protocol (i.e. it is applied for every patient) is desirable, unless there are some lower organisational targets already applied (such as those for NHS waiting times). It is therefore particularly important to note 'exceptions' in the protocol. These would be known patient groups for whom the protocol will not be applied, and there should be an adequate (evidence-based) *clinical* reason for that. Not having sufficient space or staff is not an appropriate reason, and in fact, the results of the audit might then be used to support the case for a reallocation of resources. A search for the latest evidence (preferably in the form of systematic reviews; or professional practice/organisation guidelines) is beneficial at this stage to make sure that the protocol is based on the most up-to-date, high-quality evidence available. Recommended standards, and assessment frameworks, for comprehensive low vision services are available (Wolffsohn & Karas, 2004; Dickinson et al., 2011) and specifically for services for children (Thomas et al., 2015). Having established the protocol to be followed, the performance criteria to be used to judge whether this has been met should be decided. This is likely to be in the form of information included in the patient record—for example, appropriate completion of a particular section of the record card, or the date when a particular action was performed.

An alternative data source would be from a patient questionnaire, which could be a written (postal) questionnaire, by telephone or online. Each of these formats has advantages and disadvantages, and having respondents who are visually impaired complicates this further. A written questionnaire, even in large print, may be inaccessible and may reduce responses from the most severely impaired individuals. An online questionnaire is convenient for automatic data collection but can only survey the subgroup of individuals who have internet access. Some survey formats may not be compatible with speech-reading software. The telephone questionnaire is the most accessible but requires a lot of staff time to conduct, and participants may feel inhibited to give their true opinions to someone working in the service.

For example, a service plans an audit to find out whether all patients with VI are being made aware of Charles Bonnet Syndrome (CBS) (as is recommended by various sight loss charities). The evidence for this would be (1) record of patient reporting hallucinations or definitely not, on specific questioning; (2) record of practitioner explaining condition to patient verbally; and (3) record of practitioner giving them a leaflet about the condition. All of these should be noted in the patient record if they occurred. Additional information could be gained from a questionnaire which asks patients what they know about CBS to find out whether the explanations are achieving their purpose of informing and educating the patient. Any questionnaires used should be tested for clarity of phrasing and ease of understanding by patients: online versions should be tested for compatibility with different operating systems, browsers and screen-reading software.

2. Measuring performance

It is beneficial if the whole staff team (and perhaps the wider advisory group) have been involved in the planning of the audit throughout. Without such commitment, it is unlikely that there will be sufficient motivation to undertake any change to practice which is identified during the audit process. At the very least, staff must be fully informed about what will happen in the audit at the stage where data collection will begin. When deciding what data needs to be collected, it is helpful to consider what a final report of the audit will look like and what it might say. With that in mind it should be easier to identify what information will be needed to draw the relevant conclusions. The member of staff directly responsible must have sufficient time and access to the records to gather the audit data and record it (usually on an Excel spreadsheet), making sure to protect patient confidentiality. Recording is usually very simple: the criteria were achieved (score 1), or it was not (score 0). On some occasions, a partial 0.5 score might be appropriate. The staff member should sample two to five records initially to ensure that the data are available and that the spreadsheet can be completed as expected. Following successful piloting, an agreed number of records can be audited. There is no required size for statistical significance, as might be the case in a research study. However, the sample should be large enough, or over an appropriate time period, to be representative of all patient groups seen. At the end of the audit period, the results can be analysed and presented to the staff team for discussion. If all the standards are being fully met, and there is no need for change, the next stage can be omitted.

3. Implementing change

The results of the audit, and any areas where standards are not met, need to be considered by the whole service team to identify the reasons for this, and to suggest possible means to improve compliance with the standard. The proposed changes do need to be supported by all: they are more likely to be achieved if they fit logically alongside other procedures, which might need to be adjusted to accommodate the change. To return to the CBS example, perhaps it is identified that the leaflet has not been handed out to all patients, and this is because the wording is felt not to be appropriate in all cases. So the action might be to source a different leaflet to use for those patients. Once the change has been implemented, reaudit can occur after a suitable settling-in period. The methods of reaudit should be the same as the original audit, if possible, to ensure that results are directly comparable.

4. Sustaining improvement

Even if audit (or reaudit) has shown the service to now be working to a very high standard in this aspect of care, it is important that this is sustained into the future. A plan of continuous audit can be used, where there is a periodic sampling of patient records. This might involve, for example, every 20th patient, or a particular date in each month.

PERFORMING A RESEARCH STUDY

Performing more in-depth research projects, perhaps to evaluate a new LVA or to investigate a particular aspect of visual impairment, requires careful planning and the input of a variety of professionals. Interested practitioners may want to contact a local university optometry department or teaching hospital to develop a research proposal. In the UK, the College of Optometrists can provide their members with support in planning and performing a study through their small grants scheme.

REFERENCES

Acton, J. H., Molik, B., Court, H., et al. (2016). Effect of a home visit-based low vision rehabilitation intervention on visual function outcomes: an exploratory randomized controlled trial. *Investigative Ophthalmology & Visual Science, 57*(15), 6662–6667. https://doi.org/10.1167/iovs.16-19901.

Binns, A. M., Bunce, C., Dickinson, C., et al. (2012). How effective is low vision service provision? A systematic review. *Survey of Ophthalmology, 57*(1), 34–65. https://doi.org/10.1016/j.survophthal.2011.06.006.

Bischoff, P. (1995). Long-term results of low vision rehabilitation in age-related macular degeneration. *Documenta Ophthalmologica, 89*, 305–311.

Bray, N., Brand, A., Taylor, J., et al. (2017). Portable electronic vision enhancement systems in comparison with optical magnifiers for near vision activities: an economic evaluation alongside a randomized crossover trial. *Acta Ophthalmologica, 95*(5), e415–e423. https://doi.org/10.1111/aos.13255.

Brown, J. C., Goldstein, J. E., Chan, T. L., et al. (2014). Characterizing functional complaints in patients seeking outpatient low-vision services in the United States. *Ophthalmology, 121*(8), 1655–1662. https://doi.org/10.1016/j.ophtha.2014.02.030.

Burggraaff, M., van Nispen, R. M., Hoeben, F., et al. (2012). Randomized controlled trial on the effects of training in the use of closed-circuit television on reading performance. *Investigative Ophthalmology & Visual Science, 53*(4), 2142–2150. https://doi.org/10.1167/iovs.11-8407.

Burggraaff, M., van Nispen, R. M., Knol, D., et al. (2012). Randomized controlled trial on the effects of CCTV training on quality of life, depression, and adaptation to vision loss.

Investigative Ophthalmology & Visual Science, 53(7), 3645–3652. https://doi.org/10.1167/iovs.11-9226.

College of Optometrists. (2019, November). Clinical audit in optometric practice (v4). https://www.college-optometrists.org/clinical-guidance/supplementary-guidance/clinical-audit-in-optometric-practice

Dickinson, C., Linck, P., Tudor-Edwards, R., et al. (2011). A profile of low vision services in England: the Low Vision Service Model Evaluation (LOVSME) project. *Eye, 25*(7), 829–831. https://doi.org/10.1038/eye.2011.112.

Dougherty, B. E., Kehler, K. B., Jamara, R., et al. (2011). Abandonment of low-vision devices in an outpatient population. *Optometry and Vision Science, 88*(11), 1283–1287. https://doi.org/10.1097/OPX.0b013e31822a61e7.

Ehrlich, J. R., Spaeth, G. L., Carlozzi, N. E., et al. (2017). Patient-centered outcome measures to assess functioning in randomized controlled trials of low-vision rehabilitation: a review. *Patient, 10*(1), 39–49. https://doi.org/10.1007/s40271-016-0189-5.

Euroqol Research Foundation. (n.d.). EQ-5D. Retrieved January 2, 2022, from https://euroqol.org/eq-5d-instruments/.

Goldstein, J. E., Jackson, M. L., Fox, S. M., et al. (2015). Clinically meaningful rehabilitation outcomes of low vision patients served by outpatient clinical centers. *JAMA Ophthalmology, 133*(7), 762–769. https://doi.org/10.1001/jamaophthalmol.2015.0693.

Goodrich, G. L., Mehr, E. B., Quillman, R. D., et al. (1977). Training and practice effects in performance with low-vision aids: a preliminary study. *American Journal of Optometry and Physiological, 54*, 312–318.

Hall, A., Sacks, Z. S., Dornbusch, H., et al. (1987). A preliminary study to evaluate patient services in a low vision clinic. *Journal of Vision Rehabilitation, 1*(4), 7–25.

Harper, R., Doorduyn, K., Reeves, B., et al. (1999). Evaluating the outcomes of low vision rehabilitation. *Ophthalmic and Physiological Optics, 19*(1), 3–11. https://doi.org/10.1046/j.1475-1313.1999.00411.x.

Healthcare Quality Improvement Partnership. (2020). *Best practice in clinical audit.* HQIP. https://www.hqip.org.uk/resource/best-practice-in-clinical-audit/#.YwTDiXbMLIU.

Horowitz, A., Reinhardt, J. P., & Boerner, K. (2005). The effect of rehabilitation on depression among visually disabled older adults. *Aging and Mental Health, 9*(6), 563–570. https://doi.org/10.1080/13607860500193500.

Humphry, R. C., & Thompson, G. M. (1986). Low vision aids—Evaluation in a general eye department. *Transactions of the Ophthalmological Societies of the United Kingdom, 105*, 296–303.

Kirkdale, R., Krell, J., O'Hanlon Brown, C., et al. (2010). The cost of a QALY. *QJM, 103*(9), 715–720. https://doi.org/10.1093/qjmed/hcq081.

Latham, K., & Tabrett, D. R. (2012). Guidelines for predicting performance with low vision aids. *Optometry and Vision Science, 89*(9), 1316–1326. https://doi.org/10.1097/OPX.0b013e31825bff1c.

Leat, S. J., Fryer, A., & Rumney, N. J. (1994). Outcome of low vision aid provision: The effectiveness of a low vision clinic. *Optometry and Vision Science, 71*, 199–206.

Lindsay, J., Bickerstaff, D., McGlade, A., et al. (2004). Low vision service delivery: an audit of newly developed outreach clinics in Northern Ireland. *Ophthalmic & Physiological Optics, 24*(4), 360–368. https://doi.org/10.1111/j.1475-1313.2004.00227.x.

Liu, C. J., & Chang, M. C. (2020). Interventions within the scope of occupational therapy practice to improve performance of daily activities for older adults with low vision: a systematic review. *American Journal of Occupationl Therapy, 74*(1), 1–18. https://doi.org/10.5014/ajot.2020.038372.

Liu, J., Dong, J., Chen, Y., et al. (2021). Low vision rehabilitation in improving the quality of life for patients with impaired vision: a systematic review and meta-analysis of 52 randomized clinical trials. *Medicine, 100*(19), e25736. https://doi.org/10.1097/MD.0000000000025736.

McIlwaine, G. G., Bell, J. A., & Dutton, G. N. (1991). Low vision aids—Is our service cost effective? *Eye, 5*, 607–611.

Neve, J. J., Korten, W. E. M., Jorritsma, F. F., et al. (1992). The Visual Advice Center, Eindhoven, The Netherlands. An intervenient evaluation. *Documenta Ophthalmologica, 82*, 15–23.

Nguyen, N. X., Weismann, M., & Trauzettel-Klosinski, S. (2009). Improvement of reading speed after providing of low vision aids in patients with age-related macular degeneration. *Acta Ophthalmologica, 87*(8), 849–853. https://doi.org/10.1111/j.1755-3768.2008.01423.x.

Nilsson, U. L. (1986). Visual rehabilitation of patients with advanced diabetic retinopathy. *Documenta Ophthalmologica, 62*, 369–382.

Nilsson, U. L. (1989). Visual rehabilitation of patients with advanced stages of glaucoma, optic atrophy, myopia or retinitis pigmentosa. *Documenta Ophthalmologica, 70*, 363–383.

Nilsson, U. L. (1990a). Results of low vision rehabilitation. A follow-up study of results in 295 patients and a prospective study regarding the value of educational training in the use of optical aids and residual vision (pp.144–159) [Medical Dissertations No. 313, Linkoping University].

Nilsson, U. L. (1990b). Visual rehabilitation with and without educational training in the use of optical aids and residual vision. A prospective study of patients with advanced age-related macular degeneration. *Clinical Vision Sciences, 6*, 3–10.

Pearce, E., Crossland, M., & Rubin, G. (2011). The efficacy of low vision device training in a hospital-based low vision clinic. *The British Journal of Ophthalmology, 95*(1), 105–108. https://doi.org/10.1136/BJO.2009.175703.

Rees, G., Xie, J., Chiang, P. P., et al. (2015). A randomised controlled trial of a self-management programme for low vision implemented in low vision rehabilitation services. *Patient Education and Counseling, 98*(2), 174–181. https://doi.org/10.1016/j.pec.2014.11.008.

RNIB. (2016). 10 principles of good practice in vision rehabilitation. Retrieved July 26, 2022, from https://www.rnib.org.uk/sites/default/files/10 principles of Good Practice in Vision Rehabilitation.pdf.

Rumney, N. J. (1995). Using visual thresholds to establish low vision performance. *Ophthalmic & Physiological Optics, 15*, S18–S24.

Ryan, B., Khadka, J., Bunce, C., et al. (2013). Effectiveness of the community-based Low Vision Service Wales: a long-term outcome study. *British Journal of Ophthalmology, 97*(4), 487–491. https://doi.org/10.1136/bjophthalmol-2012-302416.

Ryan, B., White, S., Wild, J., et al. (2010). The newly established primary care based Welsh Low Vision Service is effective and has improved access to low vision services in Wales. *Ophthalmic and Physiological Optics, 30*(4), 358–364. https://doi.org/10.1111/j.1475-1313.2010.00729.x.

Savage, N. S. J., Claridge, K., & Green, J. (2018). Increasing rates for certification of visual impairment at Royal Cornwall Hospital Trust: an audit series. *British Journal of Visual Impairment, 36*(2), 143–151. https://doi.org/10.1177/0264619618756471.

Shuttleworth, G. N., Dunlop, A., Collins, J. K., et al. (1995). How effective is an integrated approach to low vision rehabilitation?

Two year follow up results from South Devon. *British Journal of Ophthalmology, 79*(8), 719–723. https://doi.org/10.1136/bjo.79.8.719.

Stelmack, J. A., Tang, X. C., Reda, D. J., et al. (2008). Outcomes of the Veterans Affairs Low Vision Intervention Trial (LOVIT). *Evidence-Based Ophthalmology, 9*(4), 232–233. https://doi.org/10.1097/IEB.0b013e31818913ca.

Stelmack, J. A., Tang, X. C., Wei, Y., et al. (2017). Outcomes of the Veterans Affairs Low Vision Intervention Trial II (LOVIT II). A randomized clinical trial. *JAMA Ophthalmology, 135*(2), 96–104. https://doi.org/10.1001/jamaophthalmol.2016.4742.

Tabrett, D. R., & Latham, K. (2012). Adjustment to vision loss in a mixed sample of adults with established visual impairment. *Investigative Ophthalmology & Visual Science, 53*(11), 7227–7234. https://doi.org/10.1167/iovs.12-10404.

Taylor, J. J., Bambrick, R., Brand, A., et al. (2017). Effectiveness of portable electronic and optical magnifiers for near vision activities in low vision: a randomised crossover trial. *Ophthalmic and Physiological Optics, 37*(4), 370–384. https://doi.org/10.1111/opo.12379.

Thomas, R., Crossland, M. D., & Dahlmann-Noor, A. H. (2015). Multisource evaluation of multidisciplinary low-vision services for children and young people. *British Journal of Visual Impairment, 33*(2), 146–154. https://doi.org/10.1177/0264619615576583.

van Nispen, R. M. A., Virgili, G., Hoeben, M., et al. (2020). Low vision rehabilitation for better quality of life in visually impaired adults. *Cochrane Database of Systematic Reviews, 2020*(1). https://doi.org/10.1002/14651858.CD006543.pub2.

Virgili, G., Acosta, R., Bentley, S. A., et al. (2018). Reading aids for adults with low vision. *Cochrane Database of Systematic Reviews, 2018*(4). https://doi.org/10.1002/14651858.CD003303.pub4.

Virtanen, P., & Laatikainen, L. (1991). Primary success with low vision aids in age-related macular degeneration. *Acta Ophthalmologica, 69*, 484–490.

Vision 2020 UK. (2003). Seeing it my way. *InTech, 50*(4), 34–36.

Watson, G. R., De l'Aune, W., Stelmack, J., et al. (1997). National survey of the impact of low vision device use among veterans. *Optometry and Vision Science, 74*(5), 249–259.

Wolffsohn, J. S., & Karas, M. (2004). Clinical audit cycle of low vision rehabilitation services. *Optometry in Practice, 5*, 115–126.

Yorston, D., & Wormald, R. (2010). Clinical auditing to improve patient outcomes. *Community Eye Health Journal, 23*(74), 48–49.

The Place of Low Vision in Optometric Practice

THE ORGANISATION OF LOW VISION SERVICES IN THE UK

There is now an awareness worldwide that low vision services should aspire to adopt a holistic rehabilitative approach, rather than relying solely on providing low vision aids (LVAs). This has led to an acknowledgement that one single professional group is not best placed to deliver all aspects of such a service, and that a multidisciplinary team is required. However, there is no evidence to support the most effective model for this delivery. In the United States and Australia, there are multidisciplinary services where all the required professionals are available in a single location, but in the UK, this is extremely rare. Dickinson et al. (2011) provided profiles of the different types of low vision service (integrated and multiagency) in the UK, highlighting features of their different ways of working.

Regardless of location, those providing low vision services are always attempting to make them as inclusive as possible, with no barriers to individuals who have a need for the services (Alam et al., 2022). It is desirable that referral into the service can come from any source, including self-referral; that there are no fixed acuity or field standards which need to be met for eligibility; and that patients can refer themselves back into the service whenever required. Recommended standards for low vision clinics encompassing the built environment, staffing requirements, communication strategies and the need for audit have been published (Dickinson et al., 2011).

In the UK, the provision of optical aids for visually impaired patients by optometrists and dispensing opticians was relatively well-established prior to the increase in scope of low vision care. Therefore, a multidisciplinary approach was developed by those involved trying to improve the links between clinical services (often based in hospitals), community-based social low vision services and the voluntary sector (Ryan, 2014). Concurrently, there was a growing need to increase the availability of services to meet demand, and

in England, 'Adult Low Vision' became one of a number of enhanced clinical pathways which could be commissioned in primary care at a local level. Commissioning arrangements are negotiated via the Local Optical Committee (LOC), and sometimes practitioners require additional training and accreditation to be eligible to participate. Typically, these schemes allow for practitioners to be paid a fee for assessment and follow-up, with optical aids (from an agreed inventory) provided to the patient free of charge. Guides are available for commissioners which detail the features they should expect to find in a local scheme (College of Optometrists and the Royal College of Ophthalmologists, 2013; Clinical Council for Eye Health Commissioning CCEHC, 2017).

The Low Vision Service Wales (LVSW) is a similar government-funded primary care-based service which operates from optometric practices throughout Wales, with the advantage over the English system that it is a national rather than local scheme. The LVSW has been shown to achieve the aims intended for all such community-based provision of increasing availability of appointments and reducing travel time (Ryan et al., 2010). At the time of writing, a similar scheme is being developed in Scotland.

It should be emphasised that 'low vision care' is not an exclusive specialist area, but rather a key part of the role of any primary care optometrist (Latham & Macnaughton, 2017). Being able to offer practical advice on lighting, glare avoidance and contrast; offering a reading addition over +3.00; encouraging self-referral to social services; and signposting to charities should be a minimum requirement in any setting (although there is much more that could be done!). A brief explanation of the accessibility features of devices such as smartphones and computers and the availability of free apps is equally within the expertise of the community practitioner as it is for staff in a specialist clinic. Some of this practical advice would also be appropriate for patients who are temporarily visually impaired, such as those being referred for cataract surgery.

EQUIPMENT REQUIRED FOR LOW-VISION WORK

In fact, there is very little specialist equipment required to carry out low vision assessments, much of that required being found in any practice:

1. Mobile distance visual acuity charts, preferably ETDRS (Early Treatment of Diabetic Retinopathy Study) format (Fig. 3.4 A). Projection charts are not usually appropriate because the contrast is often lower, and it is important that the viewing distance and illumination level on the chart can be altered.

2. Trial frame and trial case lenses, preferably full aperture. A phoropter is not effective as it does not easily allow the adoption of unusual head postures, and the patient's use of eccentric viewing cannot be seen.

3. A ±1.00 DC cross-cylinder for subjective confirmation of cylindrical correction.

4. Amsler charts, preferably in the form of copies of the recording chart, showing black lines on a white background, to which diagonal lines have been added to produce a larger fixation target. These can be used for the assessment of central scotomata, and to aid in training eccentric viewing.

5. A test of (peak) contrast sensitivity such as the Mars (Fig. 3.8B) or Pelli-Robson chart. This is essential in providing full information about the patient's functional performance. It informs the prescribing of aids for reading, and when acuity in the two eyes is equal, allows the 'better' eye to be selected.

6. Reading tests for both adults and children. These must be word (rather than single letter) reading charts: one with unrelated words, such as the Bailey-Lovie (Fig. 3.12A), is best in order to avoid guessing by the patient.

7. Tape measure or metre rule to assess and compare working distance, focusing range or depth-of-field.

Additional helpful household and everyday items can be easily and inexpensively sourced:

8. A collection of materials representative of the tasks the patient may wish to perform. These might include: samples of print (magazine, map, book (standard and large print), crosswords and puzzles, newspaper, timetable, food labels and packaging, music, medication); needles and wool/cotton for knitting and sewing; and equipment for DIY (screwdriver, plug, fuse). Different types of pen (fibre-tip vs biro) and paper (dark line vs unlined), and a selection of typoscopes, would allow the patient to experience their effectiveness. All these materials could be collected together in a large tidy box (Fig. 22.1) for use when required.

9. An adjustable-position LED lamp to demonstrate the effectiveness of increased illuminance.

10. A simple demonstration of the effective use of luminance contrast, such as rice in a dark bowl, rather than a light one (Fig. 22.2).

Other more specialised items demonstrating sensory substitution could be added if the opportunity arose, and these might include: signature guides and writing frames; 'Bump-ons' to show how domestic appliances might be marked; a liquid level indicator; and a talking watch or scales. It is also helpful for the practitioner to have various apps and

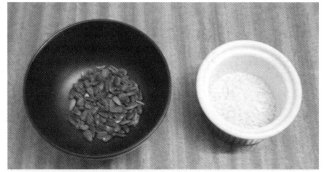
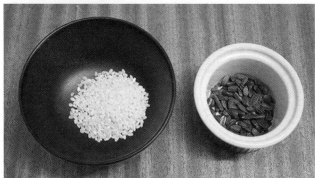

Fig. 22.2 The use of rice and sunflower seeds to demonstrate how containers can be chosen to increase luminance contrast and improve visibility: the rice is much more visible in the black bowl than in the cream bowl.

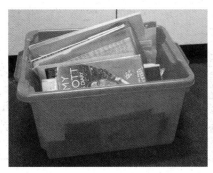
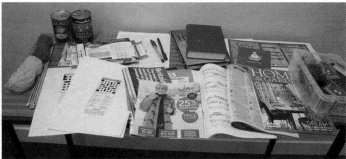

Fig. 22.1 Appropriate items can be collected in the clinic to assess the task performance of patients during low vision assessments.

accessibility settings installed on their smartphone or tablet computer for demonstration.

SELECTING A STOCK OF MAGNIFIERS

Whilst a comprehensive selection of all the LVAs available in the UK would certainly cost several thousand pounds, the majority of patients can be helped with a much more modest collection. The results of surveys in several clinics have suggested that custom-made spectacle-mounted devices are rarely used, even in specialist low vision centres, and the majority of aids recommended and dispensed are simple hand and stand magnifiers, including illuminated devices (Shuttleworth et al., 1995; Crossland & Silver, 2005).

There are, of course, major differences between practitioners and clinics in their individual prescribing preferences, but this is quite acceptable, providing that the strategy adopted fulfils the patient's requirements. The type of aid is less important than the patient being confident with the way it is to be used: nonetheless, it seems logical to prescribe simple aids where possible because they are easier to use and less expensive. The range of aids prescribed will also vary with the patient group being seen: distance telescopes were the second most common aid prescribed by Yap et al. (1990) in a clinic with a significant number of young adult patients.

Even if the majority of patients could be helped by simple hand and stand magnifiers and spectacle prescriptions, this could still involve a large number of magnifiers being stocked if every possible power is to be covered. Most patients, however, can be helped using a relatively limited range of magnifications. Leat and Rumney (1990) reported that the most common magnification prescribed is 2×, with around 70% of patients requiring 4× or less. Shuttleworth et al. (1995) prescribed aids with a magnification range of 1.5× to 20×, but the median was 3×.

Bearing this in mind, an appropriate range of magnifiers in practice would be:

1. A selection of *nonilluminated hand* magnifiers (such as the Coil 2.3×, and 3×), along with a compact folding lens which is very useful for carrying around in a pocket or handbag (such as the Eschenbach 3.5×) or can be worn on a neck-cord (Eschenbach 4×) (Fig. 22.3). *Illuminated pocket* magnifiers are useful because lighting is often unpredictable outside the home: for example, the Schweizer range (e.g. +8.00 DS, +12.00 DS, +16.00 DS) (Fig. 22.4), the Eschenbach 3× and 4× Easypocket folding illuminated magnifier.
2. A *variable-focus stand* (such as the Coil Fleximag [Fig. 7.24, right]), and a suspended 'chest' (or 'round the neck') magnifier of similar power (Fig. 22.5) are useful for DIY and needlework. Illuminated versions are available: some were designed for industrial inspection and are very robust but expensive. There are many moderately priced examples sold through craft outlets. The Daylight Company (https://daylightcompany.com/magnifying-lights-and-lamps/) sell many different types (e.g. Fig. 22.6). For best performance, it is essential that the lens

can be freely positioned and rotated, and that the base is stable (and some clamp to the worksurface). A number of these flexible- or jointed-arm magnifiers do work loose with time, and this may be a problem if you wish to use the magnifier in the practice over an extended period. A useful trial of this style of magnification can be performed easily and cheaply using a double-ended clamp which can 'convert' a hand magnifier to a stand equivalent (Fig. 7.34).

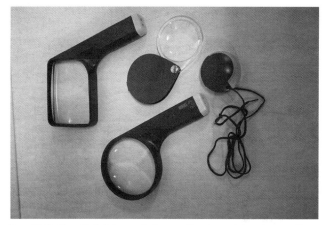

Fig. 22.3 The Coil 2.3× and 3× nonilluminated hand magnifiers; the Eschenbach 3.5× and 4× folding magnifiers: the 4× magnifier is shown with neck cord attached.

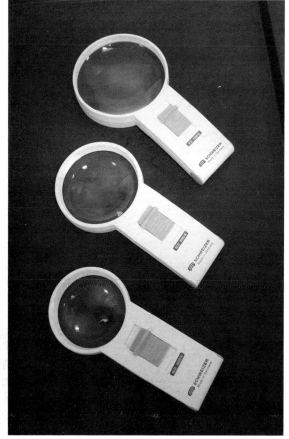

Fig. 22.4 The Schweizer +8.00 (2×) *(upper)*, +12.00 (3×) *(centre)* and +16.00 (4×) *(lower)* illuminated hand magnifiers.

3. *Nonilluminated fixed-focus stand magnifiers*, which have a wider range of magnification, (e.g. the Coil 3×, 4× and 6×) and may, in some cases, allow a pen to be used under them. Lighting is always more difficult with a stand magnifier, and the illuminated stand magnifiers such as the Eschenbach 3×, 4× and 6× magnification are extremely useful (Fig. 22.7).

4. A *flat-field magnifier*. It is limited to around 1.5× to 2× magnification but has excellent light-gathering properties and is very popular with children (Fig. 22.8).

5. *Spectacle-mounted plus lenses* can be prescribed by using standard trial case lenses mounted in a trial frame, but if possible, the patient should try out the device at home before ordering prescription spectacles. For this purpose, half-eye spectacles (and powers such as +4.00, +6.00 and +10.00 will be most useful) can be used for binocular

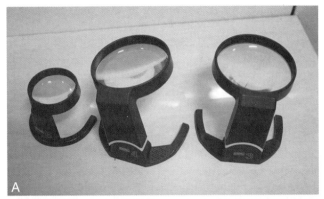

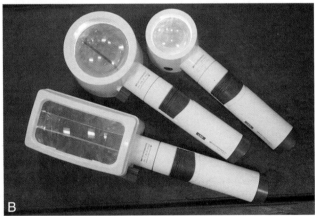

Fig. 22.7 (A) The Coil 3×, 4× and 6× nonilluminated fixed-focus stand magnifiers, which have a gap in the stand to allow the user to write under the lens. The 3× and 4× have a tilting lens for when they are to be used on a horizontal surface and can be tilted towards the user. (B) The Eschenbach 3×, 4× and 6× illuminated fixed focus stand magnifiers. The 3× has a yellow-tinted element which can be rotated in to provide additional magnification; the 4× has an optional red line guide to help with page navigation.

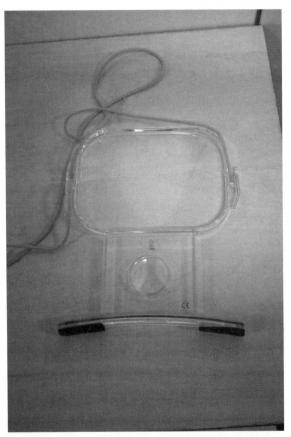

Fig. 22.5 A suspended or 'chest' magnifier, designed to be worn around the neck, and optimally positioned by altering the cord length.

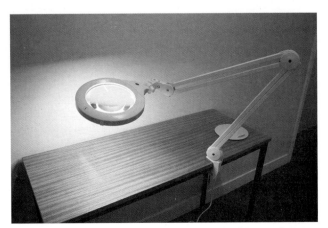

Fig. 22.6 An illuminated variable focus stand magnifier which clamps to the table.

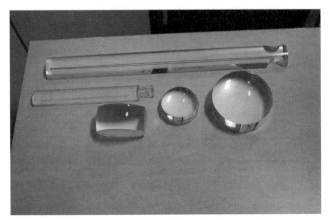

Fig. 22.8 A range of flat-field magnifiers: the 'bar style' lenses only provide magnification in one direction.

correction (Fig. 7.29). For patients with significant ametropia, clip-on lenses can be used such as the Coil Magniclip, which is available in +6.00, +10.00 and +15.00, along with a chavasse lens, which can be used to occlude the nonviewing eye (Fig. 22.9).

For higher powers, which must be monocular, the Eschenbach 4× and 7× monocular clip-on lenses can be used (see Fig. 22.9). A reading stand may be helpful to demonstrate to the patient how to use the close working distance of these aids in a comfortable position (Fig. 7.33).

6. If the range of aids stocked is to be extended to include telescopes, a 2× (MaxTV) or 3× (Eschenbach) binocular spectacle-mounted distance telescope will be the most useful aid for a sedentary task such as watching TV (Fig. 22.10A). A clip-on MaxTV is available, as well as a version for near tasks (MaxDetail). A 4× handheld focusing monocular telescope, and a 4× fixed focus telescope (Fig. 22.10B), will be the most versatile for 'spotting' outdoor tasks. Because of its ability to focus at close distance, the former can also be used for looking at supermarket shelves, shop windows and noticeboards. A spectacle mounting is available to leave the hands free whilst using this telescope for near or intermediate vision (Fig. 9.15, top left).

7. Tinted overspectacles, such as the UV Shield or NoIR filters (Fig. 22.11). Many different colours and transmissions are available but 50% and 20% transmission grey would be a good starting point.

8. A 'television reader' attached to a TV or laptop would be useful for demonstration purposes (although a magnification app on a tablet computer can be used to illustrate the principle of electronic magnification).

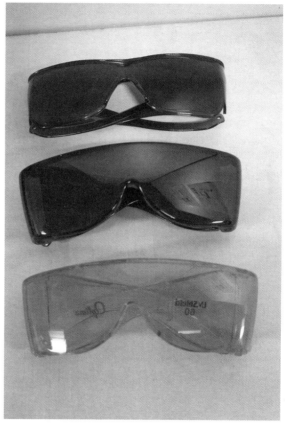

Fig. 22.11 A range of tinted overspectacles (*top*, 20% transmission grey; *centre*, 20% transmission brown; *bottom*, 60% transmission orange).

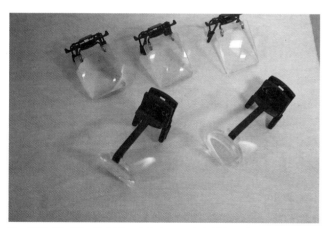

Fig. 22.9 *(Top)* The Coil Magniclip lenses (+15.00, +10.00 and +6.00). *(Bottom)* The Eschenbach monocular clip-ons (4× and 7×).

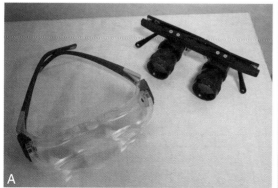
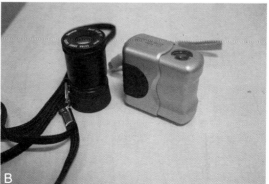

Fig. 22.10 (A) The spectacle-mounted Eschenbach MaxTV *(left)* and 3× binocular distance telescope *(right)*. (B) A 4× focusing *(left)* and a 4× fixed focus *(right)* telescope, both with carrying cords fitted.

PAYMENT FOR LOW VISION SERVICES

The usual system for the supply of LVAs in the UK is through the Hospital Eye Service (HES), where any optical aids required are provided free of charge to the patient, on permanent loan. Similar conditions for supply are allowed by the practice-based enhanced clinical pathways. Although it is not a formal exclusion, there has been a longstanding acceptance that individually prescribed magnifiers (e.g. bioptic telescopes) are not usually provided. In addition, there may be local restrictions imposed by financial constraints (e.g. a limit on the number of aids; or selecting aids from a limited inventory, or only certain suppliers). For the optometrist in community practice who is not able to refer the patient to one of these two pathways, an approach can be made to the patient's ophthalmologist on an individual basis. A letter to the ophthalmologist explaining the benefits of the particular LVAs prescribed for that patient and requesting an HES Prescription Form with which the optometrist can claim payment for the aids is a potential avenue. If the patient is entitled to a Spectacle Voucher under the General Ophthalmic Services (GOS) (either a full voucher on the basis of low income, or a lower value complex lens voucher because of the high-powered lens prescribed), this can be used towards the cost of a spectacle-mounted custom LVA.

Many aids supplied in the UK, however, are paid for privately by the individual. As suggested earlier, many patients require only simple aids and these are often modestly priced (particularly when compared to the cost of multifocal spectacles). Many are of a type that a patient may buy without having (or before having) a low vision assessment: from magazine advertisements and exhibitions aimed at patients; photographic or handicrafts shops; or online from a variety of suppliers. At the other end of the scale (in terms of both cost and complexity) are the optical aids (e.g. bioptic telescopes) or electronic aids which are not available through the NHS. In the LVSW, however, there is a single portable electronic vision enhancement system (p-EVES) device included in the inventory of aids available to practitioners.

Other sources of funding for electronic aids (and other necessary equipment/resources) are:

1. The Access to Work Scheme of the Department of Work and Pensions to help those in employment or self-employment (https://www.gov.uk/access-to-work) (GOV.UK, n.d.).
2. The Disabled Students Allowance for undergraduate and postgraduate students in Higher Education (https://www.gov.uk/disabled-students-allowance-dsa).
3. The Local Education Authority via the provisions for school students with Special Educational Needs (https://www.gov.uk/children-with-special-educational-needs).
4. Some charities may be willing to make a contribution to costs, or a device may be considered as part of a social care package provided through Social Services (https://www.nhs.uk/conditions/social-care-and-support-guide/care-services-equipment-and-care-homes/care-and-support-you-can-get-for-free/.)

If the patient is required to pay privately for an electronic aid, those individuals registered as sight impaired (SI) or severely sight impaired (SSI) are exempted from paying the VAT. Several suppliers of electronic aids will deliver the device to the patient's home and give a full demonstration and then the patient has a period of 1 or 2 weeks to decide whether to go ahead with a purchase. A scheme from another supplier involves a monthly membership fee, payment of which allows the patient to borrow any device, and then exchange or update it as required (Dickinson et al., 2017).

Being required to purchase devices certainly appeared to discourage patients from adopting many of the recommended aids in a study by Wong et al. (2011). Therefore, a loan arrangement for optical aids, or the opportunity to try on an extended basis under real-life conditions to be sure that it meets their requirements, is likely to be very beneficial. Loan of aids would also be beneficial for patients who need them for a limited time whilst awaiting treatment, or to use whilst on the waiting list for a hospital clinic appointment.

Arranging such a system would be relatively straightforward for those optometric practices which routinely operate their own existing eyecare plan. In these schemes, an individual or family pays a monthly direct debit fee to get access to, for example, regular comprehensive eye examinations, investigations that are outside the usual GOS provision (such as dry eye investigations), and discounts on spectacles and contact lenses. Provision of a low vision assessment and loan and supply of aids could easily be added to the services available in such practices.

The exact scope of such a 'loan' agreement would need to be carefully considered, because the aids need to be maintained: it must be decided whether the supply of batteries is included in the fee, and whether aids are replaced at no extra cost if broken or lost. It is important to have a signed formal agreement between the patient and the practice so that if the aid is stolen it will be covered by the patient's household insurance. Under such an eyecare scheme, the patient could be provided with access to a complete low vision service. An appropriate fee would include the initial low vision assessment, and follow-up visits including 'training' sessions if required.

REFERENCES

Alam, K., Connor, H., Gentle, A., et al. (2022). Developing consensus-based referral criteria for low vision services in Australia. *Ophthalmic and Physiological Optics*, 42(1), 149–160. https://doi.org/10.1111/opo.12902.

Clinical Council for Eye Health Commissioning (CCEHC). (2017). *Low vision, habilitation and rehabilitation framework for adults and children*, https://www.rnib.org.uk/sites/default/files/Low%20vision%2C%20habilitation%20and%20rehabilitation%20framework%20for%20adults%20and%20children%20%282%29_0.pdf.

College of Optometrists and the Royal College of Ophthalmologists. (2013). *Commissioning better eye care: Adults with low vision*, http://www.wcb-ccd.org.uk/perspectif/library/Low_vision_guidance_25_11_13_2013_PROF_263.pdf.

Crossland, M. D., & Silver, J. H. (2005). Thirty years in an urban low vision clinic: Changes in prescribing habits of low vision practitioners. *Optometry and Vision Science*, *82*(7), 617–622. https://doi.org/10.1097/01.opx.0000171336.40273.3f.

Dickinson, C., Linck, P., Tudor-Edwards, R., et al. (2011). A profile of low vision services in England: The low vision service model evaluation (LOVSME) project. *Eye*, *25*(7), 829–831. https://doi.org/10.1038/eye.2011.112.

Dickinson, C., Trillo, A. H., & Gridley, A. (2017). Electronic vision enhancement for low vision. *Optometry in Practice*, *18*(2), 93–102.

GOV.UK.(n.d.). *Access to work: Get support if you have a disability or health condition.* Retrieved January 2, 2022, from https://www.gov.uk/access-to-work

Latham, K., & Macnaughton, J. (2017). Low vision rehabilitation needs of visually impaired people. *Optometry in Practice*, *18*(2), 103–110.

Leat, S., & Rumney, N. (1990). The UWCC low vision clinic. *Optician*, *199*(5247), 12–16.

Ryan, B. (2014). Models of low vision care: Past, present and future. *Clinical and Experimental Optometry*, *97*(3), 209–213. https://doi.org/10.1111/cxo.12157.

Ryan, B., White, S., Wild, J., et al. (2010). The newly established primary care based Welsh Low Vision Service is effective and has improved access to low vision services in Wales. *Ophthalmic and Physiological Optics*, *30*(4), 358–364. https://doi.org/10.1111/j.1475-1313.2010.00729.x.

Shuttleworth, G. N., Dunlop, A., Collins, J. K., et al. (1995). How effective is an integrated approach to low vision rehabilitation? Two year follow up results from South Devon. *British Journal of Ophthalmology*, *79*(8), 719–723. https://doi.org/10.1136/bjo.79.8.719.

Wong, E. Y. H., O'Connor, P. M., & Keeffe, J. E. (2011). Establishing the service potential of secondary level low vision clinics. *Optometry and Vision Science*, *88*(7), 823–829. https://doi.org/10.1097/OPX.0b013e318218a0a2.

Yap, M., Cho, J., & Woo, G. (1990). A survey of low vision patients in Hong Kong. *Clinical and Experimental Optometry*, *73*, 19–22.

Case Studies

There are many examples which could be given, but these cases have been chosen to illustrate the use of detailed record cards specific to Low Vision Assessments (Appendix 2), with a range of the common situations, and patient characteristics, encountered. The 'prompt questions' have been removed from the history sections to save space. Patient details and the names of individuals are altered, but the names of hospitals and organisations are real. A variety of different strategies and techniques are given as examples, and all are discussed in more detail in the preceding chapters.

It is often useful to record exactly what patients say when completing the record card—direct quotes are indicated by quotation marks. It is also helpful to identify information which comes indirectly from other individuals (e.g. parent/spouse), rather than the patient themselves.

Although low vision care takes place in a variety of locations, none of the rehabilitation strategies suggested are unique to one particular setting. The records include many examples of signposting: again the precise organisations involved in offering these services may differ in different geographical locations.

CASE 1—14-YEAR-OLD

Low Vision Assessment

	Date: 25-1-2022

Patient Details

Name	Isabella Ford			DOB	20-1-2008
First visit to clinic?	Y	Referred from?	Ophthalmologist—paediatric genetics clinic	Age	14

Ocular History

Diagnosed with Stargardt disease (molecularly confirmed) 4 months ago Noticed difficulty with board over past year—increasing—went to local optom then referred Never worn spectacles	
Any change in vision in last 3 months? Yes	Which is better eye currently? Unsure

Ophthalmologist	Prof. Michaelides	Last visit	Oct 21
Hospital	Moorfields	Next visit	Today
Optometrist	J. Turner	Last eye exam	Aug 21

| Registration status (give date) | SI ☐ | SSI ☐ | Not registered ☐ |
| Contact with SS/RO? When? What was result? | Referred to Teacher for Vision Impairment—first meeting next week | | |

General Health

| Health problems | None | Medication management | None |
| GP name & address | Dr Ranj Patel, Westway Health Centre | | |

Daily Life

| **Visual Perception** |
| Can't see board from back of class
Faint colours are harder on the whiteboard—e.g. yellow/green harder than blue/purple
Colours OK in art
Reading OK although may be slower
Dad says turns on more lights in the home than she used to
Not aware of eccentric viewing |

| **Occupation/Education** |
| Year 9 at Hammersmith Academy
Favourite lessons: Science and English
Less keen on Spanish (not because of vision)
Is allowed to sit at the front of the class in all lessons
Not receiving enlarged handouts—'managing' although dad says she's holding work closer
Most homework is online—zooms in on screen and can see easily
Not had any touch typing lessons but effective at typing
Not sure about career—plan to go to university?science subject
SENCo at school (Mr Jalil) is aware of vision loss and ensures she sits at front of class
Teachers are generally quite understanding although one supply teacher made her sit at the back and accused her of 'messing around'
Has been referred to Teacher for Visual Impairment but not met them yet—first meeting next week |

| **Mobility and Travel** |
| Walks to and from school with friends—says can cross road safely—dad agrees
Sometimes gets bus with friends—can't always see number until close but 'not a problem'
Mobility OK—no trips or falls |
| Slips or trips? ☒ White cane? ☐ Walking stick or frame? ☐ Wheelchair? ☐ |

Continued

At Home
Lives with parents (good vision) and two cats in second floor flat (stairs, no lift) No difficulty with stairs No concerns at home. Good lighting. Is vegan—can't always read ingredients on snack foods, friends or family help
Sensory substitution devices? (e.g. bump-ons; talking watch; liquid level indicator) ☒

Hobbies/Interests
Likes indoor climbing—no problems with this—goes twice/week Plays drums—doesn't use music for this—no lessons/exams Meets friends in park (best friend: Maiesha) Watches videos on laptop (17″ screen) Doesn't watch much TV
Watch TV? ☐ What distance?_____Audio-description? ☐

Reading, Writing and Electronic Devices
Loves reading—favourite author: Malorie Blackman Prefers to read on screen instead of paper (always has) Uses Kindle app and library app on iPad Not tried reversed contrast Preferred print size is about 18 point—holds at 28 cm Has iPhone SE for texting and calls—enlarged font, not tried reversed contrast—holds at about 10 cm Has own laptop (17″, Windows)—manages with this although dad says gets very close
Computer? ☑   Smartphone? ☑   Duration of comfortable reading: 1–2 hours

Well-Being and Mental Health
Worried about the future Not met anyone else with vision loss Has lots of friends and talks to family, but may like to speak to someone else about this

Current Spectacles and Magnifiers
Use of Spectacles

No current spectacles

Use of Magnifiers

No current magnifiers

Other Aids/Devices or Strategies

Enlarges print on phone and zooms on laptop (Ctrl + Up)

Patient Aims

Wants to be able to see as well as her friends at school Wants to be able to keep up at school

Visual Assessment
Visions:

Right		Left	
Distance: 0.6 logMAR	Near:	Distance: 0.54 logMAR	Near:

Binocular	
Distance: 0.54 logMAR	Near: N18 fluently at 30 cm, N6 slowly at 10 cm

Reading Speed Assessment (MNREAD App)

Peak reading speed 155 words per minute
Critical print size N19
Acuity N6, holding closer

Refraction:

Rx	Right	VA	Left	VA
Distance	+0.50 DS	0.6 logMAR	+0.50 DS	0.54 logMAR

High Adds Tested

Adds do not help—'all blurred'

Contrast Sensitivity

Method: Mars chart

Right	Left	Binocular
		1.64 log units (2.3%)

This is
- [ ] Severe loss: nonsighted strategies probably indicated (Rows 1 and 2)
- [ ] Significantly reduced: optical aids may be useful (Rows 3 and 4)
- [ ] Noticeable loss: lighting and contrast need to be optimised (Rows 5 and 6)
- [x] Normal/near normal (Rows 7 and 8)

Visual Field

Central/peripheral (please delete as appropriate)
Method: Amsler and confrontation
Brief description of findings (attach plot if appropriate)

Central area 'faint' in each eye Confrontation grossly full

Other Tests:

Ishihara 21/21

Aids Demonstrated

Magnification & Description	Which Specs Used	VA	Comments on Performance	Issued
+10 D Eschenbach LED Hand Mag	n/a	N4	Fluent—likes light—would like to try for faint details/reading, e.g. thermometer in science experiments	Y
6 × 17 binoculars	n/a	0.0	Good handling. Would like to use for days out/school trips	Y
4 × 13 Microlux monocular telescope	n/a	0.1	Not sure would use—doesn't like	N

Outcomes	
Requirements Identified	Solutions Suggested
Distance	
Seeing on days out/school trips	Binoculars
Seeing in classroom	Being allowed to sit at front of class Relay system for whiteboard Having slides electronically ahead of lessons Being allowed to use iPad/laptop in class
Intermediate	
Seeing iPad at longer distance	Accessibility settings—emailed leaflet and will look at applevis.com
Near	
Seeing handouts	Enlarged handouts—suggest font 18+ Electronic handouts so Isabella can zoom in
Seeing textbooks at school Seeing faint details, e.g. on food packets	+10 D hand magnifier (can see label with this)

Action	(✓/✗)	Details
Referred to own optometrist		
Referred to GP/Consultant	✓	Report sent to consultant ophthalmologist
Referred to rehab officer/SS (LVL?)	✓	Already referred to teacher for visual impairment Report to teacher for visual impairment written – Full report of visual assessment – Suggest classroom help (e.g. relay); enlarged handouts (font 18+, A4); additional time and modified large print for exams; electronic textbooks – Explain spectacles won't help – Details of follow-up appointments in low vision and ophthalmology – Note that Isabella won't always make perfect eye contact (and this doesn't necessarily mean she is being rude or not interested) Copied to SENCo and Isabella (for her to show to e.g. supply teachers)

Referred to Access to Work		
Referred to voluntary agency	✓	Given information on VICTA for grants and social activities Given information on Stargardt's Connected for family support
Referral to counselling services/GP/other	✓	Referred to teenage/young person counsellor based in eye hospital—with consent from Isabella/parents
Info/advice given		
Leaflets given	✓	Emailed information about support, accessible technology, applevis.com
Training recommended	✓	Formal touch typing training Assessment by mobility instructor (although training may not be needed at this stage)

Recommended Action at Next Visit

Ensure school assessment has taken place Discuss modifications for exams	Date/recall period: 3 months

Commentary on Case 1

The assessment of children is often different from that of adults, particularly if the child has been visually impaired from an early age, when the role of the low vision service is habilitation rather than rehabilitation. For a congenitally visually impaired child, their activities are often matched to their capabilities: this is rather different to acquired visual loss in an adult who wishes to continue to perform the same activities in the same way as when their vision was good. Even in Case 1, where visual impairment is recent, it helps to just discuss the young person's life with them, asking about their full range of school and home activities. Some of these activities could already have been adjusted to fit in with the child: for example, the young person may be selecting an enlarged font on their electronic device. Or perhaps the school may have made sure t hat all worksheets are produced in large type (although this is often by photo-copying worksheets onto larger paper, an unwieldy solution which can also reduce text contrast). Noting the working distances used is very important, and using a short work-ing distance (relative distance magnification) can be a very effective strategy. However, it is important to assess whether accommodating to focus at these close distances is effec-tive and comfortable. In this case, it was because high adds

(which could potentially relax or replace accommodation) were not helpful.

It is also necessary to find out details of the school and teachers, so that contact can be made if required. If the school has little past experience with visually impaired pupils, then some common sense suggestions can often be made which have not been considered: sitting at the front of the class and receiving larger print are often already in place, but contrast is often not considered. Other suggestions include localised task lighting, avoidance of glare from daylight, and the use of reading stands, felt-tip pens and writing guides. Teachers can also be informed about when spectacles and tinted lenses should be worn, and requests made, for example, to wear a baseball cap in school or to sit in a particular seat (perhaps to ensure that the whiteboard is in the same direction as the null point for a child with nystagmus). Information on colour vision is useful to assess how it might affect performance in subjects such as art, geography and science.

Parents also need to be supported to learn more about the eye condition and its prognosis, and how to navigate the complex systems for financial support and education. There may be little opportunity for them to meet other parents in a similar position in their local area, and support organisations can be invaluable to facilitate this.

CASE 2—52-YEAR-OLD

Low Vision Assessment

Date: 02-12-2021

Patient Details

Name	Angela Davis			DOB	23-2-1969
First visit to clinic?	Y	Referred from?	Ophthalmology clinic	Age	52

Ocular History

Was referred to ophthalmologist for registration as SI, and then referred for Low Vision Assessment. Had a stroke 9 months ago, now discharged from Neurology clinic. Memory is affected: forgets conversations she has had until her children remind her, forgets to take medication, forgets to turn gas hob off (no accidents, kitchen just got warmer) Personal and family ocular history unremarkable

Any change in vision in last 3 months? No (although it has improved from time of stroke)	Which is better eye currently? Can't see on right side but vision is the same in both eyes

Ophthalmologist		Ms Cox	Last visit	2 months
Hospital		Manchester Royal Eye Hospital	Next visit	None planned
Optometrist		Local practice, can't remember the name	Last eye exam	Over 2 years (received reminder)

Registration status (give date)	SI ☑ 2 months ago	SSI ☐	Not registered ☐
Contact with SS/RO? When? What was result?	No contact as yet: ECLO explained what would happen when Sensory Team got in contact		

General Health

Health problems	After stroke now on several medications for high blood pressure, and blood thinning	Medication management	Sometimes forgets to take tablets in the morning but remembers later in the day
GP name & address	Dr Smith, Mandalay Medical Centre, Bolton		

Daily Life

Visual Perception
Vision good, but only on left side. Feels can't just look to right hand side to see things but has to turn whole body to compensate—she finds this very difficult when moving. No problems with light, sees colour well. No hallucinations.

Occupation/Education
Medical Secretary, but made redundant about 1 year ago (just due to reorganisation of department). Keen to get back into work but would feel 'petrified' to be going to a new place with new people. Feels she could go back into work if it was her old job with a building she knew, and the people she was friendly with who would look after her. She has heard about Access to Work.

Mobility and Travel
Had to stop driving because of vision problem—has informed the DVLA. Feels she needs someone with her outdoors and they need to walk on her right side to be a 'buffer'. This is since she went out alone and accidentally bumped into someone and they shouted at her, and this affected her confidence. In the house, often holds out her right hand to find any walls and obstacles on the right. Still tends to walk into some door frames.
Slips or trips? ☒ White cane? ☒ Walking stick or frame? ☐ Wheelchair? ☐

At Home
Lives alone. Could ask for help from friends and family if required (daughter lives nearby but is carer for autistic son and disabled partner; two sons live away but phone daily and visit at weekends). Manages cooking and cleaning, but much slower and more careful. Can't rush when moving things because has to carefully lift and then turn and then think where to put them down.
Sensory substitution devices? (e.g. bump-ons; talking watch; liquid level indicator) ☐

Hobbies/Interests
Loves reading but finds book has to be placed at arm's length and to left side (she demonstrated and is also tilting book slightly up on left side). Sometimes finds she is re-reading a paragraph already read, so uses her book mark to move down the page to keep her place. Walking the dog, but now can only go out if someone else available to go with her. Feels she has to look down constantly to check that the dog isn't walking in front of her. Used to enjoy going out with friends, but now would not even consider going out at night (in the dark).
Watch TV? ☑ What distance? Has to be on left side	Audio-description? ☐

Reading, Writing and Electronic Devices
Likes printed books, was never interested in a Kindle, or in audiobooks. Can't see small print (e.g. on labels)—has to pass to someone else to check. Uses laptop and smartphone without problems—needs to position to left.
Computer? ☑ Smartphone? ☑ Duration of comfortable reading _____

Well-Being and Mental Health
'I feel like an invalid' Was previously a very confident and independent person—would drive anywhere, do anything, without a second thought. 'It's took part of me away' Doesn't like being reliant on availability of other people for her to get out and about—feels it's not fair on them either Realises that managing her vision problems isn't just about what help she can get, but also that she needs to 'get used to it' Is annoyed when she finds herself apologising when someone else bumps into her, rather than them apologising to her

Current Spectacles and Magnifiers

Use of Spectacles

None worn previously

Use of Magnifiers

None used

Other Aids/Devices or Strategies

None

Patient Aims

Help with travelling independently

Visual Assessment

Visions:

Right		Left	
Distance: 0.1	Near:	Distance: 0.04	Near:
Binocular			
Distance:		Near: N8 at 50 cm	

Refraction:

Rx	Right	VA	Left	VA
Distance	$-0.75/+0.25 \times 90$	-0.04	$-0.25/+0.50 \times 90$	-0.02

Preferred Working Distance	Required Add	VA RE	VA LE
40 cm	+2.00	N3	N3
With 1× magnification	**Required Add**	**VA RE**	**VA LE**
Working distance 25 cm			

High Adds Tested

Not required

Contrast Sensitivity

Method: _____ Mars Letter _____

Right	Left	Binocular
1.68	1.64	1.72

This is
- [ ] Severe loss: nonsighted strategies probably indicated (Rows 1 and 2)
- [ ] Significantly reduced: optical aids may be useful (Rows 3 and 4)
- [ ] Noticeable loss: lighting and contrast need to be optimised (Rows 5 and 6)
- [x] Normal/Near Normal (Rows 7 and 8)

Visual Field

Central/peripheral (please delete as appropriate)

Method: _____   Amsler _____

Brief description of findings (attach plot if appropriate)

Each eye monocularly showed four to five squares visible to right of central spot
(Humphrey 30-2 threshold test completed for ophthalmologist assessment: shows R hemianopia to midline in upper field, but about 5° from midline in lower field).

Other Tests:

Line bisection test conducted binocularly: suggests no neglect—midpoint marked slightly to R side

Near point of convergence: using RAF rule, 8 cm, repeated three times

Aids Demonstrated

Magnification & Description	Which Specs Used	VA	Comments on Performance	Issued	Cost
40Δ base out stick-on Fresnel segments above and below RE on plano lenses			Familiarisation with prisms: patient practised looking at her hand and other objects moving from non-seeing side. Patient quickly understood that objects were not in 'correct' location. Walked around the clinic, down corridors, reporting what could be seen on non-seeing side. Was keen to try at home.	(Y)/N	

Outcomes	
Requirements Identified	Solutions Suggested
Distance	
Getting back to work	Advised px to approach the local Jobcentre Plus office about the 'Work and Health' programme which supports disabled people to find work
Walking in busy/unfamiliar environments without collisions	Peli prism (px preferred this to the alternative suggestion of explorative saccade training). Explained that this could not be used for driving in the event of seeking driving licence restoration, but px said she couldn't even imagine ever driving again at this point in time
Walking the dog	Place dog on left side so always in sight; use a dog harness/shorter lead so dog is not so free to move across in front
Remembering medication	Use smartphone app to set reminders (specific medication apps are available, or just a general reminder app)
Intermediate	
Near	
Reading	Explained that presbyopia is causing her long working distance/difficulty with small print. Suggest reading spectacles and typoscope to replace bookmark. Explained why she tilts book and encouraged to do this a little more if required.

Continued

Action	(✓/✗)	Details
Referred to own optometrist		
Referred to other university clinic		
Referred to GP/Consultant		
Referred to rehab officer/SS (LVL?)		Registration already in progress
Referred to Access to Work		Suggested contact with local Jobcentre Plus for 'Work and Health'
Referred to voluntary agency		
Referral to counselling services/GP/other		
Info/advice given		To wear prism spectacles at home and then (if feels comfortable) when out walking with companion
Leaflets given		
Training recommended		

Recommended Action at Next Visit

To assess progress with prisms. To decide whether to dispense on a distance prescription as a permanent correction. Check if Sensory Team have made contact; has patient contacted local Jobcentre Plus.	Date/recall period: 2 weeks (or sooner, when she comes to collect reading spectacles)

Commentary on Case 2

Many people who have had a stroke have visual problems, but these are not always diagnosed and managed in a timely way. There is no standard pathway for poststroke vision care, although a preferred structure for this has been proposed by Rowe et al. (2022). This patient had been referred to the ophthalmologist for registration as Sight Impaired, but it is not inevitable that all patients would be referred for Low Vision Services at that stage. It is possible that this patient could be considered at a later stage for restoration of her driving licence (although that would be likely to require deregistration), but currently would not meet the criteria of 'full functional adaptation'. In explaining eye movement training, or prism spectacles, as possible management options to the patient, it is important to make clear that the prism spectacles could not be used for driving (at least in the UK). It is important to explore any other effects of stroke (e.g. movement, speech): in this case, the stroke had not affected the patient's physical mobility but had affected her memory. Charles Bonnet syndrome tends to be linked to poor visual acuity (VA) but can also occur in cases of visual field loss: the patient should be asked about hallucinations in their non-seeing field.

The patient had not been accustomed to wearing any spectacle correction, but a reading correction is now necessary because of presbyopia. However, it was important to check that difficulties with convergence were not the reason why the patient was choosing a long working distance, and this was confirmed with a normal near point of convergence. The Amsler chart suggested 2° to 3° of macular sparing, which is likely to help with reading fluency: the positioning of the book towards the seeing side, tilting the lines to move the scotoma even further along the line, and using a typoscope are all strategies the patient had discovered for herself that can be encouraged.

At a follow-up visit, a decision can be made whether to continue with the trial distance spectacles, have a distance prescription made up and the Fresnel prisms attached to that, or a pair of spectacles ordered which have the prisms permanently attached.

It appeared that the patient's main requirement in getting back to work was to regain confidence, rather than direct practical help. The 'Work and Health' programme is designed to do that and is open to disabled individuals. It will be important at a follow-up visit, not just to check on visual requirements, but whether other suggestions and referrals have been pursued. If this has not occurred, it is important to discover why this is. It may be a practical barrier which the practitioner might be able to assist with (e.g. they may need to facilitate a contact), or the practitioner may have misjudged the patient's requirement, or the patient may have forgotten or misunderstood what was suggested.

CASE 3—75-YEAR-OLD

Low Vision Assessment

Date: 19-01-2021

Patient Details

Name	Lydia Millet			DOB	01-05-1945
First visit to clinic?	(Y)/N	Referred from?	Rang the practice enquiring about magnifiers	Age	75

Ocular History

Diagnosed with dry AMD in both eyes in 2017 Her vision has slowly deteriorated and she is having difficulties performing some day-to-day tasks She had a cataract operation on the RE in Jan 2015 and LE in Mar 2015 No other operations No other eye problems	
Any change in vision in last 3 months? Not in the last 3 months but she notices that her vision is worse than a year ago	Which is better eye currently? Both eyes feel the same

Ophthalmologist	N/A	Last visit	N/A
Hospital	N/A	Next visit	N/A
Optometrist	Dr Becker/Becker Opticians M21 9PK	Last eye exam	Jan 2020

Registration status (give date)	SI ☐	SSI ☐	Not registered ✓
Contact with SS/RO? When? What was result?	No contact with SS		

General Health

Health problems	No health problems	Medication management	Does not take any medication
GP name & address	Dr Wollstonecraft, The Withington Medical Centre, M21 9HA		

Daily Life

Visual Perception

Finds bright lights or sun overwhelming and uses plano sunglasses when it's too bright. Feel they work well. Never feels the need to use sunglasses indoors.

Doesn't notice any missing areas in vision. Can recognise faces so long as they are close.

She described seeing colours normally and was able to recognise the colours I was wearing (yellow jumper, green skirt).

CBS discussed: and no hallucinations reported.

At home she uses task lighting (LED lamp) that she can direct towards the task when she reads and writes.

Continued

Occupation/Education

Retired; was a human rights lawyer. Studied law, history and politics. Is an active member of the Women's Equality Party, writing books and articles for newspapers.

Mobility and Travel

Travels alone normally. She uses taxis when she goes to unfamiliar places, otherwise she uses the tram and the train and occasionally buses. Today, she came here by tram.
Gave up driving 2 years ago.
Sometimes is difficult for her to see bus numbers or train, tram and bus timetables. She has a smart phone (no difficulties with use) and uses it to plan routes if she needs to.
She does her shopping online, on the computer and she knows how to adjust it to magnify text if she needs too.
Her mobility in the house is good. She lives in a flat (fourth floor) and there is a lift, sometimes she uses the stairs for exercise.
She does not use a cane or any type of stick or frame to walk. She has no mobility problems and her vision is good enough to get around. She has not had any trips or falls.

Slips or trips? ☒ White cane? ☐ Walking stick or frame? ☒ Wheelchair? ☐

At Home

She lives alone in her flat.
She has hired some help for household chores such as cleaning, tidying and doing the laundry.
She likes cooking and sometimes has problems reading small print in food instructions and recipes. No difficulties setting dials on appliances or setting controls.
She is able to make hot drinks and she has not had any accidents.
There is a gardener for the block of flats where she lives. She does not do any ironing, never has done.
Does not have any SS devices such as bump-ons or others.

Sensory substitution devices? (e.g. bump-ons; talking watch; liquid level indicator) ☒

Hobbies/Interests

Likes reading political reviews and biography books and going for long walks.
Lydia likes watching BBC crime series on TV, she sits at 2 m from the TV. She does not use audio-description (although she knows what it is) because she finds it 'annoying'.
Likes going for a swim to the local swimming pool once a week. Plays the piano from memory and does not need to read the music.

Watch TV? ☑ What distance? _____ 2 m _____ Audio-description? ☒

Reading, Writing and Electronic Devices

Wants to read books and articles (political reviews and biography). She prefers reading on paper rather than on the computer when she reads books, but the reviews and articles that she reads are on the computer (laptop). She sits at about 30 cm from the computer and uses reading glasses for this and also when she is reading books or writing. Is having difficulty with some books because of the small print. She reads her own correspondence and needs good lighting for this. She also uses reading glasses for her smartphone. She does not use glasses for distance since she had her cataract operations.

Computer? ☑ Smartphone? ☑ Duration of comfortable reading _____ 1 hour if print size big enough _____

Well-Being and Mental Health
Lydia is happy because she has a 'very active life' and this is what keeps her in 'a good mood'. She used to get frustrated when she was first diagnosed and they told her that her vision would gradually deteriorate but for now things are good and she does not feel that she is missing out on anything.

Current Spectacles and Magnifiers

Use of Spectacles

Type	Date of Issue	RE Rx	VA	LE Rx	VA	Add	Near VA RE	Near VA LE
Near	Jan 2021	+3.00		+3.00			N8 @ 30 cm	N8 @ 30 cm

Use of Magnifiers

Description	Used for	Successful?
None		

Other Aids/Devices or Strategies

Description	Used for	Successful?
None		

Patient Aims

Would like some help with reading because she feels she is having trouble reading small print and can no longer read her books as easily as before with her spectacles.

Visual Assessment

Visions:

Right		Left	
Distance: 0.42 logMAR		Distance: 0.44 logMAR	
Binocular			
Distance: 0.42 logMAR			

Refraction:

Rx	Right	VA	Left	VA
Distance	+0.50/−0.50 × 180	0.40 logMAR	+0.75 DS	0.40 logMAR

Preferred Working Distance	Required Add	VA RE	VA LE
30 cm	+3.00	N8	N8
With 1× magnification	Required Add	VA RE	VA LE
Working distance 25 cm	+4.00	N6	N6

High Adds Tested

Magnification Required	Required Working Distance	Required Add	VA RE	VA LE
1.5×	~16 cm	+6.00	N4	N4

Contrast Sensitivity

Method: _____ Mars Letter Contrast Sensitivity Test _____

Right	Left	Binocular
1.20 log units (6.3%)	1.12 log units (7.6%)	1.20 log units (6.3%)

This is
☐ Severe loss: nonsighted strategies probably indicated (Rows 1 and 2)
☐ Significantly reduced: optical aids may be useful (Rows 3 and 4)
☑ Noticeable loss: lighting and contrast need to be optimised (Rows 5 and 6)
☐ Normal/near normal (Rows 7 and 8)

Visual Field

(Central)/Peripheral (please delete as appropriate)

Method: _____ Amsler grid _____
Brief description of findings (attach plot if appropriate)

No defect noticed RE or LE

Other Tests:

Aids Demonstrated

Magnification & Description	Which Specs Used	VA	Comments on Performance	Issued	Cost
Handheld illuminated Schweizer 6 D (1.5×)	No specs	N4 threshold	N8 fluent reading achieved in clinic	(Y)/N	
Stand magnifier illuminated Schweizer 8 D (2×)	Reading specs	N2.5 threshold	N5 fluent reading achieved in clinic	(Y)/N	
+6.00 (1.5×) half-eyes with prism	–	Rejected close working distance		Y/(N)	
Tinted lenses (450, 500, 550 nm)	–	Didn't find a big help	'Would look ridiculous'	Y/(N)	
				Y/N	

Outcomes	
Requirements Identified	Solutions Suggested
Distance	
Intermediate	
Near	
To read small print more fluently	(Illuminated) magnifier (spec-mounted, hand or stand, according to patient preferences)

Action	(✓/✗)	Details
Referred to own optometrist		
Referred to other university clinic		
Referred to GP/consultant		
Referred to rehab officer/SS (LVL?)		
Referred to Access to Work		
Referred to voluntary agency		
Referral to counselling services/GP/other		
Info/advice given	✓	Information about lighting—encouraged to use for other tasks Sit closer to TV if required. Amsler chart given to test herself at home Discussed using a hat as well as sunglasses to control glare
Leaflets given	✓	Information on Charles Bonnet syndrome Information about AMD and Macular Society
Training recommended		

Recommended Action at Next Visit

To ask Lydia to feedback her experiences with the magnifiers to see whether they are useful and what she is using them for. Asked her to bring an example of a task that she performs with the magnifiers to check that she is using the magnifiers optimally.	Date/recall period: 3–4 weeks

Low Vision Follow-up

Date: 16-3-2022

Patient Details

Name	Lydia Millett	DOB	01-05-1945
Date of last visit to clinic?	Feb 2021		

History Since Last Visit

Changes in vision/treatment/health: interactions with other services
Last year was provided with a stand and a handheld magnifier and when reviewed after 4 weeks she was doing very well with these. Today she has come for her annual low vision check-up but she thinks her vision has deteriorated, since magnifiers not so effective. Had a routine sight test in Jan 2022 and no change in spectacles was suggested. Referral initiated to HES. Checks each eye with Amsler chart weekly—was able to describe correct technique—no missing areas.
Progress with aids/training
Hand magnifier used in kitchen for reading labels and carries it in her bag when she goes out. Uses stand magnifier for reading books and doesn't use it outdoors.
Patient aims for today
Lydia would like stronger magnifiers that allow her to read fluently again and she would also like to know if there is anything we could do to keep her safe at home; e.g. preparing drinks, cutting vegetables, maximising the lighting at home (since she is going to refurbish and redecorate her house).

Visual Assessment

Refraction:

Rx	Right	Left
Distance	+0.50/−0.50 × 180	+0.75
Add	+4.00	+4.00

Visual Acuity:

Right		Left	
Distance: 0.76 logMAR	Near: N12 @ 25 cm	Distance: 0.86 logMAR	Near: N16 @ 25 cm
Binocular			
Distance: 0.78 logMAR			Near: N12

Issued Earlier	Magnification & Description	Specs	VA	Comments	Issued Today
Y/N	3× handheld illuminated magnifier Schweizer	No specs used	N4	N8 fluent achieved in the clinic	(Y)/N
Y/N	3× stand illuminated magnifier Schweizer	Reading specs	N4	N8 fluent reading achieved in the clinic	(Y)/N

Other Tests:

Mars Letter Contrast Sensitivity Test
RE: 1.12 log units (7.6%)
LE: 0.94 log units (11.5%)
Binocular: 1.12 log units (7.6%)

Outcomes

Action Taken
Demonstrated that new magnifiers are smaller so need to be held close to one eye for optimum field of view—RE would be best
Helped her to complete a self-referral Low Vision Leaflet (see below) so that the Social Services do an assessment of needs
Given leaflet from Thomas Pocklington Trust on lighting design for the home

Magnifiers returned: 2× handheld and stand illuminated magnifiers Schweizer	Magnifiers loaned: 3× handheld and 3× stand illuminated magnifiers Schweizer

Recommended Action at Next Visit:

Check if the magnifiers are working, and what tasks she is using them for. Check if the SS have contacted her and if so, the outcome of the visit.	Recall period/date of next visit Telephone review 2 months

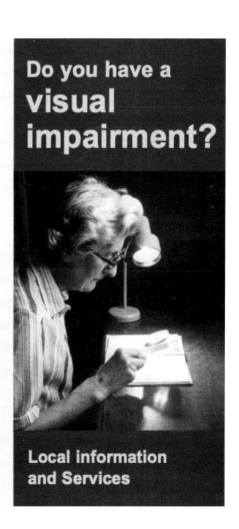

Does poor eyesight sometimes make your life difficult?

You may benefit from advice and support that your local council social services department (or its designated agency) can provide for you.

Your council has a duty to:
• Advise you of the range of services available to people with sight problems
• Carry out an assessment of your needs

These services can include:
• Supply of special equipment
• Training to manage daily tasks
• Arranging for you to be registered (if your eye specialist determines you are eligible and you consent).

Attention Driving Licence holders
In accordance with the advice shown on the driving licence, any driver with impaired vision should inform the DVLA, who will consider each case on an individual basis.

Contact the DVLA at:
Drivers Medical Branch
DVLA
Swansea
SA99 1TU
0870 600 0301

Provided by

Becker Opticians
Yew Tree Road
M21 9PK

Do you have a visual impairment?

Local information and Services

Self-referral for visual impairment

Please contact me about my sight difficulties.

My name: | Lydia Millet |

Date of birth: | 01-05-1945 |
Address: | 24 Rathem Street |

Postcode: | M21 9PL |

Telephone number and / or email address: | 07875643123 |

| lydia.millet@hotmail.co.uk |

Do you need an interpreter / translation? (tick) YES ☐ NO ☐

I would prefer information in:
| English | (language)

Do you live alone? (tick)
YES ☐ NO ☐

Do you have responsibilities as a carer? (tick) YES ☐ NO ☑

Please tick any relevant statements about the practical effects of your sight difficulties.

I have (tick):
- ☐ Difficulty getting about
- ☐ A hearing impairment
- ☐ Other conditions (specify)

I am especially concerned about (tick):
- ☑ Cooking on my own
- ☐ Crossing roads safely
- ☐ Becoming isolated
- ☐ Feelings of distress
- ☐ Coping at work
- ☐ Coping at school / college
- ☐ Reading
- ☐ Other - please specify

In the first instance, please contact (tick):
- ☑ Me   ☐ A representative
- ☐ A friend   ☐ A relative

Contact name & details:
| Lydia Millet   07875643123 |
| lydia.millet@hotmail.co.uk |

Make contact first by (tick):
- ☑ Phone   ☑ Visit
- ☐ Letter   ☐ Email

Send me information in (tick):
- ☐ Large Print   ☑ Email
- ☐ Disk   ☐ Tape

How to ask for help or advice

- Fill in the form
- Cut along the dotted line
- Keep this part for your information
- Send the form part to:

> (Social services or agent to insert details here in 16 pt size print)

If you have any difficulties in relation to these matters, you can contact:
- Citizen's Advice Bureau
- The RNIB Helpline (local call rate): **0845 766 9999**
- Your local voluntary organisation for visually impaired people.

LVL leaflet 2005

Commentary on Case 3

This patient is typical of those undergoing a first visit to a Low Vision Clinic. In this case, she is being seen in the same practice where her routine sight tests are carried out, via an enhanced clinical pathway. For the 'first time' patient, even though their requirements may be quite modest, it is necessary to explain to them the different nature of the low vision assessment and to get a full picture of their lifestyle. There are a range of issues which need to be covered, although not all will be applicable in every case. For this patient, for example, the issues of driving, digital accessibility, and advice on tinted lenses were not required. With respect to the use of electronic devices, the optometrist should check working distances carefully and ensure that the patient has an optimal refractive correction for these. Other routine advice includes task lighting (for all detailed tasks, and not just reading), sitting closer to the TV, and audio description (for theatre and visits to museums and historic sites, as well as TV). It is also important to warn patients about Charles Bonnet syndrome, even if they have not experienced hallucinations.

This patient had a mild loss of acuity, although contrast sensitivity (CS) was more severely affected. In addition, both eyes had similar performance, so binocular magnification was appropriate. With a +4.00 Add the near word VA was N6. The text size of the printed books was assumed to be N8, so allowing a 2:1 acuity reserve suggested magnification of 1.5×. At this low level of magnification, there are several different types of magnifier that could have been used: hand and stand were good options because of the built-in illumination (important because of the reduced CS), but a suspended magnifier or a flat-field magnifier would also have been possible.

Asking the patient to name colours is a very crude test of colour vision but can indicate possible functional problems the patient might experience. Loss of colour sensitivity often precedes VA loss and is a sensitive indicator of foveal function (Vemala et al., 2017). The patient was given an Amsler chart to check for any possible progression to wet age-related macular degeneration (AMD), which would have been likely to lead to distortion of the grid pattern. It is also important that patients are told what to do if they do detect distortion, and this will be based on referral pathways in that particular area.

At the Annual Review visit, Lydia had already had a recent eye examination to check on ocular health (and been referred), so the Low Vision Assessment could concentrate on rehabilitation issues. With the same target VA of N4, and a measured VA at 25 cm of N12, the magnification requirement was now 3×. Both eyes had poorer CS than previously, so the patient was advised to use the eye with better CS when using the magnifier. Using one eye will allow the eye-to-magnifier distance to be reduced and the field of view to be increased. If the patient has very strong eye dominance or is strongly left- or right-handed, it may be easier for them to use the poorer eye, so demonstrating the effect of using each eye individually is useful. As this patient has had magnifiers previously and shown good performance with them, it was decided that a telephone follow-up would be adequate, and Lydia did not need to make a visit back to the practice.

At the follow-up visit, Lydia reported difficulties at home with the preparation of food and drinks. She was also going to refurbish her flat and would like to know how to maximise lighting and optimise the environment to make the most of her vision. Information on lighting design was given to her. Although Lydia's VA did not qualify her for registration as sight impaired, the local sensory team could still visit her at home and give her advice on these issues. In this case, referral was initiated through the Low Vision Letter, but some enhanced pathways have direct referral to other agencies.

CASE 4—84-YEAR-OLD

Low Vision Assessment

Date: 20-1-2022

Patient Details

Name	Edward Vedder			DOB	12-11-1937
First visit to clinic?	(Y)/N	Referred from?	Macular Treatment Clinic (MTC)	Age	84

Ocular History

Dry AMD diagnosed at age 75, now both eyes have 'wet' AMD with regular injections in both eyes (so far RE three injections, LE six injections). Has been told he has slight cataract in both eyes, but no operation suggested.

Any change in vision in last 3 months? Both eyes have deteriorated—especially noticeable in reading vision 'magnifier not strong enough'	Which is better eye currently? Right eye

Ophthalmologist		Ms Davison	Last Visit	3 weeks ago
Hospital		Manchester Royal Eye Hospital	Next Visit	2 months
Optometrist		Specsavers	Last Eye Exam	6 months ago

Registration status (give date)	SSI ☐	SI ☑ 2019		Not registered ☐
Contact with SS/RO? When? What was result?	Told them he didn't need help when contacted at time of registration			

General Health

Health problems	High blood pressure. Arthritis—has back pain and needs to exercise regularly, and sit very straight. Holding magnifier is 'no problem'	Medication management	Has difficulty with blister packs—uses a 'pill puncher' so pills are not dropped
GP name & address	Dr Max, Littledale Medical Centre, Didsbury		

Daily Life

Visual Perception
Vision much better outdoors when it's dull. Has to use his hand to shield eyes or wear a baseball cap. Distance spectacles have photochromic lenses which do help as well. Misses numbers in a sequence—e.g. reading his credit card number when paying over the phone. Has heard about eccentric viewing (from a presentation at the Macular Society monthly meeting) but not tried it. Has some visual hallucinations in the centre of his vision (birds, flowers, especially on a white background). Not troubled by these. Had heard of Charles Bonnet syndrome from the Macular Society and has also discussed with his GP. Blinking or moving eyes makes them disappear. Task lighting used to be very effective (e.g. reading large print) but doesn't seem to help with reading now.

Occupation/Education
Retired consultant clinical psychologist but still works 1 day per week teaching about meditation and mindfulness. Has difficulty reading journals when a new paper is published.

Mobility and Travel
No difficulty at home. His wife drives him, or he travels by bus (alone). He has to ask the driver what the bus number is. His wife does the main shopping. He walks a lot and does visit local shops (he likes to achieve 10,000 steps per day with his Fitbit). He has to be careful with steps and kerbs, has had several trips but not falls. He is more worried about not seeing glass doors or windows—he once collided with a bus shelter.
Slips or trips? ☑ White cane? ☒ Walking stick or frame? ☐ Wheelchair? ☐

At Home
Lives with wife, and they share chores. He has difficulty reading food packets (even with magnifier), and setting washing machine programmes. No difficulty making hot drinks.
Sensory substitution devices? (e.g. bump-ons; talking watch; liquid level indicator) ☒

Hobbies/Interests
Goes to theatre, but difficult to see detail on stage He watches his grandson play rugby. Sits near halfway line, and asks other people about what is happening. Prefers to watch on TV when he can get really close to the screen Used to make models but stopped due to vision: not really interested in this now Walking (see previous section) Yoga exercises to help with back pain—no visual problems
Watch TV? ☑ What distance? 1.5 m (or closer if necessary) Audio-description? ☒

Reading, Writing and Electronic Devices
Would like to be able to read printed books, journals and newspapers. Currently accesses on iPad and can increase size, but it is a bit of a struggle. Likes audio books for 'fiction'. Has used the magnifier app on his phone, but it doesn't seem very effective (still struggling with reading). He finds it useful to take photos of signs and then zoom in on them. Has a keyboard with large high-contrast symbols for his laptop. Has difficulty writing in straight lines.
Computer? ☑ Smartphone? ☑ Duration of comfortable reading_   not currently

Well-Being and Mental Health
Feels a bit frustrated that his magnifier is not as good as it was, and he feels it needs to be stronger. Positive outlook—finds meditation very helpful. Has plenty of interests to keep him busy.

Current Spectacles and Magnifiers

Use of Spectacles

Type	Date of Issue	RE Rx	VA	LE Rx	VA	Add	Near VA RE	Near VA LE
Distance (photochromic)	2019	−1.50/−1.00 × 50	0.9	−1.25/−1.50 × 170	1.1			
Near (+3.25 add)	2019	+1.75/−1.00 × 50		+2.00/−1.50 × 170			N40	N40

Use of Magnifiers

Description	Used for	Successful?
4× illuminated hand magnifier	All types of reading	Used to be, but not so now. Reading very slow.

Other Aids/Devices or Strategies

Description	Used for	Successful?
(Built in) Magnifier app on phone	Labels when shopping	Not as good as magnifier

Patient Aims

A stronger magnifier for reading. Help with watching rugby matches

Visual Assessment

Visions:

Right		Left	
Distance:	Near:	Distance:	Near:
Binocular			
Distance:			Near:

Refraction:

Rx	Right	VA	Left	VA
Distance	No subjective change. Encouraged to use eccentric viewing and he said he was looking up.	0.9	No subjective change	1.1

Preferred Working Distance	Required Add	VA RE	VA LE
With 1× magnification	**Required Add**	**VA RE**	**VA LE**
Working distance 25 cm	+4.00	N40 words N20 first letter on line	N40 words N20 first letter on line

High Adds Tested

Magnification Required	Required Working Distance	Required Add	VA RE	VA LE
		+16.00 (to match current magnification)	N20 at 6 cm	

Contrast Sensitivity

Method: _____ Mars Letter _____

Right	Left	Binocular
0.88	0.64	

This is
☐ Severe loss: nonsighted strategies probably indicated (Rows 1 and 2)
☑ Significantly reduced: optical aids may be useful (Rows 3 and 4)
☐ Noticeable loss: lighting and contrast need to be optimised (Rows 5 and 6)
☐ Normal/Near Normal (Rows 7 and 8)

Visual Field

Central/~~Peripheral~~ (please delete as appropriate)
Method: _____ Amsler _____
Brief description of findings (attach plot if appropriate)

RE: central area hazy, pattern clearer down and right. Central spot was not reported to be any clearer when he looked up and left.

Other Tests:
Aids Demonstrated

Magnification & Description	Which Specs Used	VA	Comments on Performance	Issued	Cost
4× illuminated stand magnifier	Near	N20 N8 first letter	Easier to position for reading print, but no improvement	Y/(N)	
6× illuminated stand magnifier	Near	N20	'It's too small a lens'	Y/(N)	
2× spectacle mounted distance telescope	---	0.60	Handled focussing well	(Y)/N	
4× fixed focus telescope	Distance	0.32 slow	Good localisation of targets	(Y)/N	

Outcomes	
Requirements Identified	Solutions Suggested
Distance	
Watching rugby (going to theatre)	Spectacle mounted telescope; in-house commentary in sports stadium; audio-described performance in theatre
Seeing bus numbers	Handheld telescope (or holding up a card with required bus number on to alert the driver)
Intermediate	
Near	
Improvement in near word reading acuity and speed	Demonstrate that extra magnification not currently helpful, and explain why. Discuss training eccentric viewing and steady eye strategy
Help with setting appliance dials	Bump-ons: make contact with Sensory Team from Social Services to arrange home assessment (may also be able to discuss mobility issues)
Writing in straight lines	Writing frame/signature guide. Fine felt pen rather than ballpoint pen

Continued

Action	(✓/✗)	Details
Referred to own optometrist		
Referred to other university clinic		
Referred to GP/Consultant		
Referred to rehab officer/SS (LVL?)		Suggested contact Sensory Team—he has contact details.
Referred to Access to Work		
Referred to voluntary agency		
Referral to counselling services/GP/other		
Info/advice given		Try spec-mounted telescope for rugby and theatre, but if magnification not adequate try the handheld telescope instead for a short test of the VA and FOV. If this seems better, then spec-mounted telescope could be changed at next visit.
Leaflets given		
Training recommended		Given printed sheets of random words in 24-point print to practice EV and SES, using own hand magnifier. Practice two to three times each day for 5–10 minutes. Px showed good understanding of requirements. I explained that 'success' would be accurate reading, but still relatively slow.

Recommended Action at Next Visit

Assess compliance and monitor progress with EV/SES with a view to moving to more challenging practice sheets (smaller print, longer words). Test higher magnification again if required. Px to report back on telescope usefulness.	Date/recall period: 2 weeks

Commentary on Case 4

This case describes the situation of a patient for whom magnifiers do not seem to work. There are several reasons why this might be the case: the magnifier may be used incorrectly, or for an unsuitable task. In this case, however, when the visual impairment was less severe, Dr Vedder used his magnifier effectively. The most likely explanation is that the patient now has a central scotoma which has disrupted the ability to read even large print: the first letter of a word can sometimes be seen, but not the whole word. On the other hand, magnification for distance is relatively effective—eccentric viewing (EV) is often easier for the patient to keep stable and consistent for a relatively static task. In this case, the main difficulty with using a telescope is whether the field of view will be large enough to be useful for the required tasks. This is then a balance between increasing the magnification to a useful level, without compromising the field of view. A bioptic telescope may well be a useful option, although these are not supplied through the NHS in the UK.

Although EV training has not been found to be effective in a trial which investigated an unselected group of patients with macular degeneration (Dickinson et al., 2016), it can be used very effectively for patients who are not able to benefit from magnifiers because of a central scotoma. This patient was therefore given some practice reading sheets and training in EV, in conjunction with steady eye strategy (SES), beginning by reading short words in large print, letter by letter. Over a period of two to three further visits (supplemented by daily homework between), the aim would be to restore accurate reading of print, although reading may still be relatively slow, perhaps about 80 words per minute as a maximum. If EV is successfully established, then the amount of magnification required can be reviewed. His poor CS might also limit his reading speed, although reading on a high-contrast electronic device should reduce the impact of this.

Dr Vedder did experience some hallucinations but knew why he was experiencing these and was not troubled by them.

REFERENCES

Dickinson, C., Subramanian, A., & Harper, R. A. (2016). Evaluating the effectiveness of an established community-based eccentric viewing rehabilitation training model—The evaluation study. *Investigative Ophthalmology & Visual Science, 57*(8), 3640–3649. https://doi.org/10.1167/iovs.15-18458.

Rowe, F. J., Hepworth, L. R., Howard, C., et al. (2022). Developing a stroke-vision care pathway: A consensus study. *Disability & Rehabilitation, 44*(3), 487–495. https://doi.org/10.1080/0963828 8.2020.1768302.

Vemala, R., Sivaprasad, S., & Barbur, J. L. (2017). Detection of early loss of color vision in age-related macular degeneration—With emphasis on drusen and reticular pseudodrusen. *Investigative Ophthalmology & Visual Science, 58*, BIO247–BIO254. https:// doi.org/10.1167/iovs.17-21771.

APPENDIX **1**

Useful Information

EVENTS AND ORGANISATIONS

SightVillage: large trade fairs open to patients and professionals. A good place to see new low vision aids, particularly high-tech devices. Operates in several locations around the UK, with the Birmingham event being largest. https://www.qac.ac.uk/exhibitions.htm

SightCity: a larger version of SightVillage, operating annually in Frankfurt. https://sightcity.net/en/sightcity-frankfurt-english

International Society for Low Vision Research and Rehabilitation (ISLRR). Membership organisation which hosts the largest international low vision conference (every 2 years) and a semiregular newsletter. http://www.islrr.org

European Society for Low Vision Research and Rehabilitation. The European equivalent of ISLRR. https://www.eslrr.org/

PATIENT INFORMATION WEBSITES

Sight Advice FAQ. Comprehensive site about living with sight loss, developed by a combination of vision impairment charities. https://www.sightadvicefaq.org.uk/

AppleVis. Frequently updated site with information about accessibility for Apple devices. https://www.applevis.com/

AbilityNet. Help and information about accessing technology for people with vision, hearing, mobility or cognitive impairment. Includes 'my computer my way': a step-by-step guide to individual adjustments for computers, laptops, tablets and smart phones to make them easier to use. https://www.abilitynet.org.uk/

Living Made Easy (also known as the Disabled Living Foundation). Provides free impartial advice and information on solutions, gadgets, adaptations and aids to make life easier for all types of disabilities. https://livingmadeeasy.org.uk

NATIONAL CHARITIES

Royal National Institute of Blind People (RNIB). The UK's largest sight loss charity. Operates dozens of services, including a helpline, online shop for nonoptical aids, advocacy and employment advice. https://www.rnib.org.uk/

Guide Dogs for the Blind Association. Specialises in mobility, but also offers other services. https://www.guidedogs.org.uk/

Visionary. The umbrella organisation for local sight loss charities. https://www.visionary.org.uk/

VICTA (Visually Impaired Children Taking Action). Support and advice for children and young adults (<29 years) with sight loss and their families. https://www.victa.org.uk/

Fight for Sight. Major funder of low vision research in the UK. http://www.fightforsight.org.uk/

Thomas Pocklington Trust. Charity which focuses on education, employment and engagement for people with sight loss. https://www.pocklington-trust.org.uk/

Macular Society. Support and events for people with all forms of macular disease. Publishes *Sideview* journal and funds research. https://www.macularsociety.org/

Retina UK. Support for people with inherited progressive retinal disease and research into these conditions. https://retinauk.org.uk/

Albinism Fellowship UK. Volunteer-run organisation for people with albinism and their families. https://www.albinism.org.uk/

Stargardt's Connected. Small charity raising awareness of Stargardt disease and providing peer support for patients and their families. https://stargardtsconnected.org.uk/

Nystagmus Network. Charity for people with nystagmus of any cause. https://nystagmusnetwork.org/

SeeAbility. Organisation for people with learning disability, autism and sight loss. https://www.seeability.org/

Blind Veterans UK. Charity supporting people with sight loss who served in the armed forces. https://www.blindveterans.org.uk/

Look UK. An organisation supporting young people with visual impairment and their families. https://www.look-uk.org

Esme's Umbrella. An organisation raising awareness of Charles Bonnet Syndrome and offering assistance to individuals with the condition. https://charlesbonnetsyndrome.uk/

Sightline Telephone Befriending Service. https://www.sightline.org.uk/

Talking News Federation. Provides local newspapers in audio format. https://tnf.org.uk/ (for national newspapers and magazines see https://www.rnib.org.uk/newsagent)

British Blind Sport. A charity that makes sport and recreational activities accessible to people who are visually impaired. https://britishblindsport.org.uk/

LOCAL CHARITIES

The RNIB Sightline Directory has details of local services and can be searched by town or postcode or by type of organisation. https://www.sightlinedirectory.org.uk/

Some of these organisations serve a wide geographic area; for example, Henshaws in the North of England (https://www.henshaws.org.uk), Blind Aid in London (https://www.blindaid.org.uk) and Sight Scotland (https://sightscotland.org.uk)

LOW VISION AID MANUFACTURERS AND DISTRIBUTORS

Associated Optical: https://www.associatedoptical.com/
Edward Marcus: https://www.edwardmarcus.co.uk/
Optima Low Vision: http://www.optimalowvision.co.uk/
Optelec: https://uk.optelec.com/
Sussex Vision: https://www.sussex-vision.co.uk/
Sight and Sound: https://www.sightandsound.co.uk/
Oxsight: https://oxsightglobal.com/
GiveVision: https://www.givevision.net/
Vision Aid: https://www.visionaid.co.uk

PODCASTS AND RADIO PROGRAMMES

In Touch—on BBC Radio 4 on Tuesday evenings at 8:40 p.m., and online at BBC Sounds.
Tech Talk—on RNIB Connect Radio and available as a podcast.

APPS

Unless otherwise specified, these are available on Android and Apple devices.

Magnification

SuperVision +

Text-to-Speech, Scene Recognition and Object Identification

SeeingAI (Apple only)
EnvisionAI
KNFB reader
Supersense

BeMyEyes
TapTapSee
Aira

Talking Books and Newspapers

Dolphin EasyReader
Audible

Mobility and Navigation

Soundscape (Apple only)
Lazarillo
GoodMaps Explore
RNIB Navigator
RightHear
Super Lidar (Apple only)
BlindSquare

Other

Audio Game Hub
Ellie (dating app for disabled people, fully accessible)

Sample Record Sheets

Some practitioners prefer to use blank pages or electronic records for low vision assessments, but those who prefer to use record cards may wish to use the following examples.

FIRST VISIT ASSESSMENT RECORD CARD

Low Vision Assessment
Patient Details

Name			DOB	
First visit to clinic?	Y/N	Referred from?	Age	

Ocular History

Any change in vision in last 3 months?		Which is better eye currently?		
Ophthalmologist			Last visit	
Hospital			Next visit	
Optometrist			Last eye exam	

Registration status (give date)	SI ☐	No ☐	Not registered ☐
Contact with SS/RO? When? What was result?			

General Health

Health problems		Medication management	
GP name & address			

Daily Life (Prompt Questions—Choose Appropriately)

Visual Perception	
Open Questions	**Follow-Up Questions**
Do you see better when it's bright or dull? Do you have any problems with bright light? Do you notice any missing areas of your vision? Do you miss some letters in a word/words on the line? Do you see colours normally? Do you ever see coloured lights/shapes? Do you think your eyes are playing tricks with you?	Do you wear tinted spectacles/sunglasses? Just outdoors, or indoors as well? Do you have task lighting at home? Do things disappear when you look straight at them? Do you think you see better if you look to one side?

Occupation/Education	
Open Questions	**Follow-Up Questions**
What do you do for a living? What were you trained as? What have you retired from? Are you studying?	Are you aware of Access to Work scheme? Does your employer know about your eye condition? Reason for retirement/loss of job—vision related? What course are you studying? Where? What provision is made for exams?

Mobility and Travel

Open Questions	Follow-Up Questions
How do you usually get around? How did you get here today? Do you usually use the bus/train/taxis? Do you go anywhere unaccompanied? What difficulties do you have when you go out? How do you do your shopping? Do you use a white cane?	Why? How do you feel about going to new places? Can you see bus numbers/train departure boards? What apps or technology do you use for route planning? Do you have problems with: Curbs, crossings, signs, bus numbers, steps, people's faces, cars? Have you ever had any slips or trips while out and about? How is your mobility in the house?

Slips or trips? ☐ White cane? ☐ Walking stick or frame? ☐ Wheelchair? ☐

At Home

Open Questions	Follow-Up Questions
Who do you live with? Are you in a house or a flat? Ground floor or upstairs? With a lift? Who does the housework? Who does the cooking? Are there any appliances you have problems with? Do you have any gadgets to help you?	What kinds of things can you cook? Can you make hot drinks? Can you read cooking labels? Do you garden, iron, vacuum, dust, do the washing?

Sensory substitution devices? (e.g. bump-ons; talking watch; liquid level indicator) ☐

Hobbies/Interests

Open Questions	Follow-Up Questions
What do you do for fun? What are your interests? Have you recently given up any interests? (Vision related?) Do you have any hobbies? Do you watch TV? (At what distance?)	Do you watch sport, go to the theatre/cinema/bingo, play cards, eat out? Do you have any hobbies that involve close work like sewing, knitting, model making, electronics, puzzles? Do you play music?

Watch TV? ☐ What distance? _____ Audio-description? ☐

Reading, Writing and Electronic Devices	
Open Questions	**Follow-Up Questions**
What types of thing do you read? What would you LIKE to be able to read? Is larger print easier for you to read? How do you deal with correspondence? Do you use a computer? Do you use a mobile phone?	Do you read books? Do you read newspapers? Large print? Kindle/e-books? Audiobooks? Do you read/write letters? If not, why not? Have you downloaded any apps? Do you prefer reading on paper or on screens? Why? Do you prefer white-on-black or black-on-white?

Computer? ☐ Smartphone? ☐ Duration of comfortable reading ————

Well-being and mental health	
Open Questions	**Follow-Up Questions**
Does your vision loss get you down? Do you feel frustrated by not being able to do things? Do you have people you can talk to/who help you?	Have you spoken to your doctor about this? Have you received any treatment for this? Would you like me to refer you to someone you can talk to about this?

Current Spectacles and Magnifiers
Use of Spectacles

Type	Date of Issue	RE Rx	VA	LE Rx	VA	Add	Near VA RE	Near VA LE

Use of Magnifiers

Description	Used For	Successful?

Other Aids/Devices or Strategies

Description	Used For	Successful?

Patient Aims

Visual Assessment

Visions:

Right		Left	
Distance:	Near:	Distance:	Near:
Binocular			
Distance:		Near:	

Refraction:

Rx	Right	VA	Left	VA
Distance				

Preferred working distance	Required Add	VA RE	VA LE
With 1× magnification	Required Add	VA RE	VA LE
Working distance 25 cm			

High Adds Tested

Magnification Required	Required Working Distance	Required Add	VA RE	VA LE

Contrast Sensitivity

Method _____

Right	Left	Binocular

This is

☐ Severe loss: nonsighted strategies probably indicated (Row 1 and 2)
☐ Significantly reduced: optical aids may be useful (Row 3 and 4)
☐ Noticeable loss: lighting and contrast need to be optimised (Row 5 and 6)
☐ Normal/near normal (Row 7 and 8)

Visual Field

Central/peripheral (please delete as appropriate)
Method _____
Brief description of findings (attach plot if appropriate)

Other Tests:

Aids Demonstrated

Magnification & Description	Which Specs Used	VA	Comments on Performance	Issued	Cost
				Y/N	
				Y/N	
				Y/N	
				Y/N	
				Y/N	

Outcomes	
Requirements Identified	Solutions Suggested
Distance	

Intermediate	
Near	

Action	(✓/✗)	Details
Referred to own optometrist		
Referred to other university clinic		
Referred to GP/consultant		
Referred to rehab officer/SS (LVL?)		
Referred to Access to Work scheme		
Referred to voluntary agency		
Referral to counselling services/GP/other		
Info/advice given		
Leaflets given		
Training recommended		

Recommended Action at Next Visit

FOLLOW-UP VISIT RECORD CARD

Low Vision Follow-up
Patient Details

Name		DOB	
Date of last visit to clinic?			

History Since Last Visit

Changes in Vision/Treatment/Health: Interactions With Other Services
Progress With Aids/Training
Patient Aims for Today

Visual Assessment
Refraction:

Rx	Right	Left
Distance		
Add		

Visual Acuity:

Right		Left	
Distance:	Near:	Distance:	Near:
Binocular			
Distance:		Near:	

Issued Earlier	Magnification & Description	Specs	VA	Comments	Issued Today
Y/N					Y/N
Y/N					Y / N
Y/N					Y/N
Y/N					Y/N
Y/N					Y/N

Other Tests:

Outcomes

Action taken	
Magnifiers returned:	Magnifiers loaned:
Recommended action at next visit	Recall period/date of next visit

Patient Literature

These sheets give examples of written information which might be given to patients after their appointment. They can be emailed to the patient after the appointment, or printed in **an appropriate font size** and handed out at the end of the low vision assessment.

GOOD LIGHTING

Magnification alone is not sufficient: no magnifier will work effectively if there is not enough light.
Light should not be directed into your eyes.
Use lights to supplement natural daylight, even during the day.
Keep the level of light constant throughout the house—it takes longer to adapt from light to dark areas and vice versa.
Have stairs and doorways well lit.
Change lampshades if necessary to direct the light where you need it, and stop the shade from blocking the light.

How to Improve Lighting Conditions at Home

Make good use of daylight:
- Draw the curtains well back
- Clean the windows regularly
- Avoid nets, but blinds can be helpful to avoid glare
- Pale walls and ceilings to reflect light
- Chair placed sideways near to the window

Task Lighting

LED lamps are best.
Helps with reading—brightness is important to improve reading.
Cost-effective: cheaper than ceiling light and gives more brightness.
If you halve the distance, you get four times the brightness.
WHEN to use it:
- Reading
- Writing
- Hobbies
- Working in the kitchen
- Eating meals

Stick-on LED lights in strips can be fitted underneath wall cupboards, or inside a wardrobe.

Carry a torch for seeing detail anywhere that the lighting is poor.

HOW to use it:

- Light pointing at the task, away from your eyes
- Lamp next to your forehead, not shining on the magnifier so there are no annoying reflections

TYPE of lamp:

- LED is best so it does not get too warm—it will be very close to your face
- Flexible or joint arm—needs to be adjusted to different angles
- Heavy base or clamp fitting—so it cannot topple over

Where do I buy a lamp?

Local DIY stores

The Partially Sighted Society

Telephone: 01302 965195

https://www.partsight.org.uk/shop/lighting-lamps

Royal National Institute of Blind People (RNIB)

https://shop.rnib.org.uk/house/lighting

Optima Low Vision Services Ltd

Telephone: 01803 864218 www.optimalowvision.co.uk

The Daylight Company

Telephone: 0800 055 77 11

https://daylightcompany.com/reading-lamps-and-lights/

TINTS, SUNGLASSES AND VISORS

Is light sometimes too bright for you?

Does light sometimes reduce your vision? In bright light, do objects appear:

- washed out,
- faded and
- poor contrast?

If the answer to the above questions is yes, you may be suffering from glare.

Getting Rid of Glare

Indoors:

- Move your chair so it is not facing the window
- Use curtains or blinds to block direct sunlight
- Move the computer or TV screen so that light does not fall directly on it

Out and about:

- Walk on the shaded side of the road/street
- Wear an eyeshade
- Use a hat with a brim or a cap

Tinted lenses or sunglasses can make you more comfortable, but your vision will be reduced if they are too dark.

- Photochromic lenses (that darken in the sun) may not be dark enough outdoors and too slow to fade coming indoors.
- Overspectacles may be a better option: wear over your spectacles whenever required, and remove as you move into lower brightness areas.

Different colour tints are available: experiment to find the best colour and density (how dark the tint is). A grey tint which transmits between 20% and 40% of the light is a good place to start.

ELECTRONIC MAGNIFIERS

Electronic (video) magnifiers are stronger than optical magnifiers. You can sit at a comfortable distance from the screen, and look with both eyes, whilst wearing your ordinary spectacles. You will probably see more letters at once than with a normal magnifying glass. This probably means you can read for longer without getting tired, although the speed may be the same as with the optical magnifier. You can also use some of them for writing and handicrafts. They can make things brighter, dimmer and bolder, and sometimes you can change the colour of what you are looking at, which might be more comfortable.

People usually have optical magnifiers as well for some tasks, and for back-up in case of breakdowns.

A DESKTOP ELECTRONIC MAGNIFIER with a large screen is not portable, needs to be used on a table and takes up quite a lot of space. It also takes more practice to reach the best performance—do not be disheartened if you cannot read very quickly the first time you use it. These magnifiers are expensive to buy (£1500 upwards).

PORTABLE ELECTRONIC MAGNIFIERS have a much smaller screen and are powered by rechargeable batteries. Some are small and light enough for you to carry around in your pocket and take out shopping or to a restaurant. The screen is only a few inches in size, so the amount of information displayed and the magnification are limited. Costs start at about £150, but those with larger screens are more expensive.

TELEVISION READERS are the cheapest electronic magnifiers (£100–£300). They consist of a handheld camera which can be plugged in to your own TV or computer. The might not have as many options as more expensive electronic magnifiers. The camera itself is small and easily portable, and because it can be used with different devices, you could move it from work to home or take it on holiday with you.

Buying an Electronic Magnifier

Electronic low vision aids are not usually available through the NHS. They are provided by the local education authority for **children** who need one for school, and **university students** can use Disabled Students Allowance to buy one. People who need an electronic magnifier **at work** can have this provided through the 'Access to Work' Scheme (https://www.gov.uk/access-to-work).

If you are **registered** as severely sight impaired (SSI) or sight impaired (SI), you do not need to pay **VAT** on electronic magnifiers.

Charities

If you are not eligible for any of the help aforementioned schemes, some charities may be able to assist. You may also approach a local group such as Round Table, Lions or Rotary Club; or you may be eligible for help from an ex-service (Blind Veterans UK) or occupational charity.

Finding a Supplier

Most suppliers will have products in each of the three categories described earlier. You can often get a very similar device from several different suppliers.

You should think about more than just the cost when deciding who to purchase from:
1. Will they refund your money if you do not find the device helpful?
2. What sort of warranty and after-sales service is offered?
3. Will they come to your home to demonstrate and/or install the electronic magnifier?
4. How much training will they give you in learning to use it—is this included in the cost?

Some suppliers attend exhibitions and conferences (e.g. those organized by the Macular Society https://www.macularsociety.org) and these are useful for you to compare different models.

The leading exhibition of electronic aids for the visually impaired each year is 'Sight Village': it takes place every year in different locations around the UK and is free to attend.

https://www.qac.ac.uk/exhibitions.htm

MAKING YOUR COMPUTER EASIER TO SEE

1. Good lighting
2. Light should not shine directly onto screen
3. Try not to have a window behind the screen
4. Large monitor bigger image
5. Closer to screen also bigger image
6. Adequate spectacles for computer distance
7. Consider learning to touch type, using a keyboard with larger letters (available in different colours—yellow, white, black-on-white), or keyboard stickers to make the keyboard more visible
8. Customization of your computer:
   - 'Magnifier' can increase the size of a screen area (Windows)
   - 'Narrator' can read the letters as you type (Windows)
   - A built-in screen reader, screen and cursor magnification, and Dictation—Accessibility (Mac)

   Examples of more complete screen reader programmes are as follows:
   - SuperNova
   - Zoomtext Magnifier/Reader
   - JAWS

   Apple computers and portable devices include a built-in complete screen reader called VoiceOver.
   More information on these can be found here:

   SuperNova
   http://www.dolphinuk.co.uk/
   Telephone: 01905 754 577

   Zoomtext Magnifier/Reader and JAWS
   http://www.aisquared.com/zoomtext/more/zoomtext_magnifier_reader/

   Sight & Sound Technology
   Welton House North Wing
   Summerhouse Road
   Moulton Park
   Northampton
   NN3 6WD
   Telephone: 0845 634 7979
   Telephone: +44 1604 798070
   Fax: +44 1604 798090
   http://www.sightandsound.co.uk
   Visit www.applevis.com for details on accessibility options on all Apple devices.

INFORMATION ABOUT REGISTERING AS SIGHT IMPAIRED OR SEVERELY SIGHT IMPAIRED

What Is Registration?

If your sight cannot be improved by wearing glasses, you can ask your optometrist to refer you to a consultant ophthalmologist (your GP can also do this for you). If your sight cannot be improved medically, the consultant may tell you about registering as sight impaired with your local council. When you register your sight impairment, it will be easier to access some of the help and support you need.

There are two levels of registration:
- SSI (used to be called blind)
- SI (used to be called partially sighted)

Being registered does not necessarily mean that you will lose all your sight; nine out of ten people who are registered have some useful sight.

Why Should I Register?

If you are registered, there is a range of benefits to which you may be entitled. Some benefits are only available to those registered as SSI.
- Financial benefits such as Disability Living Allowance, Personal Independence Payments or Attendance Allowance, depending on age and circumstances.
- Employment and Support Allowance.
- Additional personal tax allowance (SSI only).
- Free local public transport.
  Disabled Persons Railcard
  Disabled parking permit ('blue badge')
- Free sight tests
- Reduction in TV licence fee (SSI only).
- Cinema exhibitors card for reduced cinema tickets.
- Other benefits from some local theatres, sports grounds and museums.
- VAT exemption when buying electronic aids designed to help with sight impairment.

Being registered will allow you easier access to help with home life, mobility—getting around in your community, work and education.

How Do I Register?

The consultant will decide whether you are eligible for registration by measuring your distance vision and your field of vision; that is, how far you can see and how much you can see from the side of your eye when you are looking straight ahead.

If you meet the criteria, the consultant will register you as SI or SSI by completing the Certificate of Vision Impairment (CVI). The form gives details of the assessment of your vision. It also gives other relevant information about your circumstances and your preferred format for correspondence.

What Happens to the Certification Form?

You will be asked to sign the form to agree that a copy can be sent to your local council's Social Services Department, your GP and the Department of Health. The hospital keeps a copy and you will be given a copy for yourself.

Your name will be put on a list held by your Social Services Department, or in some areas, the local society for blind and partially sighted people. Social Services will carry out an assessment of needs, during which they work with you to identify what changes could be made to your living situation to help you adjust to your sight loss. This varies from region to region, so ask your optometrist, GP, consultant ophthalmologist, or Eye Clinic Liaison Officer for details of how the procedure works in your area.

Can I Get Help Before I Am Registered?

Usually, once you know that your eyesight cannot be improved by wearing glasses, you can begin to receive help from your local Social Services team or local society for people with sight loss. This can be requested before you are registered. Hospital eye clinics can fill in a form, Referral of Vision Impairment (RVI), with your consent, to request help from Social Services. Alternatively, you can ask your optometrist for a Low Vision Leaflet (LVL), which tells you where to go for help, and includes a tear-off form which you can fill in and send to Social Services yourself to ask for an assessment.

If you would like to talk to someone about registration, get in touch with RNIB on **0303 123 9999**, email **helpline@rnib.org. uk** or say: **'Alexa, call RNIB Helpline'** to an Alexa-enabled device.

INFORMATION SHEET—HAND MAGNIFIER

This sheet was prepared for

NAME: _____DATE:_____

YOU WERE SEEN IN THE CLINIC BY_____

<u>GENERAL ADVICE</u>

USE YOUR VISION to make the most of it, and when you get tired, have a short rest. Using your eyes can in no way harm your vision. If necessary sit very close to the television, so that you can reach and touch the screen. This will not harm your eyes in any way, but will make the picture much larger and clearer to you. The screen on your electronic devices (e.g. TV, computer or phone) can seem 'glary' when viewed in a darkened room, so keep the room light switched on as well. If you have a lamp on top of the television, you should keep it switched off when you are watching, and if there is a window behind the television, then draw the curtains across.

In general, when reading or doing close work you should have a reading lamp which throws light directly onto your work from a close distance. You may need this extra lighting even during the daytime. Using an LED lamp is best, because it does not get warm in use.

If your circumstances change in the future, or you have any problems or queries, please make another Clinic appointment (Telephone: 0111 222 3333). We will also write to you every 3 months to check that your aid is still achieving what you want.

<u>INSTRUCTIONS FOR THE USE OF YOUR (NONILLUMINATED) HANDHELD MAGNIFIER</u>

This aid should be used with/without* your distance/near/bifocal/varifocal* spectacles.

Use your _____eye/both eyes* to read.

delete whichever not applicable

Adjust the light as you were shown in the Clinic, getting it close to the page, but not shining into your eyes. If possible, place the lamp so it is lower than the magnifier, and does not give reflections on the lens surface. If the magnifier is held at the wrong distance from the page, you will not see clearly. Start with the magnifier flat on the page and then gradually bring it towards you until the print is as big and clear as possible. If you bring the magnifier too far, the print will blur and distort, and you should go back and try again.

It is impossible to make powerful magnifiers which are also large enough to cover a full page. In order to see as many words as possible through the magnifier, place your eye close to the magnifier (or bring the magnifier up close to your eye) whilst still keeping the magnifier at the correct distance from the page. You can move the magnifier across the page, but you may find it better to keep the magnifier still and move the page instead.

If you are reading a newspaper, fold it into four to get it to a manageable size, and place a firm piece of card or board behind it to keep it flat. Practice every day for a few minutes, as you have been shown, and you will find reading becoming easier and less tiring. Try not to get discouraged—using a magnifier properly is a skill, and it will take time and patience to acquire.

The magnifier lens can be cleaned with a damp cloth and dried with a soft towel.

If the aid needs any repair or adjustment, please contact the clinic.

INFORMATION SHEET—(ILLUMINATED) STAND MAGNIFIER

This sheet was prepared for

NAME: _____ DATE:_____

YOU WERE SEEN IN THE CLINIC BY_____

<u>GENERAL ADVICE</u>

USE YOUR VISION to make the most of it, and when you get tired have a short rest. Using your eyes can in no way harm your vision. If necessary sit very close to the television, so that you can reach and touch the screen. This will not harm your eyes in any way, but will make the picture much larger and clearer to you. The screen on your electronic devices (e.g. TV, computer or phone) can seem 'glary' when viewed in a darkened room, so keep the room light switched on as well. If you have a lamp on top of the television, you should keep it switched off when you are watching, and if there is a window behind the television, then draw the curtains across.

In general, when doing close work you should have a lamp which throws light directly onto your work from a close distance. You may need this extra lighting even during the daytime.

If your circumstances change in the future, or you have any problems or queries, please make another Clinic appointment (Telephone: 0161 200 3860). We will also write to you every 3 months to check that your aid is still achieving what you want.

<u>INSTRUCTIONS FOR THE USE OF YOUR STAND MAGNIFIER</u>

This aid should be used with/without* your distance/near/bifocal/varifocal* spectacles.

Use your _____eye/both eyes* to read.

*delete whichever not applicable

Your magnifier has a light inside it, so you should not need extra lighting. However, leave the normal room lighting on, but check there are no distracting reflections on the lens surface.

If you are reading a newspaper, fold it into four to get it to a manageable size, and place a firm piece of card or board behind it to keep it flat. If the magnifier is held at the wrong distance from the page, you will not see clearly through it. This magnifier is designed to touch the page, and if it does not, the print will be blurred. It is impossible to make powerful magnifiers which are also large enough to cover a full page. In order to see as many words as possible through the magnifier, bring it close to your eye, whilst still keeping the magnifier touching the page. To read long lines of text you can move the magnifier across the page, but you may find it better to keep the magnifier still and move the page instead.

Practice every day for a few minutes, as you have been shown, and you will find reading becoming easier and less tiring. Try not to get discouraged—using a magnifier properly is a skill, and it will take time and patience to acquire.

Clean the magnifier lens with a damp cloth and dry with a soft towel. If the magnifier has a light inside it <u>DO NOT IMMERSE IT IN WATER.</u>

If the aid needs any repair or adjustment, please contact the clinic.

INFORMATION SHEET—TELESCOPIC DISTANCE AID

This sheet was prepared for

NAME: _____ DATE:_____

YOU WERE SEEN IN THE CLINIC BY _____

<u>GENERAL ADVICE</u>

USE YOUR VISION to make the most of it, and when you get tired have a short rest. Using your eyes can in no way harm your vision. If necessary sit very close to the television, so that you can reach and touch the screen. This will not harm your eyes in any way, but will make the picture much larger and clearer to you. The screen on your electronic devices (e.g. TV, computer or phone) can seem 'glary' when viewed in a darkened room, so keep the room light switched on as well. If you have a lamp on top of the television, you should keep it switched off when you are watching, and if there is a window behind the television, then draw the curtains across.

In general, when reading or doing close work you should have a reading lamp which throws light directly onto your work from a close distance. You may need this extra lighting even during the daytime.

If your circumstances change in the future, or you have any problems or queries, please make another Clinic appointment (Telephone: 011 222 3333). We will also write to you every 3 months to check that your aid is still achieving what you want.

<u>INSTRUCTIONS FOR THE USE OF YOUR DISTANCE AID</u>

You have been given a _____ (*insert name of aid*) _____.

Use your _____ eye/both eyes*

This aid should be used with/without* glasses

*This aid is for distance viewing only, at a distance of _____, and its focus cannot be adjusted.

*This aid is for use at a distance of _____, but it can also be focussed as close as _____.

*delete/complete as applicable

This aid should <u>NOT</u> be used whilst walking, because you will only see a small area of the object at any one time, but it should be useful for _____

Practice using the aid every day for a few minutes, as you have been shown. Start by 'spotting' and focusing on stationary objects around the room whilst you are sitting down. Then move on to focusing on objects you are viewing across the street or garden, whilst standing at the window. You will find that you can then manage to follow moving objects with practice. Try not to get discouraged—using a magnifier properly is a skill, and like any new skill it takes time and patience to acquire.

Clean the aid by wiping the front and back surfaces with a soft moist cloth. <u>DO NOT ALLOW THE AID TO BECOME WET, OR IMMERSE IT IN WATER</u>.

If the aid needs any repair or adjustment, please contact the clinic.

WHAT TO EXPECT FROM THE LOW VISION ASSESSMENT

If you have not had an eye examination/sight test recently, within the past year we will book you in for full sight test before your low vision (LV) assessment. This is required to check your spectacle prescription and the health of your eyes. The Low Vision Clinic does not offer medical or surgical treatment for any eye diseases. If, after assessment, it is felt that such treatment might be appropriate, or further medical investigation of your eye condition is needed, then you will be referred to an eye specialist—an ophthalmologist—via your GP.

When you attend the Low Vision appointment:

Please bring all the glasses you are currently using. Please bring all the magnifiers and/or Low Vision Aids you are currently using.

What to expect from the low vision assessment:

The Low Vision Clinic offers help and advice if you are unable to see adequately with ordinary spectacles.

The optometrist will be asking you a series of questions to determine the state of your vision, how you feel about it and the problems that you are having in your daily life, such as seeing colours, going shopping, walking around, seeing people, your job, studies and hobbies.

Following these questions, your optometrist will check your distance and near vision and will work out what help they can give you to maximise the use of your remaining vision.

The help offered by your optometrist will come in the form of magnifiers, telescopes for distance and near, electronic visual enhancers and many other optical and nonoptical devices, as well as advice regarding illumination and contrast. We are also able to prescribe aids if your vision problems are due to a limited visual field—either a hemianopia (a loss of vision on one side) or tunnel vision (a very small remaining central island of vision).

A first visit will usually take about 1 1/2 hours, but follow-up appointments are often shorter.

At the end of the low vision assessment we may recommend that you try a magnifier, a lamp or a special pair of spectacles to allow you to see more clearly. Low vision aids are used in a different way to 'ordinary' spectacles, and it takes a little time and effort to get used to using them. You will be instructed in the use of the aid, and then take it home to practice. You will then be followed up after 2 to 3 weeks to make sure that the aid is successful. We may suggest that you practice reading and using your eyes in a different way, in order to make the best use of your remaining vision.

FIRST VISIT QUESTIONNAIRE

The Low Vision Clinic offers help and advice if you are unable to see well enough with ordinary spectacles. We carry out a full assessment of your vision at the present time, a thorough investigation of the problems you are experiencing, a discussion of your requirements, and then attempt to meet these, using high-powered or tinted spectacles, telescopes, magnifiers, lighting and other simple gadgets. Your first appointment will take around 1½ hours, but follow-up appointments are shorter.

At the end of the Low Vision Assessment we may recommend that you try a magnifier, a lamp or a special pair of spectacles to allow you to see more clearly. Low vision aids are used in a different way to 'ordinary' spectacles, and it takes a little time and effort to get used to using them. You will be shown how the aid works, instructed in the use of the aid, and then take it home to practice. You will then be followed up after 2 to 3 weeks to make sure that the aid is successful. We may also suggest that you practice reading and using your eyes in a different way, in order to make the best use of your remaining vision.

If you have ANY spectacles or magnifiers at the moment (even if you do not use them or do not think they are useful) it is VERY IMPORTANT that you bring them along with you to the appointment.

PLEASE TURN THE PAGE OVER AND COMPLETE THE QUESTIONS:

PATIENT'S NAME ------------

To help to identify your requirements, tick on the list below any items which you would like to be able to see better:

READING:

Books   _____

Newspapers/magazines   _____

Letters   _____

Bills and Bank Statements   _____

SHOPPING:

Labels and instructions   _____

Prices   _____

Items on Shelves   _____

WRITING:

Form filling   _____

Letters   _____

Crosswords and puzzles   _____

Bingo   _____

OTHER ACTIVITIES:

Sewing   _____

Knitting   _____

DIY   _____

Music   _____

Mobile phone   _____

Computer   _____

TV   _____

TRANSPORT:

Bus numbers   _____

Station/airport information   _____

Timetables   _____

4 | APPENDIX

Examples of Clinic Letters

REFERRAL TO TEACHER FOR VISUAL IMPAIRMENT

Ada Lovelace
Specialist Teacher for Visual Impairment
Ambridge Town Hall
Borchester
BC1 1AA

Dear Ms Lovelace,
Re: Ellen Wilkinson, DOB 16-8-2017

Please can I refer Ellen to the visual impairment team? Ellen's parents have given their permission for this referral.

She is a 4-year-old girl with oculocutaneous albinism. She is under the care of Professor Archer, Consultant Ophthalmologist and is registered as sight impaired.

Ellen will be starting at Ambridge Primary School in September. She currently attends Lower Loxley nursery 3 days per week, where she is managing well.

Ellen's visual acuity today was 0.6 logMAR (6/24). This means that things in the distance need to be about four times larger, or Ellen needs to be about four times closer, for her to see them as well as someone with perfect sight. She could see pictures of font size 8 at 20 cm. Her colour vision appears normal, but she is sensitive to bright light.

Ellen has some nystagmus which is reduced when she looks to her left, so I think it would help if she sits on the right hand side of the classroom (so the teacher and whiteboard are to her left).

Ellen has some glasses which she needs to wear all of the time. She has a pair of sunglasses which she will need to wear in bright light. She should also be allowed to wear a hat when she is outdoors, for example, at playtime and for PE.

Today I have prescribed her a dome magnifier. In the clinic she was able to see magazine pictures well with this. She also has some 6 × 17 binoculars for days out and school trips.

I will see Ellen again in the low vision clinic in 6 months.

Yours sincerely,
A.N. Optometrist, MSc, MCOptom, ProfCertLV
Low Vision Clinic
Borsetshire General Hospital

CC: Parents
CC: Reception teacher, Ambridge Primary School
CC: SENCo, Ambridge Primary School
CC: Professor Archer, Consultant Ophthalmologist, Borsetshire General Hospital

REPORT FOR TEACHER OF VISUAL IMPAIRMENT

Ada Lovelace
Specialist Teacher for Visual Impairment
Ambridge Town Hall
Borchester
BC1 1AA

Dear Ms Lovelace,
Re: Amelia Jones, DOB 31-10-2010

I saw Amelia in the low vision clinic again this morning. As you know, Amelia has vision impairment caused by Stargardt disease for which she sees Professor Archer. She is registered as severely sight impaired and has an Education and Health Care Plan.

Amelia is in Year 8 at Borchester High School. She enjoys school, particularly maths. She is less keen on geography. She has lots of friends.

I am pleased to report that her vision is stable, at 1.0 logMAR (6/60) with her glasses on and both eyes open. This means that things in the distance need to be about 10 times larger, or Ellen needs to be about 10 times closer, for her to see them as well as someone with perfect sight. The MNREAD test showed that she could read fluently—at 128 words per minute—for print of Font 14 or larger from 30 cm. She could read smaller print but this was slower and she had to hold the test closer.

Amelia has good support at school including receiving enlarged print, being allowed to sit where she needs to in the classroom, a portable electronic magnifier and an iPad relay system for the board. She can touchtype and has received some mobility training.

Amelia told me that her teachers are generally understanding, although her music teacher often forgets to enlarge the work before the lesson. I wonder if you could remind her music teacher to ensure that enlarged print is always available for her?

Amelia told me that she is not very confident walking in unfamiliar environments. She has not received any mobility training for 3 years and is keen for some top-up mobility training as she becomes more independent.

Today I have updated Amelia's glasses. As she is short-sighted, she can read without her glasses and should be allowed to take them off for reading if she wishes. A sloping desk may help her to see her work at a close distance.

I have prescribed her a folding 24 D LED illuminated hand magnifier for shop prices and menus, although she usually prefers to use her phone to magnify things. I have also replaced her 8×20 binoculars as she had lost her last pair.

I will see Amelia again in 1 year, but if she has any problems before then she will email me on anoptometrist@nhs.net.

I hope this report is helpful to you.

Yours sincerely,
A.N. Optometrist, MSc, MCOptom, ProfCertLV
Low Vision Clinic
Borsetshire General Hospital

CC: Parents
CC: Head of Year 8, Borchester High School
CC: SENCo, Borchester High School
CC: Professor Archer, Consultant Ophthalmologist, Borsetshire General Hospital

REPORT FOR GP

Dr Jehan Sadat
Ambridge Health Centre
High Street
Ambridge
BC1 1CB

Dear Dr Sadat,
Re: Elizabeth Fry, DOB 21-12-1949, NHS number: 555 122 1234

Thank you for referring Ms Fry for a low vision assessment. She attended the clinic this morning.

As you know, she has age-related macular degeneration. She is seen in the macular clinic at Borsetshire General Hospital every 12 weeks. She has received multiple intravitreal injections to both eyes and thinks her vision is currently stable.

Ms Fry is a retired teacher. She is a parish councillor and has struggled to read all of the minutes from her meetings. She no longer drives, because of her vision, and she has a bus pass. She is a carer for her husband, who has dementia. Her daughter lives a few doors away and helps Ms Fry with shopping and reading correspondence. Ms Fry has not fallen because of her vision.

Her visual acuity today was R. 0.5 logMAR (6/19), L. 1.3 logMAR (3/60). She could read N18 print fluently and N10 print slowly at 35 cm. Her contrast sensitivity was reduced at 5.8%.

Today I have prescribed some stronger reading glasses for Ms Fry to use with her parish council minutes. She will have to hold the page closer with these glasses—at 20 cm—but seemed comfortable with this in the clinic. She knows not to walk around in these glasses.

I demonstrated the importance of good lighting for reading. She will move her reading lamp from her husband's study to the dining table, where she deals with her correspondence. I have also suggested she moves her armchair so she is a little closer to the television.

Ms Fry told me that she sometimes experiences low mood because of her poor sight and caring for her husband. I have given her some information about carer's breaks arranged by the Borsetshire Carers' Association and the details of the Macular Society support line. I have encouraged her to speak to you if her mood worsens or she has any other concerns.

I have not arranged to see Ms Fry again in the low vision clinic, but she should continue to attend the macular clinic and her local optometrist for regular eye examinations.

Yours sincerely,
A.N. Optometrist, MSc, MCOptom, ProfCertLV
Low Vision Clinic
Borsetshire General Hospital

CC: Elizabeth Fry
CC: Consultant Ophthalmologist, Macular Clinic, Borsetshire General Hospital

REPORT FOR OPHTHALMOLOGIST

Professor Archer
Consultant Ophthalmologist
Borsetshire General Hospital
The Hill
Borchester
BC1 9QQ

Dear Professor Archer,
Re: Carol Hanisch, DOB 14-3-1961, Hospital number: 1555665, NHS number: 555 121 2232

Thank you for asking me to see Dr Hanisch. She attended the low vision clinic this afternoon. She is struggling with her work as a history lecturer, particularly for reading.

I am afraid I was not able to improve her vision further with refraction:

R. $+2.50/-1.75 \times 95$	1.1 logMAR (6/76)
L. $+3.00/-2.50 \times 100$	1.1 logMAR (6/76)
Add $+4.00$	N20 at 25 cm

Her contrast sensitivity was reduced at 9%. Her visual field was full to confrontation.

I have prescribed her an 8 × 20 monocular telescope and a +28 D illuminated hand magnifier.

Today I demonstrated different types of electronic magnifier. She could read very fluently with a desktop electronic vision enhancement system, preferring white on black print. I also showed her some text-to-speech devices including SeeingAI (for her iPhone) and Orcam.

She met with the Eye Clinic Liaison Officer this afternoon to discuss the Access to Work scheme.

Dr Hanisch is coming to see you again at the end of October. Please could you register her as sight impaired at that visit?

Yours sincerely,
A.N. Optometrist, MSc, MCOptom, ProfCertLV
Low Vision Clinic
Borsetshire General Hospital

CC: Carol Hanisch
CC: GP

REFERRAL TO REHABILITATION WORKER FOR VISUAL IMPAIRMENT

Susan Anthony
Rehabilitation Officer
Sensory Support Services
Ambridge Town Hall
Borchester
BC1 1AA

Dear Ms Anthony,
Re: Louise Weiss, DOB 8-1-1948
14 Lake Street, Ambridge, BC2 2NB
Tel: 01234 444332

Please can I ask you to make contact with Louise Weiss? She was in touch with your services in 2001 but her vision is far poorer now.

Ms Weiss has advanced glaucoma and is registered as severely sight impaired.

Her visual acuity today was 0.8 logMAR (6/38) with her glasses on and both eyes open. She has approximately 5 degrees of visual field in her right eye. Her left eye sees hand movements only.

Ms Weiss lives alone and is struggling with cooking and household tasks. She also struggles with crossing the road, and has recently stopped going out alone. Her son lives in London and visits most weekends to help with her correspondence and shopping.

I think Ms Weiss would benefit from a home visit and further advice from your service. She has given me permission to make this referral.

With many thanks.

Yours sincerely,
A.N. Optometrist, MSc, MCOptom, ProfCertLV
Low Vision Clinic
Borsetshire General Hospital

CC: Louise Weiss
CC: GP

Page numbers followed by '*f*' indicate figures, '*t*' indicate tables.